S0-BRB-755

TEXTBOOK OF

VETERINARY HISTOLOGY

TEXTBOOK OF VETERINARY HISTOLOGY

H. DIETER DELLMANN

Docteur-Vétérinaire, Habil.
Clarence Hartley Covault Distinguished Professor Emeritus in Veterinary Medicine
Professor Emeritus of Veterinary Anatomy
Department of Biomedical Sciences
Iowa State University College of Veterinary Medicine
Ames, Iowa

JO ANN EURELL, DVM, PHD

Associate Professor of Morphology
Department of Veterinary Biosciences
University of Illinois
Urbana, Illinois

Fifth Edition

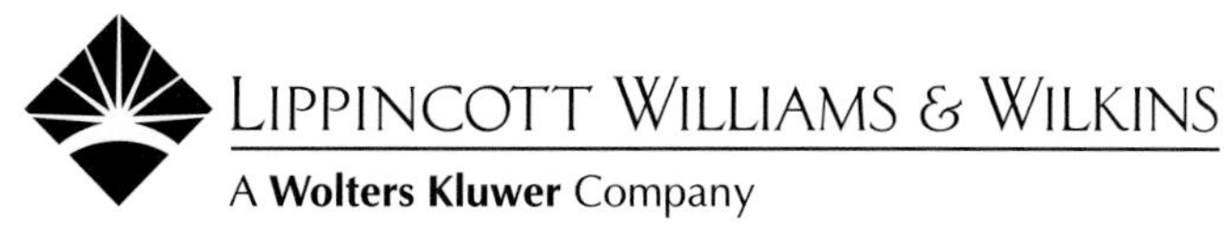

Philadelphia • Baltimore • New York • London
Buenos Aires • Hong Kong • Sydney • Tokyo

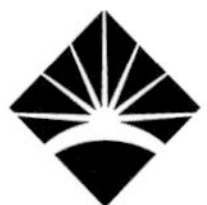

Editor: Carroll Cann
Managing Editor: Joanne Husovski
Marketing Manager: Diane Harnish

351 West Camden Street
Baltimore, Maryland 21201-2436 USA

Rose Tree Corporate Center
1400 North Providence Road
Building II, Suite 5025
Media, Pennsylvania 19063-2043 USA

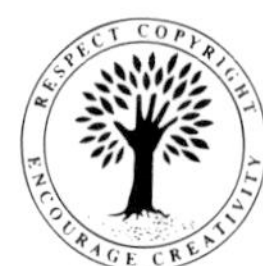

Accurate indications, adverse reactions and dosage schedules for drugs are provided in this book, but it is possible that they may change. The reader is urged to review the package information data of the manufacturers of the medications mentioned.

Printed in the United States of America

First Edition,

Library of Congress Cataloging-in-Publication Data

Textbook of veterinary histology / [edited by] H. Dieter Dellmann, Jo Ann Eurell. — 5th ed.
p. cm.
Includes bibliographical references and index.
ISBN 0-683-30168-3
1. Veterinary histology. I. Dellmann, Horst-Dieter. II. Eurell, Jo Ann Coers.
SF757.3.T49 1998
636.089'10189—dc21 98-4762
CIP

The publishers have made every effort to trace the copyright holders for borrowed material. If they have inadvertently overlooked any, they will be pleased to make the necessary arrangements at the first opportunity.

To purchase additional copies of this book, call our customer service department at **(800) 638-0672** or fax orders to **(800) 447-8438**. For other book services, including chapter reprints and large quantity sales, ask for the Special Sales department.

Canadian customers should call **(800) 665-1148**, or fax **(800) 665-0103**. For all other calls originating outside of the United States, please call **(410) 528-4223** or fax us at **(410) 528-8550**.

Visit Williams & Wilkins on the Internet: **http://www.wwilkins.com** or contact our customer service department at **custserv@wwilkins.com**. Williams & Wilkins customer service representatives are available from 8:30 am to 6:00 pm, EST, Monday through Friday, for telephone access.

99
2 3 4 5 6 7 8 9 10

Preface

The concept of providing a concise textbook for veterinary medical students continued to guide us in the editing of the fifth edition. Chapters have been rewritten extensively, new and important material has been incorporated, and some material included in the previous editions, which we believe to be beyond the scope of this text, has been deleted to provide a more concise coverage of topics relevant to the basic science studies of veterinary students and veterinarians. Many new illustrations have been added.

We hope that colleagues and students alike will continue to share their concerns and suggestions for future improvement of both text and illustrations.

H. Dieter Dellmann
Ames, Iowa
Jo Ann Eurell
Urbana, Illinois

Acknowledgments

We thank the contributors for their acceptance of most of our editorial suggestions and for critical revision of their chapters. They have facilitated our editorial tasks and made them enjoyable. We welcome J.A. Eurell, G. Flottorp, B. Frappier, R. Leiser, and Ch. McL. Press as new contributors.

Contributors to the fourth edition who have not participated in the revision for the fifth edition are no longer listed. We gratefully acknowledge previous contributions by N. Björkman (Chapter 14), E. Brown (Chapters 2, 3, 8, and 18), M.L. Calhoun (Chapters 2 and 10), G.H. Cardinet III (Chapter 5), L.L. Collier (Chapter 17), L. Nicander (Chapter 8), C.G. Plopper (Chapter 9), A.W. Stinson (Chapters 2 and 10), and J.H. Venable (Chapters 5 and 7).

Appreciation and thanks are expressed to Dean Biechler for his imaginative suggestions for and skillful production of new illustrations and for his incredible patience; to Joanne B. Messick for the micrographs for the color plates in Chapter 4; to Joan Thompson for excellent technical assistance in slide preparation, and to Robert Myers and Elaine Estes for assistance with computer imaging and slide production (Chapters 3, 4, and 5); to R. DenAdel for his photographic talents (Chapters 1, 3, 6, 8, 12, 15, and 17); to H.A. Wilson for his skills in photomicrography and darkroom printing, for his advice, and for his attention to detail that few can match (Chapter 10); to Jill Verlander for providing electron micrographs; to Janell Gerhartz for artwork and photographic assistance; to Gail Loughridge for fine computer graphics; and to Joty Koshla for carefully prepared histologic sections (Chapter 11).

Last, but certainly not least, we wish to thank Carroll Cann and, especially, Joanne Husovski, from Williams & Wilkins, for their many suggestions and excellent editorial input.

Contributors

Donald R. Adams, PhD
University Professor
Department of Biomedical Sciences
Iowa State University
College of Veterinary Medicine
Ames, Iowa

Vibeke Dantzer, DVM, Dr. Vet Sci
Associate Professor
Department of Anatomy and Physiology
Royal Veterinary and Agricultural University
Copenhagen, Denmark

Ahmed Deldar, DVM, PhD
Senior Clinical Pathologist
Lilly Research Laboratories
Eli Lilly and Company
Greenfield, Indiana

H. Dieter Dellmann, Docteur-Vétérinaire, Habil.
Clarence Hartley Covault Distinguished Professor Emeritus in Veterinary Medicine
Professor Emeritus of Veterinary Anatomy
Department of Biomedical Sciences
Iowa State University
College of Veterinary Medicine
Ames, Iowa

Jo Ann Eurell, DVM, PhD
Associate Professor of Morphology
Department of Veterinary Biosciences
University of Illinois
Urbana, Illinois

Thomas F. Fletcher, DVM, PhD
Professor of Veterinary Anatomy
Department of Veterinary Pathobiology
College of Veterinary Medicine
University of Minnesota
St. Paul, Minnesota

Gordon Flottorp, DS, PhD
Audiophysicist Emeritus
The Institute of Audiology
Oslo, Norway

Isak Foss, DVM, MS
Associate Professor
Department of Morphology, Genetics, and Aquatic Biology
Norwegian College of Veterinary Medicine
Oslo, Norway

Brian L. Frappier, PhD
Clinical Assistant Professor
Department of Veterinary Biomedical Sciences
College of Veterinary Medicine
University of Missouri
Columbia, Missouri

Charles Henrikson, PhD
Senior Lecturer
Department of Comparative Biosciences
School of Veterinary Medicine
University of Wisconsin–Madison
Madison, Wisconsin

Thor Landsverk, Dr. med. vet.
Professor
Department of Morphology, Genetics, and Aquatic Biology
Norwegian College of Veterinary Medicine
Oslo, Norway

Rudolf Leiser, Dr. med. vet.
Professor
Institut f. Veterinär-Anatomie, -Histologie und–Embryologie
Justus–Liebig–Universität Giessen
Giessen, Germany

Nancy A. Monteiro-Riviere, PhD
Professor of Investigative Dermatology and Toxicology
Companion Animal and Special Species
Cutaneous Pharmacology and Toxicology Center
College of Veterinary Medicine
North Carolina State University
Raleigh, North Carolina

Charles McL. Press, BSc (Vet.), BVSc, PhD
Research Fellow
Department of Morphology, Genetics, and Aquatic Biology
Norwegian College of Veterinary Medicine
Oslo, Norway

Jánis Priedkalns, BVSc, PhD
Elder Professor Emeritus of Anatomy and Histology
Department of Anatomy and Histology
Faculty of Medicine
The University of Adelaide
Adelaide, South Australia

David C. Van Sickle, DVM, PhD
Professor
Department of Anatomy
Purdue University School of Veterinary Medicine
Adjunct Professor
Department of Basic Medical Sciences
Indiana University School of Medicine
West Lafayette, Indiana

Karl-Heinz Wrobel, Dr. med. vet., Dr. rer. nat.
Professor
Institut für Anatomie
Universität Regensburg
Regensburg, Germany

Contents

1

Cytology

H. DIETER DELLMANN

The cell is the smallest structural unit of living material of a multicellular organism. Surrounded by the cell membrane, the cell is composed of a nucleus and cytoplasm that contains organelles and inclusions. These are suspended in the cytoplasmic matrix or cytosol, which consists of a fluid phase within a three-dimensional network of microtubules, microfilaments, and intermediate filaments collectively referred to as the cytoskeleton.

Cellular shape, size, and structure vary widely and express adaptations for the specific functions of each cell in specialized tissues and organs. Despite varying degrees of functional differentiation and thus variation in cell structure, most cells share general structural characteristics (Fig. 1.1).

CELL MEMBRANES

The cell membrane (plasma membrane or plasmalemma) is the membrane surrounding the cell. The nucleus, most organelles, and inclusions are likewise bounded by similarly structured membranes that participate in numerous cell functions, such as protein synthesis, secretion, phagocytosis, respiration, and transmembrane transport.

The cell membrane measures 8 to 10 nm in width and thus is too thin to be resolved with the light microscope. In routine histologic preparations, cell membranes are, however, visible when sectioned tangentially, when enough of the extrinsic cell coat is exposed to stain, or when the membrane—coat complex is thick enough to absorb stain (e.g., in adjacent epithelial cells).

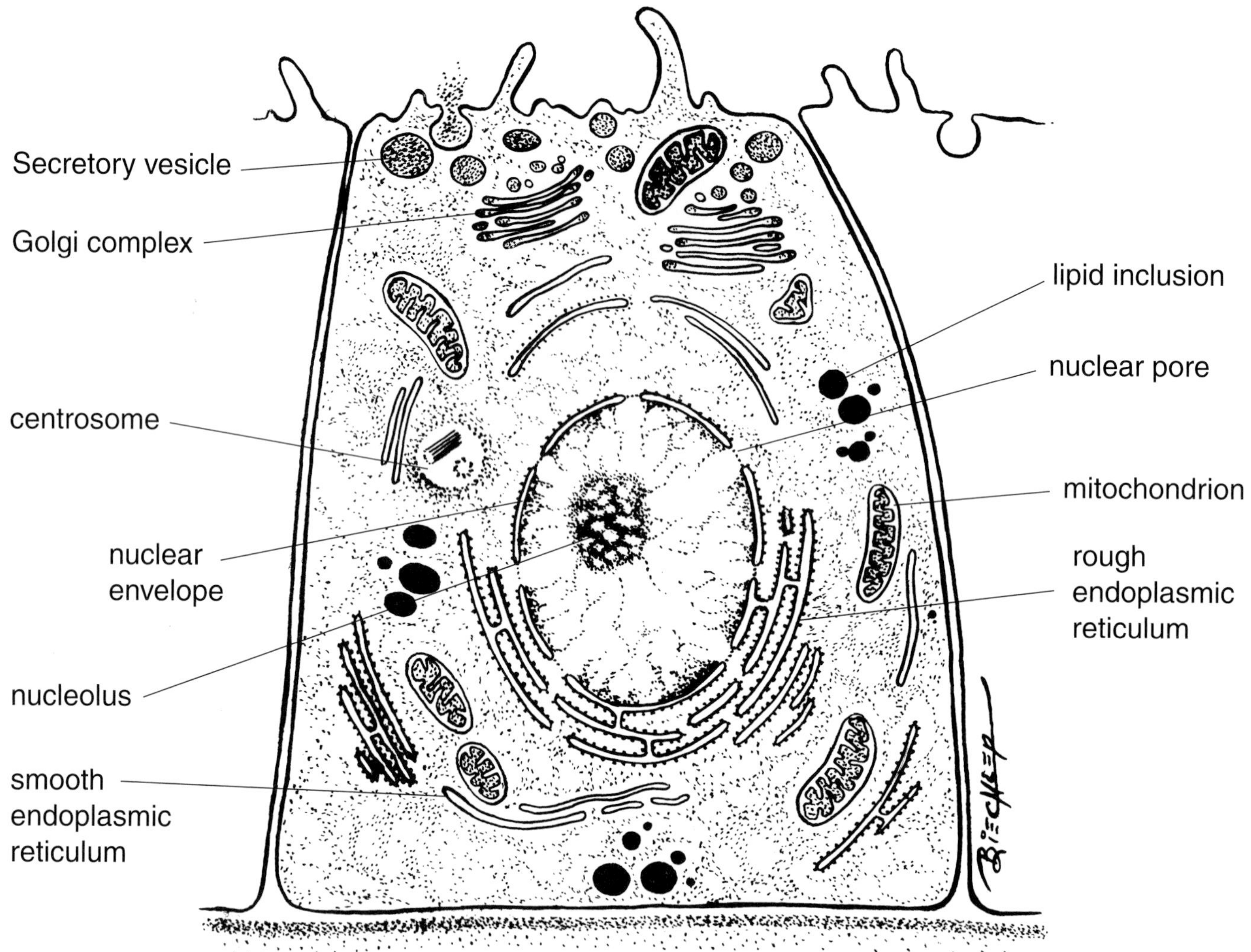

Figure 1.1. *Schematic drawing of the general organization of a cell.*

At the fine-structural level, the cell membrane is characteristically trilaminar. It consists of an outer and an inner electron-dense lamina, each approximately 2.5 nm thick, and an electron-lucent intermediate lamina approximately 3 nm thick (Fig. 1.2).

Irrespective of their differing functions, all cell membranes have a common basic structure. Each cell membrane consists of two leaflets composed primarily of phospholipid molecules that are arranged perpendicularly to the cell surface (Fig. 1.3). The lipids are amphipathic; therefore, polar, hydrophilic heads of these molecules face both the cytoplasmic and extracellular surfaces. Their nonpolar, hydrophobic tails (fatty acids) oppose each other in the center of the membrane, which is likewise the preferential site of cholesterol molecules. Additionally, glycolipids are present only in the external leaflet of the cell membrane.

Proteins associated with the lipid bilayer may be classed as **integral membrane proteins** or **peripheral membrane proteins.** Many of the integral proteins are amphipathic **transmembrane proteins**, i.e., they extend through the membrane and protrude at both surfaces. Peripheral membrane proteins are present at one or the other surface in contact with underlying integral proteins or the polar ends of the phospholipid molecules.

Membrane lipids and proteins are not necessarily in a fixed position but may change their location within the plane of the membrane; however, the lipids seem to be confined largely to their own monolayer.

Carbohydrates are attached to the membrane lipids or proteins at the external surface of the plasma membrane and at the luminal aspect of the membrane of organelles. Oligosaccharides are bound to membrane proteins (glycoproteins) and lipids (glycolipids), polysaccharides are bound to proteins only (proteoglycans). They form an extrinsic cell coat, referred to as **glycocalyx** (Fig. 1.4), which is present on all cells. It protects cells from mechanical and chemical damage, prevents undesirable interactions with other cells and extracellular components, and is responsible for a variety of transient cellular interactions.

The cell membrane plays an essential role in cell function. The lipid bilayer is permeable to a variety of molecules, such as water, ethanol, O_2, and CO_2; lipid-soluble substances rapidly diffuse across the bilayer. Membrane transport proteins form carriers and channels that transfer polar and water-soluble molecules such as amino acids, ions, and sugars across cell membranes. Most **channels** are present in the plasma membrane; they are hydrophilic pores through which passive transport of specific ions occurs. Ion channels are gated, i.e., they open in response to a stimulus such as a change in the electric potential of the membrane (voltage-gated channel) or the binding of a ligand (ligand-gated). Most **carriers** actively pump (active transport) solutes, such as sodium, potassium, and calcium, across the membrane, whereas some carriers also transport solutes passively. Some carriers belong to the family of transport adenosinetriphosphatases (ATPases), present in the membrane of the endoplasmic reticulum, which actively transport a variety of peptides into the lumen of

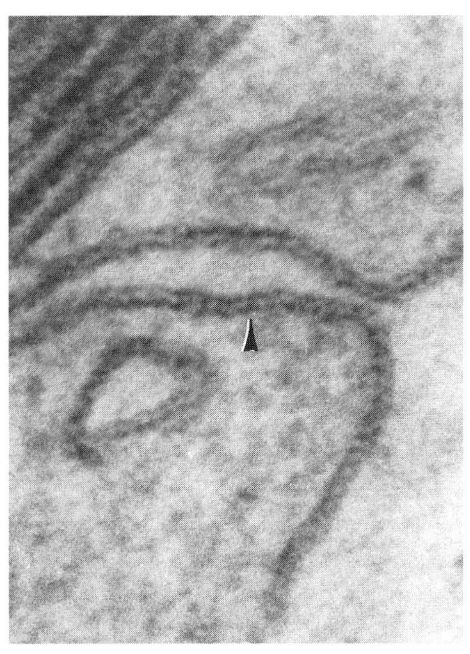

Figure 1.2. *Trilaminar plasma membrane (arrow) of a neurolemmocyte (×415,000).*

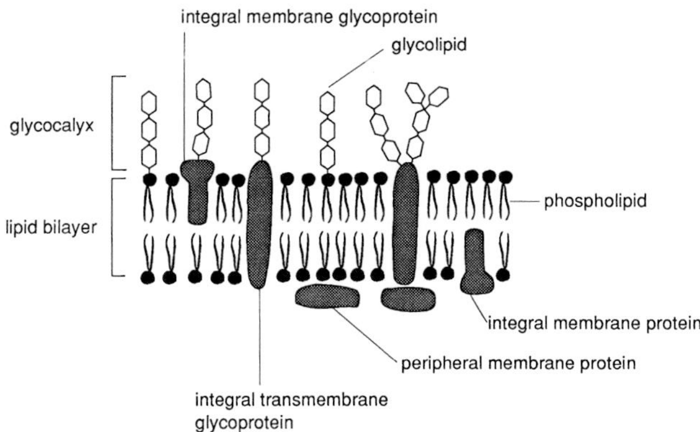

Figure 1.3. *Schematic drawing of the organization of the cell membrane.*

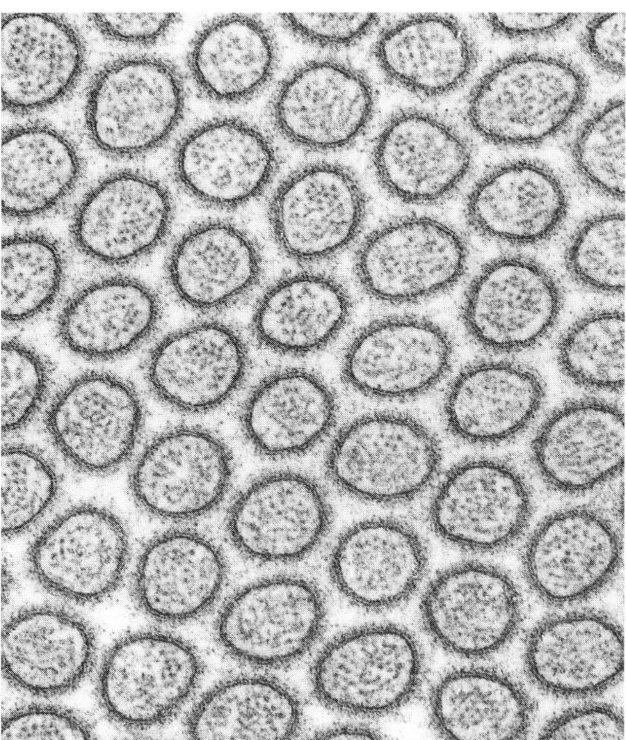

Figure 1.4. *Cross section through microvilli of a small intestinal absorptive cell. Note the distinct glycocalyx and the cross sections of numerous actin filaments (×99,000).*

the endoplasmic reticulum (ER). Specific cell surface receptor proteins mediate diverse functions, such as receptor-mediated endocytosis (phagocytosis), and antigen recognition. Hormone-activated cellular events likewise depend on special surface receptors. Cell—cell adhesion is mediated by integral membrane proteins, referred to as cell adhesion molecules (CAMs), i.e., immunoglobulin family members, cadherins, integrins, and selectins.

NUCLEUS

The nucleus is the largest cellular organelle. Most commonly, nuclei are spherical to ovoid (Fig. 1.5), but they may also be spindle-shaped (smooth muscle), bean- or kidney-shaped (monocytes), or multilobulated (neutrophilic leukocytes) (Fig. 1.6). Usually, cells contain only one nucleus, but certain cell types, such as skeletal muscle cells and osteoclasts, normally have several nuclei. Mammalian erythrocytes lack a nucleus. Nuclear size, shape, and location within the cell vary within wide limits and are influenced by a variety of factors, such as functional stage, circadian rhythms, and type of tissue.

Cells are most commonly observed during interphase of the cell cycle, when they perform their various specialized functions. The interphase nucleus is bounded by the nuclear envelope and contains chromatin, one nucleolus or several nucleoli, and a nuclear matrix.

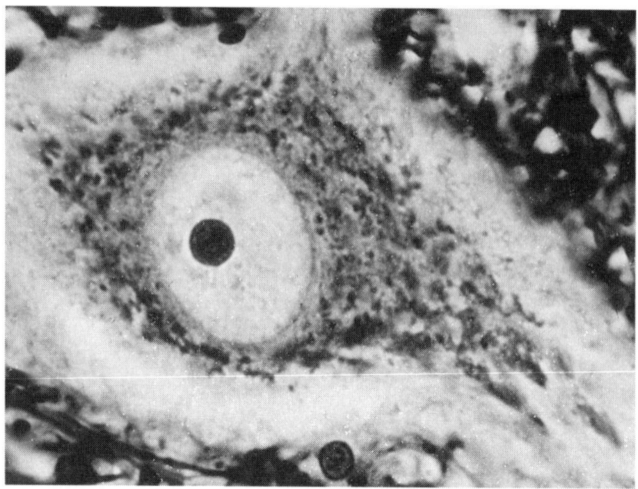

Figure 1.5. *Motor nerve cell from the spinal cord. The ergastoplasm or chromatophilic substance is visible as dark, pleomorphic masses throughout the cytoplasm. The euchromatic nucleus contains a distinct nucleolus (Cresyl violet Luxol fast blue, ×1100).*

Nuclear Envelope

The nuclear envelope consists of two concentric membranes separated by a 25-nm-wide perinuclear space. The outer nuclear membrane usually is studded with ribosomes, and it is continuous with the membranes of the rough ER (Fig. 1.7). At the inner surface of the inner membrane, a fibrous lamina is present. It is composed of nuclear lamins, which are bound to membrane proteins and to which specific sites of (hetero-) chromatin are attached. A layer of intermediate filaments surrounds the nuclear envelope.

The nuclear envelope is interrupted by numerous nuclear pore complexes, comprising a central aqueous channel (the nuclear pore), an outer ring of proteins, and fibrils that project into the cytosol and nuclear matrix. Through the aqueous channel, water-soluble molecules diffuse passively into and out of the nucleus. The pores mediate selective and active transport into the nucleus of proteins (e.g., histones, gene regulatory proteins) that are essential for the function of the nucleus. The transport of messenger ribonucleic acid (mRNA), transfer RNA (tRNA), and ribosomal subunits out of the nucleus is also selective and active.

Chromatin

Chromatin represents chromosomal material and is composed of deoxyribonucleic acid (DNA), basic proteins called histones, and nonhistone chromosomal proteins. Nucleosomal histones are structural proteins around which strands of DNA are wrapped to form nucleosomes; adjacent nucleosomes are linked by short regions of linker DNA. With the help of non-nucleosomal histones, nucleosomes are usually packed together in regular arrays, interrupted by short nucleosome-free regions, to form 30-nm-diameter chromatin fibers. During mitosis, these fibers are further coiled and folded, in association with other proteins, and become highly condensed chromosomes.

Chromatin occurs in two forms: heterochromatin and euchromatin. **Heterochromatin** is visible as irregular electron-dense or basophilic clumps or threads, often preferentially located at the nuclear periphery (see Fig. 1.12), scattered throughout the nucleus, or in association with the nucleolus (nucleolus-associated chromatin). Heterochromatin consists of the tightly coiled portions of chromosomes that lie entangled within the nucleus. Here, genes are repressed and transcription does not take place. Heterochromatin is the predominant form of chromatin in relatively inactive cells. The remainder of the chromatin is **euchromatin**. It is uncoiled and, therefore, less condensed than heterochromatin, electron-lucent, and essentially unstained (Fig. 1.5). Approximately 10% of this euchromatin is active chromatin, whereas the rest is transcriptionally inactive. Euchromatin is particularly abundant in active cells, characterized by light nuclei.

Most mammalian nuclei are sexually dimorphic, because one of the paired X chromosomes remains heterochromatic during interphase in the female. This **sex chromatin** (Barr body) appears either as an almost spherical chromatin condensation underneath the nuclear envelope of most cells of females or as a prominent nuclear appendage in neutrophilic leukocytes (see Fig. 1.6).

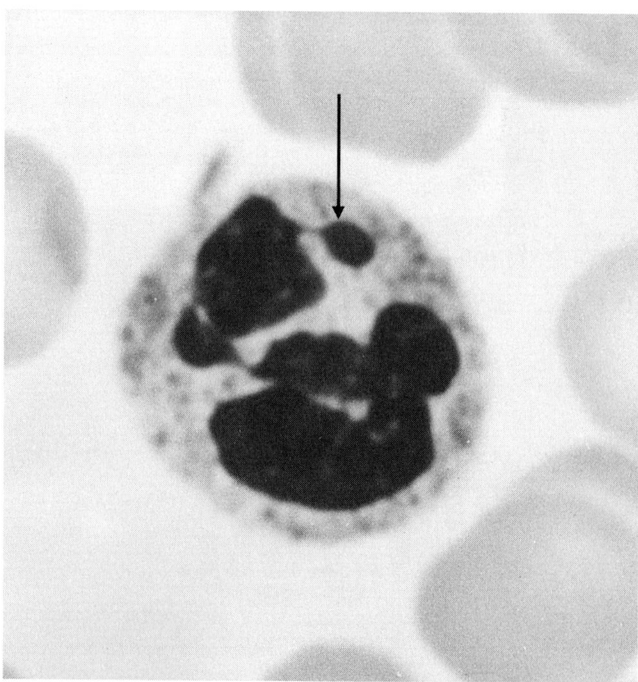

Figure 1.6. *Sex chromatin (arrow) in the nucleus of a polymorphonuclear leukocyte (×3800).*

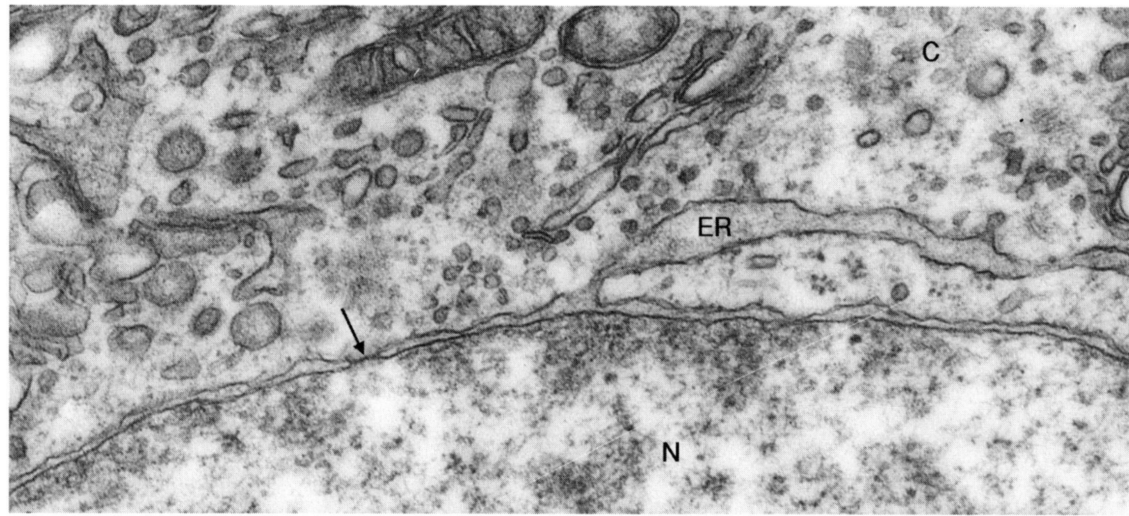

Figure 1.7. *Part of the nucleus (N), with electron-dense heterochromatin and electron-lucent euchromatin, and the cytoplasm (C) of a neurohypophysial glial cell. The nuclear envelope is pierced by pores (arrow). The perinuclear space between the inner and outer nuclear membranes is continuous with a cisterna of the endoplasmic reticulum (ER) (×67,000).*

Nucleolus

The nucleolus is a conspicuous, spherical, basophilic organelle (see Fig. 1.5). The nucleolus contains loops of DNA from several chromosomes; each loop contains a group of ribosomal RNA (rRNA) genes, called the nucleolar organizer region. In the nucleolus, a primary rRNA transcript and ribosomal proteins imported from the cytoplasm are combined to form large ribonucleoprotein particles. These are processed into immature small and large ribosomal subunits that are exported into the cytoplasm, where they become functional when they are assembled into ribosomes.

The number and size of the nucleoli are activity-dependent. Cells with pronounced protein synthesis require more ribosomes than less active cells and, therefore, have large and sometimes multiple nucleoli.

With the electron microscope, three regions are identified in the nucleolus. The granular region (pars granulosa) contains maturing ribosomal precursor particles. The pale-staining fibrillar center contains transcriptionally inactive DNA. The dense fibrillar region (pars fibrosa) corresponds to transcripts of rRNA genes.

Nuclear Matrix

The nuclear matrix is the insoluble material that is left in the nucleus after a series of biochemical extraction steps. It consists mainly of proteins that bind to specific DNA sequences and may participate in DNA transcription and replication.

ORGANELLES OF PROTEIN SYNTHESIS

Protein synthesis begins in the nucleus with the transcription of DNA, yielding three types of RNAs, which are subsequently exported into the cytoplasm. Here, they participate in the synthesis of proteins. Proteins to be used intracellularly are synthesized on free ribosomes, those destined for the plasma membrane, or lysosomes, or secretory vesicles are synthesized in conjunction with endoplasmic reticulum and Golgi complex.

RNA Molecules

rRNAs are combined with cytoplasmic proteins in the nucleus to form immature ribosomal subunits, which form ribosomes when protein synthesis is to begin (see p. 5). Ribosomes move along the mRNA and translate successive codons into amino acid sequences.

mRNAs are RNA transcripts that direct the synthesis of protein molecules. mRNA comprises varying numbers of codons, i.e., groups of three nucleotides that specify one amino acid to be produced.

tRNAs have one set of nucleotides that form anticodons, i.e., groups of three nucleotides that base-pair to complimentary nucleotides of mRNA codons; another set of nucleotides is attached to an amino acid specific for that codon.

Ribosomes

Ribosomes are small electron-dense cytoplasmic particles (15 × 25 nm in diameter, and thus not visible with the light microscope) composed of a large and a small subunit. Before protein synthesis, these two subunits exist as separate entities. Protein synthesis at the ribosome begins with the positioning of an initiator tRNA on the small ribosomal subunit with the help of initiation factors; the initiator tRNA then moves along the mRNA, and when it recognizes an initiation codon on that mRNA, the initiation factors dissociate from the small ribosomal subunit and a large ribosomal subunit binds to it. Thus, a functional ribosome is formed, which then begins the synthesis of a protein chain.

Both free and membrane-bound ribosomes occur either singly or in groups, called **polyribosomes** or **polysomes**, which simultaneously translate the same mRNA.

In some cells, such as early-developing erythrocytes (rubriblasts) and neurons, which synthesize large amounts of intracellular proteins, large numbers of free ribosomes occur and confer distinct basophilia to the cytoplasm.

Rough Endoplasmic Reticulum

The **rough endoplasmic reticulum** (rER) consists of a continuous network of tubes and flat and wide sacs, referred to as cisternae (see Figs. 1.8 and 1.10), bounded by a membrane in which the cytosolic surface is studded with ribosomes (thus the designation rough). Aggregates of rER appear as basophilic regions within many cells, such as nerve cells (Fig. 1-5) and pancreatic acinar cells. These regions are referred to as the ergastoplasm or chromidial substance.

The rER functions primarily in the biosynthesis of many various proteins destined for either extracellular or intracellular use (i.e., secretory proteins, lysosomal proteins, membrane proteins). The translation of such a protein begins with the assembly of a functional ribosome, as described previously. The mRNA then encodes an ER signal peptide. A cytosolic signal recognition particle (SRP) then binds to the ER signal peptide and the ribosome to form a complex that attaches to an SRP receptor in the ER membrane. The ribosome then becomes bound to the ER membrane via a ribosome receptor, at which time the SRP is released into the cytosol for reuse. During translation, the protein enters the rER lumen through a hydrophilic pore. The signal peptide is removed, and the protein is eventually released into the cisternal lumen. At that time, the ribosome becomes detached from both mRNA and ER membrane and disassembles into its subunits.

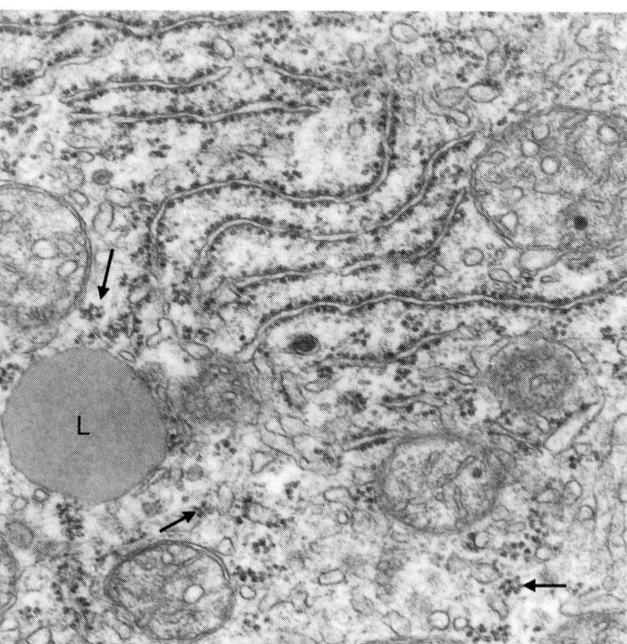

Figure 1.8. *Cisternae of rough endoplasmic reticulum with their characteristic ribosomes; also notice polyribosomes (arrows) and a lipid droplet (L). Luteal cell (×30,000).*

In the cisternal lumen, ER-resident proteins help in the folding of proteins and the formation of disulfide bonds. N-linked oligosaccharides are added to most proteins.

Membrane proteins are also synthesized by the rER, whereas membrane lipids are synthesized by the smooth ER, catalyzed by enzymes in which active sites are facing the cytosol.

Golgi Complex and Associated Vesicles

After their synthesis in the rER, proteins are transferred to the Golgi complex, in which they are modified and packaged.

When stained with silver salts or osmium, the Golgi complex appears as a black network of cisternae. In routine light-microscopic preparations, it may be visible as a lighter-stained region called the negative Golgi image.

At the fine-structural level, the Golgi complex consists of parallel membrane-bounded flattened cisternae, called Golgi stacks, and associated tubules and vesicles at the lateral surfaces and at either face of the stacks (Figs. 1.9 and 1.10). Each stack comprises a cis-cisterna, one or several medial cisternae, and a trans-cisterna. Both the cis-cisternae and trans-cisternae are joined to a compartment of interconnected tubules and cisternae, called the cis-Golgi and trans-Golgi networks, respectively.

Incorrectly assembled and folded proteins remain in the rER. Only proteins that have been correctly assembled and folded in the rER are packaged into transport vesicles that bud off from transitional elements, i.e., ribosome-free regions of the rER. These vesicles deliver the proteins to the cis-Golgi network (Fig. 1.10). The proteins then move, via transport vesicles, to the cis-cisterna, the medial cisterna, the trans-cisterna, and finally to the trans-Golgi network.

Three groups of functions are performed in the Golgi complex. Proteins are modified by addition of oligosaccharides (N- and O-linked glycosylation) and sugars, glycosaminoglycan chains to form proteoglycans, phosphorylation, and sulfation. Proteins are modified by initiation of enzymatic proteolysis (e.g., prohormones begin to be broken down into active forms) and by removal of sugars. These various functions take place in the Golgi stack, in which each cisterna is considered to have its specific set of processing enzymes. Proteins are sorted in the trans-Golgi and cis-Golgi networks. In the

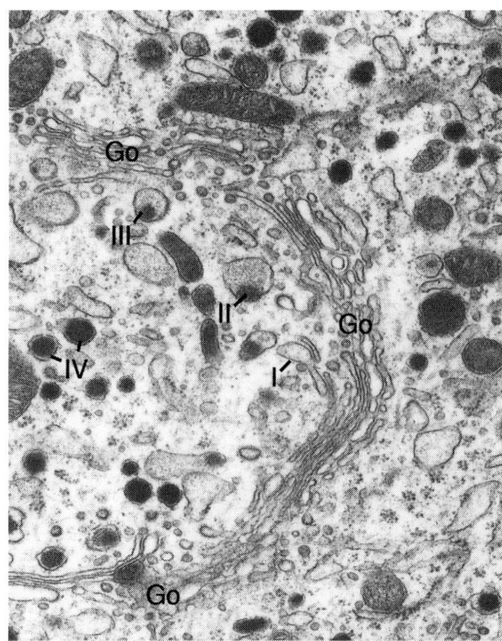

Figure 1.9. *Electron micrograph of the Golgi complex (Go) and surrounding cytoplasm of an adenohypophysial cell. As the secretory granules mature, they move away from the concave (trans) side of the Golgi complex and their content becomes more electron-dense. Sequence of the maturation process of the secretory vesicles (I, II, III, IV) (×23,700).*

trans-Golgi network, lysosomal proteins destined for late endosomes are sorted from those of the constitutive and regulated secretory pathways and packaged into separate sets of vesicles. ER-resident proteins that happen to escape to the cis-Golgi network are sorted here, or in later Golgi cisternae, and are returned to the ER.

Three types of vesicles derive from the Golgi complex: transport vesicles destined to late endosomes; transport vesicles of the constitutive secretory pathway destined to the plasma membrane; and secretory vesicles of the regulated secretory pathway destined to the plasma membrane (Fig. 1.10).

Clathrin-coated transport vesicles containing lysosomal enzymes bud off the trans-Golgi network, shed their clathrin coat, and move toward and fuse with late endosomes (see p. 7).

Constitutive secretion involves the continuous transport of membrane proteins and lipids and proteins for secretion (e.g., extracellular matrix proteins) to the plasma membrane of the appropriate cell surface. Transport vesicles release their content through exocytosis.

Secretory vesicles (also referred to as secretory granules, dense core vesicles, or condensing vacuoles) bud off the trans-Golgi network as clathrin-coated vesicles, containing secretory proteins. These proteins become greatly condensed, and proteolytic processing that began in the trans-Golgi network is completed. Upon detachment from the trans-Golgi network, the vesicles shed their coat and, in response to an extracellular stimulus, migrate toward the cell surface, where they are discharged from the cell by exocytosis (Figs. 1.9 and 1.10).

Exocytosis of secretory vesicles and the discharge of the contents of transport vesicles involve fusion of the vesicular membrane with and incorporation into the plasmalemma or the endosomal membrane. This process would lead to enlargement of the cell surface or endosomal compartment, if it were not balanced by membrane retrieval. The membrane of secretory vesicles of the regulated pathway is internalized through **endocytosis** and moves in vesicular form to the trans-Golgi network, to be reused in the secretory process. After insertion of new membrane into the plasmalemma in the constitutive secretory pathway, old membrane is endocytosed for recycling or degradation. From endosomes, vesicles bud off and shuttle back to the Golgi complex.

OTHER MEMBRANOUS ORGANELLES

Endosomes and Lysosomes

There are two distinct types of **endosomes:** early endosomes and late endosomes. These are polymorphic membrane-bounded tubes and vesicles. **Early endosomes** are usually located close to the plasma membrane and are a sorting compartment for endocytotic vesicles (Fig. 1.10). After these vesicles have delivered their cargo to early endosomes, most ligands dissociate from their receptors, and the receptors are shuttled back to the plasma membrane via transport vesicles (Fig. 1.10). Other ligands remain bound to their receptors and are either conveyed to a different part of the cell surface (transcytosis) or are degraded in lysosomes. Transport from early endosomes to late endosomes takes place through endosomal carrier vesicles (multivesicular bodies). **Late endosomes** lie in the vicinity of the Golgi complex and nucleus and receive materials for digestion from early endosomes or fuse with heterophagosomes or autophagosomes (Fig. 1.10). Eventually, they become lysosomes (see p. 9).

Materials destined for digestion reach lysosomes via three routes: endocytosis, phagocytosis, and autophagy.

Endocytosis refers not only to membrane internalization of secretory vesicles but also to the uptake of macromolecules into endocytotic vesicles and their selective transport within or across the cell (transcytosis; Fig. 1.11). If fluids are ingested via small vesicles, the process is referred to as **pinocytosis**, if the ingestion involves large particulate matter, it is called **phagocytosis**.

Pinocytosis comprises fluid phase endocytosis and receptor-mediated endocytosis. **Fluid phase endocytosis** is constitutive; it involves internalization of extracellular fluid and substances dissolved in it. The process begins with the formation of clathrin-coated pits, their invagination into the cell, and detachment, thus forming coated vesicles (Fig. 1.10). These vesicles shed their coats and fuse with early endosomes. **Receptor-mediated endocytosis** is the binding of macromolecules (ligands) to specific receptors and their uptake via coated

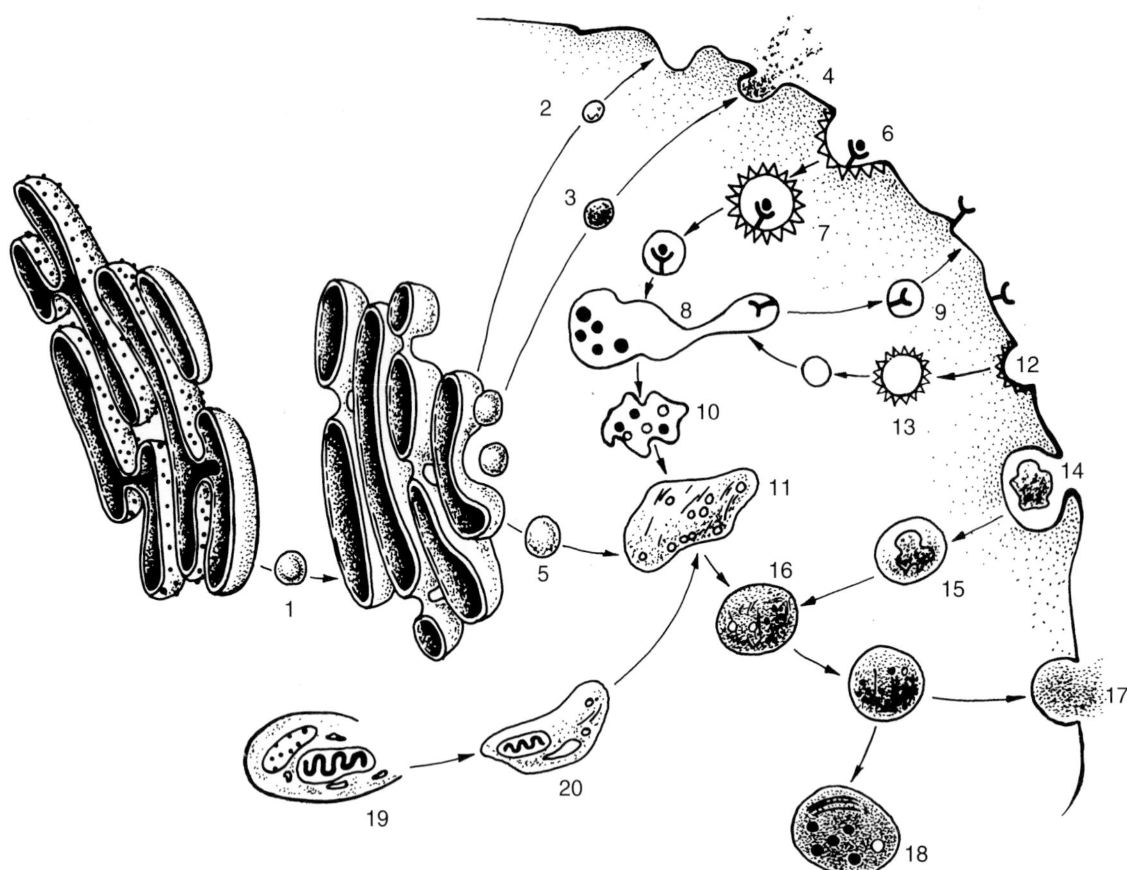

Figure 1.10. *From the ribosome-free transitional elements of the rER, transport vesicles (1) join the cis-Golgi network. Three types of vesicles originate from the trans-Golgi network: transport vesicles of the constitutive secretory pathway (2); secretory vesicles of the regulated secretory pathway (3), the contents of which are released by exocytosis (4); and transport vesicles that carry lysosomal enzymes to late endosomes (5). Ligands are taken up by receptor-mediated endocytosis (6) into endocytotic coated vesicles (7) that merge with early endosomes (8), in which they dissociate from their receptors; receptors are returned to the cell surface (9), and ligands are transported via endosomal carrier vesicles (10) to late endosomes (11) for lysosomal processing. In fluid-phase endocytosis (12), fluid is taken up into coated vesicles (13) that shed their coats and merge with early endosomes (8). Phagocytosis (14) gives rise to heterophagosomes (15) that fuse with late endosomes or lysosomes (16) from which the end products of digestion diffuse into the cytoplasm; indigestible materials are either released (17) or permanently stored as lipofuscin (18). Obsolete cellular organelles become enclosed by sER membranes (19) and become an autophagosome (20) that merges with a late endosome (11) or lysosome (16), in which the organelles are digested.*

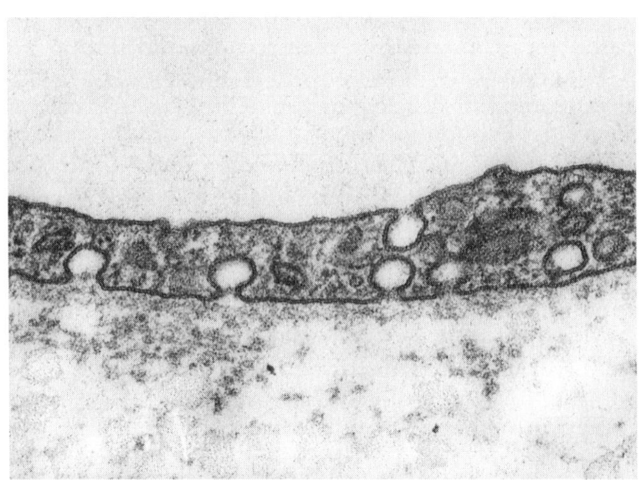

Figure 1.11. *Transcytotic vesicles are forming at the surfaces and are present within the cytoplasm of this capillary endothelial cell (×76,000).*

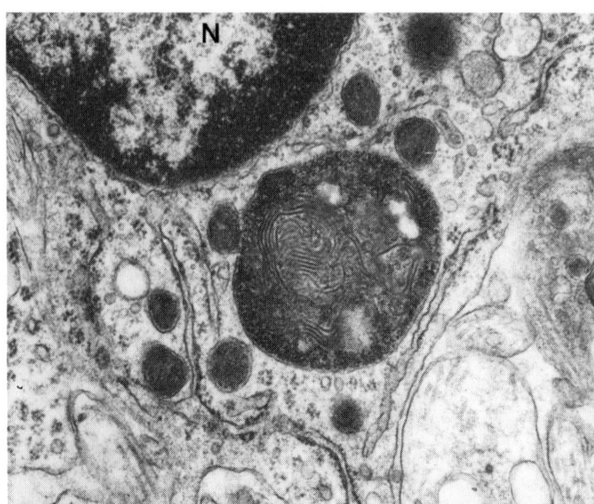

Figure 1.12. *Large dense lamellar body in an adenohypophysial cell. Nucleus (N) with peripheral accumulations of heterochromatin and light-staining areas of euchromatin (×25,300).*

pits into endocytotic vesicles (Fig. 1.10). After loss of their coats, endocytotic vesicles merge with early endosomes (Fig. 1.10).

Phagocytosis is a regulated endocytotic process during which specialized cells, primarily macrophages and neutrophils, take up particulate matter such as microorganisms, senescent (e.g., erythrocytes) and damaged cells, or cellular debris. During this process, which is called **heterophagy**, the plasma membrane invaginates, detaches, and forms a phagosome (also called heterophagosome) that fuses with a late endosome or lysosome, in which degradation of the ingested matter takes place (Fig. 1.10). Indigestible materials remain in the cell as residual bodies.

When cellular organelles become obsolete, they are disposed through **autophagy**, during which they are enclosed by ER membranes to form an autophagosome, which in turn fuses with a late endosome or lysosome (Fig. 1.10). The process of removal of aged, damaged, or excess secretory vesicles is called **crinophagy**.

Laminated concentric membrane-bounded structures represent the indigestible residues of lysosomal activity and are variably referred to as **dense lamellar bodies**, **myelinated bodies**, or **residual bodies** (Fig. 1.12); they may also occur as **vacuolated dense bodies** (Fig. 1.13). Their contents may either be released from the cell or remain permanently within the cell as **lipofuscin** pigment (see Figs. 1.10 and 1.13).

The absence of one or more lysosomal enzymes, a result of genetic defects, causes lysosomal storage diseases, such as gangliosidosis, in which undigested substrates accumulate in lysosomes and eventually interfere with normal cell function.

Lysosomes are membrane-bounded vesicles that contain a variety of hydrolytic enzymes, e.g., nuclease, proteases, lipases, that function optimally at a pH of 5, which is maintained by an adenosine 5′-triphosphate (ATP)-driven H^+ pump. In addition, phagocytosed microorganisms, extracellular debris, or effete organelles are present. Characteristically, the membrane prevents leakage of enzymes into the cytosol and permits the end products of digestion to be released into the cytosol. The permeability of the bounding membrane may change, however, under certain circumstances, such as lack of oxygen, regression of the mammary gland, or involution during embryonic development. The enzymes are then liberated into the cytoplasm and the cells are destroyed.

Lysosomal enzymes are sorted in the trans-Golgi network and become sequestered into clathrin-coated transport vesicles. As these vesicles move away from the Golgi complex, they shed their clathrin coat and move toward and fuse with late endosomes. Lysosomal hydrolases are released, and transport vesicles bud from the late endosome to return to the trans-Golgi network. Late endosomes, in which the digestive process begins at an initial approximate pH of 6, become lysosomes through an unknown process involving changes in membrane characteristics and a decrease in pH (pH = 5).

Smooth Endoplasmic Reticulum

The smooth endoplasmic reticulum (sER) consists of a network of tubules that, in most cells, are the ribosome-free terminal portions of rER, referred to as transitional elements. These tubules give rise to transport vesicles that carry molecules synthesized within the rER to the cis-Golgi network (Fig. 1.10). In cells involved in lipid metabolism (e.g., intestinal absorptive cells, hepatocytes, steroid hormone synthesizing cells) and ion movements (e.g., striated muscle cells), the sER performs major cell functions and is more abundantly developed. The sER in these cells consists of single vesicles and an anastomosing network of tubules of rather uniform size, often in an irregular, tortuous, and entangled arrangement (Fig. 1.14). In these cells, the sER may be

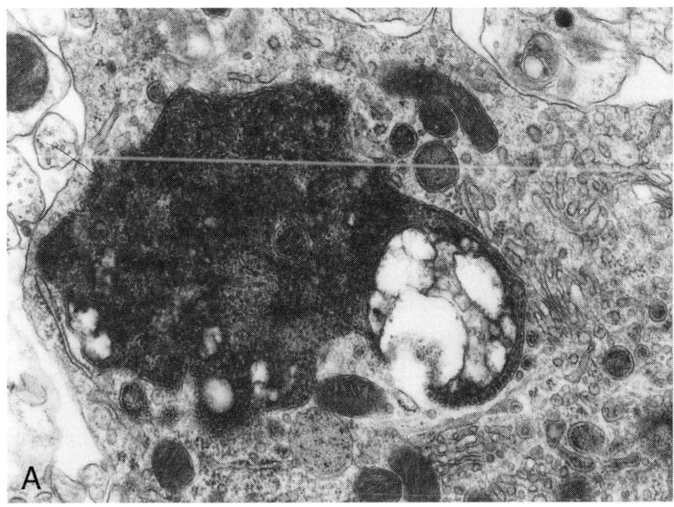

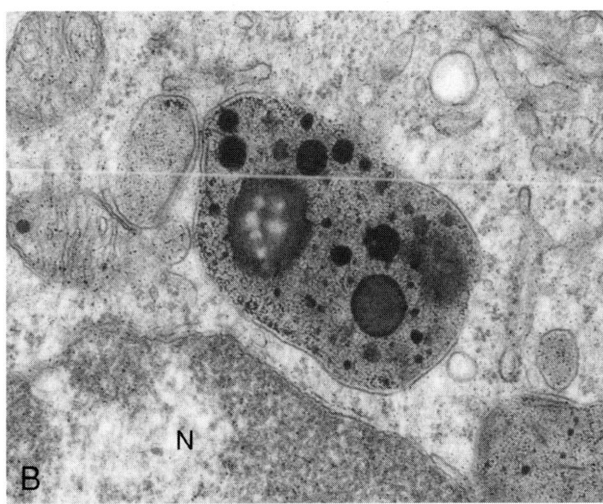

Figure 1.13. ***A.***, *Vacuolated dense body in a glial cell (×22,800).* ***B.***, *Lipofuscin granule in an adenohypophysial cell. Nucleus (N) (×29,850).*

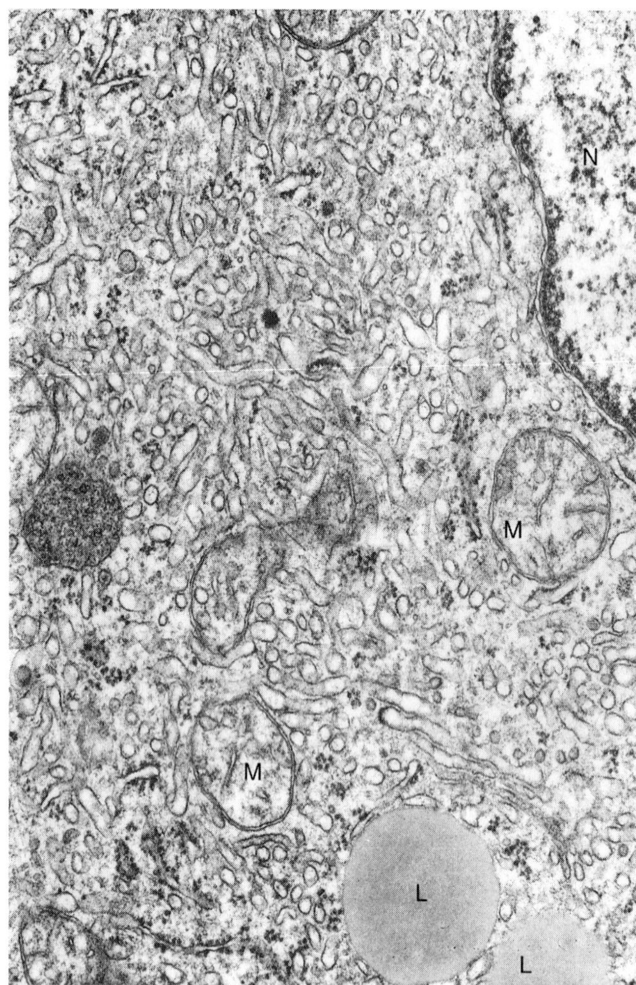

Figure 1.14. *This adrenal cortical cell contains an abundant smooth endoplasmic reticulum, mitochondria (M), and lipid droplets (L) in the vicinity of the nucleus (N) (×27,000).*

visualized at the light-microscopic level with silver impregnation methods.

The sER participates in a variety of functions. The enzymes for synthesis of cholesterol, sex steroids (androgens, estrogens, progesterone), glucocorticoids, and mineralocorticoids are located on the membranes of sER. Reconstitution of triglycerides from monoglycerides and fatty acids in intestinal absorptive cells takes place in the sER. A variety of compounds, e.g., alcohol, opiates, and lipid-soluble drugs such as barbiturates, are metabolized by the sER of hepatocytes. Expansion of the sER occurs in response to the presence of these compounds; after they are metabolized, excess sER is removed by autophagy. In muscle cells, the sER (sarcoplasmic reticulum) regulates muscle contraction by release and reuptake of calcium ions.

Annulate Lamellae

Stacks of membrane-bounded cisternae with numerous pore complexes, identical to isolated nuclear envelopes, are present in germ cells and cells with high protein synthesis. Their functional significance is unknown.

Peroxisomes

Peroxisomes are small membrane-bounded organelles that vary in size and shape. They have a finely granular electron-dense content and frequently contain crystalline electron-dense inclusions. Peroxisomes are particularly abundant in hepatocytes and in the epithelial cells of the proximal convoluted tubule of the kidney. Peroxisomes perform oxidative reactions. They produce H_2O_2; catalase uses this H_2O_2 to oxidize a variety of substances. The energy derived from oxidations is either used for metabolic processes or is dispersed as heat. Peroxisomes detoxify certain substances, such as ethanol, and play a role in gluconeogenesis.

Mitochondria

When living cells are stained with supravital dyes, such as Janus Green B, mitochondria become visible as small rods or spheres approximately 0.2 μm in diameter and up to 12 μm in length. Mitochondria are the chief source of ATP (energy) for the cell and are thus partic-

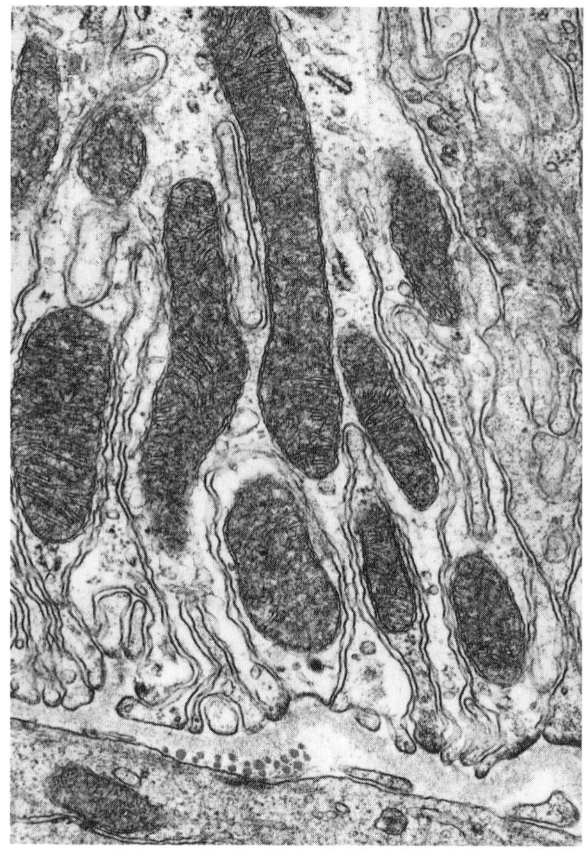

Figure 1.15. *The inner membrane of the mitochondria in the interdigitating processes of the cells of the proximal convoluted tubule of the kidney is thrown into folds (×28,000).*

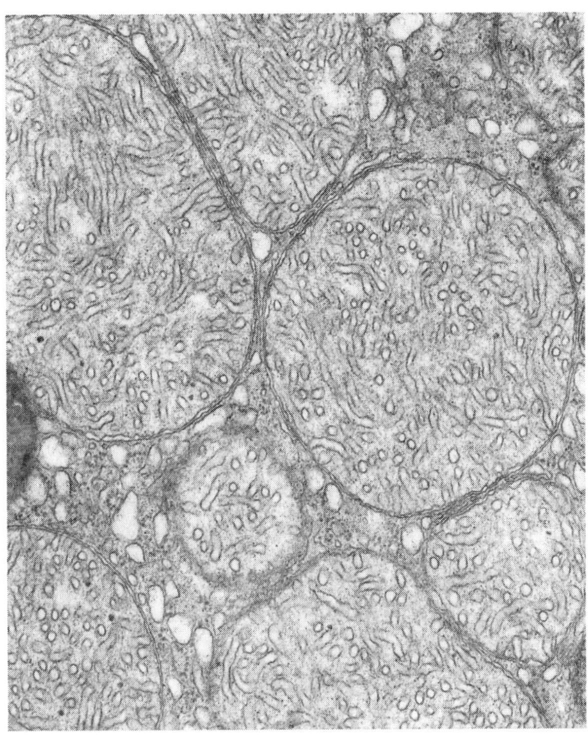

Figure 1.16. *The inner membrane of these mitochondria in the adrenal cortex forms cylindric tubules that project into the mitochondrial matrix (×28,500).*

ularly numerous in cells with high metabolic activity. In many cells, mitochondria seem to be distributed randomly and change their location continually, whereas in others, they are stationary at sites of high energy consumption, such as in the basal processes of the epithelial cells of the convoluted tubules of the kidney (Fig. 1.15).

At the fine structural level, mitochondria comprise an outer bounding and an inner membrane (Figs. 1.15 and 1.16), an intermembranous space, and a matrix space. The **outer membrane** is a smooth, saclike structure, permeable to molecules below 5000 D. The **inner membrane** is impermeable to most small ions and is thrown into folds (cristae) (Fig. 1.15) or cylindric or prismatic tubules (tubuli) (Fig. 1.16) that project into the interior of the mitochondrion. The enzymes of the respiratory chain are located in the inner membrane.

The main function of mitochondria is to perform most cellular oxidations and to produce ATP and heat. This is accomplished in the citric acid cycle by enzymatic oxidation of pyruvate and fatty acids. In the citric acid cycle, large amounts of nicotinamide adenine dinucleotide (NADH) are produced. In a process called oxidative phosphorylation, reactive electrons from NADH react with molecular oxygen (O_2) in the respiratory chain to produce ATP from adenosine 5′-diphosphate (ADP) and inorganic phosphate. This ATP is rapidly transported into the cytoplasm, in exchange for ADP produced by ATP hydrolysis in the cytosol.

The **intermembranous space** contains enzymes that use ATP passing out of the matrix to phosphorylate other nucleotides. The inner membrane encloses a space occupied by the **matrix**, which contains occasional granules that are binding sites of calcium and other divalent cations. In addition, many enzymes, including those that oxidize fatty acids and pyruvate, and those required for the citric acid cycle are present. The mitochondrial matrix also contains mitochondrial DNA and enzymes required for their transcription, tRNAs and mRNAs, and mitochondrial ribosomes.

Mitochondria do not replicate by de novo synthesis but grow and divide. This process involves two protein synthesis machineries, that of the mitochondrion and that of the cytosol, from which proteins are transported into the mitochondrial matrix through the mitochondrial membranes.

CYTOSKELETON

A variety of cellular functions are performed or mediated by microfilaments, intermediate filaments, and microtubules. Together with a variety of proteins that interconnect these structures or link them to other structures, such as the plasma membrane or secretory granules, they make up the **cytoskeleton**. The cytoskeleton is a dynamic structure, the components of which are continuously assembling and disassembling. All three components of the cytoskeleton are involved in changes of the cell shape, muscle contraction, and intracellular movements, such as axoplasmic transport, chromosome migration during cell division, and traffic of vesicles, mitochondria, endosomes, and lysosomes. Microtubules and microfilaments are ubiquitous and their fundamental structure is the same in all cells. Intermediate filaments are heterogenous, and their composition varies in different cell types.

Microfilaments

Microfilaments are ~8 nm in diameter and are helices (F actin) of globular G actin monomers. Only approximately half of the cellular actin is present in filamentous form; the other half is monomeric. Actin-binding proteins cross-link actin filaments into parallel bundles (e.g., in filopodia and microvilli; Figs. 1.4 and 1.17), contractile bundles (e.g., in dividing cells), and gel-like networks beneath the cell membrane (cell cortex). Various types of myosin can link adjacent actin filaments, mediating their movements against each other, or they can link actin filaments and a membrane, moving membrane-bounded organelles or causing movements of the cell membrane (e.g., during phagocytosis). In muscle cells, actin filaments slide against myosin, mediating cellular contraction.

Intermediate Filaments

Intermediate filaments measure 8 to 10 nm in diameter. These filaments are helical arrays of tetrameres, each composed of elongated filamentous protein

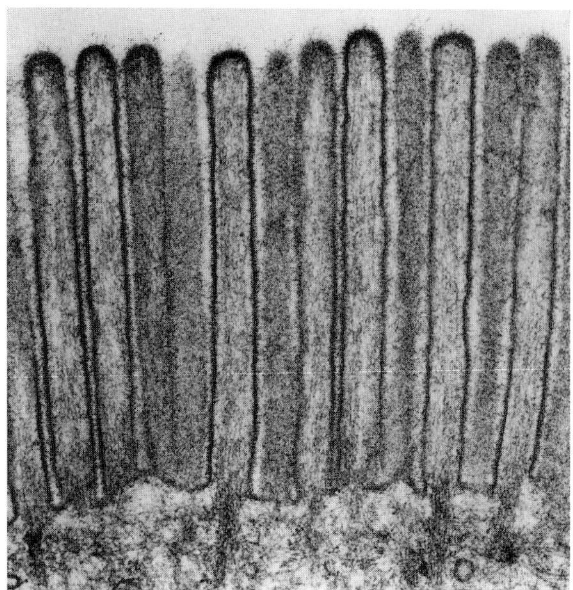

Figure 1.17. *The microvilli at the apical surface of a small intestinal absorptive cell contain numerous microfilaments that project into the terminal web (×51,000).*

monomers. Although present in almost all cells, where they form perinuclear networks that extend to the plasma membrane, intermediate filaments are especially abundant in cells subjected to mechanical stress, such as epithelial cells, muscle cells, and peripheral nerve fibers.

On the basis of their chemical composition, distinctive function, and distribution, six major types of intermediate filaments have been identified. **Keratin filaments**, also referred to as tonofilaments, occur primarily in epithelial cells. These filaments are chemically and functionally diverse; they are particularly abundant in stratified squamous epithelial cells, where they are linked to other structural proteins, subserving barrier functions; keratin filaments provide mechanical stability by being attached to special structural proteins at desmosomes and hemidesmosomes. **Desmin filaments** are abundant in smooth muscle cells, supporting thin filaments and transmitting their contractile forces to the cell surface; in striated muscle cells, desmin filaments link adjacent myofibrils and connect them to the plasma membrane. **Vimentin filaments** are present in many cells of mesodermal origin and are particularly concentrated around the nucleus. **Glial filaments**, composed of glial fibrillary acid protein (GFAP), are the major cytoskeletal filaments of astrocytes and neurolemmocytes (Schwann cells). **Neurofilaments** support nerve cell processes, especially the long axons (Fig. 1.18). **Nuclear lamins** form a fibrous lamina on the inner surface of the nuclear envelope (see p. 4).

Microtubules

Microtubules are hollow tubules of variable length that measure 25 nm in diameter. The microtubule wall is composed of 13 linear protofilaments bundled in parallel to form a cylinder. Each protofilament is in turn made of alternating heterodimers of globular α- and β-tubulin subunits (see Fig. 1.22).

Microtubules are polar structures with a plus and a minus end; microtubules are in a continuous state of polymerization at the fast-growing plus end and depolymerization at the minus end, unless stabilized. Microtubule growth is initiated in various locations throughout the cytosol, the major one being the centrosome, also called cell center or cytocentrum (Fig. 1.1). The centrosome contains a pair of centrioles and an electron-dense pericentriolar matrix, where polymerization begins.

Microtubules provide binding sites for microtubule-associated proteins (MAPs), which prevent depolymerization and mediate interaction with other cell components. Cytoplasmic dyneins and kinesins are also called microtubule motor proteins. These are MAPs that actively move organelles, such as secretory, transport, and endocytotic vesicles, ribosomes, and mitochondria along the microtubules.

Microtubules play an essential role in cell division (mitotic spindle). Antimitotic drugs, such as colchicine and vincristine, inhibit cell division by preventing the addition of tubulin heterodimers to existing microtubules and by inducing microtubule depolymerization. Microtubules are the major structural components of cilia, basal bodies (see p. 16), and centrioles. Each **centriole** is a cylindrical structure, ~ 0.1 μm in diameter and ~ 0.3 μm in length, that is barely visible with the light microscope. The centriolar wall comprises nine groups of three microtubules in longitudinal and parallel arrangement. Each triplet is composed of one complete microtubule that is fused with two incomplete microtubules; triplets are interconnected through stabilizing linker proteins.

Microtubules determine the distribution of microfilaments and intermediate filaments within the cell, thereby specifying their polarity. Microtubules function in the maintenance of shape of erythrocytes and platelets. They are essential for the growth of processes in developing nerve cells as well as for anterograde and retrograde axonal transport of various organelles (see chapter 6) (Fig. 1.18).

CYTOPLASMIC INCLUSIONS

Cytoplasmic inclusions are either transitory cellular structures that do not participate in cellular metabolism or permanent ones that do play metabolic roles. Some of these inclusions are exogenous (e.g., phagocytosed material, residual bodies). Most inclusions are endogenous and include glycogen, lipid, pigments, and protein crystals.

Glycogen

Glycogen, the major storage form of carbohydrate, is particularly abundant in liver and in cardiac and skeletal muscle cells. In routine histologic sections, glycogen

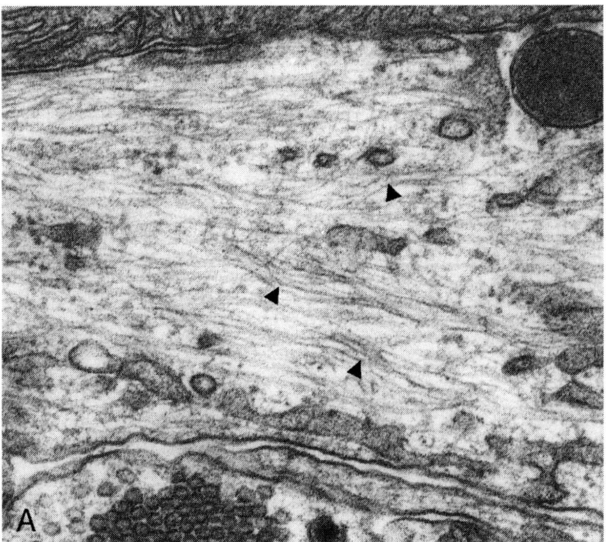

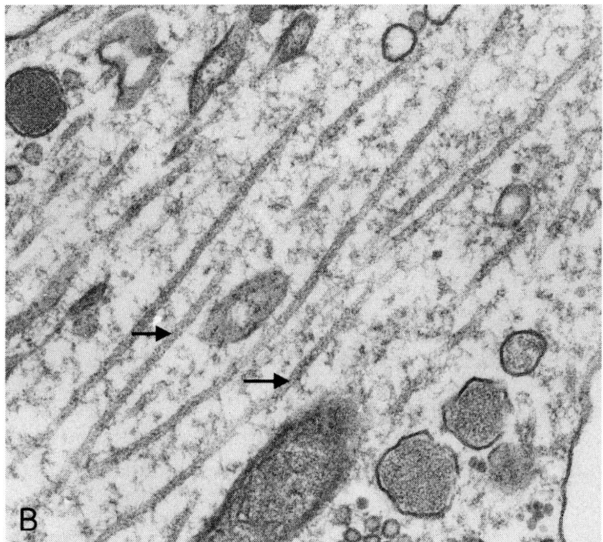

Figure 1.18. *Intermediate filaments (arrowheads) and microtubules (arrows) in axons of neurosecretory neurons (×63,000).*

remains unstained, but it can be demonstrated selectively by the periodic acid-Schiff (PAS) reaction or Best s carmine stain. At the fine-structural level, glycogen occurs either as single electron-dense granules 10 to 40 nm in diameter (β-particles) or as larger assemblies of these granules, forming rosette configurations called α-particles.

Lipid

Fat is stored primarily in adipose cells but is also present in a variety of other cells, e.g., steroid hormone-producing cells. It is an important energy reserve. Because most routine histologic techniques involve the use of fat solvents, lipids are demonstrated only with special techniques, such as osmic acid fixation, which renders fat resistant to extraction, or in Sudan III-stained frozen sections. With the electron microscope, lipid is seen in the form of droplets devoid of a bounding membrane (see Figs. 1.8 and 1.14).

Melanin

Melanin is a dark brown to black pigment that occurs primarily in the pigment epithelium of the retina, in the leptomeninx of the central nervous system, and in the integument. It is synthesized by melanocytes and forms membrane-bounded granules (melanosomes) that may be transferred to other cells, such as the keratinocytes in the stratum basale of the skin.

Hemosiderin

Hemosiderin is the result of hemoglobin degradation after phagocytosis of erythrocytes in the spleen, liver, bone marrow, and hemal nodes. This golden brown pigment occurs as granular cytoplasmic inclusions in phagocytes. It contains iron, which permits its distinction from other pigments of similar color (e.g., lipofuscin). With the electron microscope, hemosiderin is seen to be composed of accumulations of particles of ferritin, an iron-containing protein.

Lipofuscin

Lipofuscin is a golden brown pigment, stainable with certain fat dyes, that is commonly found in cardiac muscle, liver, and some nerve cells. It is composed of the indigestible residues of phagocytosis, autophagy, and crinophagy and is thus the morphologically heterogeneous end product of lysosomal activity. The amount of pigment increases with the age of the animal and accumulates in the form of residual bodies (Figs. 1.10, 1.13).

CYTOPLASMIC MATRIX

The cytoplasmic matrix, also called cytosol, fills the spaces of the three-dimensional cytoskeletal reticulum that stretches between the cell surface and organelles and inclusions. The fluid matrix contains water and electrolytes, enzymes, cytoskeletal molecules, proteins, ribosomes, glycogen, and lipids. It is the site of protein synthesis and intermediary metabolism. Diffusion of molecules (e.g., thyroxine, end products of lysosomal digestion) throughout the cell takes place in the matrix. Temporarily, the matrix may change from a fluid state to a gel-like consistency and vice versa (sol—gel transformation), facilitating or impeding intracellular diffusion.

SPECIALIZATIONS OF THE CELL SURFACE

The following paragraphs describe cell structures as they relate to specific cell functions. Thus, repetitious descriptions are avoided in the histology and organol-

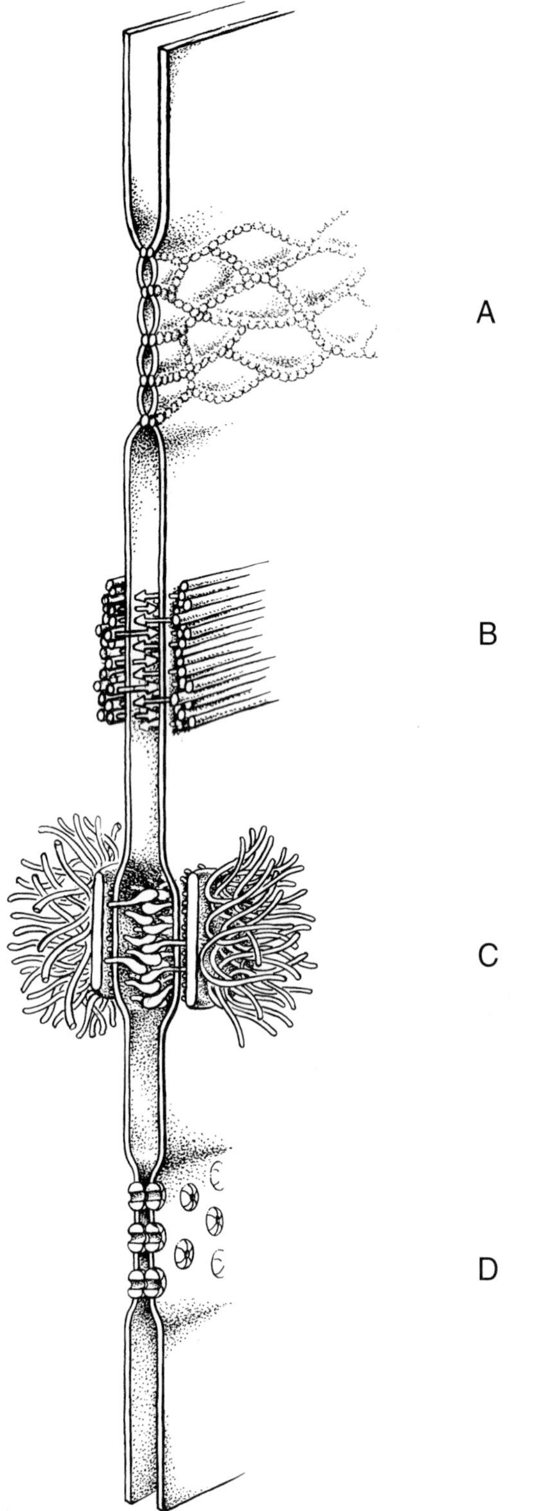

Figure 1.19. *Diagrams of intercellular junctions: tight junction (A), zonula adherens (B), macula adherens (C), gap junction (D). (Modified and redrawn from Cormack DH. Ham s histology. 9th ed. Philadelphia: JB Lippincott, 1987; and Alberts B, Bray D, Lewis J, et al. Molecular biology of the cell. New York: Garland,*

ogy chapters, in which only those differences that reflect specialized functions of certain cells are reviewed.

Intercellular Junctions

Most cells in the mammalian organism are attached to other cells to form tissues and organs. Specializations of the cell surface provide not only a means of attachment between cells but also a way of communication.

There are three major types of morphologically and functionally distinct intercellular or cell-to-cell junctions: tight or occluding junctions form a barrier between lumen and intercellular space; adhering or anchoring junctions hold adjacent cells together or attach them to the extracellular matrix; gap or communicating junctions mediate movement of molecules between cells (Fig. 1.19).

TIGHT JUNCTIONS

Tight (or occluding) junctions are unique to epithelial cells. They consist of irregularly anastomosing ridges that seal neighboring cells together in a beltlike fashion (Fig. 1.19). The number of ridges varies according to the types of epithelium. At these ridges, transmembrane proteins of adjacent cells make contact across the intercellular space. Tight junctions constitute a barrier that prevents the passage of water-soluble molecules from the lumen to the basolateral intercellular space and vice versa. Tight junctions, however, may be selectively permeable to certain substances. They also maintain cell polarity by preventing the basolateral movement of apical membrane proteins (e.g., enzymes).

ADHERING (ANCHORING) JUNCTIONS

In adhering junctions, the cytoskeletal elements of one cell are connected to those of a neighboring cell or to the extracellular matrix. Three types of junctions are classified as adhering junctions: zonula adherens, desmosome, and hemidesmosome.

The **zonula adherens** is also referred to as belt desmosome or intermediate junction. It is located below the tight junction and surrounds epithelial cells in a beltlike fashion (Fig. 1.19). Zonulae adherentes in adjacent cells are directly apposed. They are held together by transmembrane linker proteins, of the cadherin family of cell-to-cell adhesion molecules (cCAMs). A bundle of actin filaments runs parallel to the junctional cell membrane; via intracellular attachment proteins, it is attached to the transmembrane linker proteins. Zonulae adherentes are prominent in the lining cells of the intestine, where contraction of the actin filament bundle causes protrusion of the cell surface and splaying of the microvilli, thereby enhancing absorption. In the developing organism, zonulae adherentes are believed to play a role in the folding of epithelial sheets into tubes.

A **desmosome**, also called spot desmosome or macula adherens, is a disklike structure approximately 200 to

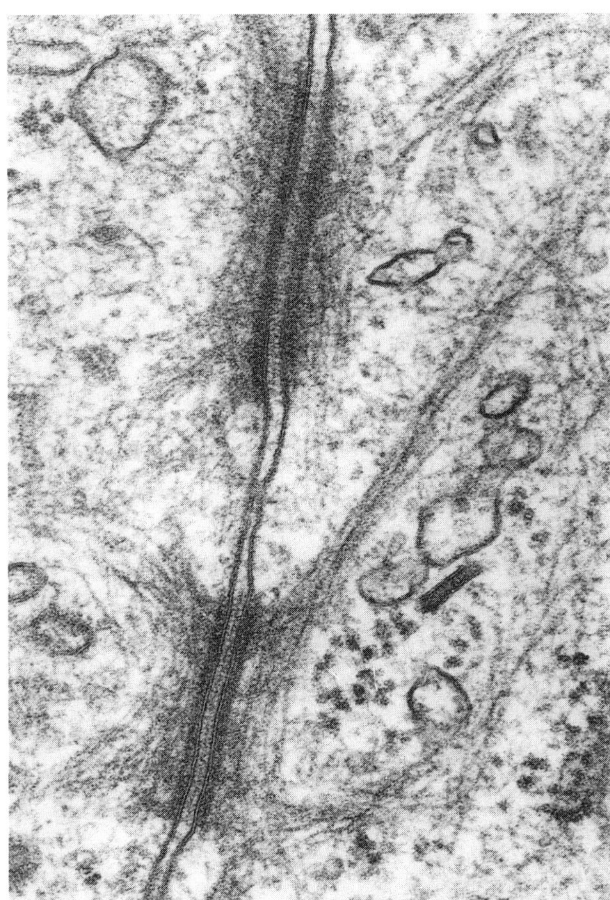

Figure 1.20. *Desmosomes between two neurohypophysial glial cells. Notice the distinct central electron-dense lines and the intermediate filaments that form hair pin loops (×87,500).*

400 nm in diameter (Figs. 1.19 and 1.20), that has a counterpart in a neighboring cell. Transmembrane linker proteins, also belonging to the cadherin family of cCAMs, hold together adjacent membranes. In the intercellular space, often a central electron-dense line is visible, caused by the apposition of the oligosaccharide moieties of the cadherins. The transmembrane linker proteins, in turn, are connected to a set of intracellular attachment proteins that form an electron-dense attachment plaque beneath the plasma membrane. Intermediate filaments are attached to this plaque, forming hairpin loops. Desmosomes effectively link the cytoskeleton of adjacent cells, especially in epithelia, and enable them to resist mechanical stress and maintain their integrity.

Small desmosomelike contacts occurring at multiple sites between cells (e.g., ciliary epithelium) are called **puncta adherentia**.

Hemidesmosomes resemble desmosomes, but they do not connect adjacent cells to the basal lamina. The transmembrane linker proteins are integrins that attach to extracellular matrix proteins on the one hand and to intracellular attachment proteins on the other. The latter form a dense subplasmalemmal plaque, which is the point of termination of intermediate filaments.

COMMUNICATING JUNCTIONS

Gap junctions are communicating junctions that permit the direct passage of inorganic ions and other small water-soluble molecules from cell to cell. At their level, the intercellular space is narrowed to approximately 2 nm (Fig. 1.21). This space is bridged by six transmem-

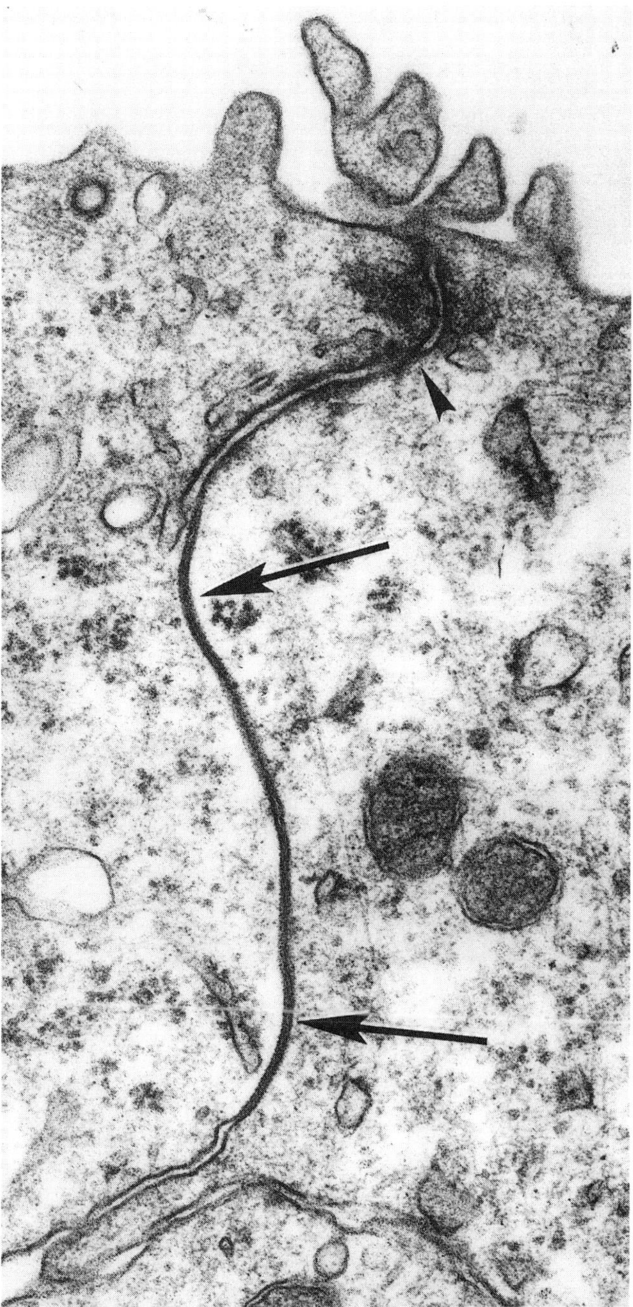

Figure 1.21. *Zonula adherens (arrowhead) and extensive gap junctions (arrows) between two ependymal cells (×60,000).*

brane proteins of the apposed membranes, which are complementary and interlock, and which are called connexons. The proteins of two adjacent connexons constitute the wall of a hydrophilic channel, 1.5 nm in diameter (Fig. 1.19). Gap junctions permit the conduction of electrical impulses, and possibly synchronization of function, and metabolic cooperation (nutrient transfer) of cells. Gap junctions are thus of considerable functional importance and are absent only in skeletal muscle, spermatozoa, and circulating blood cells.

Specializations of the Free Surface

CILIA AND FLAGELLA

Ciliated cells are commonly found in the respiratory system, where they function in the movement of a mucous film. They also occur in the male and female reproductive systems, where they promote the propulsion of spermatozoa and oocytes. Several hundred cilia may be found on a single cell (see Figs. 9.4 and 9.5). Cilia are approximately 0.2 μm in diameter and between 5 and 15 μm in length and thus are visible with the light microscope. At the fine-structural level, cilia consist of an axoneme surrounded by the plasma membrane (Fig. 1.22). The axoneme is composed of nine doublet microtubules around two central single microtubules. The two central microtubules are complete. In each outer doublet, one microtubule is complete (circular cross section) and the other is partial (C-shaped cross section). The wall of the partial microtubule is made of only 10 protofilaments and is fused to that of the complete microtubule. At regular intervals, pairs of dynein side arms project from the microtubules; adjacent doublets are linked by an elastic protein, nexin. From each of the nine doublets, radial spokes extend to the central sheath that surrounds the two central microtubules. The tubules extend throughout the entire length of the cilium, from the apex to the **basal body**. The basal body is located at the base of the cilium, and its structure is identical to that of centrioles. The two central tubules terminate at the base plate, an electron-dense disk; the peripheral doublets are continuous with the inner pair of microtubules of the triplets of the basal body.

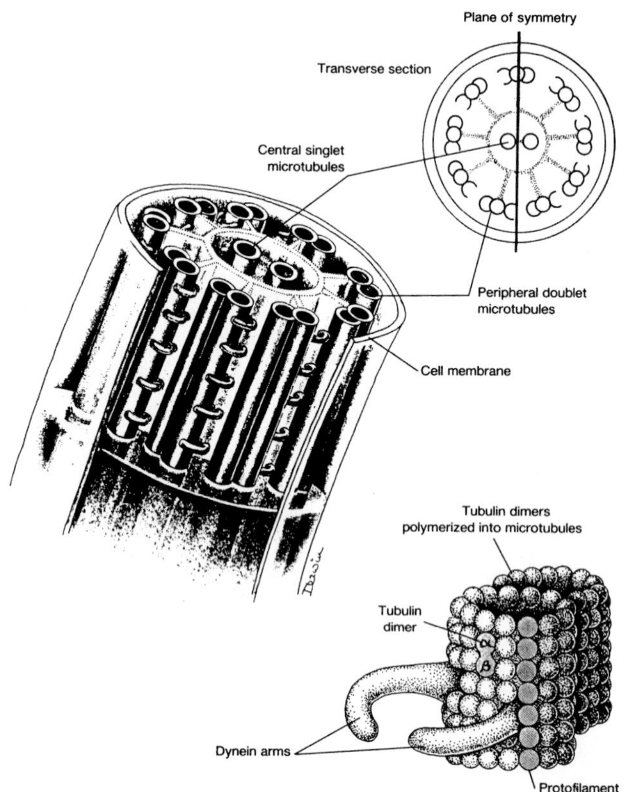

Figure 1.22. *Diagram of the structure of a cilium. (From Cormack DH. Ham's histology. 9th ed. Philadelphia: JB Lippincott, 1987.)*

Cilia are rigid during their effective stroke, e.g., when propelling mucus, and become flexible during their return, or recovery, stroke. They function in a metachronal rhythm, in which each row of cilia beats in sequence. During ciliary movement, doublets of microtubules slide in relation to one another, using energy provided by the splitting of ATP through ATPase located within the dynein arms.

A single long cilium is referred to as a **flagellum**. The most prominent example of a flagellated cell is the mammalian spermatozoon, the flagellum of which may be several hundred micrometers long; it uses undulatory movements for its propulsion.

MICROVILLI

In cells in which the principal function is absorption, the free surface is considerably increased by a varying number of cytoplasmic evaginations called microvilli (Fig. 1.17). These are observable with the light microscope when they are particularly numerous and densely packed, as in the small intestine (striated border) and the proximal convoluted tubule of the kidney (brush border). With the electron microscope, the microvilli are seen to be slender cylindric processes, approximately 0.1 μm in diameter and of variable length. The villus core is made of 20 to 30 parallel actin filaments (Fig. 1.4), which extend from their attachment to a region of amorphous material at the tips of the microvilli into the terminal web, which is composed of spectrin and myosin molecules. The actin filaments are attached to the plasma membrane by myosin molecules that mediate upward movement of the plasma membrane over the core of the microvillus. In vitro, microvilli have been shown to contract as a result of the interaction of microvillous actin filaments with myosin in the terminal web.

Another variety of microvilli are those present at the luminal surface of the epithelial lining of the epididymis. They are slender and often branching cytoplasmic processes of varying length. They contain actin filaments that extend into the apical cytoplasm. The tips of these microvilli are usually entwined.

STEREOCILIA

The hair cells of the spiral organ, or organ of hearing (Corti), and the receptor cells in the vestibular sensory receptors of the inner ear have long, rigid microvilli that are commonly referred to as stereocilia. They differ from other microvilli in that they are narrower at the base than at the tip. They contain actin filaments that confer rigidity to these structures and enable them to detect minute movements of their fluid environment.

CELL CYCLE

Most cells in the organism are subject to cyclic events that reoccur at regular intervals, referred to as the cell cycle. In a somatic cell (as opposed to a reproductive or germ cell), this cycle is divided into two phases. It begins with the dividing phase, referred to as M phase or mitosis, continues with the interphase, during which cells perform their specific functions and grow, and terminates with a new cell division.

Interphase

Interphase is subdivided into three phases. The G_1 (gap 1) or **preduplication phase** is the period between the previous mitosis and the beginning of DNA duplication. Most cells are in this stage while they perform their particular functions. The duration of this phase varies within wide limits. In adult nerve cells, which never divide, it lasts for the lifetime of the organism.

During the following S or **synthesis phase**, DNA replication occurs, resulting in two chromosomes, each of which consists of 50% original (parental) and 50% replicated (new) DNA. These chromosomes are referred to as sister **chromatids**. Each chromatid contains a specific DNA sequence, the centromere, that is necessary for ultimate proper segregation of the chromatids. Duplication of the centrioles takes place, and daughter centrioles begin to grow. S phase lasts between 6 and 8 hours.

After completion of the S phase and before mitosis (M phase) begins, the cell passes through a rather short G_2 (gap 2) or **postduplication phase**. During this phase, the elongation of daughter centrioles is completed. The duration of the G_2 phase is between 1 and 2 hours.

M Phase

M phase is also referred to as the cell-division phase and comprises mitosis, i.e., nuclear division, and cytokinesis, i.e., cytoplasmic division. M phase lasts between 30 and 90 minutes. Although a continuous event, it is divided into six consecutive phases: (*1*) prophase, (*2*) prometaphase, (*3*) metaphase, (*4*) anaphase, (*5*) telophase, and (*6*) cytokinesis.

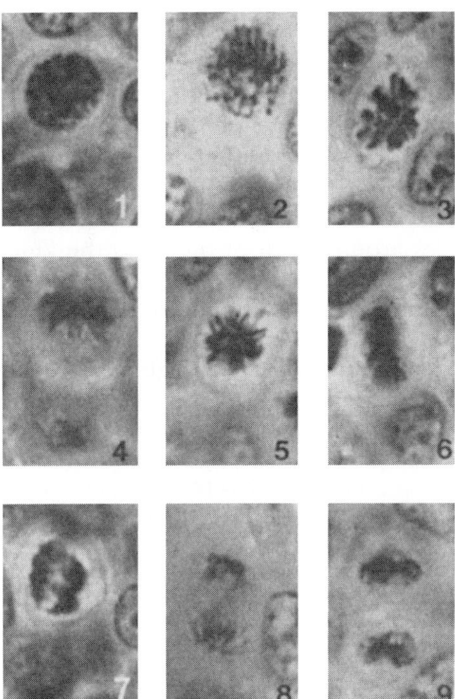

Figure 1.23. *Mitotic divisions in the epithelial cells of the epiglottis.* ***1–3:*** *Prophase,* ***4–6:*** *metaphase;* ***7, 8:*** *anaphase;* ***9:*** *telophase. Hematoxylin and eosin (×1250). (Courtesy of A. Hansen.)*

Upon entering **prophase**, the cell hypertrophies and assumes a spherical shape by retracting its processes and losing surface differentiations (Fig. 1.23). The chromosomes become visible, and as prophase proceeds, they shorten, thicken, and coil and are seen to consist of two sister chromatids. The pairs of centrioles begin to move to the opposite poles of the cell; microtubules of the cytoskeleton disassemble and those of the mitotic spindle assemble.

Prometaphase begins with the disintegration of the nuclear envelope and the disappearance of the nucleolus. The cell becomes more elongated. Centrosomes at opposite poles of the cell form spindle poles. Spindle microtubules enter the nuclear region. On each centromere, a kinetochore forms, to which kinetochore microtubules attach. Other spindle microtubules are referred to as polar microtubules and those outside the spindle are called astral microtubules.

When the chromosomes are arranged with all their centromeres in the same plane, the metaphase or equatorial plane, the cell is in **metaphase** (Fig. 1.23). The chromosomes are held in place by the kinetochore microtubules, which are attached to opposite spindle poles. The arms of the bent chromosomes are directed toward the poles of the cell.

The addition of colchicine to rapidly dividing cells in culture inhibits spindle formation and causes arrest of mitosis. The chromosomes also become more condensed, and because of their characteristic shapes, they can be used to establish the karyotype of an individual.

During **anaphase**, the kinetochore of each chromosome splits, and the sister chromatids, now called (daughter) chromosomes, are pulled to the opposite spindle poles of the cell by the shortening kinetochore microtubules. As the polar microtubules elongate, the spindle poles move farther apart (Fig. 1.23).

In **telophase**, each group of chromosomes are at the poles of the cell (Fig. 1.23), and the nuclear envelope reassembles around each of them. As the kinetochore microtubules disappear, the chromosomes decondense. At the same time, the nucleoli are reconstituted. This marks the end of mitosis.

During **cytokinesis**, the cleavage furrow, a constriction that began to develop late in anaphase, deepens at the equator of the elongated cell by contraction of a contractile ring composed of actin and myosin. Thus, a slender cytoplasmic bridge is formed, referred to as the midbody, that contains tightly packed microtubules. The bridge eventually breaks, and the two separate daughter cells round up, thus completing cytokinesis.

Meiosis

In contrast to the somatic cells, which have a diploid set of chromosomes, the male and female germ cells (spermatozoon and oocyte) possess a haploid number of chromosomes. Because they derive from diploid precursors, these germ cells undergo a special type of division, during which the number of chromosomes is reduced by one-half. This process is referred to as **meiosis** and is described in detail in Chapter 12.

REFERENCES

Alberts B, Bray D, Lewis J, et al. Molecular biology of the cell. New York: Garland Publishing, 1994.

Bershadsky A, Vasiliev JM. Cytoskeleton. New York: Plenum Press, 1988.

Bittar EE, Bittar N, eds. Cellular organelles and the extracellular matrix. Principles of medical biology. London: Jai Press Inc., 1995;3.

Cantin M, ed. Cell biology of the secretory process. Basel: Karger, 1983.

Chiechanover AJ, Schwartz AL, eds. Cellular proteolytic systems. New York: Wiley-Liss, 1994.

Dustin P. Microtubules. Berlin: Springer-Verlag, 1984.

Goodenough DA, Goliger JA, Paul DL. Connexins, connexons and intercellular communication. Annu Rev Biochem 1996;65:475.

Kanno Y. Intercellular communication through gap junctions. New York: Elsevier, 1995.

Krstic RV. Ultrastructure of the mammalian cell. Berlin: Springer Verlag, 1979.

Lipowski R, Sackmann E. Structure and dynamics of membranes. Handbook of biological physics. Amsterdam: Elsevier Science B. V., 1995;1.

Porter KR, Bonneville MA. An introduction to the fine structure of cells and tissues. 4th ed. Philadelphia: Lea & Febiger, 1973.

Robinson MS, Watts C, Zerial M. Membrane dynamics in endocytosis. Cell 1996;84:13.

Smith CA. Cell biology. 2nd ed. New York: Chapman and Hall, 1996.

Tager JM, Azzi A, Papa S, et al., eds. Organelles in eukaryotic cells. Molecular structure and interaction. New York: Plenum Press, 1989.

Thilo L. Endocytosis: aspects of organellar processing. Ann N Y Acad Sci 1994;710:209.

2

Epithelium

BRIAN L. FRAPPIER

INTRODUCTION

Cells, Tissues, and Organs

Epithelium is a **tissue**. A **tissue** is an aggregation of cells and intercellular substances specialized to perform particular functions. Despite its structural and functional complexity, the animal body is composed of only four basic types of tissue: **epithelium, connective tissue, muscle**, and **nervous tissue** (Table 2.1). **Organs** consist of various arrangements of the four basic tissues.

Main Characteristics of Epithelium

Epithelium exists in two major forms: **surface epithelium** and **glandular epithelium**. **Surface epithelium** consists of sheets of aggregated cells of similar type that cover or line all of the external and internal surfaces of the body. **Glandular epithelium**, the secretory cells of endocrine and exocrine glands, results from the proliferation of surface epithelial cells into underlying connective tissue.

All three embryonic germ layers take part in the formation of epithelium. **Ectoderm** is the origin of the epithelium of the external body surfaces. Most of the lining epithelium of the digestive and respiratory systems originates from **endoderm**, and **mesoderm** gives rise to the lining of the vascular system, the serous membrane body cavities, and parts of the urogenital system.

At the basal surface of all epithelial cells that make contact with underlying connective tissue, a thin sheet of extracellular matrix, the **basement membrane**, is present. The basement membrane usually is not visible in routine light-microscopic sections but can be demonstrated with the periodic acid-Schiff (PAS) technique or silver stains. As seen with the electron microscope, the basement membrane invariably consists of two distinct layers: the **lamina lucida**, a low density layer next to the epithelial cell membrane, and the underlying electron-dense **lamina densa** (**lamina basalis**). These two laminae are synthesized by the epithelial cells and are composed principally of proteoglycans, primarily heparan sulfate, as well as laminin, fibronectin, and type IV collagen. In most basement membranes, a third component, the **sub-basal lamina** is present. The sub-basal lamina is composed principally of reticular fibers and connects the lamina densa to the subepithelial connective tissue. In addition to providing attachment for the epithelium, the sub-basal lamina permits stretching and recoil of the epithelium in distensible organs.

Table 2.1.
The Basic Tissues

Epithelium
Muscle
Connective tissue
Nervous tissue

Table 2.2.
Characteristics of Epithelium

Derive from all three embryonic germ layers
Contact a basement membrane
Cover body surfaces (surface epithelium)
Form secretory cells of glands (glandular epithelium)
Are avascular
Possess functional diversity
Are capable of mitosis

In addition to underlying all epithelia-contacting connective tissue, a basement membrane is found between epithelia in the renal corpuscle and between epithelia in the lung alveolus. In these locations, the sub-basal lamina is absent. A basement membrane is also found around smooth muscle cells, skeletal muscle cells, and cardiac muscle cells, as well as around adipocytes and neurolemmocytes.

Basement membranes serve in a variety of capacities, e.g., as ultrafilters in capillaries, particularly those of the renal corpuscle, as selective barriers to exchange of macromolecules, and as a guide to epithelial cell movements. Because blood and lymph vessels do not penetrate the basement membrane, epithelial cells must receive their nutritional support by diffusion from capillaries located in the underlying connective tissue.

Epithelial cells are specialized for a variety of different functions, among which are protection, absorption, secretion, excretion, and formation of barriers for selective permeability. Epithelial cells continuously proliferate via mitosis to replace cells lost through attrition. The main characteristics of epithelium are summarized in Table 2.2.

CLASSIFICATION

The classification of the various surface epithelial types is based on: *(a)* the number of layers present, and *(b)* the shape of the epithelial cells. A surface epithelium consisting of a single layer of cells resting on the basement membrane is described as a **simple epithelium**. A **stratified epithelium** is composed of two or more layers of cells with only the basal cell layer resting on the basement membrane. The names given to the various types of stratified epithelia are based **on the shape of the surface cells** without regard to the shape of those within the deeper layers. A surface epithelium is considered **pseudostratified** if all of its cells contact the basement membrane but not all extend to the free surface. As a result, nuclei are located at different levels within a pseudostratified epithelium, giving the false impression of being stratified.

MICROSCOPIC STRUCTURE

Simple Squamous Epithelium

Simple squamous epithelium consists of a single layer of thin, flat, scalelike cells. On surface view (Figs. 2.1A and 2.2), the cells have an irregular shape with a slightly serrated border. They fit together to form a continuous sheet. A spherical to oval nucleus, near the center of the cell, gives a slightly elevated appearance to this area. On cross section, the cell appears thicker in the area of the nucleus and has thin attenuated strands of cytoplasm on either side (Fig. 2.2).

Simple squamous epithelium lines moist internal surfaces, such as the serous membrane of body cavities, the internal surface of the heart, and the luminal surface of blood and lymph vessels. The simple squamous epithelium lining the serous membrane of body cavities (pleural, pericardial, and peritoneal cavities) is referred to as **mesothelium**; that lining the heart, blood vessels, and lymph vessels is referred to as **endothelium**. Simple squamous epithelium is also found lining the pulmonary alveoli, the anterior chamber of the eye, the internal surface of the tympanic membrane, the membranous labyrinth of the internal ear, the glomerular capsule, and a portion of the loop of the nephron.

Simple Cuboidal Epithelium

Simple cuboidal epithelium is a single layer of cells, the width and height of which are approximately equal. These cells appear as squares in cross sections but are more hexagonal when seen from the surface (Figs. 2.1B and 2.3). When the height is slightly less than the width of a cell, it is known as **low cuboidal epithelium**, and when the height is slightly greater than the width, the epithelium is called **tall cuboidal epithelium**. The classification of epithelia is not always clear-cut; however, and many times, intermediate forms require some subjective judgment regarding classification.

Simple cuboidal epithelium can be found lining the ducts of many glands and the collecting ducts of the kidney, as a component of the choroid plexus and ciliary body, and lining the follicles of the thyroid gland. The epithelium of the lens and the retinal pigment epithelium are also examples of simple cuboidal epithelium.

Simple Columnar Epithelium

Simple columnar epithelium consists of tall, narrow cells with considerably greater height than width (Figs. 2.1C and 2.4). Usually, the nuclei are oval and are located near the base of each cell. Generally, simple columnar epithelium lines organs that perform absorp-

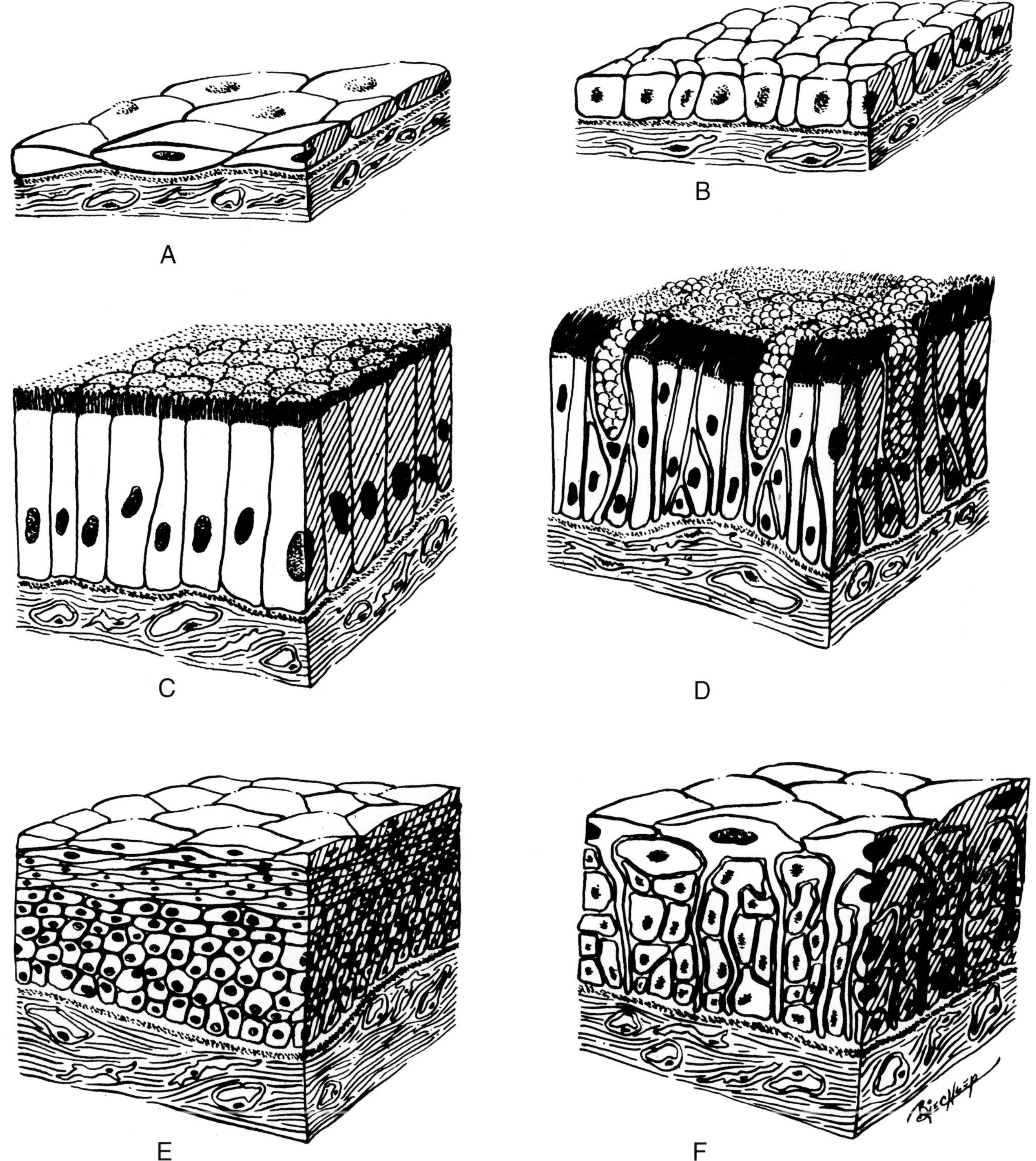

Figure 2.1. *Schematic drawings illustrating the major types of surface epithelia.* ***A.****, Simple squamous epithelium.* ***B.****, Simple cuboidal epithelium.* ***C.****, Simple columnar epithelium bearing microvilli.* ***D.****, Pseudostratified columnar epithelium with cilia and goblet cells.* ***E.****, Stratified squamous epithelium, nonkeratinized.* ***F.****, Transitional epithelium.*

tive or secretory functions, e.g., the glandular stomach, the small and large intestines, and the gallbladder in the digestive system; the bulbourethral gland in the male reproductive system; and the uterus and uterine tube in the female reproductive system.

Pseudostratified Columnar Epithelium

Pseudostratified columnar epithelium is composed of a single layer of cells, but because the cells are irregular in shape and size, their nuclei are located at various lev-

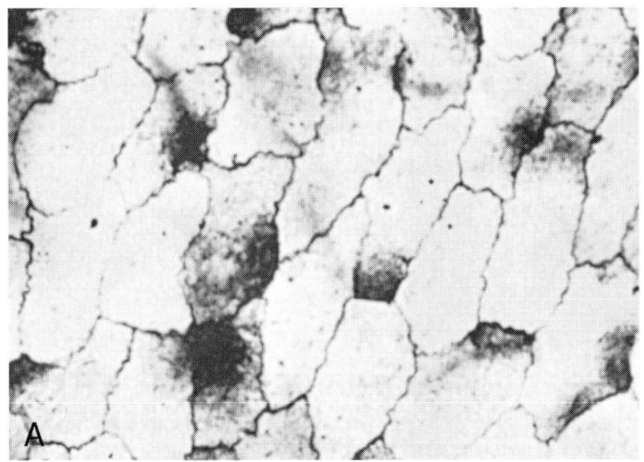

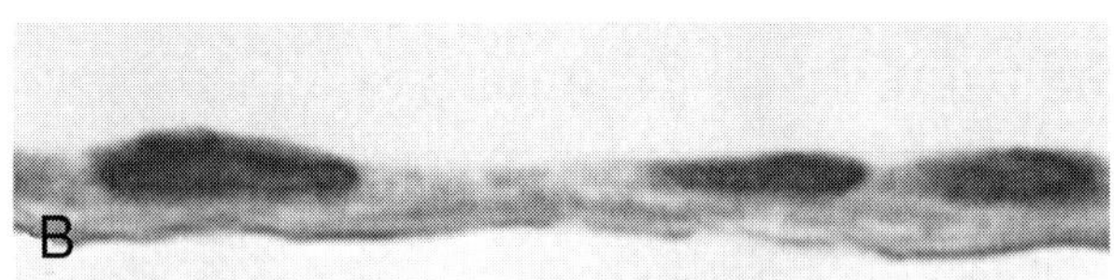

Figure 2.2. *Simple squamous epithelium. **A.**, Surface view of silver-impregnated mesothelium, mesentery. Silver stain (×500). **B.**, Cross section of mesothelium, peritoneum on the surface of the urinary bladder. Hematoxylin and eosin (×1200). (**B**: from Stinson AW, Brown EM. Veterinary histology slide sets. East Lansing, MI: Michigan State University, Instructional Media Center, 1970.)*

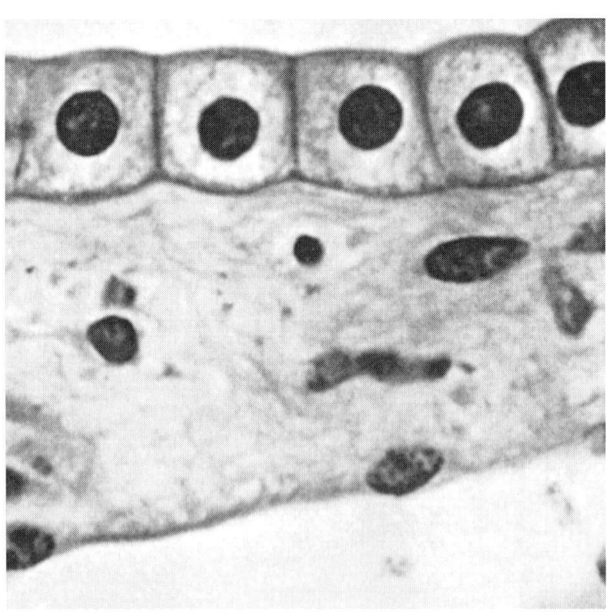

Figure 2.3. *Simple cuboidal epithelium, collecting duct, kidney (horse). Hematoxylin and eosin (×900).*

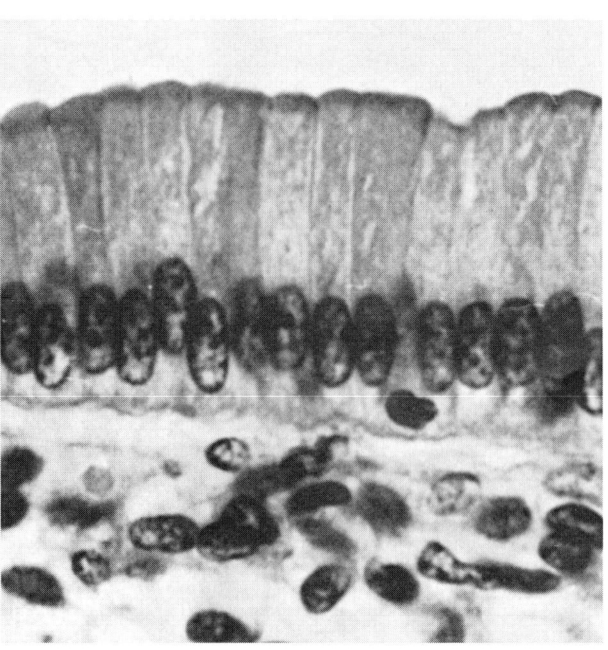

Figure 2.4. *Simple columnar epithelium, lining of gallbladder (pig). Hematoxylin and eosin (×900).*

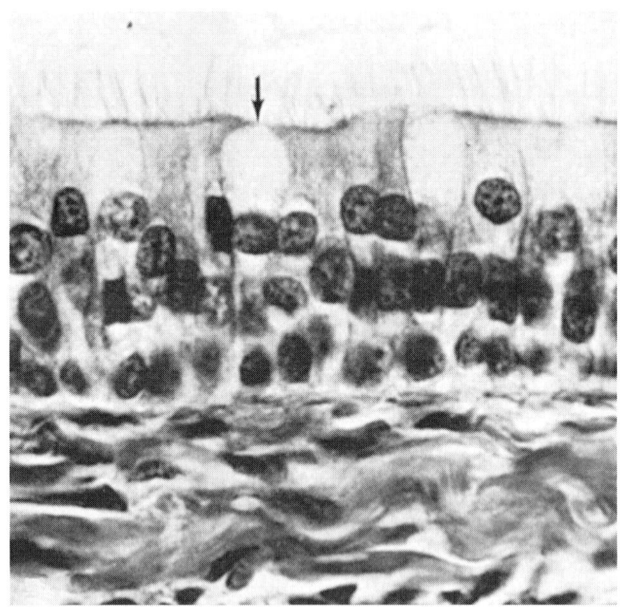

Figure 2.5. *Pseudostratified columnar epithelium with cilia and goblet cells, trachea (dog). The arrow points to a goblet cell. Hematoxylin and eosin (×1200).*

els. Therefore, the epithelium appears to have several layers (Figs. 2.1D and 2.5). In this type of epithelium, all cells rest on the basement membrane but not all reach the surface. Those cells that reach the surface of the epithelium are **ciliated** or **nonciliated epithelial cells** and **goblet cells** (unicellular mucous glands). **Basal cells** are attached to the basement membrane but do not reach the surface of the epithelium. By division and differentiation, basal cells replace other epithelial cell types lost by attrition.

Ciliated, pseudostratified columnar epithelium with goblet cells lines the greater part of the nasal cavity, paranasal sinuses, and nasopharynx, as well as the auditory tubes, the trachea, and the bronchi. In the respiratory system, the goblet cells produce a thin mucous film over the epithelium. Dust particles in the inhaled air become trapped in this mucus, and the current created by the ciliated cells moves the dust-laden mucus to the body openings. A pseudostratified columnar epithelium possessing long branched microvilli (stereocilia) and lacking goblet cells is found lining the duct of the epididymis and the ductus deferens.

Stratified Squamous Epithelium

Stratified squamous epithelium consists of several layers of cells; only the superficial cells have a squamous shape (Fig. 2.1E). Two types of stratified squamous epithelia are recognized (Fig. 2.6). **Keratinized stratified squamous epithelium** has cells on the surface layer that have lost their nuclei and are filled with keratin, a water-resistant protein that forms a protective barrier against the destructive forces of the environment. In **nonkeratinized stratified squamous epithelium**, the flattened superficial cells retain their nuclei.

Three to five distinct cell layers are present in stratified squamous epithelium (see also Chapter 16). The deepest layer of cells next to the basement membrane is the **stratum basale** (Figs. 2.1E and 2.6), which is a single layer of cuboidal to columnar cells. The next layer is the **stratum spinosum** (Fig. 2.6), composed of a varying number of layers of polyhedral cells tightly adhered to each other by numerous **desmosomes** (maculae adherentes). In ordinary histologic preparations, the cytoplasm between the desmosomal attachments shrinks, and wherever the cells remain attached, small spiny processes radiate from the surface of the cells. This appearance gives rise to the name of the layer, stratum spinosum, or spiny layer. Actually, these spiny processes contain **tonofilaments** condensed at the site of the desmosomes (see Fig. 16.4).

As the cells of the stratum spinosum move toward the surface, they become more flattened and accumulate **keratohyalin and lamellar granules** in their cytoplasm. This layer of cells is the **stratum granulosum** and is not present in all stratified squamous epithelia. It is absent in nonkeratinized stratified squamous epithelium as well as in the keratinized forms that produce hard keratin, such as those found in the wall of the hoof and in the horn of ruminants.

The **stratum lucidum** occurs only in nonhairy skin regions (Fig. 2.6). This layer of flattened keratinized cells between the stratum granulosum and the stratum corneum has a translucent appearance because it contains **eleidin**, a protein similar to keratin but with a somewhat different staining affinity.

The outermost layer of keratinized stratified squamous epithelium is the **stratum corneum**. It consists of dead, keratinized cells that are fairly resistant to environmental irritants. During keratinization, the nuclei become pyknotic and subsequently disappear, along with virtually all cytoplasmic organelles. Groups of cells in the outermost layer of the stratum corneum become loose and separate. This process gives rise to the descriptive term **stratum disjunctum**.

A stratum corneum is not present in nonkeratinized stratified squamous epithelium found on moist surfaces. In these locations, the cells do indeed contain keratin but retain their nuclei. This layer is termed the **stratum superficiale**.

In areas where stratified squamous epithelium is keratinized, the cells undergo a series of transformations as they move from the stratum basale to the stratum

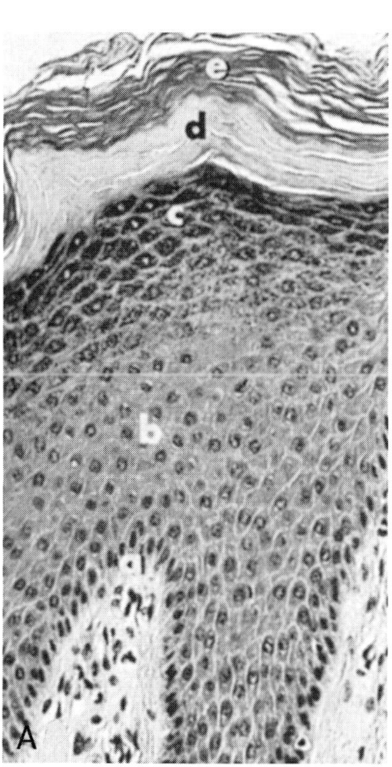

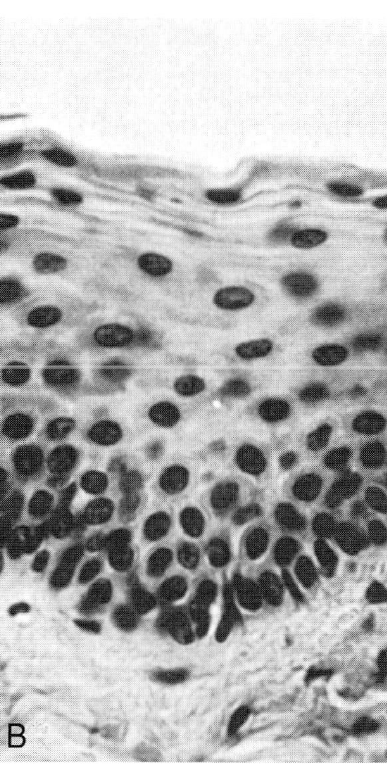

Figure 2.6. *Stratified squamous epithelium.* ***A.,*** *Keratinized stratified squamous epithelium, skin of teat (cow). Stratum basale (a), stratum spinosum (b), stratum granulosum (c), stratum lucidum (d), stratum corneum (e). Hematoxylin and eosin (×150).* ***B.,*** *Nonkeratinized stratified squamous epithelium, lip (cat). Hematoxylin and eosin (×380).*

corneum. The process of keratinization involves the gradual disappearance of Golgi complexes, mitochondria, and nuclei, and a decreased lysosomal activity with a concurrent accumulation of **tonofilaments**. Stratum basale cells are rich in polyribosomes that are concerned with the synthesis of tonofilaments. As these germinative cells move up into the stratum spinosum, the tonofilaments condense into bundles (tonofibrils) and become attached to desmosomes. The cells in the stratum granulosum are flat and contain numerous nonmembrane-bounded keratohyalin granules, which are readily visible with the light microscope. With the electron microscope, the tonofilaments are seen to extend into the periphery of the cell, intermingling with the granules. The cells of the stratum granulosum also contain unique, oval, membrane-bounded granules (100 to 500 nm) composed of alternating light and dark lamellae. These Golgi-derived **lamellar granules** (membrane-coating granules) are located at the cell periphery. By the time the cells reach the stratum lucidum, they are more elongated and flattened and all the organelles are gone. With the light microscope, only the cell outlines are visible, and the cytoplasm appears homogeneous. Ultrastructural examination reveals densely packed filaments embedded in a dense matrix, probably derived from the keratohyalin granules. In the stratum corneum, the contents of membrane-coating granules are secreted by exocytosis, thereby giving rise to the intercellular substance between stratum corneum cells. This substance is a major component of the barrier properties of the epithelium. Cells in the stratum corneum appear lifeless, and as those on the surface dry, they desquamate.

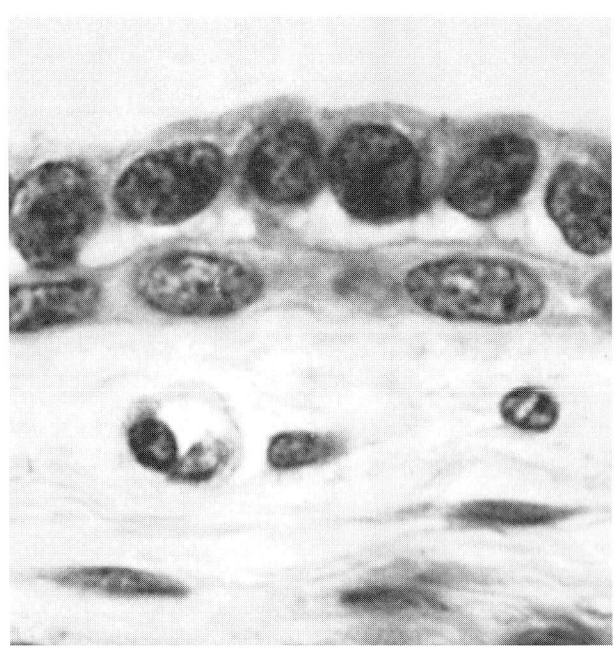

Figure 2.7. *Stratified (two-layered) cuboidal epithelium, duct of carpal gland (pig). Hematoxylin and eosin (×1400).*

Stratified Cuboidal Epithelium

Stratified cuboidal epithelium consists of two or more layers of cells with a surface layer of typical cuboidal cells. Frequently, it occurs as a distinct two-layered epithelium (Fig. 2.7) lining the excretory ducts of glands.

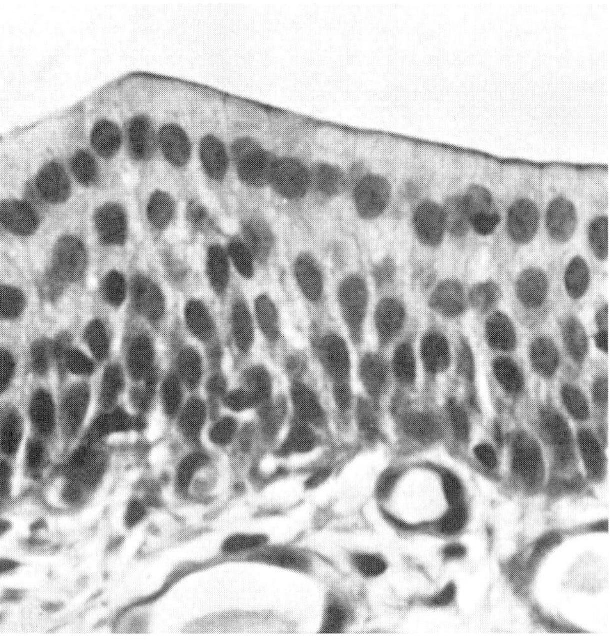

Figure 2.8. *Stratified columnar epithelium, penile urethra (horse). Hematoxylin and eosin (×620). Note that the surface cells are columnar and the nuclei form a fairly regular row.*

Stratified Columnar Epithelium

Stratified columnar epithelium consists of several layers of cells. The superficial layer of tall, prismatic cells does not extend to the basement membrane (Fig. 2.8). The deeper layers are composed of smaller polyhedral cells that do not reach the surface. This type of epithelium may be found in the distal portion of the urethra, as circumscribed areas in a transitional epithelium, in the parotid and mandibular ducts, and in the lacrimal sac and duct.

Transitional Epithelium

Transitional epithelium, a pseudostratified type with a wide variety of appearances, lines hollow organs capable of considerable distention, such as the renal pelvis and calices, ureter, urinary bladder, and urethra. Transitional epithelium may also be seen in the palpebral conjunctiva, larynx, and nasopharynx. The shape of the epithelial cells depends on the degree of organ distention at the time of fixation. When the epithelium is under little tension, the surface cells are large and pillow-shaped, whereas the deeper cells are smaller and irregularly shaped (Figs. 2.1F and 2.9). The cells in-

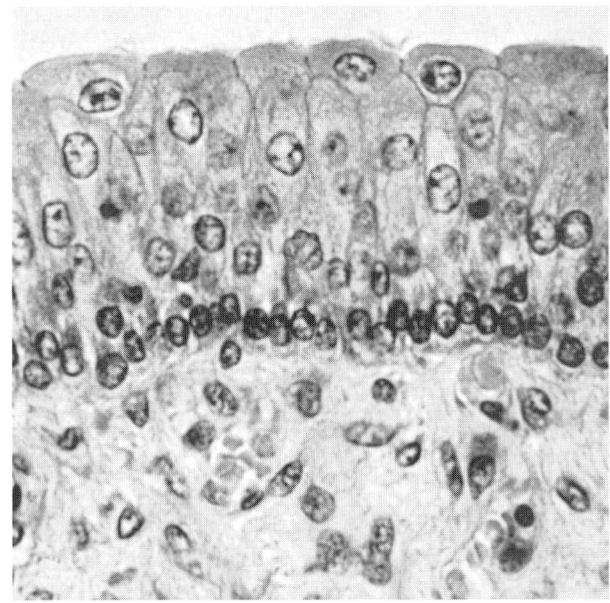

Figure 2.9. *Transitional epithelium, urinary bladder (pig). Hematoxylin and eosin (×480). Note occasional pillow-shaped surface epithelial cells and that the cells increase in size as they approach the free surface.*

crease in size from the basal layers to the superficial layers. When the epithelium is stretched, the cells become flattened and elongated, and the total height of the epithelium decreases.

The luminal surface of transitional epithelial cells appears relatively smooth with the light microscope. On electron micrographs, however, areas of thickened plasmalemma (plaques) anchored by numerous cytoplasmic filaments are seen on the luminal plasmalemma (cell membrane). The region between the membrane plaques is a normal cell membrane, and when the bladder contracts, the plaques fold together much like a hinge, producing typical transitional epithelial surface ridges. Upon distention, they unfold, allowing expansion of the luminal surface.

The surface epithelium of the urinary bladder is a barrier to the diffusion of water from the subepithelial tissue to the hypertonic urine stored in the lumen. Morphologic evidence of this diffusion barrier includes: *(a)* the increased thickness of the outer lamina of the trilaminar cell membrane compared to the inner lamina; *(b)* a concentration of tonofilaments immediately beneath the luminal surface; and *(c)* junctional complexes located between the adjacent surface cells that prevent intercellular diffusion.

Detailed studies of developing transitional epithelium indicate that when the epithelium becomes multilayered and the cells elongate and overlap each other, all remain attached to the basement membrane by slender cytoplasmic processes, much like the attachment in pseudostratified epithelium (Fig. 2.1F). This type of attachment allows the cells to form a parallel alignment when the urinary bladder is distended; thus, fewer layers of cells are seen.

SPECIAL CHARACTERISTICS OF EPITHELIAL CELLS

The location of cellular organelles and variations in luminal, basal, and lateral cell membranes characterize a definite polarized organization of epithelial cells. These special morphologic and functional features are described in detail in Chapter 1 (page 13) and in connection with the organs in which those epithelia occur.

GLANDS

The secretory cells of endocrine and exocrine glands constitute **glandular epithelium**. These cells derive from the proliferation of surface epithelial cells into underlying connective tissue. A **gland** is a structure that may consist exclusively of glandular epithelium or may include a complex duct system, lined by surface epithelium, and a supportive framework of connective tissue, the **stroma**. Glands are found, in one form or another, in most organs of the body.

Classification

Glands are classified based on **morphologic characteristics**, the **nature of the secretory** product, and the **mode of release of the secretory product** (Table 2.3).

MORPHOLOGIC CHARACTERISTICS

Unicellular glands consist of a single secretory cell in a nonsecretory epithelium. An example of this type of gland is the goblet cell. It is a specialized epithelial cell

Table 2.3.
Classifications of Glands

Based on Morphologic Characteristics
- Unicellular glands
- Multicellular glands
  - Intraepithelial
  - Extraepithelial
  - Endocrine
  - Exocrine
    - Simple
      - Tubular—straight, coiled, branched
      - Acinar/Alveolar—single, branched
      - Tubuloacinar/Tubuloalveolar
    - Compound
      - Tubular
      - Acinar/Alveolar
      - Tubuloacinar/Tubuloalveolar

Based on the Nature of the Secretory Product
- Serous
- Mucous
- Seromucous (mixed)

Based on the Mode of Release of the Secretory Product
- Merocrine (eccrine)
- Apocrine
- Holocrine
- Cytocrine

that produces mucinogen, which is released onto the epithelial surface. As this secretory material is synthesized, it fills and expands the apical portion of the cell and forces the nucleus into the slender basal portion, thus giving the cell a distinct goblet shape (see Figs. 2.5 and 10.50).

Multicellular glands are composed of more than one cell, and most glands belong in this classification. They may occur as a cluster of only a few secretory cells within a surface epithelium, forming **intraepithelial glands**, or as large accumulations of cells that have proliferated into the underlying connective tissue, forming **extraepithelial glands**.

Endocrine glands are multicellular glands that do not have a system of ducts to convey their secretory product to sites of utilization. Instead, the secretory products, often referred to as **hormones**, are released directly into the intercellular fluid, from which they are transported to a site of action by the blood and lymph.

Exocrine glands are multicellular glands with a system of ducts through which their secretory products are transported to the sites of utilization. Exocrine glands are either **simple glands**, consisting of one to several secretory units connected to the surface through an **unbranched duct**, or **compound glands**, with many secretory units emptying into a **branched** duct system.

Simple glands

Simple exocrine glands have secretory units of various shapes and dispositions. These morphologic character-

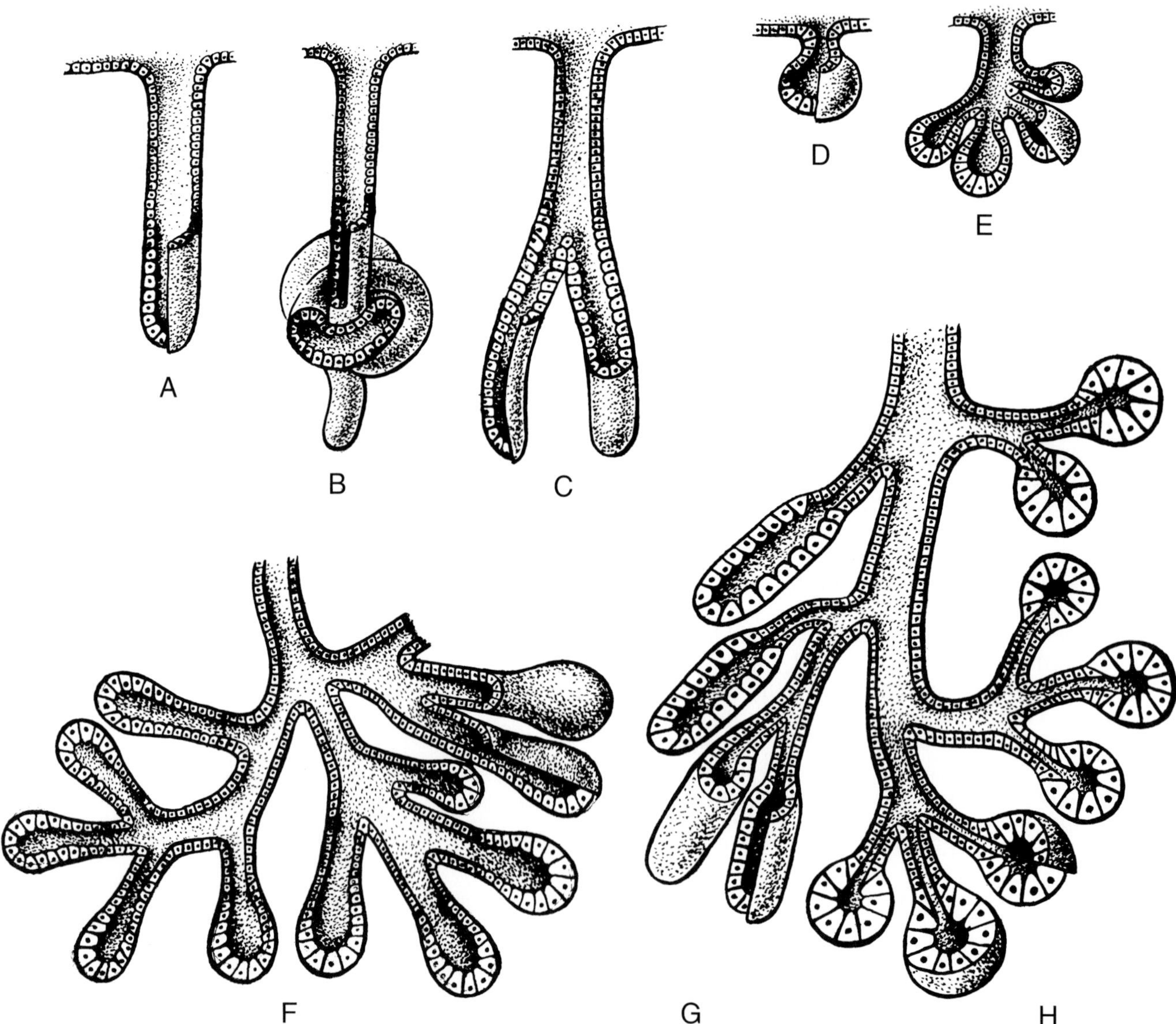

Figure 2.10. *Schematic drawings illustrating the types of exocrine glands.* ***A.***, *Simple tubular gland.* ***B.***, *Simple coiled tubular gland.* ***C.***, *Simple branched tubular gland.* ***D.***, *Simple acinar/alveolar gland.* ***E.***, *Simple branched acinar/alveolar gland.* ***F.***, *Compound tubuloacinar/tubuloalveolar gland.* ***G.***, *Compound tubular gland.* ***H.***, *Compound acinar/alveolar gland.*

istics form the basis for the following types of glands. **Simple straight tubular glands**, such as those in the large intestine, pursue a straight, unbranched course in the surrounding tissue and open directly onto the surface (Figs. 2.10A and 2.11). The terminal portion of **simple coiled tubular glands** is disposed in coils or convolutions. In histologic sections, the secretory unit appears as a cluster of cross-sectional profiles (Figs. 2.10B and 2.12). Sweat glands of the skin are good examples of this type. **Simple branched tubular glands** have a branched terminal portion (Figs. 2.10C and 2.13). The branches converge into a single duct near the opening onto the surface, and both portions are lined with secretory cells. The glands of the stomach are typical simple branched tubular glands.

Simple acinar and **simple alveolar glands** are similar because they have an enlarged, spherical secretory unit connected to the surface by a constricted duct (Figs. 2.10D and 2.14). The lumen of the **acinus** is small and narrow, but that of the **alveolus** is large and distended (Fig. 2.15). Simple acinar and simple alveolar glands are rare; some of the sebaceous glands are of the simple acinar type, whereas the simple alveolar type is found in the respiratory system of the chicken. **Simple branched acinar** and **simple branched alveolar glands** are more common than unbranched glands. In these branched types, two or more acini or alveoli occur together, and their secretory product empties through a common duct (Fig. 2.10E). Many of the larger sebaceous glands

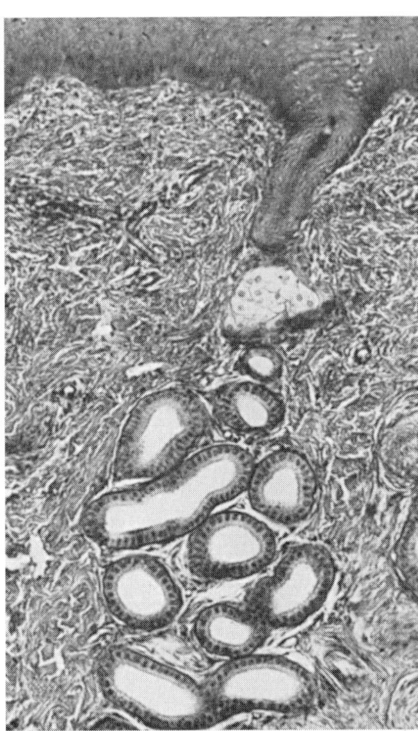

Figure 2.12. *Simple coiled tubular gland. Ceruminous gland, ear canal (cow). Hematoxylin and eosin (×120).*

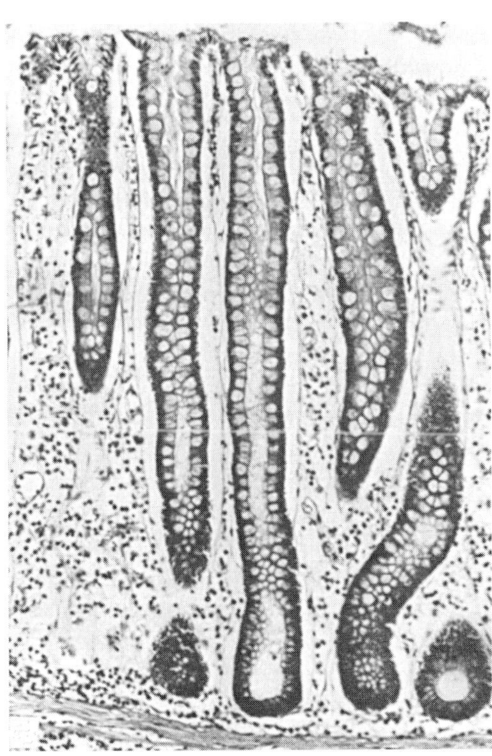

Figure 2.11. *Simple tubular glands. Large intestine (dog). Hematoxylin and eosin (×120).*

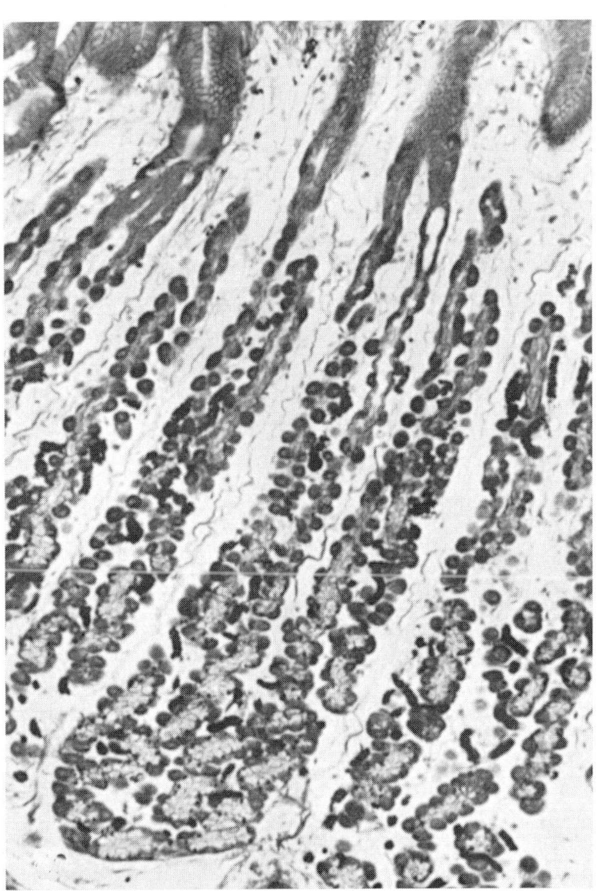

Figure 2.13. *Simple branched tubular glands. Fundic stomach (dog). Hematoxylin and eosin (×120).*

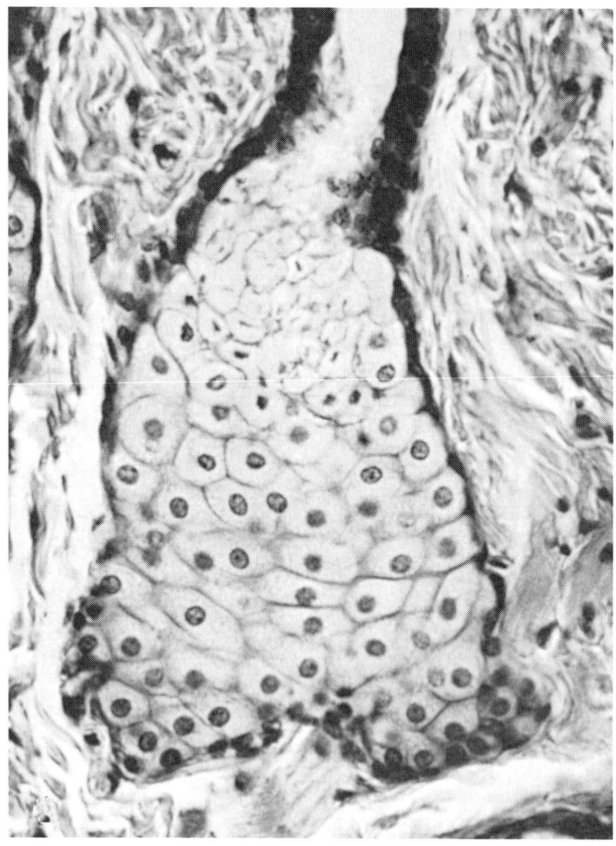

Figure 2.14. *Simple acinar gland. Sebaceous gland, nostril (horse). Hematoxylin and eosin (×300).*

of the skin are of the simple branched acinar type. Simple branched alveolar glands are found in the respiratory system of the chicken.

Simple tubuloacinar and **tubuloalveolar glands** have secretory units composed of both a tubular portion with a terminal acinus or alveolus and occur only in the branched form. The minor salivary glands that empty into the oral cavity are classified as this type.

Compound glands

Compound glands contain the same types of secretory units as those of the simple glands but have **elaborate duct systems that branch repeatedly**. Compound glands are classified into tubular, acinar, alveolar, tubuloacinar, and tubuloalveolar types. For example, a gland with a highly branched duct system in which secretory units consist of tubules of glandular epithelium would be classified as **compound tubular**, whereas a **compound tubuloacinar gland** contains either a mixture of acinar and tubular secretory units or tubular secretory units with terminal acini. The various types of secretory units and ducts found in compound glands are illustrated in Figures 2.10F, 2.10G, and 2.10H and Figure 2.16.

PARENCHYMA. Compound glands are composed of secretory units and ducts, collectively termed **parenchyma**; the supportive or connective tissue elements comprise the **stroma**. Large glands are partly or completely divided into **lobes**, which are large, easily recognized structural units. The lobes are further subdivided by connective tissue into **lobules**, which in turn are composed of numerous **secretory units** (Fig. 2.16). Some of the smaller compound glands have only lobules and secretory units. The various segments of the duct system of compound glands are identified by their location within the gland.

Secretory product produced in **tubules**, **acini**, or **alveoli** of a compound gland flows first into an **intralobular duct**, usually located in the center of the lobule. Intralobular ducts continue as **interlobular ducts** as they emerge from the lobule to enter the interlobular connective tissue. Interlobular ducts converge to form large **lobar ducts**, the ducts that drain individual lobes of the gland. The **main duct** is formed by the convergence of the lobar ducts (Fig. 2.16).

In some glands, such as the parotid salivary gland, portions of the intralobular ducts also contribute to the secretory product and, thus, are called **secretory ducts**. These ducts are also called **striated ducts**, because their cells contain many mitochondria oriented perpendicularly to the long axis of the cell and located between infoldings of the basal plasmalemma, thus giving the cells

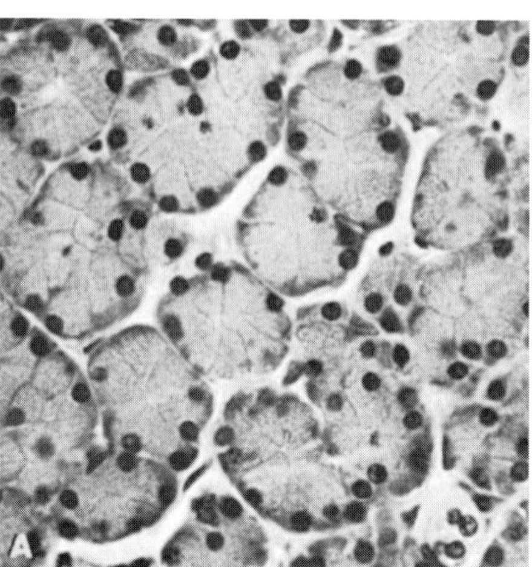

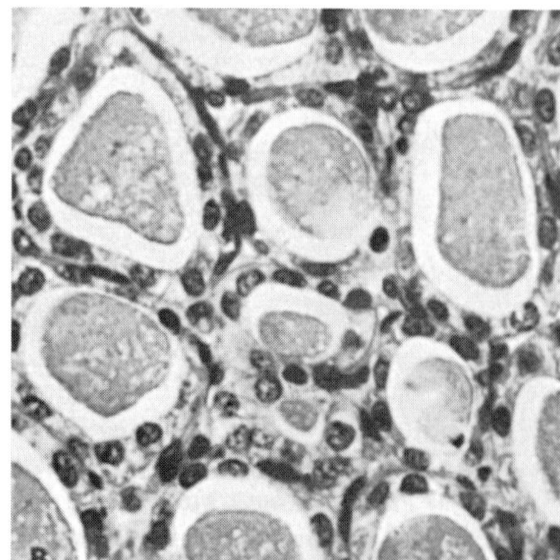

Figure 2.15. *Types of secretory units.* ***A.****, Acini, characterized by a small lumen, parotid salivary gland (horse). Hematoxylin and eosin (×480).* ***B.****, Alveoli, mammary gland (sow). Note the large lumen. Hematoxylin and eosin (×480).*

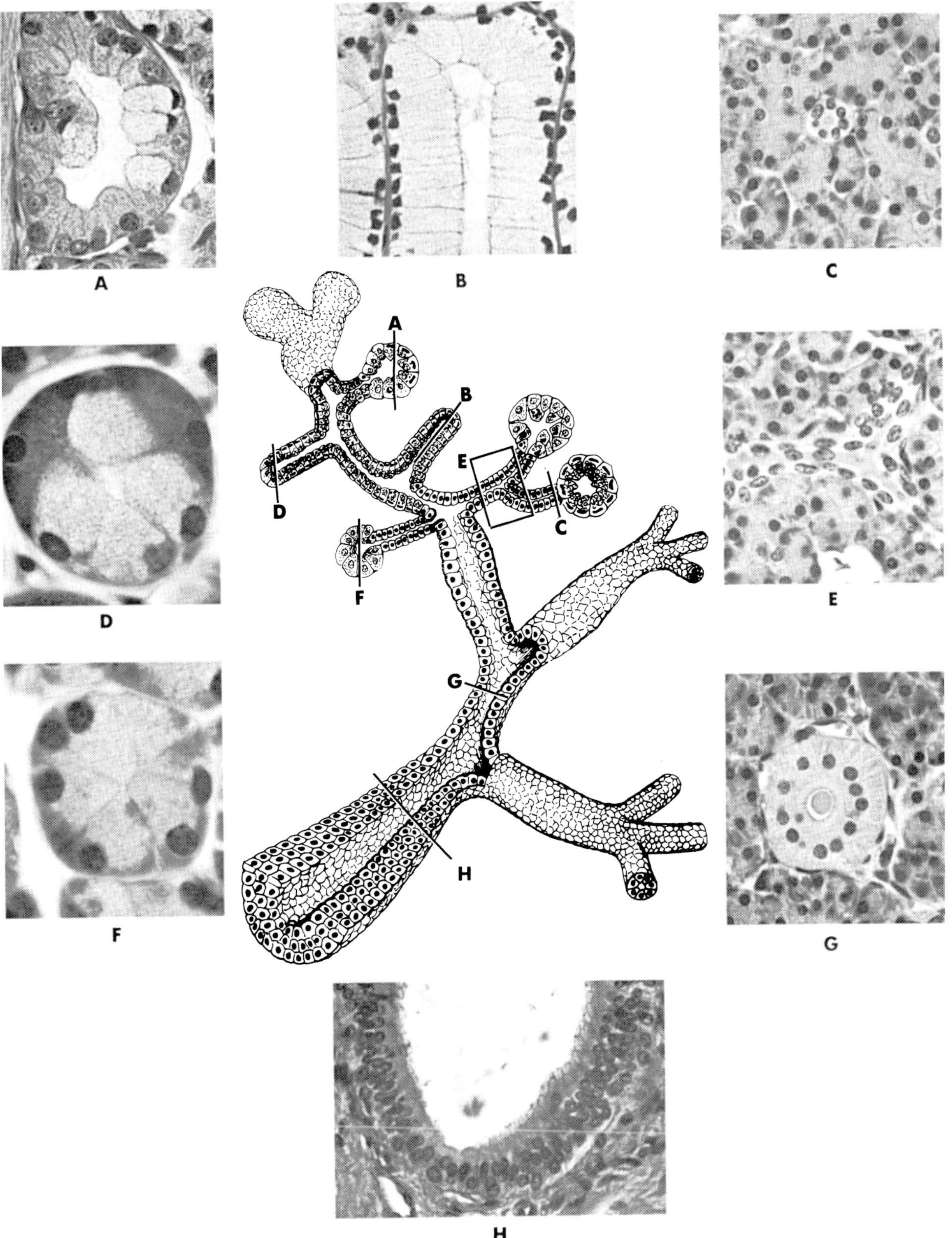

Figure 2.16. *Schematic composite drawing and photomicrographs of the duct system and secretory units of a compound gland. The photomicrographs correspond to the areas labeled A through H.* ***A.***, *Seromucous alveolus, trachea (pig). Trichrome (×600).* ***B.***, *Mucous tubular secretory unit, bulbourethral gland (bull). Hematoxylin and eosin (×480).* ***C.***, *Cross section of intercalated duct, parotid salivary gland (horse). Hematoxylin and eosin (×480).* ***D.***, *Mucous acinus with serous demilunes, seromucous salivary gland (horse). Hematoxylin and eosin (×1000).* ***E.***, *Longitudinal section through intercalated duct, parotid salivary gland (horse). Hematoxylin and eosin (×480).* ***F.***, *Serous acinus, parotid salivary gland (horse). Hematoxylin and eosin (×1200).* ***G.***, *Striated intralobular duct, parotid salivary gland (horse). Hematoxylin and eosin (×480).* ***H.***, *Interlobular duct, mandibular salivary gland (dog). Hematoxylin and eosin (×300). (Drawing from Stinson AW, Brown EM. Veterinary histology slide sets. East Lansing, MI: Michigan State University, Instructional Media Center, 1970.)*

a striated appearance (Fig. 2.16G). **Intercalated ducts** are small, nonsecretory intralobular ducts that connect the secretory units with the secretory (striated) duct (Figs. 2.16C and 2.16E). Intercalated ducts are prominent in the parotid salivary gland and are also present in the mandibular and sublingual salivary glands, as well as in the pancreas.

The general term **excretory duct** describes any of the previously mentioned ducts that function only to transport the secretory product to the site of utilization. They do not contribute to the secretory product as do the secretory ducts.

STROMA. The **stroma** of compound glands includes the capsule and the internal supportive framework. The **capsule**, composed of collagen, elastic, and reticular fibers, completely surrounds the gland and gives rise to connective-tissue sheets (**septa**) or strands (**trabeculae**) that extend well into the parenchyma. Septa clearly define the lobes and lobules and provide support for the various lobar and interlobular ducts. Fine **reticular fibers** encircle the individual secretory units.

NATURE OF THE SECRETORY PRODUCT

Both simple and compound glands may be classified as mucous, serous, or seromucous (mixed), based on the type of secretory product. **Serous glands** produce a thin, watery product. The cells of the secretory units usually have spherical nuclei near the center of the cells, and the apical cytoplasm is filled with small secretory granules (Fig. 2.16F). These granules are precursors of enzymes produced by many of the serous glands and are called **zymogen granules**. The parotid salivary gland and the exocrine part of the pancreas are typical serous glands.

Mucous glands produce a thick, viscous secretion (**mucin**) that contributes to a protective coating over the lining of hollow organs that communicate with the outside of the body (Fig. 2.16B). This protective coating is termed **mucus** and contains cast-off epithelial cells and leukocytes, in addition to mucin. The cells of the mucous-secreting units are filled with **mucinogen**, the precursor of **mucin**, which stains light with hematoxylin and eosin. The nuclei are displaced toward the basal part of the cell and are usually flattened against the cell membrane.

Glands that contain both mucous and serous cells are described as **seromucous**, **mucoserous**, or simply **mixed**. The combinations of these two types of cells vary considerably from one gland to another. In seromucous glands, the arrangement of the serous and mucous cells is variable. Some secretory units contain both serous and mucous cells intermixed (Fig. 2.16A). Other seromucous glands are composed of a mixture of all-mucous acini and all-serous acini, rather than each acinus containing some serous and some mucous cells. Most commonly, the serous cells are located at the periphery of the mucous secretory unit and are half-moon- or crescent-shaped cells called **serous demilunes** (Fig. 2.16D). They empty their serous secretory product into the lumen of the secretory unit by way of intercellular canaliculi, i.e., minute extracellular channels. Some seromucous tubuloacinar glands have a mucous tubular unit with a terminal serous acinus.

MODE OF RELEASE OF THE SECRETORY PRODUCT

The mode by which the secretory product is released from the cell forms the basis for a third classification of

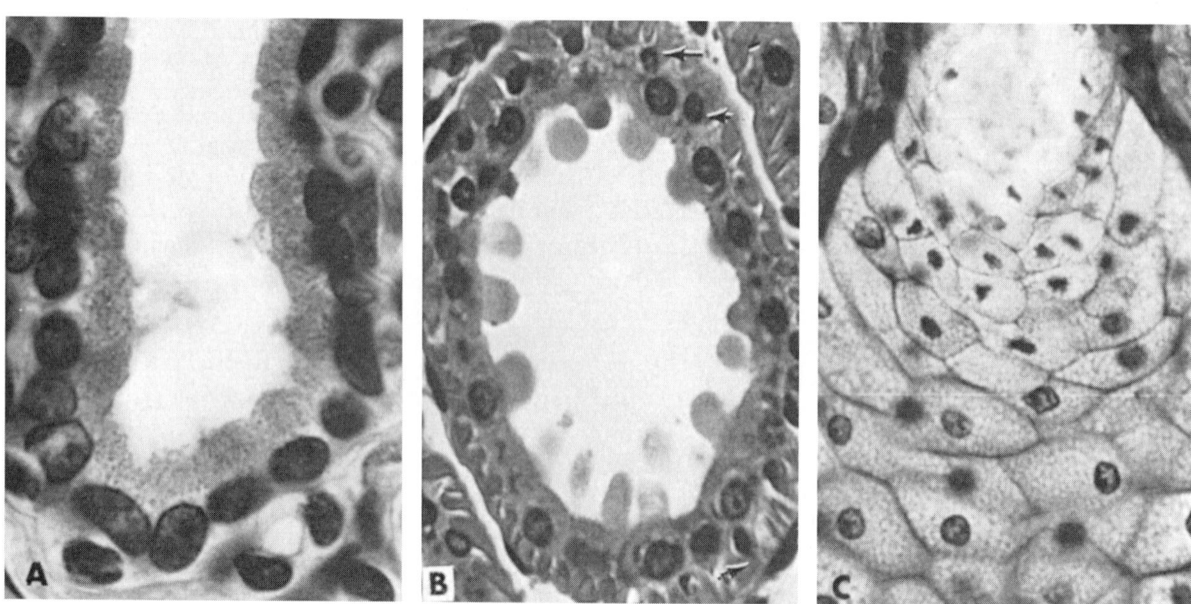

Figure 2.17. *Secretory units illustrating the various modes of release of the secretory product.* ***A.***, *Merocrine (eccrine) gland, prostate (dog). Hematoxylin and eosin (×1200).* ***B.***, *Apocrine sudoriferous gland, skin (pig), with myoepithelial cells at arrows. Hematoxylin and eosin (×610).* ***C.***, *Holocrine gland, sebaceous gland (horse). Hematoxylin and eosin (×480).*

glands. There are four modes of secretion: merocrine, apocrine, holocrine, and cytocrine.

During the **merocrine** (sometimes called **eccrine**) mode of secretion, the contents of small **secretory granules** are released as the secretory product (Fig. 2.17A). The secretory granules are usually enclosed within a membrane. When the secretory granule reaches the cell surface, its membrane fuses with the plasmalemma, thereby discharging the secretory product via **exocytosis**.

In the **apocrine** mode of secretion, a large, single, intracellular secretory granule is also surrounded by a membrane. As the secretory granule migrates into the cell apex, the plasmalemma, and a portion of the neighboring cytoplasm, surround the granule. Eventually, the plasmalemma constricts beneath the granule, causing the granule, and some surrounding cytoplasm, to bulge into the gland lumen (Fig. 2.17B). Constriction of the plasmalemma proceeds until the membrane-bounded granule, together with a rim of cytoplasm and plasmalemma, is released, leaving the cell plasmalemma intact. Apocrine glands in the secretory state are easily recognized; however, when they are in a resting phase with no secretory droplets, their differentiation from merocrine glands is difficult. Examples of apocrine glands include the mammary gland and the general body sweat glands.

In the **holocrine** mode of secretion, entire cells are released as the secretory product (Fig. 2.17C). The sebaceous glands of the skin are typical holocrine glands. The cells become filled with lipid granules and move toward the duct; the cells then disintegrate, and their contents are extruded into the duct.

In the **cytocrine** mode of secretion, secretory material is transferred from one cell to the cytoplasm of another cell. It is exemplified in the epidermis, where melanocytes transfer the brown pigment, melanin, into the cytoplasm of the keratinocytes.

Myoepithelial Cells

In some glands, **myoepithelial cells** are interposed between the base of the secretory cells and the basement membrane. As their name suggests, myoepithelial cells possess characteristics of both muscle cells (actin and myosin microfilaments) and epithelial cells (cytoplasmic keratin). These cells, when stimulated, contract and force the secretory product into the duct system. Myoepithelial cells are especially well developed in sweat and mammary glands (Fig. 2.17B). In the mammary gland, myoepithelial cells are stimulated by oxytocin.

REFERENCES

Bharadwaj MB, Calhoun ML. Histology of the urethral epithelium of domestic animals. Am J Vet Res 1959;20:841.

Hashimoto K. The eccrine and apocrine glands and their function. In: Jarret A, ed. The physiology and pathophysiology of the skin. New York: Academic Press, 1978;5.

International Committee on Veterinary Gross Anatomical Nomenclature. Nomina anatomica veterinaria. 4th ed. Ithaca, NY: International Committee on Veterinary Gross Anatomical Nomenclature, 1994.

International Committee on Veterinary Histological Nomenclature. Nomina histologica. 2nd ed. (revised). Ithaca, NY: International Committee on Veterinary Histological Nomenclature, 1994.

Martin BF, Wong YC. Development and maturation of the bladder epithelium of the guinea pig. Acta Anat 1981;110:359.

Petry G, Amon H. Licht- und elektronenmikroskopische Studien ber Struktur und Dynamik des bergangsepithels. Z Zellforsch 1966;69: 587.

Phillips SJ, Griffin T. Scanning electron microscope evidence that human urothelium is a pseudostratified epithelium. Anat Rec 1985;211:153A.

Severs JJ, Hicks RM. Analysis of membrane structure in transitional epithelium of rat urinary bladder. 2. The discoidal vesicles and Golgi apparatus: their role in luminal membrane biogenesis. J Ultrastruct Res 1979;69:279.

3

Connective and Supportive Tissues

JO ANN C. EURELL
DAVID C. VAN SICKLE

Connective and supportive tissues connect other tissues, provide a framework, and support the entire body by means of cartilage and bones. These tissues also play an important role in thermoregulation and in defense and repair mechanisms.

A common characteristic of most connective and supportive tissues is their mesodermal origin. The ectoderm of the head region, however, also participates in the formation of connective and supportive tissues. Embryonic connective tissue, or mesenchyme, arises from the mesodermal somites and lateral layers of the somatic and splanchnic mesoderm. Subsequently, all other connective and supportive tissues are derived from mesenchyme.

All connective and supportive tissues are composed of cells, fibers, and amorphous ground substance (proteoglycans, glycosaminoglycans, and interstitial fluid) in varying proportions. Mesenchyme, however, lacks fibers during early development.

Based on occurrence, connective and supportive tissues are classified as embryonic or adult with several subgroups.

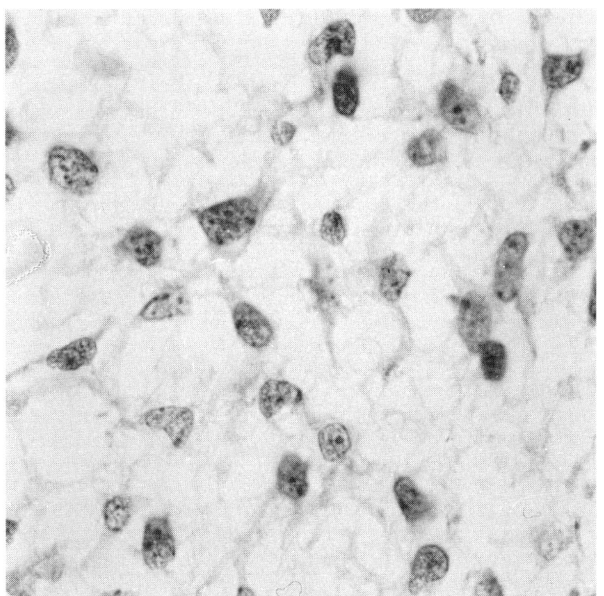

Figure 3.1. *Mesenchyme (rat embryo). Note the stellate mesenchymal cells in an amorphous ground substance. Hematoxylin and eosin (×800).*

CONNECTIVE TISSUE CELLS

The cells of connective tissue remain as resident cells in a fixed location within the tissue or they enter the tissue and move around as immigrant or wandering cells. In response to certain stimuli, some resident cells, such as the macrophage, can become immigrant cells.

Resident Cells of Connective Tissue

MESENCHYMAL CELLS

Mesenchymal cells are irregularly shaped with multiple processes (Fig. 3.1). These pluripotential, undifferentiated cells are usually found adjacent to blood vessels. They are smaller than fibroblasts and have fewer cytoplasmic organelles. The nucleus is the most prominent feature of this cell. The mesenchymal cell population serves as a reservoir of cells that can differentiate into other types of connective tissue cells as needed.

FIBROCYTES AND FIBROBLASTS

The most common cell of connective tissue is the **fibrocyte** (Fig. 3.2A). Fibrocytes are generally elongated and spindle-shaped, with processes that contact adjacent cells and fibers. Their heterochromatic nucleus is surrounded by a scant amount of pale cytoplasm. Secretory vesicles in the cytoplasm discharge their contents (e.g., procollagen, proteoglycans, proelastin) into the surrounding microenvironment. At the electron microscopic (EM) level, the cytoplasm has sparse rough endoplasmic reticulum (rER) and a small Golgi complex.

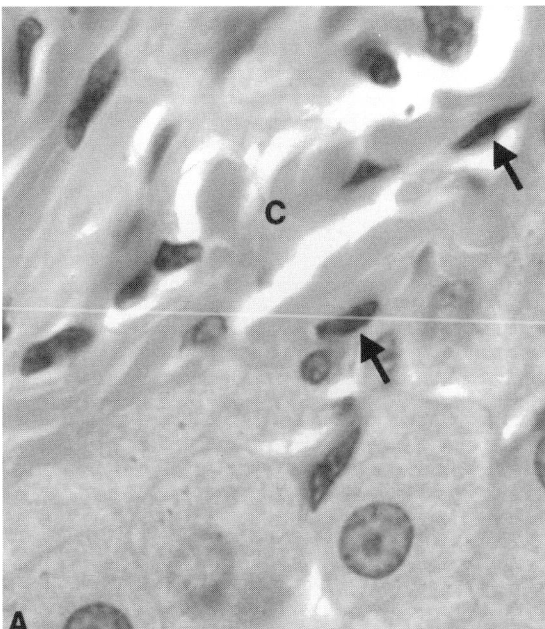

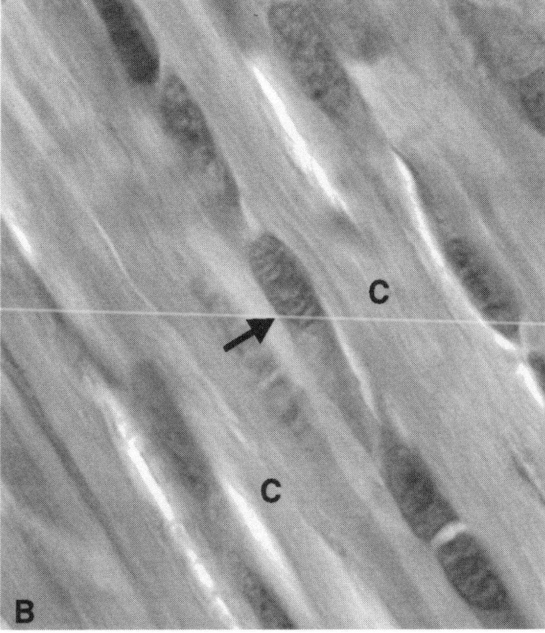

Figure 3.2. *A.*, Fibrocytes (arrows), collagen fibers (C), connective tissue, liver (dog). **B.**, Fibroblasts (arrow), tendon (young puppy). The cells are located between collagen fibers (C). Hematoxylin and eosin (×1520).

Free ribosomes, mitochondria, lysosomes, and vesicles are also present. Actin filaments occur as bundles in the cell processes. Fibrocytes are responsible for forming the fibers and ground substance of connective tissue.

The **fibroblast** has a larger, more euchromatic nucleus and more abundant, basophilic cytoplasm than the fibrocyte (Fig. 3.2B). At the EM level, abundant rER and a prominent Golgi complex are present in the cytoplasm. These structural characteristics indicate more active connective tissue matrix production in comparison to the fibrocyte. Fibroblasts may arise directly from undifferentiated mesenchymal cells or are transformed from fibrocytes under the influence of microenvironmental factors (e.g., cytokines).

Myofibroblasts are fibroblasts that contain actin filaments associated with dense bodies and therefore also resemble smooth muscle cells. It is believed that myofibroblasts play a role in contraction during wound healing.

RETICULAR CELLS

Reticular cells are similar in appearance to the fibrocyte (Fig. 3.3). They are stellate-shaped cells with a spherical nucleus and basophilic cytoplasm. Reticular cells produce **reticular fibers**, which form the fine structural network of organs such as the lymph nodes, spleen, and bone marrow. These cells are fixed in the tissue and are capable of phagocytosis. Reticular cells should not be confused with the reticulocyte, an immature erythrocyte.

ADIPOCYTES

Adipocytes are also referred to as **fat cells** or **adipose cells** (Fig. 3.4). Individual adipocytes or clusters containing multiple cells are normal components of loose connective tissue, but when the fat cells outnumber other cell types, the tissue is called **adipose tissue** (see more on adipose tissue later in this chapter). Mature **unilocular adipocytes** are spherical or polyhedral cells that measure up to 120 μm in diameter. Most of the cell is occupied by a single, large nonmembrane-bounded lipid droplet surrounded by a thin layer of cytoplasm. The cell nucleus is displaced to the periphery by the lipid droplet, which is surrounded by cytoplasm that contains a small Golgi complex, mitochondria, rER, and microfilaments.

In contrast, mature **multilocular adipocytes** contain a more centrally located nucleus with multiple lipid droplets in the cytoplasm (Fig. 3.5). Both the Golgi complex and rER are rather inconspicuous, but many mitochondria are present. The high concentration of cytochromes in the mitochondria is primarily responsible for the brown color of aggregates of multilocular

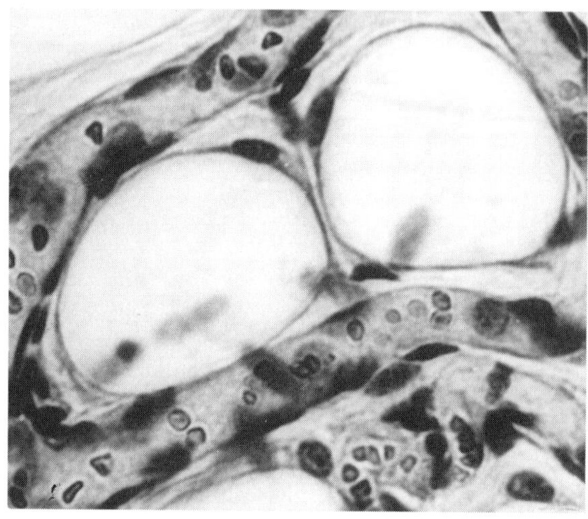

Figure 3.4. *Two white adipocytes surrounded by capillaries. Hematoxylin and eosin (×630). (Courtesy of A. Hansen.)*

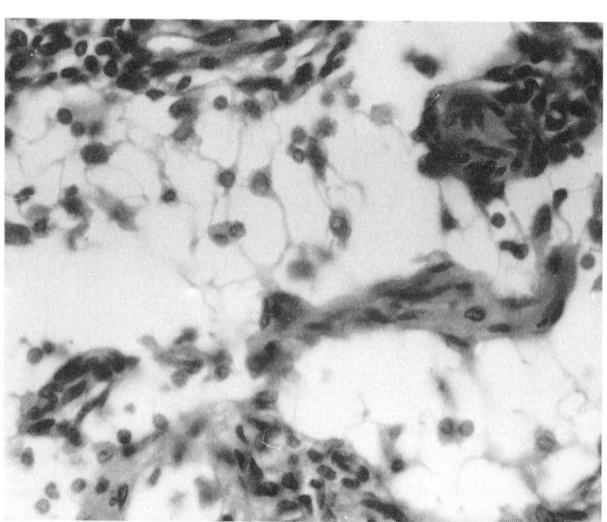

Figure 3.3. *Reticular connective tissue, lymph node (sheep). Note the numerous interconnected reticular cells, which form a three-dimensional network. Hematoxylin and eosin (×600).*

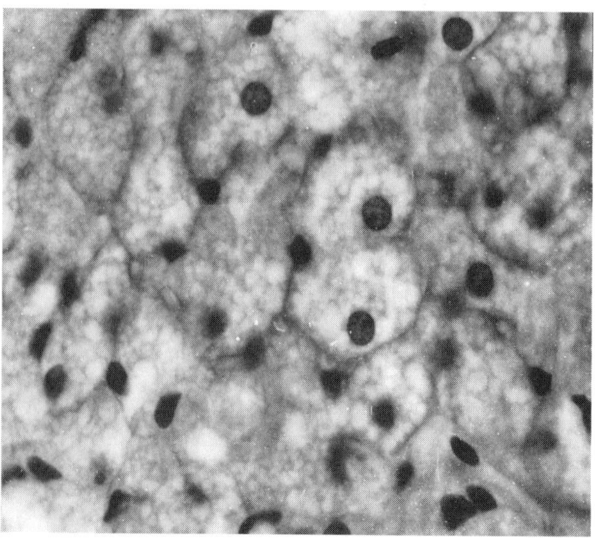

Figure 3.5. *Brown adipose tissue. Note the numerous small lipid inclusions in the multilocular adipocytes. Hematoxylin and eosin (×600).*

adipocytes, which are referred to as brown fat (described below). Unilocular adipocytes produce chemical energy, whereas multilocular adipocytes metabolize lipid to produce heat.

Because fat is rapidly dissolved by most of the dehydration and/or clearing agents commonly used for the preparation of histologic sections, the lipid droplets appear as clear spaces surrounded by cytoplasm (Fig. 3.4). When rapidly processed, the lipid can be preserved and stained with certain dyes, such as osmium tetroxide or Sudan III.

PERICYTES

Pericytes are elongated cells that are located adjacent to the endothelium lining small blood vessels. The cells are surrounded by the basal lamina of the blood vessel and make frequent contact with the underlying endothelial cells. Pericytes resemble fibrocytes in appearance but have contractile filaments similar to smooth muscle. Their function is uncertain.

MAST CELLS

Mast cells are common in loose connective tissue, especially that of the skin and intestine, and are often particularly abundant around blood vessels. They are large, polymorphic, spherical or ovoid cells that contain a prominent, centrally located nucleus. Numerous secretory granules are present in the cytoplasm (Fig. 3.6). These cells can be identified with immunocytochemistry or a **metachromatic stain,** which has the capacity to stain different elements of a cell in different colors or shades (e.g., toluidine blue, a blue dye that stains heparin-containing granules red). At the EM level, the mast cell granules are membrane-bounded and have crystalline, lamellar, or fine granular characteristics. The remaining cytoplasm is occupied by an extensive Golgi complex, cisternae of rER, free ribosomes, and mitochondria.

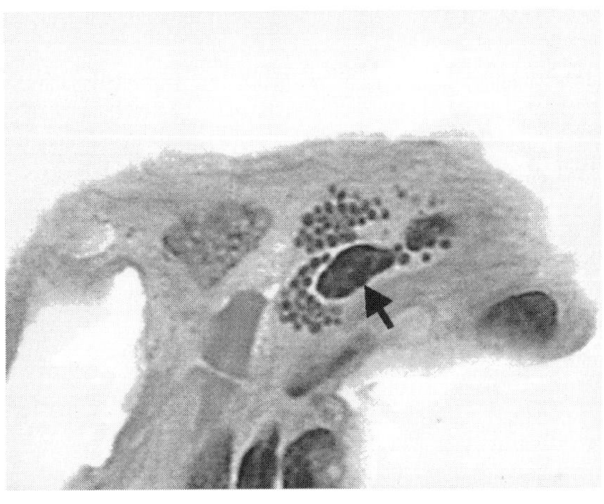

Figure 3.6. *Mast cell (arrow), lung (rabbit). Note the characteristic granules. Hematoxylin and eosin, plastic section (×1200).*

Mast cells are rich in **histamine**, **heparin**, and proteases. Histamine is a vasoconstrictor that causes increased permeability of small venules, thereby permitting leakage of plasma resulting in tissue edema. This localized inflammatory reaction is designed to dispose of foreign antigens rapidly. Histamine also stimulates smooth muscle contraction in small airways. Heparin acts as an anticoagulant and is believed to stimulate angiogenesis. In allergic and anaphylactic reactions, the interaction of circulating antigens with antibodies on the surface of sensitized mast cells induces release of granules by exocytosis. Proteases can destroy nearby cells, tissue matrix, and activate complement components. Inflammatory mediators (e.g., eicosanoids) and cytokines (e.g., interleukin-2 [IL-2], interleukin-3 [IL-3], and tumor necrosis factor alpha [TNF-α]) are also produced by the mast cell after the antigen-antibody interaction.

The mast cell and the basophil both have basophilic cytoplasmic granules that contain similar inflammatory products. Basophils, however, are not normally found in connective tissues but may infiltrate under the influence of lymphocytes. Although the basophil and mast cell have some attributes in common, the exact relationship between them is unclear.

MACROPHAGES

Macrophages are phagocytic cells that can be fixed (e.g., histiocytes) or freely mobile in tissues. They are derived from monocytes that migrate across blood vessel walls into the connective tissue. Histochemical stains for lysosomal enzymes, such as acid phosphatase, facilitate the identification of macrophages. Macrophages are large, ovoid, or spherical cells that contain cytoplasmic vacuoles and are readily distinguishable with the light microscope (Fig. 3.7). At the EM level, they are charac-

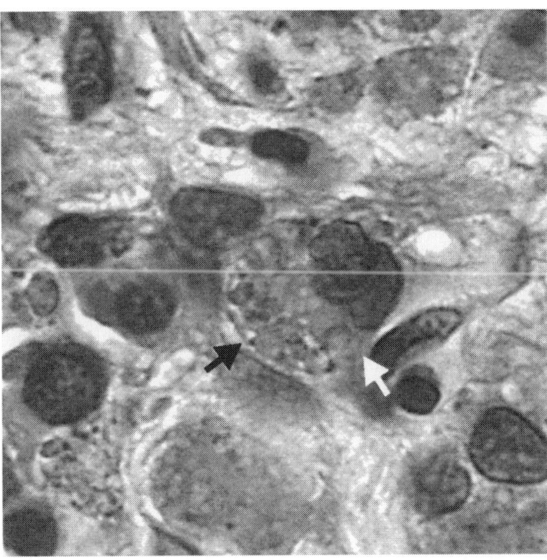

Figure 3.7. *Macrophage (arrows), connective tissue. Note the numerous cytoplasmic vacuoles and phagolysosomes. Hematoxylin and eosin (×1200).*

terized by numerous lysosomes, phagosomes, phagolysosomes, and pseudopodia (footlike extensions of the cell membrane) (Fig. 3.8). Abundant ribosomes, rER, smooth endoplasmic reticulum (sER), mitochondria, and a Golgi complex are also present.

A variety of chemotactic stimuli (e.g., infectious agents, cytokines) cause macrophages to migrate to locations in the body where foreign material must be removed. Macrophages engulf material by pinocytosis and phagocytosis. Phagocytosis may be indiscriminate (e.g., dust particles in the lung) or may involve specific interaction with receptors on the macrophage surface (e.g., Fc receptors and immunoglobulin G [IgG] and immunoglobulin M [IgM]).

Inflammation can be characterized as acute or chronic based on the relative proportion of neutrophils to macrophages. Acute inflammation has more neutrophils than macrophages, whereas chronic inflammation has more macrophages than neutrophils. **Multinucleated giant cells** or foreign-body cells (Fig. 3.9) arise during chronic inflammation and are a result of the fusion of several macrophages in response to the presence of foreign material. Macrophages also act as **antigen-presenting cells**, which process and display foreign substances so that lymphocytes can recognize and respond more effectively to the challenge.

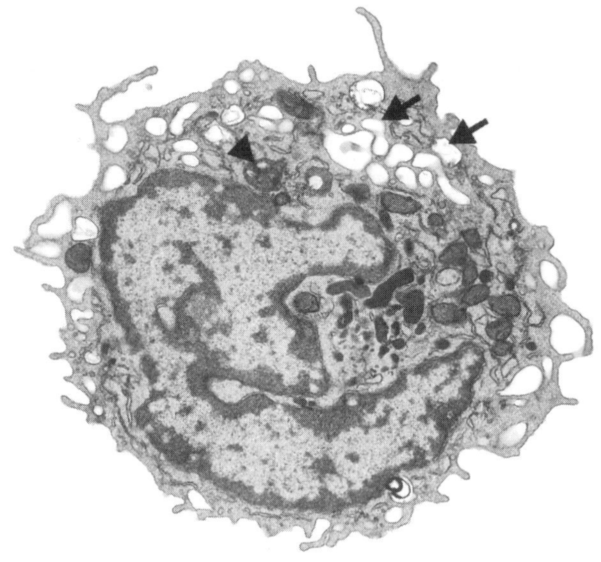

Figure 3.8. *Macrophage containing abundant pinocytotic vacuoles (arrows) and phagolysosomes (arrowhead) (×8000). (Courtesy of J. Turek.)*

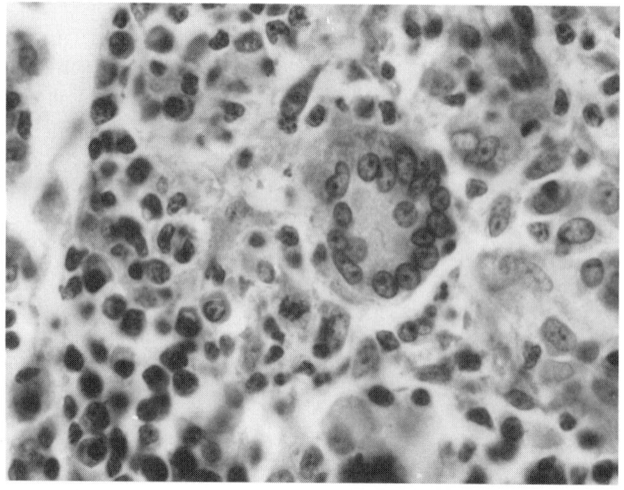

Figure 3.9. *Multinucleated giant cell, lymph node (sheep). Crossman s trichrome (×435).*

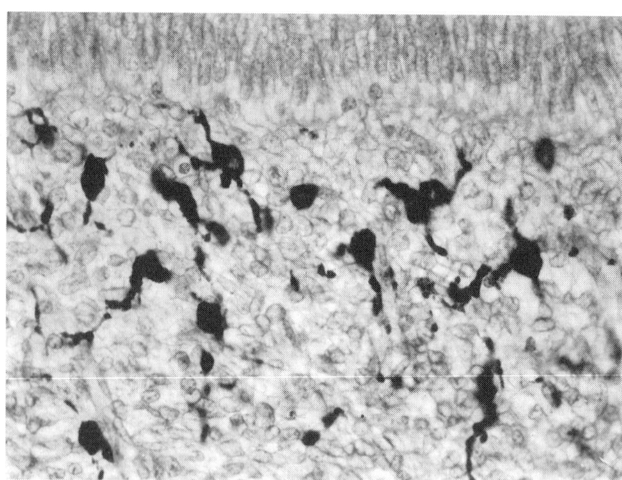

Figure 3.10. *Pigment containing cells in the lamina propria of a uterine caruncle (sheep). Hematoxylin and eosin (×325).*

Macrophages synthesize and secrete many substances that are a reflection of their multiple functions. These substances include enzymes such as lysozyme, which lyses the wall of many bacteria; cytokines (interferons and interleukin); complement components (C2, C3, C4, and C5); coagulation factors; and reactive chemical species (hydrogen peroxide, hydroxyl radicals, nitric oxide), which are important components of the bactericidal and cytocidal (e.g., tumor cells) activities of macrophages.

PIGMENT CELLS

Cells in connective tissue may contain pigments, including melanin in domestic animals or pteridines and purines in fish and amphibians (Fig. 3.10). When present in large numbers, the cells impart color to the connective tissue. They occur in various locations such as the dermis, uterine caruncles of sheep, meninges, choroid, and iris. Their significance is described in connection with these organs.

Immigrant Cells of Connective Tissue

PLASMA CELLS

Plasma cells are spherical, ovoid, or pear-shaped cells with a spherical, eccentric nucleus. The chromatin is often arranged in peripherally located clumps or in cen-

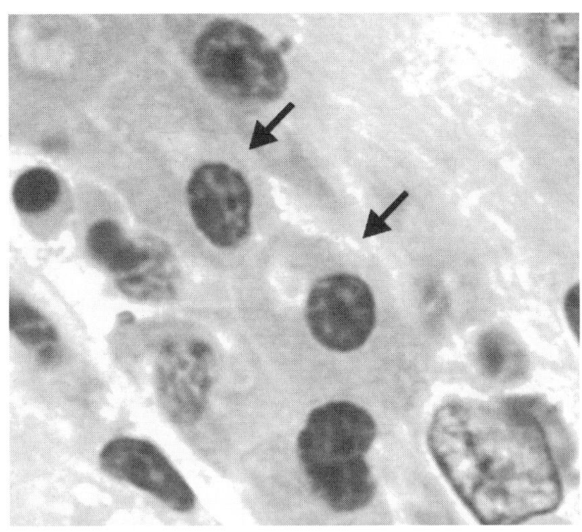

Figure 3.11. *Plasma cells (arrows), connective tissue, duodenum. Hematoxylin and eosin (×900).*

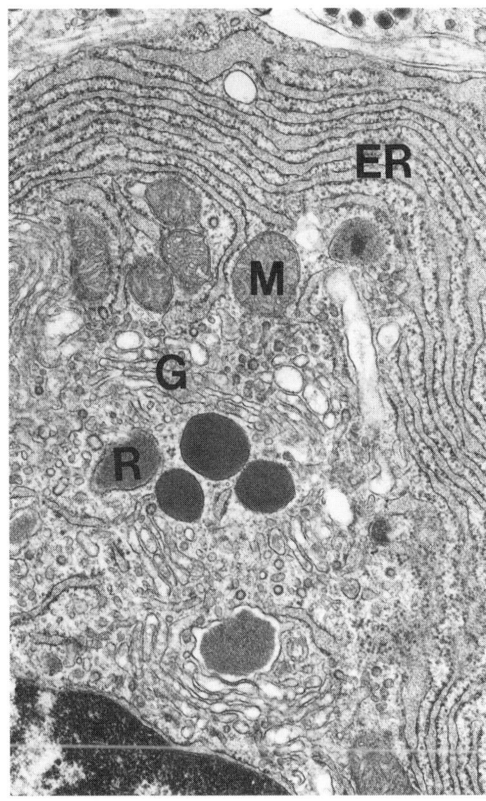

Figure 3.12. *Part of a plasma cell with abundant rough endoplasmic reticulum (ER), mitochondria (M), extensive Golgi complex (G), and Russell bodies (R) (×19,500).*

trally converging strands that give the nucleus a cartwheel appearance (Fig. 3.11). The cytoplasm is intensely basophilic, and a negative Golgi image is usually present. At the fine-structural level, in addition to an extensive Golgi complex, the cytoplasm has abundant rER with dilated cisternae containing slightly granular and moderately electron-dense material and spherical inclusions referred to as Russell bodies (Fig. 3.12). Russell bodies give a positive reaction for immunoglobulin. Free ribosomes and mitochondria are also present in the cytoplasm.

Plasma cells are most numerous in lymphatic tissue, especially in the center of medullary cords of lymph nodes. They are also particularly abundant in bone marrow, the loose connective tissue of the lamina propria of the gastrointestinal tract, the respiratory system, and the female reproductive system.

Plasma cells do not originate in loose connective tissue but develop from B lymphocytes that immigrate from the blood; they produce circulating or humoral antibodies (see Chapter 8).

OTHER FREE CELLS OF LOOSE CONNECTIVE TISSUE

Depending on its location and various other factors (infestation by parasites, presence of bacteria, and the like), loose connective tissue may contain a varying number of lymphocytes, monocytes, and granulocytes (especially eosinophils and neutrophils). The structure and function of these free cells are described in the section on blood (see Chapter 4).

Globule leukocytes are mononuclear cells with acidophilic and metachromatic cytoplasmic granules. These cells are found in connective tissues of the respiratory, digestive, reproductive, and urinary systems. Globule leukocytes are believed to be a subpopulation of T lymphocytes, but origination from mast cells has also been proposed. Their function is unknown.

CONNECTIVE TISSUE FIBERS

Structural connective-tissue fibers include collagen, reticular, and elastic fibers. In addition, **fibrous adhesive proteins** such as fibronectin and laminin bind structural fibers together or help cells attach to the connective tissue matrix.

Collagen Fibers

Collagen is the principal fiber type in mature connective tissue. The turnover rate of collagen is tissue-specific and can vary within the same tissue. Most collagen digestion occurs through the action of metalloproteinases (e.g., collagenase) and serine proteases.

Collagen polypeptide chains are synthesized in the rER as pro-α chains that contain extension peptides (propeptides) at both ends (Fig. 3.13). To date, 25 α chains have been recognized. Within the rER cisternae, these pro-α chains assemble into triple helices to form **procollagen** molecules. The molecules are then transferred to the Golgi complex, packaged into secretory vesicles, and released by exocytosis. At this point in syn-

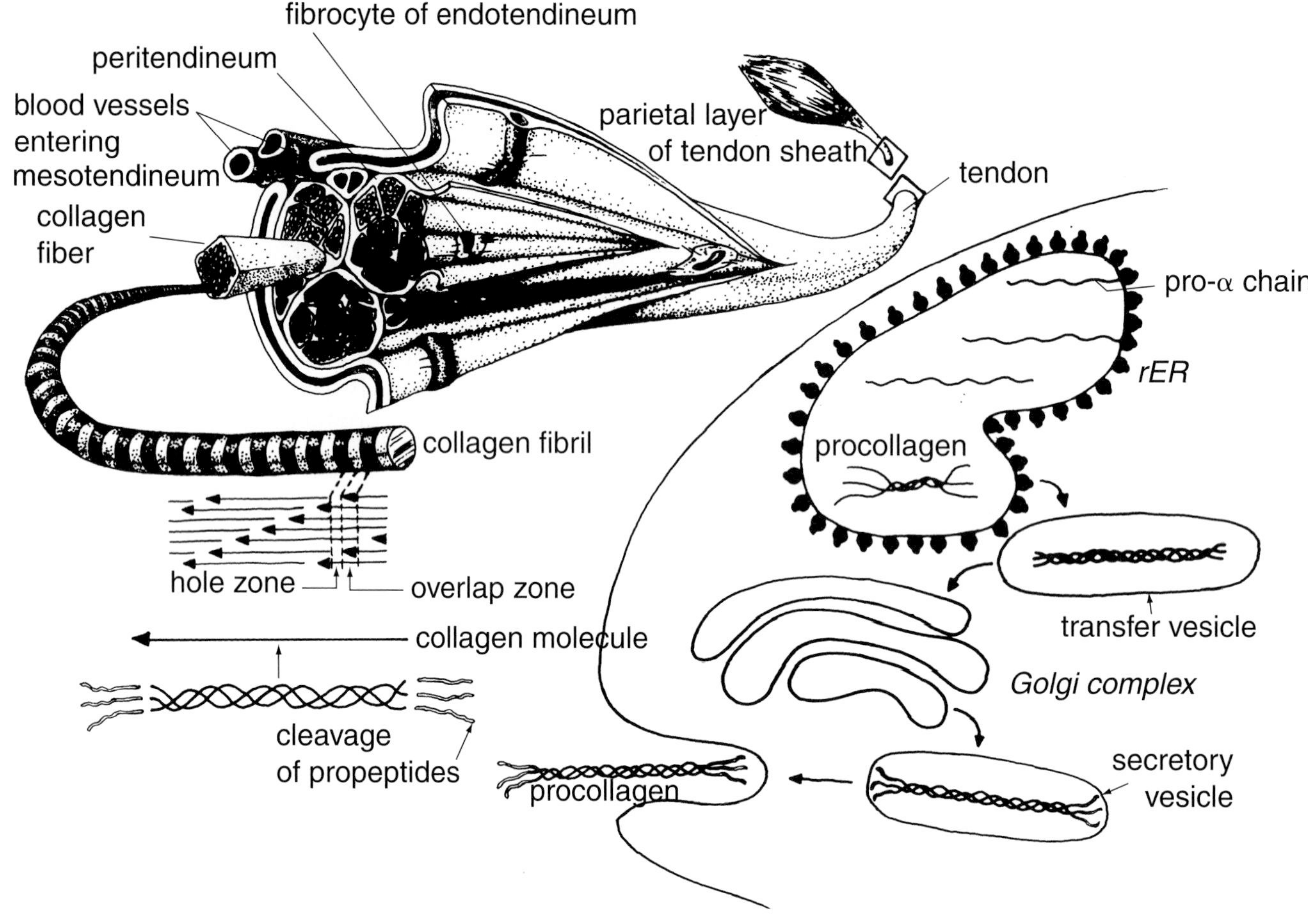

Figure 3.13. *Collagen polypeptide chains are synthesized within the cell and released into the extracellular space as procollagen. In fibril-forming collagen, peptides are then cleaved from the procollagen, resulting in a collagen molecule. The collagen molecules are assembled in such a way that hole zones are created, which stain dark, in contrast to overlap zones, which exclude stain. Bundles of light- and dark-banded fibrils form collagen fibers. In a tendon, individual collagen fibers are surrounded by endotendineum and bundles of fibers are bound by peritendineum. In this drawing, the sheath surrounding the tendon is reflected to show the collagen fiber bundles (fascicles) inside. Blood vessels pass through the mesotendineum to supply the tendon.*

thesis, collagen can be classed as fibril-forming, network-forming, or fibril-associated collagen. Approximately 15 total collagens are recognized within the three classes.

Fibril-forming collagen then undergoes extracellular enzymatic cleavage of the propeptides to yield collagen molecules. These molecules in turn assemble in the extracellular matrix (ECM) to form **collagen fibrils**. The fibrils are only visible with the electron microscope, are up to several micrometers in length, and vary in diameter (10 to 300 nm) with characteristic cross-striations repeated at 67-nm intervals (Figs. 3.13 and 3.14). Bundles of these fibrils form **collagen fibers** that are visible by light microscopy (Fig. 3.2B). Fibril-forming collagen includes types I, II, III, V, and XI. Fibers composed of type I collagen account for 90% of the body collagen. Fresh collagen fibers are white, and in histologic preparations, they stain with acid dyes. Thus, they are red to pink in hematoxylin and eosin (H&E)-stained sections, red with van Gieson s method, and blue in Mallory s and Masson s triple stains (green when light green stain is used). The fibers are flexible and can adapt to the movements and changes in size of the organs with which they are associated. Collagen fibers are characterized by a high tensile strength and a poor shear strength and can be stretched only to approximately 5% of their initial length. Consequently, they are found wherever high tensile strength is required, such as in tendons, ligaments, and organ capsules.

Network-forming collagen is not cleaved by enzymes outside the cell. The intact terminal regions of the collagen molecule interact, and the collagen forms a flexible framework for the basal lamina of epithelia. Network-forming collagen includes types IV and VII.

Fibril-associated collagen also is not cleaved after secretion. These collagens bind periodically to the surface of fibril-forming collagen and may mediate the interactions of fibrils with one another and with other matrix components. Collagen types IX and XII are believed to perform this function.

Reticular Fibers

In routine histologic preparations, reticular fibers cannot be distinguished from other small collagen fibers. These fibers can be identified only with certain silver impregnations (thus the term **argyrophilic** or **argentaffin fibers**) or with the periodic acid-Schiff (PAS) reagent (Fig. 3.15). These fibers are actually individual collagen fibrils (type III collagen) coated by proteoglycans and glycoproteins. This coating increases the affinity for silver salts. When individual reticular fibers are bundled to form collagen fibers, the coating is supposedly displaced and the argyrophilia decreases.

Reticular fibers form delicate, flexible networks around capillaries, muscle fibers, nerves, adipose cells, and hepatocytes, and serve as a scaffolding to support cells or cell groups of endocrine, lymphatic, and blood-forming organs. They are an integral part of basement membranes.

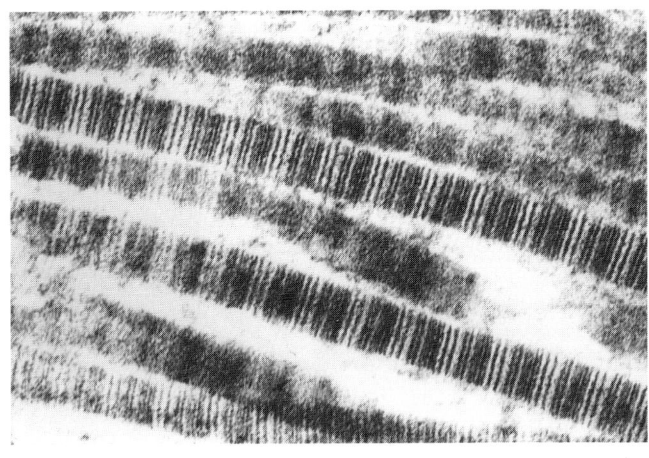

Figure 3.14. *Electron micrograph of collagen fibrils with characteristic cross striations (×88,000).*

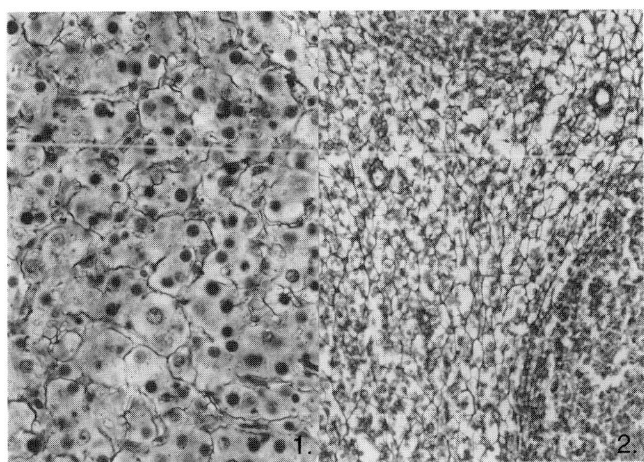

Figure 3.15. *Reticular fibers. **1.**,* Liver (pig). Achucarro silver impregnation (×435). **2.**, Lymph node (dog). Palmgren silver impregnation (×230).

Elastic Fibers

Elastic fibers and/or sheets (laminae) are present in organs in which normal function requires elasticity in addition to tensile strength. Elastic fibers can be stretched as much as two and one-half times their original length, to which they return when released. Elastic fibers are found in the pinna of the ear, vocal cords, epiglottis, lungs, ligamentum nuchae, dermis, aorta, and muscular arteries.

Elastic fibers usually occur as individual, branching, and anastomosing fibers. Their diameters vary within a wide range, from 0.2 to 5.0 μm in loose connective tissue to as large as 12 μm in elastic ligaments, such as the ligamentum nuchae (Fig. 3.16). In H&E-stained histologic sections, the larger elastic fibers in elastic ligaments are readily distinguished as highly refractile, amorphous, light pink strands; they are stainable by certain selective dyes, such as orcein and resorcin-fuchsin.

The main component of elastic fibers is **elastin**, an amorphous protein of low electron density. Elastin is rich in proline and glycine but contains little hydroxyproline. One theory of elastin structure is that the molecules are randomly coiled and joined by stable, covalent crosslinks. The fiber coils can stretch and then recoil as needed. Elastin is synthesized by fibroblasts and smooth muscle cells as tropoelastin, i.e., single polypeptide chains that are transformed into elastin, crosslinked, and assembled in the extracellular space.

The secondary component of elastic fibers is 10-nm microfibrils that cover the elastin core (Fig. 3.17). The microfibrillar material is composed of a glycoprotein, **fibrillin**, which is necessary for elastic fiber integrity. The microfibrils are secreted before elastin and provide a scaffolding on which elastin forms fibers and sheets. Developmentally, the elastic fiber is the last fiber to appear in organs (e.g., lung) or connective tissue.

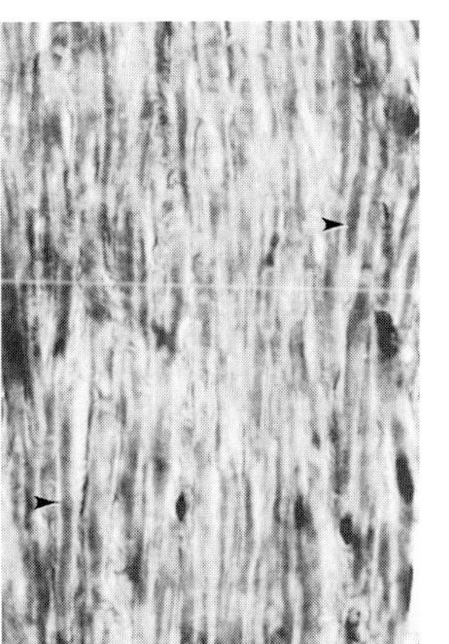

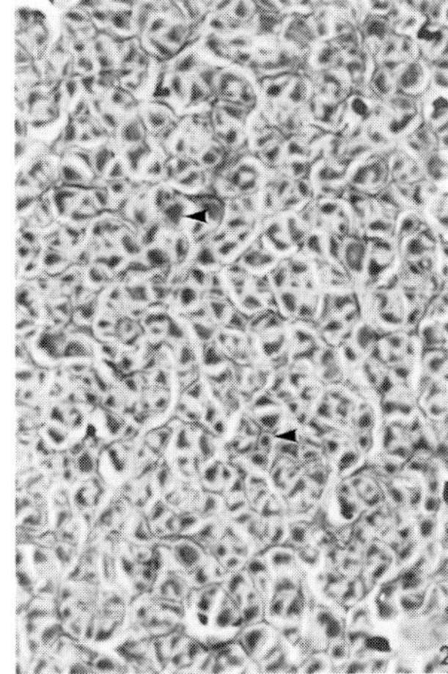

Figure 3.16. *Ligamentum nuchae, large ruminant. **1.**,* Longitudinal section; **2.**, cross section. Note that the large elastic fibers (arrows) are surrounded by networks of collagen fibers. Crossman s trichrome (×600).

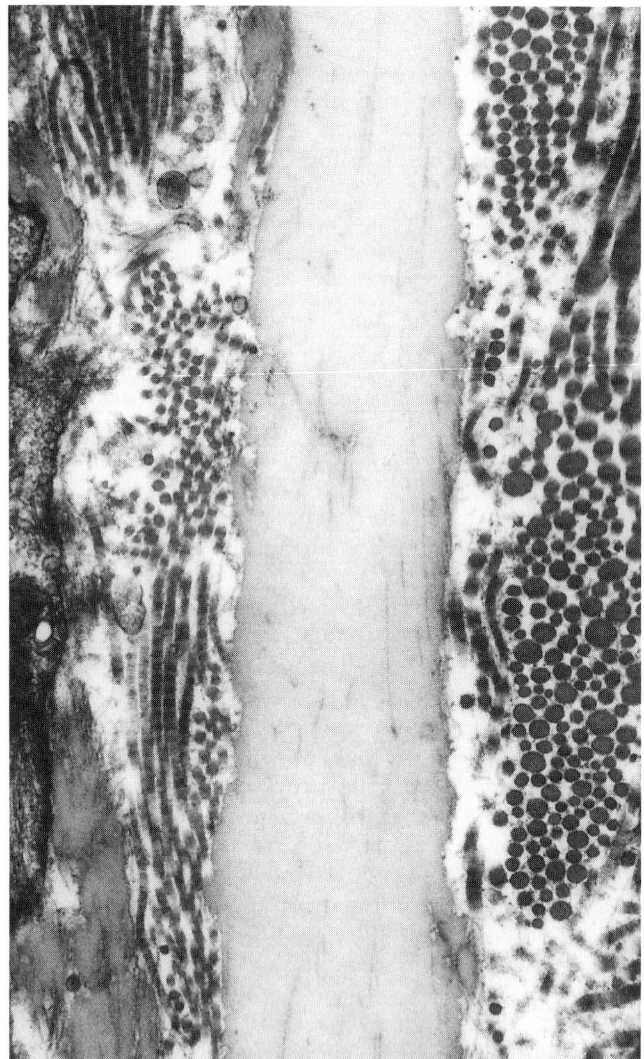

Figure 3.17. *Electron micrograph of an elastic lamina between collagen fibrils (longitudinal and cross sections). The electron-dense thin lines in the elastic lamina are microfibrils (×21,000).*

Fibrous Adhesive Proteins

The extracellular matrix contains noncollagenous fibrous proteins that play a role in organizing the matrix and help cells to adhere to it. **Fibronectin**, a major product of mesenchymal cells, is a fibril-forming protein that binds to various structures, including the cell membrane, collagen, elastin, and proteoglycans, and probably mediates the connection between the cytoskeleton and the extracellular matrix. Fibronectin plays a role in a variety of processes, such as cell adhesion, cell differentiation, cell growth, and phagocytosis.

Laminin is a large glycoprotein. It is the major constituent of basal laminae and is synthesized by the cells that are in contact with it (e.g., epithelial cells, smooth muscle cells, neurolemmocytes). Laminin is present in the lamina lucida (lamina rara) and specifically attaches the cell to the lamina densa (basal lamina), in which type IV collagen forms a network of considerable strength and flexibility (Fig. 16.6).

GROUND SUBSTANCE

The cells and fibers of connective tissue are embedded in an amorphous ground substance composed of **glycosaminoglycans** (GAGs) and **proteoglycans**. The ground substance forms a hydrated gel that, by virtue of its high water content, has unique properties of resiliency.

Seven major types of GAGs can be distinguished. **Hyaluronic acid** is a nonsulfated GAG. It is a large, long molecule that forms networks with spaces that are filled with tissue fluid. The resulting gel is particularly abundant in the vitreous humor of the eye and in synovial fluid; it is also found in the umbilical cord, loose connective tissue, skin, and cartilage. Hyaluronic acid also serves as the core of proteoglycan aggregates. **Chondroitin-4-sulfate** and **chondroitin-6-sulfate** are abundant in cartilage, arteries, skin, and cornea. A smaller amount is found in bone. **Dermatan sulfate** is found in skin, tendon, ligamentum nuchae, sclera, and lung. **Keratan sulfate** is present in cartilage, bone, and cornea. **Heparan sulfate** is found in arteries and the lung, whereas **heparin** is found in mast cells, the lung, liver, and skin. The latter six GAGs are of the sulfated variety.

Proteoglycans are formed by covalently linking GAGs to a protein core and range in size from small molecules (decorin, m.w. 40,000) to large aggregates (aggrecan, m.w. 210,000) (Fig. 3.18). In addition to filling space in the connective tissue matrix and imparting its unique biomechanical properties, proteoglycans may regulate the passage of molecules and cells in the intercellular space. They are also believed to play a major role in chemical signaling between cells and may bind and regulate the activities of other secreted proteins.

Proteoglycans in low concentrations are not detected in H&E-stained sections, but when present in higher concentrations, as in hyaline cartilage, they stain with basophilic dyes. When stained with toluidine blue or crystal violet, a metachromatic reaction occurs, i.e., the amorphous ground substance stains a different color from that of the dye solution.

EMBRYONIC CONNECTIVE TISSUES

Mesenchyme

Mesenchyme is composed of irregularly shaped mesenchymal cells and amorphous ground substance (Fig. 3.1). The cell processes contact adjacent cells and thus form a three-dimensional network. Mesenchymal cells undergo numerous mitotic cell divisions and continuously change their shape and location to adapt to the transformations that occur during embryonic growth. During early development, mesenchyme does not con-

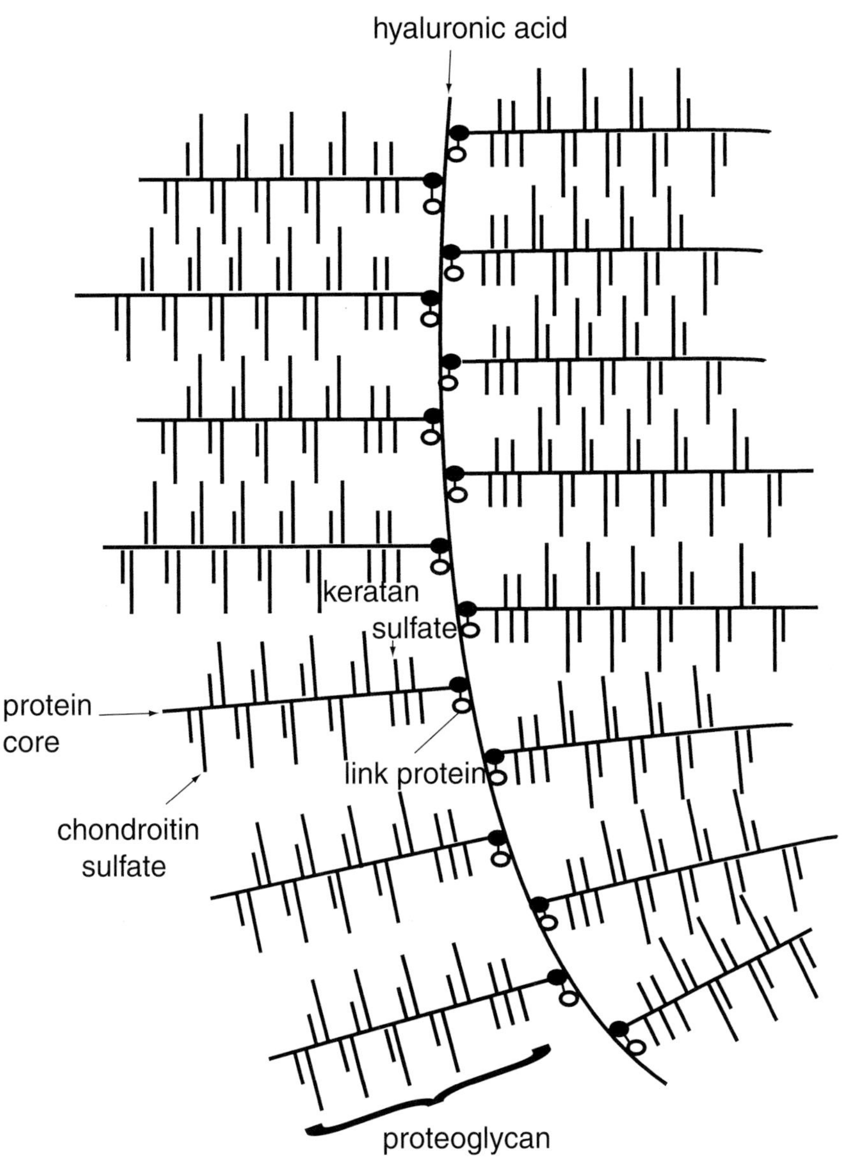

Figure 3.18. *The matrix of cartilage contains aggrecans, which are composed of proteoglycans bound to a hyaluronic acid chain by link proteins. The proteoglycans are composed of glycosaminoglycans, such as chondroitin and keratan sulfate, bound to a protein core.*

tain fibers, and the abundant amorphous ground substance fills the wide intercellular spaces.

Mesenchyme gives rise to various types of adult connective tissues, as well as blood and blood vessels. As mesenchyme differentiates into other types of connective tissue, some of the transitional forms are not easily distinguished.

Mucous Connective Tissue

Mucous or gelatinous connective tissue is found primarily in the embryonic hypodermis and umbilical cord (Fig. 3.19). It is characterized by stellate fibroblasts that form a network. The intercellular space is occupied by a viscous, gel-like amorphous ground substance that has a positive reaction for glycosaminoglycans or proteoglycans. Collagen fibers are also present. In the adult organism, gelatinous connective tissue occurs in the papillae of omasal laminae and reticular folds, the bovine glans penis, and the core of the rooster comb.

ADULT CONNECTIVE TISSUES

Adult connective tissues are classified based on the variation of quantity and arrangement of fibers within the matrix. The properties of cell structure and the biochemical composition of fibers and ground substance are similar across connective tissue types.

Loose Connective Tissue

Loose, irregularly arranged, or areolar connective tissue is the most widely distributed type of connective tissue in the adult animal (Fig. 3.20A). The cells and fibers of loose connective tissue are widely separated by spaces filled with ground substance. Compared to other types of connective tissue, the cells in loose connective tissue are more abundant and include both fixed and immigrant populations. All three fiber types (reticular, collagen, and elastic) are present. The relative abundance and orientation of fibers vary widely and depend primarily on the location and specific function of the tissue. In cases of injury, the stage of healing also causes variation in fiber arrangement.

The amorphous ground substance of loose connective tissue is composed of proteoglycans that bind a significant quantity of tissue fluid. This fluid has limited ability to circulate. Substances dissolved in the tissue fluid can diffuse through the amorphous ground substance and thus have ready access to connective tissue cells. Circulating tissue fluid is formed at the arterial end of capillaries and absorbed by either venous or lymphatic capillaries.

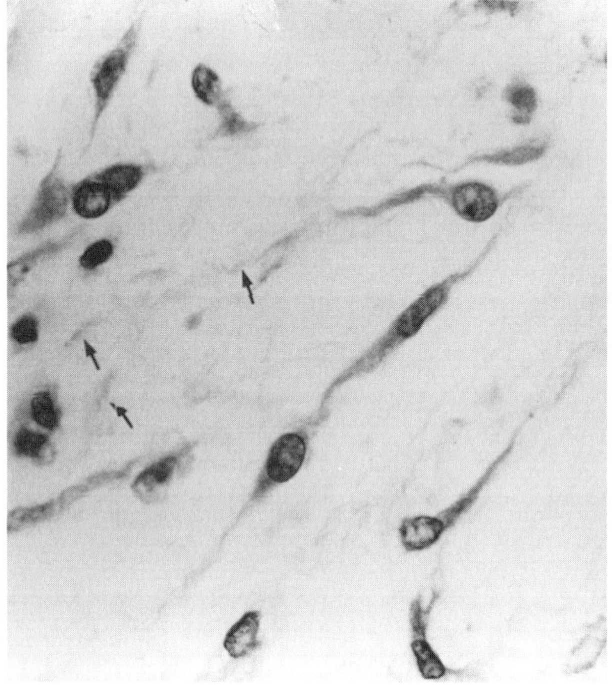

Figure 3.19. *Gelatinous connective tissue, umbilical cord (pig). Fine collagen fibers (arrows) are present. Hematoxylin and eosin (×800).*

Loose connective tissue is present beneath many epithelia, where it provides support and a vascular supply and makes up the interstitial tissue in most organs, thereby allowing easy movements and shifting of organs. Loose connective tissue is present around nerve and skeletal muscle bundles as named tissue layers (e.g., epineurium) and found between the layers of smooth musculature of hollow organs. The pia mater and arachnoid of the brain are also composed of loose connective tissue.

Many important functions are performed by loose connective tissue. They range from the purely mechanical, such as support and dampening biomechanical effects in various locations (e.g., hypodermis), to more sophisticated functions, such as participation in tissue repair and defense activities (inflammation).

Dense Connective Tissue

The fibers in dense connective tissue are more abundant than cells and amorphous ground substance. Dense connective tissue is commonly classified as either **dense irregular connective tissue**, with a seemingly random orientation of the fiber bundles, or **dense regular connective tissue**, in which fibers are oriented in a regular pattern.

DENSE IRREGULAR CONNECTIVE TISSUE

Fibrocytes are the predominant cell population in **dense irregular connective tissue** (Fig. 3.20B). Collagen fibers are generally arranged in bundles that cross each other at varying angles. In thin aponeuroses or muscle fasciae, these bundles are located in a single layer. In heavier aponeuroses, organ capsules, or dermis, the bundles are superimposed in several layers and interlace with one another in multiple planes. This irregular configuration allows adaptation to changes in the size of an organ or the diameter of a muscle, and stretching forces can be withstood in any direction. Continuation of surface connective tissue into the organ or muscle enhances strength, and overstretching becomes rather dif-

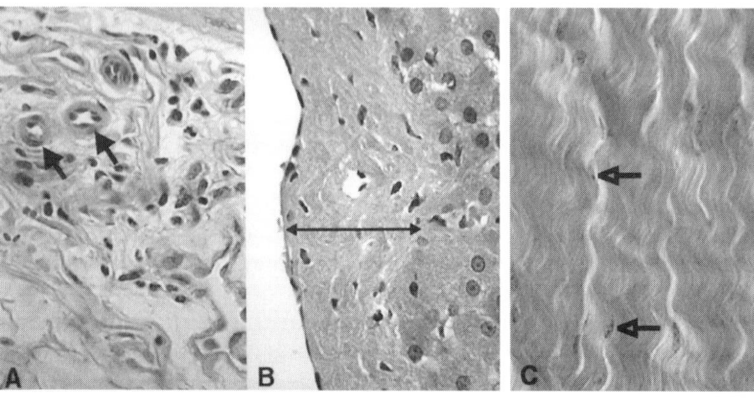

Figure 3.20. ***A.**, Loose connective tissue with blood vessels (arrows), liver (dog). **B.**, Dense irregular connective tissue (arrow), liver (dog). **C.**, Dense regular connective tissue with fibrocytes (arrows), tendon. Hematoxylin and eosin (×600).*

ficult. The presence of elastic networks facilitates a fast return to resting conditions.

Dense irregular connective tissue is found in a variety of locations, such as the lamina propria of the initial portions of the digestive system, the capsule of the lung (visceral pleura) and other organs (spleen, liver, kidney, testis), fasciae, aponeuroses, joint capsules, pericardium, and dermis. Special functional and morphologic features are described with the various organ systems.

DENSE REGULAR CONNECTIVE TISSUE

Dense regular connective tissue occurs as collagenous tendons and ligaments or elastic ligaments (Fig. 3.20C). In both types, all fibers are arranged in the same plane and direction, according to specific functional requirements.

Collagenous tendons and ligaments

The great tensile strength of collagenous tendons is reflected in their structure. They consist of fascicles of parallel collagen fibers (Fig. 3.13). Individual collagen fibers are surrounded by fibrocytes, which form the **endotendineum**. These fascicles are bound together by sparse, loose connective tissue (the **peritendineum**) that forms a protective sheath around the blood vessels and nerves of the tendon. The peritendineum is continuous with the **epitendineum**, the dense irregular connective tissue around the entire gross tendon. Repair of a severed tendon is effected by the fibroblasts of associated connective tissue.

The fibrocytes between the collagen fibers of the tendon are long, flat cells of varying shape. Winglike cytoplasmic processes extend between adjacent collagen fibers and give the fibrocytes a stellate appearance in cross sections of tendon.

The typical tendon structure may be altered at points of insertion into bone or cartilage or where the tendon courses around bones. Wherever tendons or ligaments insert on bone or cartilage, the dense regular collagenous tissue of the tendon gradually changes to fibrocartilage and then to mineralized fibrocartilage before the point of osseous penetration. Collagen fibers from the tendon or ligament are embedded in the bone matrix as **penetrating fibers** (Sharpey s fibers). The function of this arrangement is to gradually transmit biomechanical forces from a flexible fibrous unit to a stiffer osseous unit. In areas where tendons course around bones, they are subject not only to tension but also to compression, which causes the cells to enlarge and to become encapsulated such that the tissue appears similar to fibrocartilage.

The mobility of the tendon is ensured either by the surrounding epitendineum or the **tendon sheaths**, which consist of a visceral and a parietal portion (Fig. 3.13). The visceral portion is tightly anchored to the tendon and is separated from the parietal portion by a fluid-filled synovial cavity. Both the parietal and the visceral portions of the tendon sheath comprise dense irregular connective tissue and a synovial layer, the structure of which is similar to that of synovial membranes. Blood vessels supplying the tendon pass through a gap between the opposing edges of the synovial sheath known as the **mesotendineum**.

Collagenous ligaments contain a lower percentage of ground substance than tendons and the collagen fibers are organized more randomly. Named connective tissue layers are not assigned to ligaments.

Elastic ligaments

Large elastic fibers that branch and interconnect predominate in **elastic ligaments**. The fibers are surrounded by loose connective tissue (Fig. 3.16). The ligamentum nuchae and some dorsal ligaments of the spinal column are examples of elastic ligaments

Reticular Connective Tissue

The stroma of all lymphatic organs (spleen, lymph node, hemal lymph node, hemal node, tonsils), diffuse lymphatic tissue, solitary lymphatic nodules, and bone marrow is made of reticular connective tissue. This tissue is composed of stellate reticular cells and a complex three-dimensional network of reticular fibers (Fig. 3.15) (see Chapter 8).

Adipose Tissue

Adipose tissue, or fat, is a specialized type of connective tissue that, in addition to performing insulating and mechanical functions, plays an important role in the metabolism of the organism. One of the most important functions of adipose tissue is its participation in fat metabolism. The turnover of intracellular fat is rapid, with a continuous cycle of withdrawal and deposit, even if the organism has to draw on its fat reserves to supplement food intake.

Intracellular lipids are synthesized mainly from fatty acids but also from carbohydrates and proteins. The fatty acids necessary for lipid synthesis are derived from the enzymatic breakdown by lipoprotein lipase of the triglycerides contained in blood chylomicrons or lipoproteins; after their uptake by the adipocytes, the fatty acids are resynthesized to triglycerides.

Under hormonal (insulin) or nervous (norepinephrine) control, intracellular enzymatic hydrolysis of triglycerides takes place, and fatty acids and glycerol are released into the blood and catabolized in energy-yielding reactions. In brown adipocytes, mitochondrial respiration is uncoupled from adenosine 5′-triphosphate (ATP) synthesis; thus, the oxidation of stored fat generates heat rather than ATP, causing a rise in body temperature in arousing hibernating mammals.

In mammalian subcutaneous connective tissue, the adipose-tissue component serves as a thermal and mechanical insulator. In the foot pads and digital cushions, adipose tissue is associated with bundles of collagen and elastic fibers. This combination of fibers and fat cells allows the adipose tissue to act as a dampening cushion, and at the same time, the cells are protected by the great tensile strength of the collagen fibers. After deformation, the elastic fibers allow the adipose cells to return to normal shape.

Two types of adipose tissue, white and brown, are distinguished in most mammals by differences in color, vascularity, structure, and function.

WHITE ADIPOSE TISSUE

The cells of **white fat** are separated by septa of loose connective tissue into clusters of adipose cells referred to as lobules. Each adipose cell is surrounded by a delicate network of collagen and reticular fibers that supports a dense capillary plexus and nerve fibers (Fig. 3.4). In addition, the narrow intercellular spaces contain a few fibrocytes, mast cells, and sparse amorphous ground substance.

BROWN ADIPOSE TISSUE

Brown adipose tissue (brown fat) is composed of aggregates of multilocular adipocytes (Fig. 3.5). The intercellular connective tissue consists of fibrocytes, collagen, and reticular fibers. Capillaries form a dense plexus, and the adipocytes are directly innervated by adrenergic axons.

Brown adipose tissue is particularly common and abundant in rodents and hibernating mammals. It is located primarily in the axillary and neck regions (interscapular fat body), along the thoracic aorta and in the mediastinum, in the mesenteries, and around the aorta and vena cava dorsal to the kidney. It may also be found in the same locations in other domestic mammals.

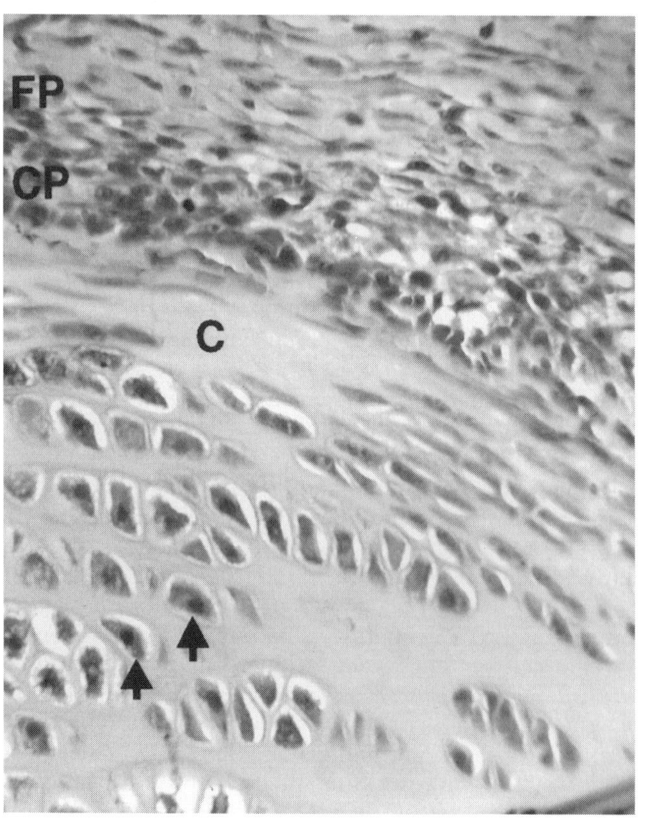

Figure 3.21. *Immature hyaline cartilage (dog). The fibrous layer (FP) and cellular layer (CP) of the perichondrium border the cartilage (C) containing chondroblasts (arrows). Hematoxylin and eosin (×300).*

ADULT SUPPORTIVE TISSUES

Cartilage

Cartilage is specialized for a supportive role in the body. It possesses considerable tensile strength because the intercellular substance is laced with collagen and/or elastic fibers, and the firm but pliable ground substance enhances its weightbearing ability. In general, this tissue is avascular, alymphatic, and aneural; however, blood vessels may penetrate cartilage structures greater than 3 mm in dimension (e.g., cartilaginous epiphyses of developing bones).

CARTILAGE CELLS

Two cell types are recognized in cartilage: the **chondroblast** and the **chondrocyte.**

Chondroblast

The **chondroblast** is found in growing cartilage (Fig. 3.21). The cell is oval-shaped with a spherical nucleus and a prominent Golgi apparatus. The cytoplasm is basophilic as a result of large quantities of rER. The chondroblast actively forms the matrix of cartilage that surrounds the perimeter of the cell.

Chondrocyte

After cartilage matrix formation is complete, the chondroblast becomes a less active cell, the **chondrocyte** (Fig. 3.22). The chondrocyte varies from elongate to spherical in shape, depending on the location within the cartilage. Each chondrocyte is located within a **lacuna,** a cavity within the semirigid cartilage matrix. In living cartilage or at the fine-structural level, the cell fills the lacuna. Short cytoplasmic processes extend into the intercellular substance. In most light microscopic preparations, the cell surface appears separated from the lacunar walls because of shrinkage. The chondrocyte has a spherical nucleus with one or more nucleoli and abundant rER and Golgi complex. Glycogen and lipid accumulate in old chondrocytes, and in routine preparation, the cells appear vacuolated. Although considered a less active cell than the chondroblast, the chondrocyte is responsible for continual ongoing maintenance of the surrounding matrix.

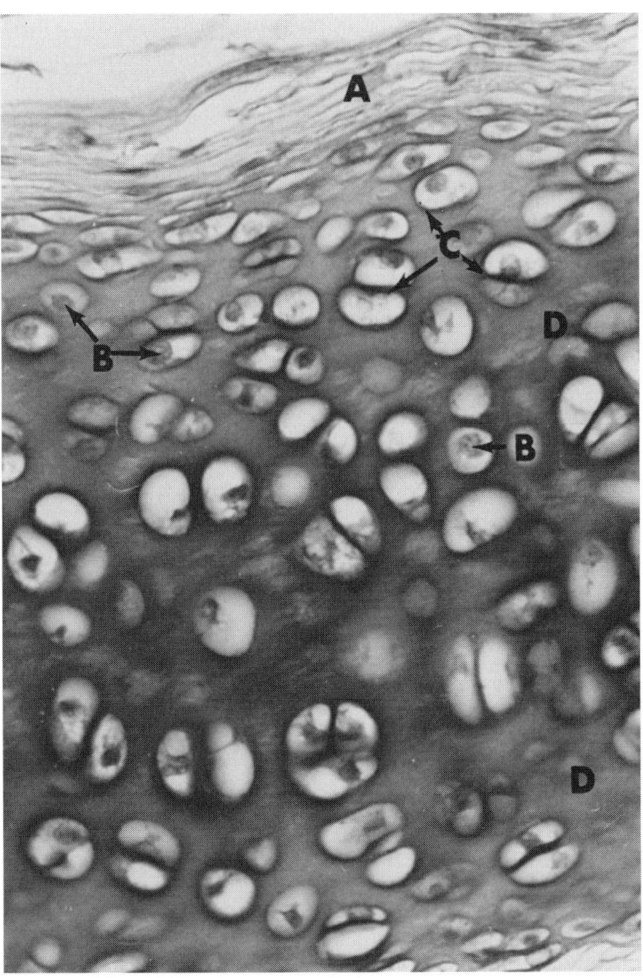

Figure 3.22. *Mature hyaline cartilage (dog). The fibrous perichondrium (A) surrounds the cartilage mass. The chondrocytes (B) lie in lacunae. The territorial matrix (C) is darker than the interterritorial matrix (D). Hematoxylin and eosin (×425).*

CARTILAGE MATRIX

The matrix of cartilage is composed of fibers and ground substance as found in other connective tissues, but the **cartilage matrix** has unique biomechanical properties. Collagen forms the framework of the matrix. The major cartilage collagen is type II, but type I predominates in fibrocartilage and other collagen types are known to be present in cartilage.

The ground substance contains the GAGs chondroitin sulfate, keratan sulfate, and hyaluronic acid, all of which play an important role in transporting water and electrolytes, as well as in binding water to give hyaline cartilage its resiliency. The GAGs complex with proteins to form proteoglycans (Fig. 3.18). **Aggrecan** is formed by joining proteoglycans to a hyaluronic acid core with link proteins. The proteoglycans are also bound to adjacent collagen fibers, thereby forming a loose network that functions as a molecular sieve, limiting movement of larger molecules.

Additional components of the cartilage matrix include the adhesive molecules, **chondronectin**, **anchorin CII**, and **fibronectin**, which are involved in the interaction between collagen and chondrocytes. The matrix is mineralized by **hydroxyapatite** in the deep region of the articular cartilage and in the zone of hypertrophy of the physis.

Overall, the matrix is slightly basophilic when stained with H&E, reacts positively with PAS, and exhibits a marked metachromasia with metachromatic stains. Staining intensity varies across the matrix due to variations in matrical biochemical composition.

CLASSIFICATION OF CARTILAGE

On the basis of different structural characteristics of the matrix, three types of cartilage are distinguishable: **hyaline cartilage**, **elastic cartilage**, and **fibrocartilage**.

Hyaline cartilage

Hyaline cartilage is found on the articulating surfaces of bones and provides support in the nose, larynx, trachea, and bronchi. It forms most of the entire appendicular and axial skeleton in the embryo.

The chondrocytes in mature hyaline cartilage vary in size (Fig. 3.22). Chondrocytes near the surface of cartilage are small, and their lacunae are elliptic, with their long axes parallel to the surface. Deep within the cartilage, the cells are larger and more polyhedral. Some lacunae contain only one cell; others contain two, four, or sometimes six cells. These multicellular lacunae are called **cell nests** or **isogenous cell groups**.

The amorphous ground substance of hyaline cartilage is a firm gel laced with type II collagen fibers. Because the fibers have the same refractive index as the amorphous ground substance, they cannot be seen in standard preparations. Surrounding each chondrocyte is a thin layer of **pericellular matrix** that contains proteoglycans but lacks collagen. The **territorial matrix** surrounds the pericellular matrix and is composed of a network of fine collagen fibers and ground substance. The **interterritorial matrix** lies outside the territorial matrix and fills the remaining matrix space. This matrix region contains large collagen fibers and abundant proteoglycans. Differences in collagen and proteoglycan content account for the staining differences between regions as observed under the light microscope.

At the ultrastructural level, **matrix granules** are present adjacent to the chondrocytes. These granules are proteoglycans secreted by the chondrocytes and represent early stages of matrix production. The proteoglycans later become components of aggrecan in the surrounding matrix.

Except on articular surfaces, hyaline cartilage is surrounded by connective tissue called the **perichondrium**, which is composed of two distinct layers (Fig. 3.21). The layer immediately adjacent to the cartilage is composed of chondroblasts and a network of small blood vessels; it is called the **cellular** or **chondrogenic layer**. The outer **fibrous layer** of the perichondrium is made of irregularly arranged collagen fibers and fibroblasts.

Elastic cartilage

Elastic cartilage is found where elasticity, as well as some rigidity, is needed, such as in the epiglottis and external auditory canal. It is also part of the corniculate and cuneiform cartilages of the larynx.

In addition to all of the structural components of hyaline cartilage, elastic cartilage possesses a dense network of elastic fibers that are visible in ordinary H&E preparations (Fig. 3.23). The elastic fibers are few in number near the perichondrium but form a dense network within the cartilaginous mass. Chondrocytes located away from the surface of elastic cartilage contain many fat vacuoles.

Fibrocartilage

Of the three cartilage types, **fibrocartilage** occurs least frequently. It is often interposed between other tissues and hyaline cartilage, tendons, or ligaments. Fibrocartilage is found in the intervertebral disks and makes up the menisci of the stifle joint. In dogs, the atrial and ventricular heart muscles are joined together by fibrocartilage.

The most striking characteristic of fibrocartilage is the presence of prominent type I collagen fibers in the matrix (Fig. 3.24). The microscopic appearance of fibrocartilage may vary with location. Fibrocartilage that attaches ligaments and tendons to bone has large collagen fiber bundles dispersed in a plane parallel to the direction of the pulling forces, with rows of small lacunae containing chondrocytes between collagen bundles (Fig. 3.24A). In the fibrocartilaginous cardiac skeleton of the dog, the chondrocytes and collagen fibers are distributed more randomly (Fig. 3.24B). The amorphous ground substance is most abundant in the vicinity of the cells, whereas the remainder of the matrix contains primarily collagen fiber bundles. Fibrocartilage lacks a distinct perichondrium, although it is surrounded by col-

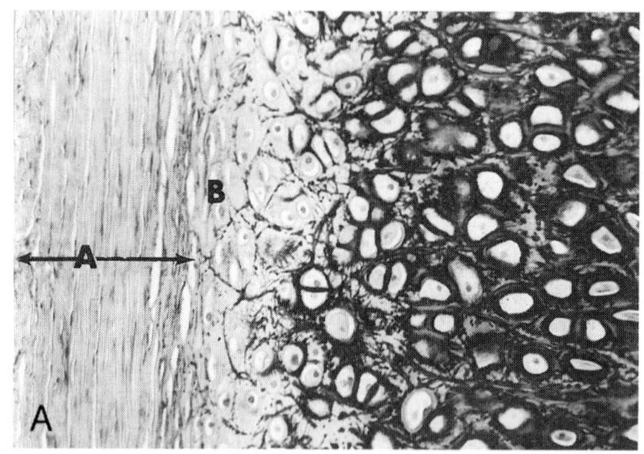

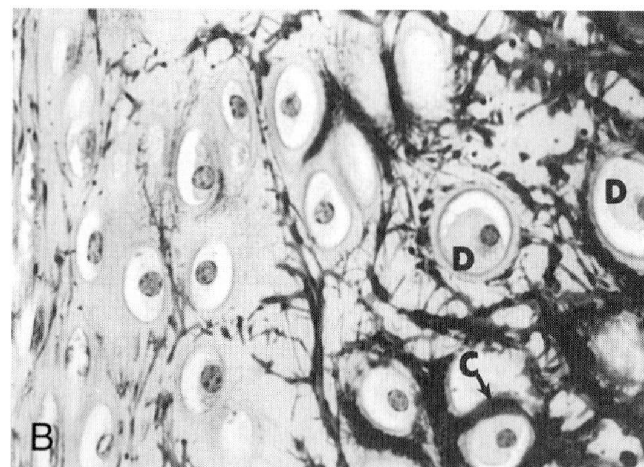

Figure 3.23. *Elastic cartilage, external ear (dog).* ***A.***, *Perichondrium (A) with sparse elastic fibers (black) penetrating the cellular layer (B) (×80).* ***B.***, *High-power magnification illustrates elastic fibers (C) coursing through the matrix. The chondrocytes (D) nearly fill the lacunae. Verhoeff s stain (×425).*

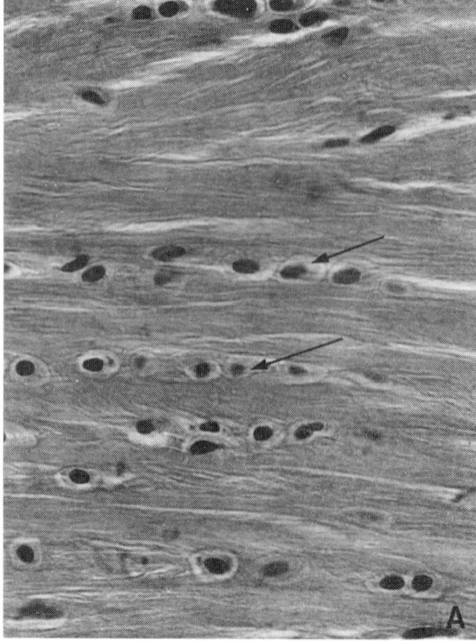

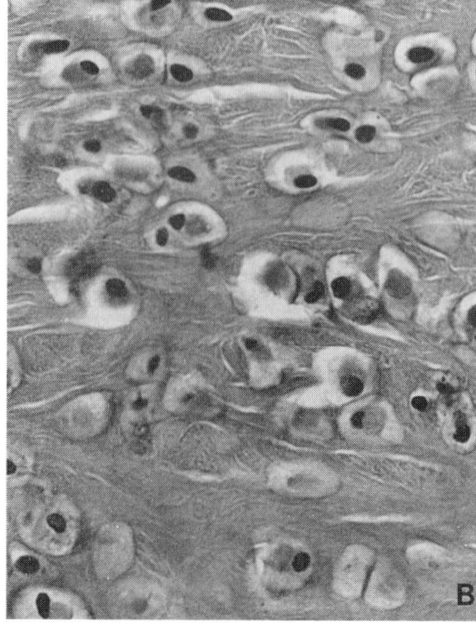

Figure 3.24. ***A.***, *Fibrocartilage at ligament insertion on bone (dog). The lacunae (arrows) are oriented in the plane of pulling forces. Hematoxylin and eosin (×300).* ***B.***, *Cardiac skeleton (dog). The lacunae and collagenous fibers are randomly arranged. Hematoxylin and eosin (×570).*

lagen fibers in some locations. A cellular chondrogenic layer is absent.

DEVELOPMENT OF CARTILAGE

The first indication of cartilage formation within the embryo is a clustering of mesenchymal cells. These cells enlarge, withdraw their processes, and synthesize and secrete amorphous ground substance and procollagen (type II). They are then referred to as chondroblasts, and the cell clusters are called **centers of chondrification**. As the intercellular matrix increases, the cells become spherical and isolated from each other in lacunae; at this point, they are called **chondrocytes**.

Chondroblasts undergo several mitotic divisions, and after each division, new intercellular ground substance separates the two daughter cells. This process leads to substantial expansion of the cartilage from within and is referred to as **interstitial growth**. Concurrently, the mesenchyme surrounding the cartilage primordium differentiates into the perichondrium. Chondroblasts from the cellular layer of the perichondrium divide and secrete additional matrix on the surface of the cartilage. The process is called **appositional growth**. The ability of the chondrogenic layer to produce cartilage persists into adult life, but it is dormant until a need arises for new cartilage.

During the development of elastic cartilage, fibroblasts initially produce undifferentiated fibrils that later become elastic fibers. The fibroblasts later transform into chondroblasts and secrete a more typical cartilage matrix.

NUTRITION OF CARTILAGE

Unlike other connective tissues, most cartilage is avascular. Therefore, the chondrocytes must depend on diffusion of nutrients through the gelled intercellular substance. These nutrients diffuse from capillaries outside the perichondrium or from synovial fluid bathing the cartilage surface. When the intercellular matrix becomes calcified, diffusion is no longer possible, and the chondrocytes die. This phenomenon occurs in aging and is natural in endochondral bone development.

If cartilage exceeds 3 mm^3 in size, then vessels may penetrate the matrix. An example of vascularized cartilage is the hyaline cartilage of developing epiphyses of long bones, which contain blood vessels in cartilage canals.

Bone

Bone is a connective tissue with cells and fibers embedded in a hard, unbending substance that is well suited for supportive and protective functions. The organ-bone-gives internal support to the entire body and provides attachment of the muscles and tendons necessary for movement. It protects the brain and organs in the thoracic cavity and contains the bone marrow within its medullary space. Bone functions metabolically by providing a source of calcium to maintain proper blood calcium levels and various growth factors (e.g., transforming growth factor beta [TGF-β]) that play a role in remodeling.

Bone is a dynamic tissue that is renewed and remodeled throughout the life of all mammals. Its construction is unique because it provides the greatest tensile strength with the least amount of weight of any tissue.

BONE CELLS

Osteoblast

The **osteoblast** is the cell responsible for active formation and mineralization of bone matrix. The cells range from columnar to squamous in shape and are located on surfaces of bone where new bone is being deposited (Figs. 3.25 and 3.26). The nucleus is located in the basal region of the intensely basophilic cytoplasm. The Golgi apparatus and rER are prominent between the nucleus and the secretory surface of the osteoblast. The cell deposits **osteoid** (collagen I and proteoglycans), the unmineralized matrix of bone.

Osteocyte

As matrix secretion approaches completion, approximately 10% of the osteoblasts surround themselves with osteoid and modulate into osteocytes. The **osteocyte** is the principal cell in mature bone and resides in a **lacuna**

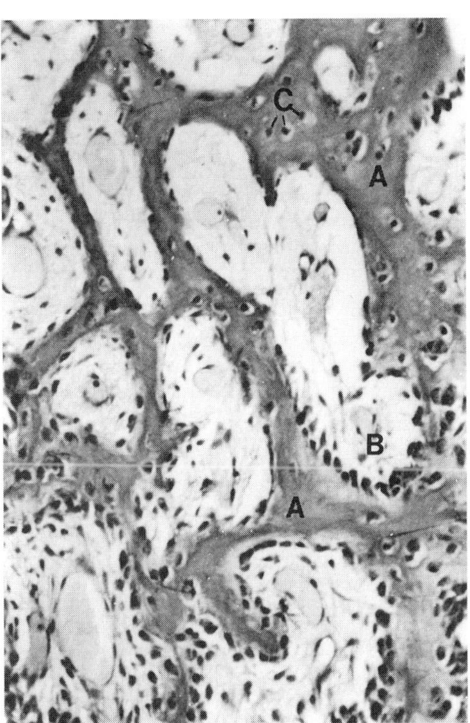

Figure 3.25. *Trabecular bone (A) of intramembranous osteogenesis has osteoblasts (B) and osteocytes (C) within lacunae. Note the prominent blood vessels in the mesenchyme. Hematoxylin and eosin (×175).*

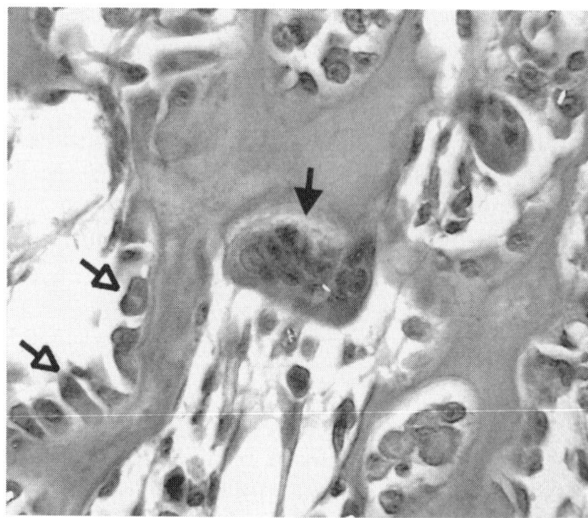

Figure 3.26. *Osteoclast, in an erosion lacuna (arrow), resorbing bone. Osteoblasts (open arrows) are forming bone (B). Hematoxylin and eosin (×475).*

surrounded by calcified interstitial matrix (Fig. 3.25). Numerous long, slender processes extend from the cell body into the **canaliculi** within the matrix, and gap junctions are present where the cell contacts processes of an adjacent osteocyte. Young osteocytes resemble osteoblasts, but as they mature, the Golgi complex and rER are less prominent and lysosomes increase in number.

The exact way in which osteocytes preserve the integrity of bone matrix is not completely understood. The long cellular processes are able to shorten and lengthen. This activity may serve as a pump to move fluid through lacunae and canaliculi to transfer metabolites from the surface of the bone. The lysosomal enzymes in osteocytes may help to maintain the mineral content of the matrix, but their function in calcium release is probably minimal, because the osteoclast (described below) plays the major role in bone resorption. Osteocytes are also believed to remove and replace perilacunar bone, a 1-μm layer immediately adjacent to the osteocyte. Because perilacunar bone has a lower mineral content, it is more soluble and thus can exchange minerals with the surrounding extracellular fluid. Therefore, perilacunar bone may be a mineral reservoir, with little contribution to the structural integrity of bone. Perilacunar bone removal is called **osteocytic osteolysis**. The extent to which this process normally occurs is unclear. The perilacunar space and walls of the canaliculi are covered with GAGs. The maintenance of this covering by osteocytes is important to maintain the integrity of this tissue. Osteocytes are essential in preserving bone structure because upon their death, osteoclasts immediately move to the area and resorb the bone.

Osteoclast

The **osteoclast** is a large, multinucleated cell located on the surface of bone (15 to 30 nuclei per cell, which is 40 to 100 μm in diameter) (Fig. 3.26). Occasional mononuclear osteoclasts are not easily recognized. The cytoplasm is acidophilic and contains a small amount of rER, ribosomes, numerous smooth vesicles, and mitochondria.

The activated osteoclast has a ruffled border created by extensive infoldings of the cell membrane that sweep across the bony surface. The cell secretes acid and lysosomal enzymes into this region. The cell membrane immediately surrounding the ruffled border adheres tightly to the bony surface, thereby sealing the area of active bone resorption. As the osseous matrix is enzymatically digested, an **erosion lacuna** (Howship s lacuna) is formed. The lacuna remains after the osteoclast is no longer present, thus indicating prior areas of resorption. Osteoclasts may also be found in bone remodeling units as part of a cellular complex that remodels cortical bone in the adult (described later in this chapter). In addition to the release of mineral and protein components of bone, osteoclasts are also responsible for the release and activation of TGF-β.

Osteoclasts are derived from pluripotent cells of the bone marrow, which also give rise to monocytes and macrophages.

BONE MATRIX

The matrix of bone is composed of type I collagen fibers and small quantities of ground substance produced by the osteoblasts. Mineralization of the osteoid occurs as hydroxyapatite crystals that are deposited in the osteoid framework.

The organic intercellular substance of bone contains sulfated glycosaminoglycans, glycoproteins, and collagen. The collagen fibers in each osteonal lamellae course in a spiral direction with respect to the long axis of the central canal. In addition to their spiral orientation, the collagen fibers alternate at right angles to those in each adjacent lamella. This arrangement imparts considerable strength to each osteon.

The inorganic component of bone consists of submicroscopic hydroxyapatite crystals deposited as slender needles within the collagen fiber network. Such an efficient arrangement enhances the tensile strength that is characteristic of bone. The principal ions in bone salt are Ca, CO_3, PO_4, and OH, and the amounts of Na, Mg, and Fe are substantial. Bone, then, is a major storehouse for calcium and phosphorus, which are mobilized whenever they are needed.

STRUCTURAL AND FUNCTIONAL CHARACTERISTICS

Bone is distinguished from cartilage by the presence of both a canalicular system and a direct vascular supply. The growth process of bone also differs from cartilage.

Adult cartilage depends entirely on diffusion for nourishment; bone, however, has a unique lacunar-canalicular system for supplying the bone cells with metabolites in a mineralized matrix in which diffusion is

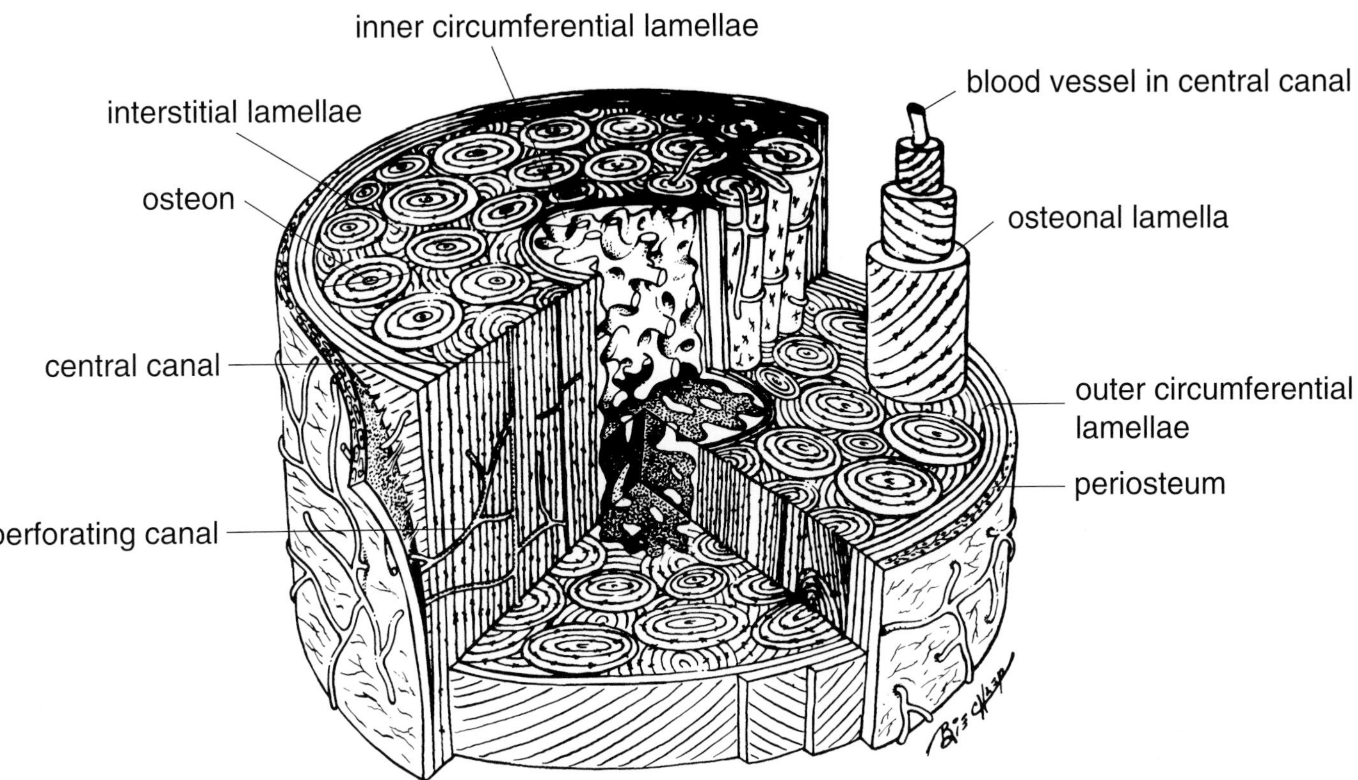

Figure 3.27. *The structural unit of compact bone is the cylindrical osteon. In this drawing, an osteon is telescoped to show the concentric osteonal lamellae that surround the central canal. Blood vessels reach the central canal through perforating canals from either the periosteal or endosteal surface. The space around adjacent osteons is filled by interstitial lamellae, and inner and outer circumferential lamellae form the surfaces of compact bone.*

not an option (Figs. 3.27 and 3.28). Canaliculi extend from one lacuna to another and to the bone surface, where they open into the connective tissue surrounding the capillaries. The canalicular system provides a conduit system for nourishment of the mature osteocytes.

The extensive capillary supply of bone further enhances the efficiency of the canalicular system. In fact, osteocytes are not more than one-tenth of a millimeter away from a capillary.

Unlike cartilage, bone grows by apposition only. Because the intercellular substance mineralizes so rapidly, interstitial growth of bone is not possible. Therefore, bone increases in size and changes shape by adding layers to one or more of its existing surfaces and by removing bone from other surfaces.

Macroscopic structure

An adult long bone (e.g., humerus) cut in half longitudinally consists of enlarged ends (**epiphyses**) connected by a hollow cylindrical shaft (**diaphysis**) (see Fig. 3.32). The ends of the epiphyses are covered by a thin layer of hyaline cartilage (**articular cartilage**), whereas the remainder of the external surface of the bone is covered by a vascular fibrous membrane (**periosteum**) (Figs. 3.27 and 3.29). Each region of the bone is composed of lamellar bone, but it is arranged differently to best perform its biomechanical function. The epiphyses have a thin shell of compact bone (subchondral bone) under the articular cartilage with a network of **trabeculae** extending from this structure and terminating near the beginning of the diaphysis. The wall of the diaphysis

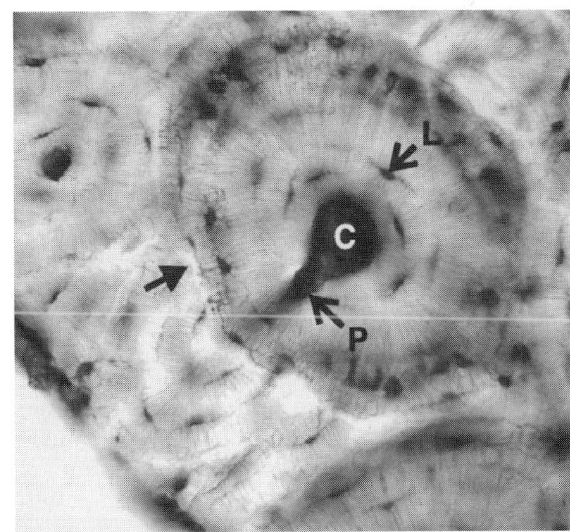

Figure 3.28. *Osteon of ground bone surrounded by a light cement line (solid arrow). The central canal (C) carries blood vessels, lymphatics, nerves, and branches into a transverse perforating canal (P). Lacunae (L) are located between lamellae of compact bone that surround the central canal. Fine canaliculi extend from each lacuna. Unstained (×230).*

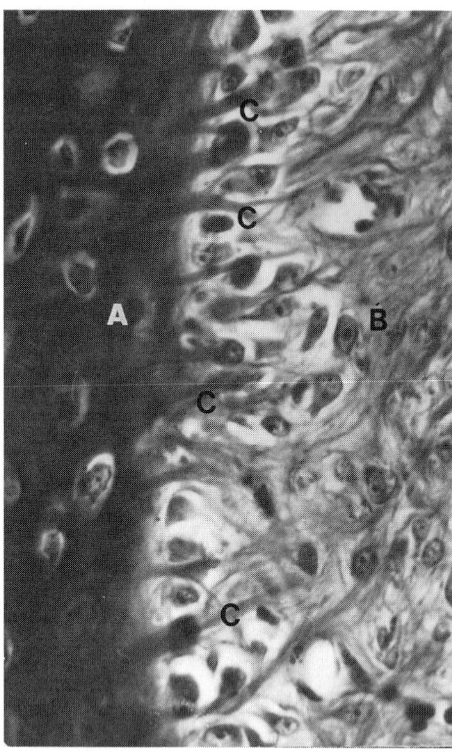

Figure 3.29. *Decalcified bone (cat). Bone (A) with periosteum (B) attached by perforating fibers (C). Hematoxylin and eosin (×500). (Courtesy of A. Hansen.)*

is composed of **compact bone** and rarely contains trabeculae. The inner (medullary) cavity of the epiphysis and diaphysis is lined by **endosteum** and contains adipose tissue or red (hemopoietic) or yellow (adipose) bone marrow, depending on the age of the animal or the region of the bone.

In the growing animal, the diaphysis and epiphysis are separated by the **physeal metaphyseal** region. This region consists of a specialized hyaline cartilage plate named the **physis**, which is responsible for the animal s bone growth in length, and the **metaphysis**, where temporary trabeculae are converted to permanent trabeculae (see Figs. 3.32 and 3.37). Upon cessation of growth, the physis undergoes ossification, thus leaving a transverse yet perforated plate of bone (epiphyseal scar), and the metaphysis becomes the metaphyseal area of the diaphysis.

Thus, in the midshaft or **diaphysis**, the wall of the hollow cylinder is composed of compact bone that encloses the **medullary** or **marrow cavity**. The ends of long bones, the **epiphyses**, are composed primarily of spongy or trabecular bone. The communicating spaces, which are filled with marrow, are continuous with the marrow cavity of the diaphysis. In an immature animal, the diaphysis and epiphysis are separated by a cartilaginous physis located adjacent to the metaphysis. The articulating epiphyseal surfaces are covered with hyaline cartilage, the **articular cartilage**.

Histologic preparation

Because of its dense mineral deposits, bone is difficult to section and process for histologic procedures. Decalcification before histologic processing removes the mineral from the bone, leaving behind the organic matrix and the bone cells for study (Fig. 3.30). If examination of osseous mineral content is required, undecalcified sections can be prepared using special techniques (Fig. 3.28).

Microscopic structure

The outermost layers of the shaft of a long bone consist of compact bone arranged as **outer circumferential lamellae** (2 to 8 μm thick). Inside the outer circumferential lamellae are **osteons** (Haversian systems) formed by concentric lamellae surrounding longitudinally oriented vascular channels (**central canals**) (Fig. 3.27). Basophilic **cement lines**, composed of mineralized matrix deficient in collagen, delimit each osteon and interstitial system (Fig. 3.28). Scalloped or irregular cement lines result from bone resorption followed by bone formation during normal bone turnover. Between the osteons are many irregularly shaped groups of lamellae called **interstitial lamellae**. Internal surfaces of compact bone from adult animals are composed of **inner circumferential lamellae** encircling the medullary cavity.

Lacunae are located between each lamella of the compact bone (Fig. 3.28). Radiating from the lacunae are the branching canaliculi that penetrate and join canaliculi of adjacent lamellae (Fig. 3.28). Thus, the lacunae and canaliculi form an extensive system of interconnecting passageways for the transport of nutrients.

The **central canal** of each osteon contains capillaries, lymphatic vessels, and nonmyelinated nerve fibers, all supported by reticular connective tissue. Central canals are connected with each other and with the free surface

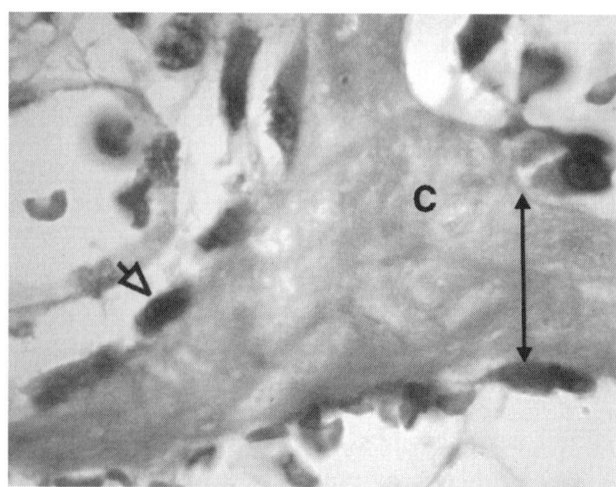

Figure 3.30. *Intramembranous bone development. Bone spicule (arrow) is formed by osteoblasts (open arrow) surrounding the immature bone. Irregularly arranged collagen fibers (C) are present in bony matrix, thus it is considered woven bone. Hematoxylin and eosin (×900).*

by transverse or horizontal channels called **perforating canals** (Figs. 3.27 and 3.28). Classical terminology describes the central canal as the Haversian canal, and the perforating canal is known as Volkmann s canal.

Most bones are invested with a tough connective tissue layer, the **periosteum** (Fig. 3.27). It has two layers: an inner **osteogenic** layer that provides cells necessary to form bone, and an outer **fibrous** layer made of irregularly arranged collagen fibers and blood vessels. The vessels branch and enter the perforating canals and ultimately reach the central canal of the osteons. The cellular layer is more evident in young animals than in adults. The periosteum is attached firmly to the bone by bundles of coarse collagen fibers that have been incorporated into the outer circumferential and interstitial lamellae of the bone. These fibers are called **perforating (Sharpey s) fibers** (Fig. 3.29). A periosteum is absent on the articulating surfaces of bone, which are covered with hyaline cartilage, and at sites where tendons and ligaments insert on bones.

The marrow cavity and osteonal canals are lined with a layer of squamous cells (lining cells), osteoblasts, and osteoclasts called the **endosteum**. Bone-lining cells have osteogenic capacity and are joined to each other by gap junctions between the long cell processes. Some cells send processes into canaliculi to join those of nearby osteocytes. Recently, the possibility has been suggested that these cells form an ion barrier so that the fluid flowing through the lacunae and canaliculi is separated from the interstitial fluid. In addition, endosteal cells may play a role in mineral homeostasis by regulating the flow of calcium and phosphate in and out of bone fluids, thus maintaining an optimum microenvironment for the growth of bone crystals.

OSTEOGENESIS

Bone is classified by the arrangement of collagen fibers in the matrix (woven versus lamellar bone) or by the type of precursor connective tissue (intramembranous versus endochondral ossification).

Woven bone has collagen fibers that are arranged in an irregular anastomosing fashion (Fig. 3.30), whereas **lamellar bone** has a more organized matrix, which is deposited in layers (Fig. 3.28). Woven bone is formed rapidly and is considered to be an immature form of bone; it is usually replaced by the lamellar bone. Woven bone is found in developing bone, fracture repair sites, and certain bone tumors.

Regardless of the site, bone develops by a process of transformation from an existing connective tissue. The two different types of bone development depend on specific cells differentiating within two different microenvironments. When bone forms directly from connective tissue, the process is termed **intramembranous ossification** (Fig. 3.30). This term arose because the soft tissue located where bone will form is arranged in a layer and, hence, is membranous. The process of bone formation in preexisting cartilage models is termed **endochondral** or **intracartilaginous ossification** (Fig. 3.31). During this process, calcified cartilage is replaced by bone. The terms intramembranous and endochondral indicate the type of microenvironment in which the bone forms and do not relate to a given type of adult bone.

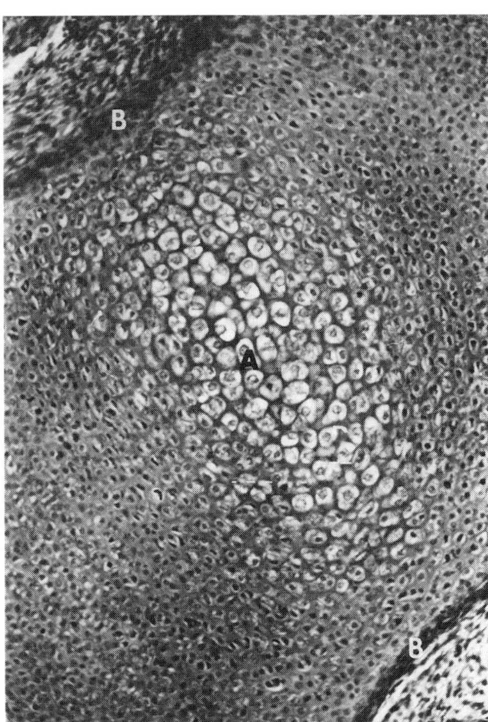

Figure 3.31. *Endochondral ossification of a long bone (dog). Hypertrophied cartilage cells (A) are in the center of the model. Note the thin mineralized cartilage remnants between enlarged lacunae; perichondrium (B). Hematoxylin and eosin (×80).*

Intramembranous ossification

The process of intramembranous ossification takes place within well-vascularized connective tissue, such as found in the developing calvarium of the skull. **Osteoprogenitor cells** differentiate into osteoblasts. These cells begin to synthesize and secrete osteoid. The first secreted component of osteoid is collagen, and the remaining constituents of the ground substance are produced somewhat later. During early intramembranous osteogenesis, osteoblasts become surrounded by a partially mineralized matrix containing visible collagen fibers (Fig. 3.30). Gradually, more osteoid is produced, followed by complete mineralization. As a result, some osteoblasts become trapped within their lacunae and become osteocytes. These small, isolated pieces of developing bone within the connective tissue are called the **centers of ossification**, which ultimately radiate in several directions to form **trabeculae** (Fig. 3.25). Such bone is called **trabecular**, **spongy**, or **cancellous** bone.

As the osteoblasts synthesize and secrete the organic matrix, plasmalemma buds, called **matrix vesicles**, form along the cell margin adjacent to the osteoid and pinch off. Matrix vesicles contain lipid, accumulate calcium ions, and have alkaline phosphatase activity, all of which are required to initiate and maintain the process of mineralization.

The bony trabeculae increase in width and length by the addition of new lamellae, forming a primary spongiosa of trabecular bone. In areas of the spongiosa where compact bone forms, the mesenchymal space between trabeculae fills with osseous tissue except for a central canal containing the vasculature of the new osteon. In regions where spongy bone persists, the mesenchymal soft tissue located between trabeculae becomes bone marrow.

Endochondral ossification

Bones of the extremities, vertebral column, pelvis, and base of the skull are formed initially as hyaline cartilage models that are replaced by bone in the developing embryo.

PRIMARY CENTER OF OSSIFICATION. As the cartilage model grows both in width and in length, it reaches a stage when most of the remaining growth occurs at the ends of the model. The chondrocytes in the midsection mature and enlarge, so that the intercellular substance between the hypertrophied cells becomes extremely thin (Figs. 3.31 and 3.32). At the same time, these chondrocytes release matrix vesicles, similar to those of osteoblasts, that promote calcification of the surrounding cartilage matrix. This calcification prevents the hypertrophied chondrocytes from receiving adequate nutrition and results in their degeneration and death.

In the meantime, the perichondrium is invaded by numerous capillaries. This event changes the microenvironment of the chondrogenic layer to one that favors osteogenesis on the surface of the cartilage model. The osteoprogenitor cells of this layer differentiate into osteoblasts and form a thin shell of bone around the midsection of the cartilage model. This **periosteal band** or **bony collar** forms by intramembranous ossification, and the perichondrium becomes the periosteum. Blood vessels are essential in activating the osteogenic potential of the inner layer of the perichondrium, the cells of which retain the ability to differentiate into either chondroblasts or osteoblasts throughout their life. This ability is especially significant in fracture healing, during

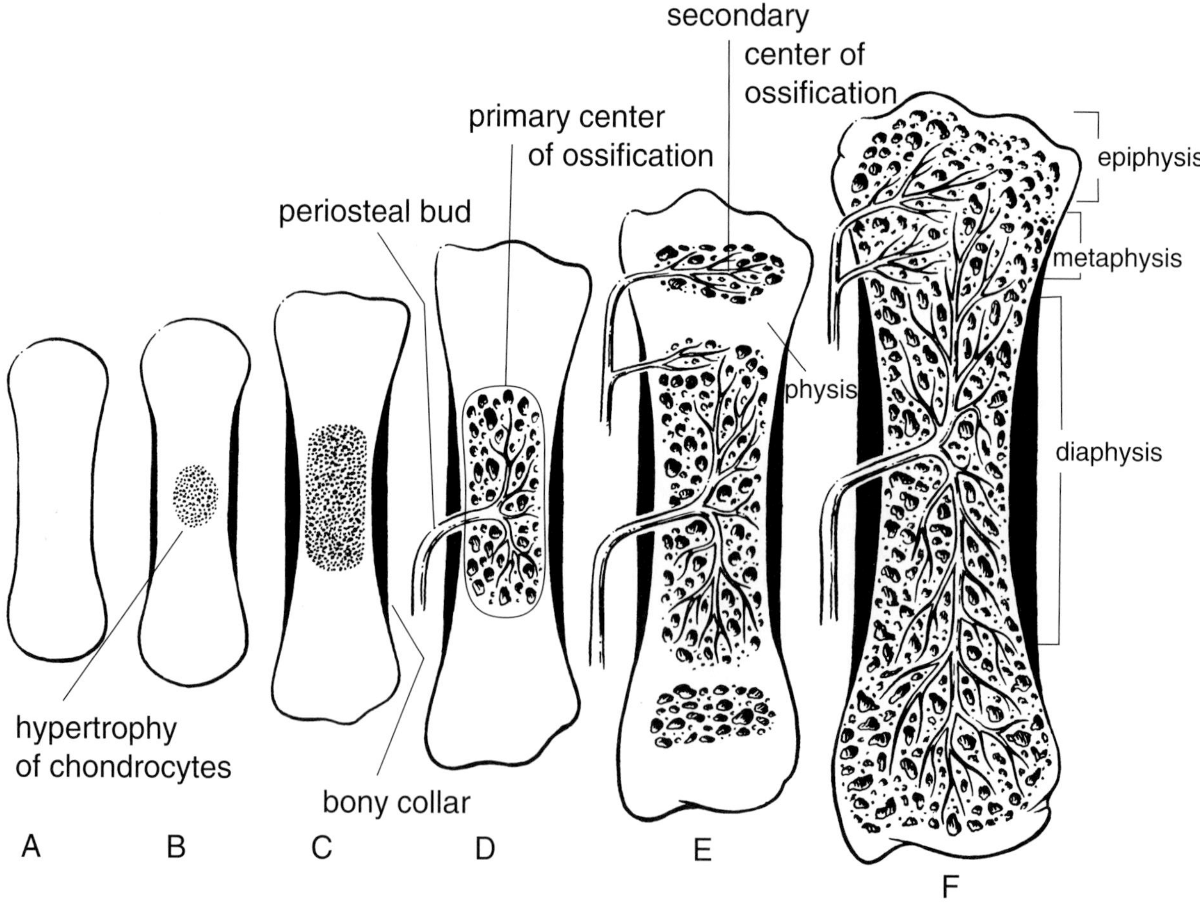

Figure 3.32. *The stages of endochondral ossification of a long bone.* ***A.,*** *A hyaline cartilage model forms initially.* ***B.,*** *The chondrocytes in the center of the model hypertrophy.* ***C.,*** *A bony collar begins to form around the cartilage model.* ***D.,*** *Blood vessels from the periosteum (periosteal bud) invade the cartilage model, bringing bone-forming cells to initiate the primary center of ossification.* ***E.,*** *The physis and secondary centers of ossification are established.* ***F.,*** *The growth plate closes in the mature bone and a confluent marrow cavity from the epiphysis to the diaphysis is formed.*

which cartilage forms in areas that are relatively devoid of capillaries, but endochondral ossification occurs as soon as capillaries grow into the area (see p. 58).

After the bony collar forms around the midsection of the model, blood vessels from the periosteum invade the area of the degenerating hypertrophied chondrocytes, thereby raising the oxygen level (Figs. 3.32 and 3.33). Pericytes, osteoprogenitor cells from the periosteum, and undifferentiated mesenchyme cells all accompany the invading capillaries. These blood vessels and their associated cells constitute the **periosteal bud**. When the periosteal bud reaches the interior of the midsection of the cartilage model, the **primary center of ossification** is established. Under the influence of inductive bone-forming factors in the blood plasma, the osteoprogenitor cells that accompany the capillaries differentiate into osteoblasts. These cells cluster around fragments of the calcified cartilage, begin to synthesize and secrete osteoid, and somewhat later contribute to the mineralization process. Such osteoblastic activity continues until bone trabeculae containing cores of calcified cartilage are formed.

While the primary center of ossification is forming, the cartilage at each end of the model continues to proliferate by interstitial growth, resulting in an increase in the length of the model. The capillaries from the primary center of ossification invade the model toward both epiphyses, where their associated cells initiate endochondral bone formation at the medullary edge. The chondrocytes undergo the same sequence of changes as described previously. The bony collar continues to increase in thickness, hence the primitive bone in the primary center is no longer needed for support. Therefore, most of the bone in the primary center is resorbed by osteoclasts, thus forming the marrow cavity, which becomes filled with hemopoietic tissue developed from the undifferentiated mesenchymal cells brought in with the periosteal bud.

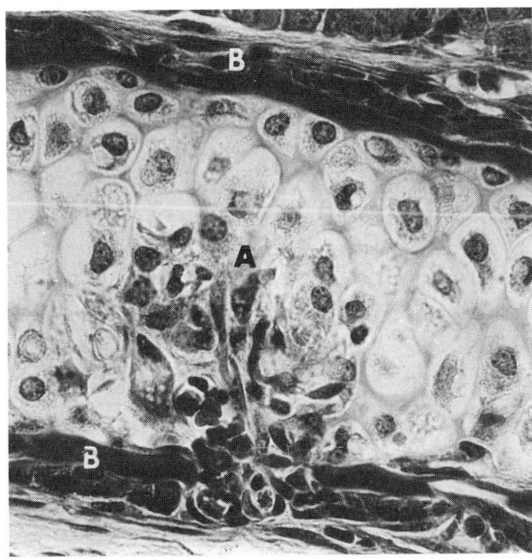

Figure 3.33. *Primary center of ossification (cat). Periosteal bud (A) entering hypertrophied cartilage. Perichondrium (B). Crossman s trichrome (×570).*

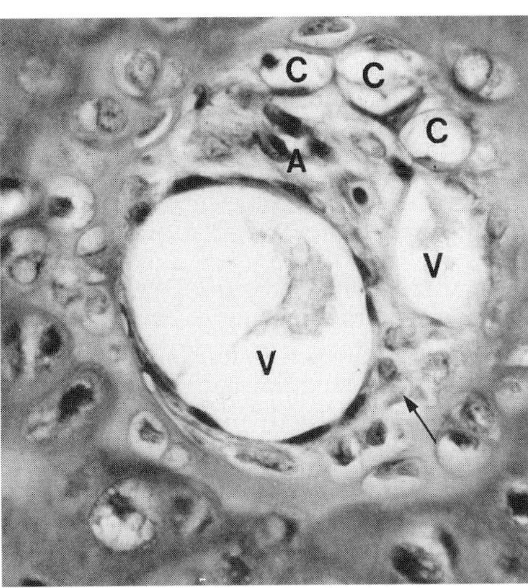

Figure 3.34. *Cartilage canal in epiphysis of a 1-day-old puppy containing an arteriole (A), venules (V), and glomerular capillaries (C). Degenerating cartilage at arrow.*

SECONDARY CENTERS OF OSSIFICATION. The cartilaginous epiphyses of the larger long bones develop additional centers of ossification referred to as **secondary centers** (Fig. 3.32). The epiphyseal cartilage of newborn animals is well supplied with cartilage canals containing arterioles, venules, and nonmyelinated nerve fibers, all surrounded by connective tissue (Fig. 3.34). These canals arise from the perichondrium and are evenly spaced throughout the epiphysis, providing nutrients to a given area. The vessels do not enter the epiphyseal plate or penetrate the future articular cartilage. The arterioles of these canals end in a capillary glomerulus, and the initial sites of ossification occur as multiple foci adjacent to the glomeruli. When ossification begins, the chondrocytes next to the glomerulus of the cartilage canal hypertrophy and degenerate, and the surrounding matrix calcifies. This process is followed by circularly oriented layers of hypertrophic and dividing chondrocytes. Thus, this cellular arrangement resembles that of the growth zones in the physis. Because the connective tissue in the cartilage canals is continuous with the perichondrium, these cells have the same osteogenic potential for bone formation. Ultimately, these foci fuse into a single secondary center of ossification, forming spongy bone in the epiphysis.

Ossification does not replace all of the epiphyseal cartilage. Enough cartilage remains to serve as a template for enlarging the end of the bone, as well as serving as the articular cartilage. A transverse plate of cartilage is left between the diaphysis and each epiphysis. In domestic animals, this physis persists until puberty, and then it too is replaced by bone.

Growth in length

The physis and metaphysis function to lengthen bone and to provide a scaffolding for constructing metaphyseal cancellous bone. Continued interstitial growth of the cartilage cells in the physis, involving chondrocytic hyperplasia, synthesis of proteoglycans, and chondrocyte hypertrophy, serves to lengthen the long bones.

Five zones or regions are present in a longitudinal section through the physis (Fig. 3.35). From the epiphysis to the metaphysis, the following zones are present:

1. The **reserve zone** (resting zone) is adjacent to the bone and marrow cavity of the epiphysis (Fig. 3.36). Here, the small chondrocytes are dispersed in an irregular pattern and are nourished by epiphyseal blood vessels, which are arranged in glomeruli. **Matrix vesicles**, membrane-bounded structures similar to those produced by osteoblasts, are produced by chondrocytes in this zone, but matrix mineralization does not occur until deeper in the physis.
2. In the **zone of proliferation**, the chondrocytes are somewhat larger and tend to form rows or columns at right angles to the epiphysis (Fig. 3.36). New cells are produced through cell division at the top of the columns. The cells in the columns possess all the organelles necessary for synthesis of matrix and each cell is separated from the adjacent cell by a layer of matrix.
3. As maturation progresses in the **zone of hypertrophy**, the cells increase in size and begin to accumulate calcium. The cellular calcium is released into the matrix of the deep hypertrophic zone and matrix vesicles begin calcium uptake. The action of alkaline phosphatase and neutral proteases released from matrix vesicles causes a local increase of phosphate. Accumulation of calcium in the vesicles and the increase in phosphate leads to mineralization and the last two or three hypertrophied cells are bordered by a wall of calcified matrix. Transverse septa between the cells do not calcify. Some of these hypertrophied cells become shrunken, and their pyknotic nucleus appears to attach to the transverse septum.
4. The metaphyseal capillaries make a sharp U-shaped bend in the **zone of resorption** and return to the medullary circulation (Figs. 3.37 and 3.38). Individual capillary loops and perivascular connective tissue invade the lacunae of the degenerating hypertrophic chondrocytes located at the base of the cell columns.
5. In the **zone of ossification**, osteoblasts differentiate from cells accompanying the invading capillaries. These cells deposit bone on the remains of the calcified walls of the chondrocytic lacunae. The resulting trabeculae of bone with calcified cartilage centers are known collectively as the **primary spongiosa** (Figs. 3.37 and 3.39).

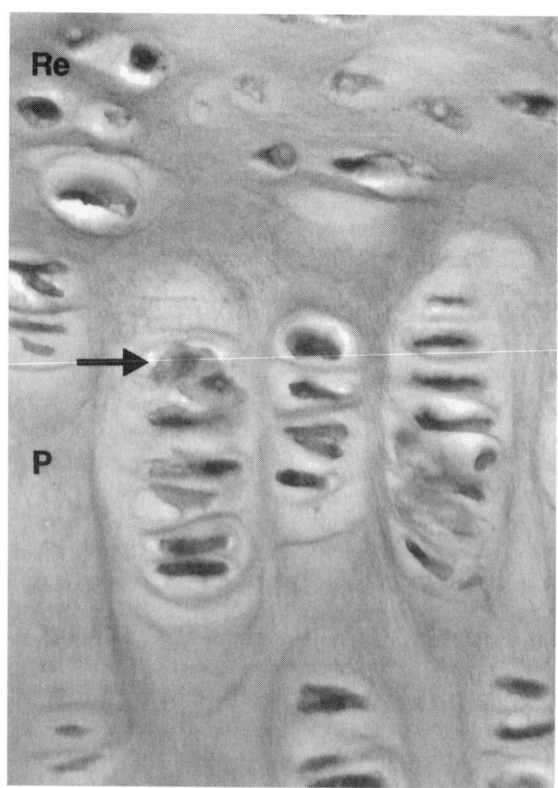

Figure 3.36. *Chondrocytes of the reserve zone (Re) are scattered and spherical. New cells are produced at the top of the columns (arrow) in the zone of proliferation (P). Hematoxylin and eosin (×550).*

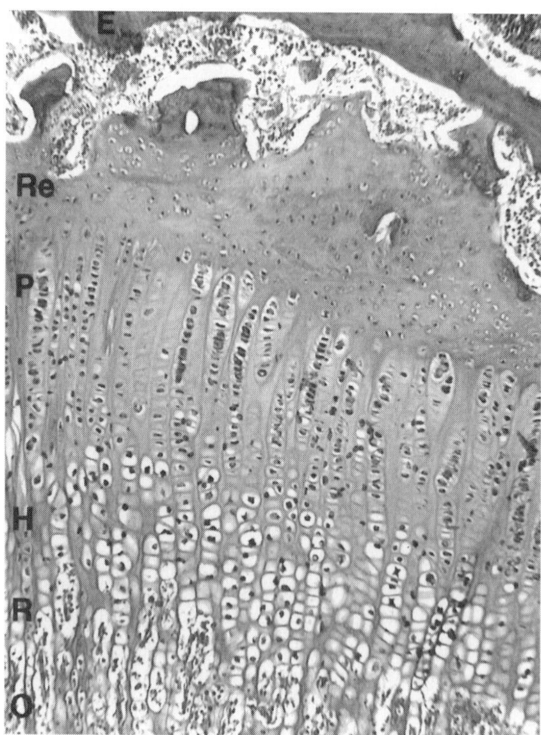

Figure 3.35. *The physis is anchored to epiphyseal bone (E). Chondrocytes in the reserve zone (Re) are scattered in the matrix. In the zone of proliferation (P), chondrocytes are arranged in columns. The cells increase in size in the zone of hypertrophy (H). Metaphyseal capillaries enter the zone of resorption (R), and bone is formed on the cartilage remnants of the physis in the zone of ossification (O). Hematoxylin and eosin (×200).*

The surface of numerous trabeculae of the primary spongiosa are covered with osteoclasts for a short dis-

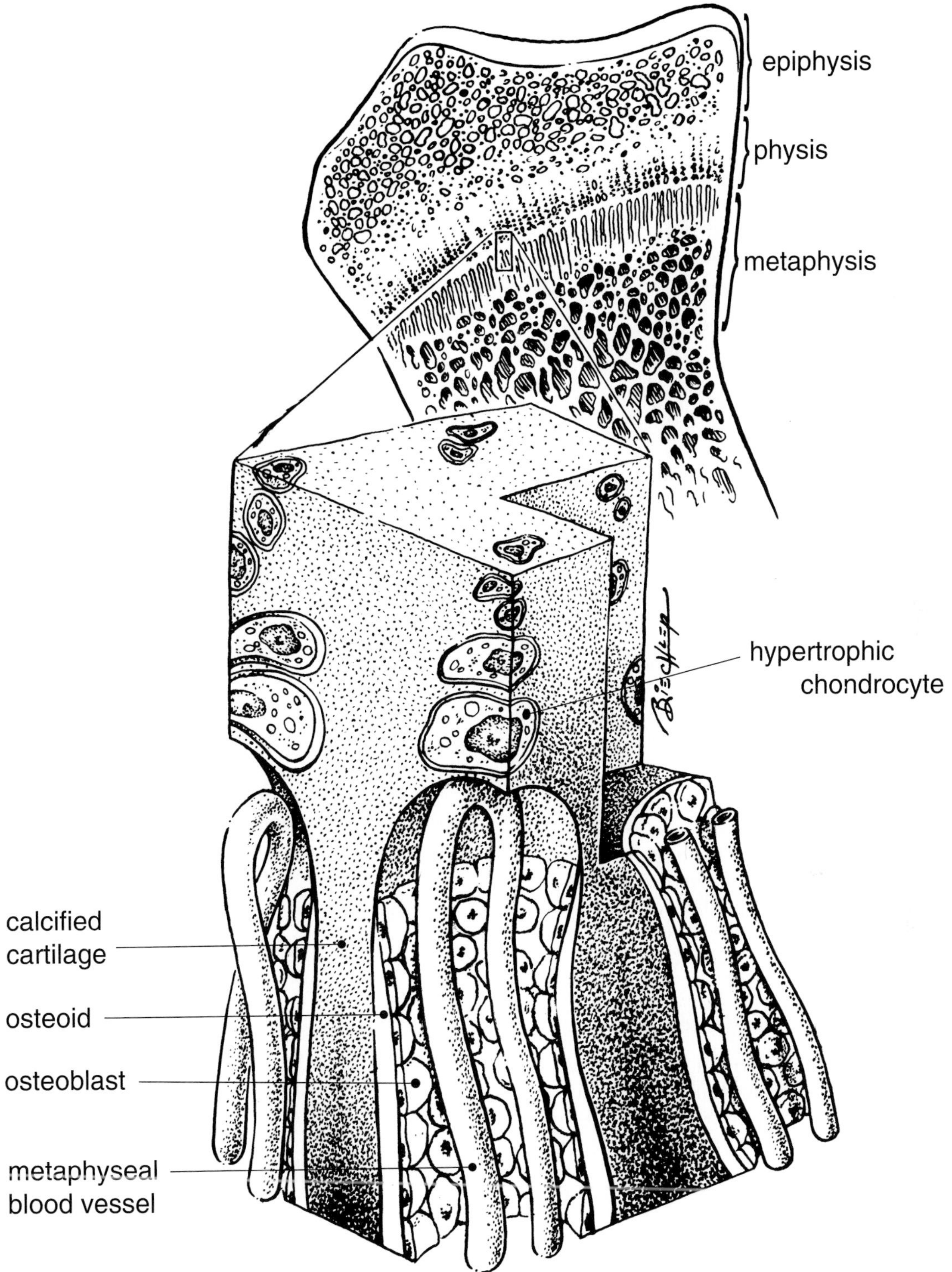

Figure 3.37. *Metaphyseal blood vessels make a sharp bend in the zone of resorption. Capillary loops invade the lacunae of the degenerating hypertrophic chondrocytes. Osteoblasts form bone on the remnants of the calcified physeal cartilage.*

tance into the metaphysis. Precursors of these osteoclasts arrive with the invading metaphyseal vessels. The osteoclasts actively resorb bone from the surface of the trabeculae.

Because the cartilage cores are continuous with the cartilaginous intercellular substance of the physis, the new bony trabeculae are anchored firmly to the physis. In longitudinal sections through the growth plate, the bony trabeculae and their cartilage cores resemble separate stalks attached to the growth plate. In a cross section taken through the metaphyseal side of the physis, however, each trabecula is actually a wall between adja-

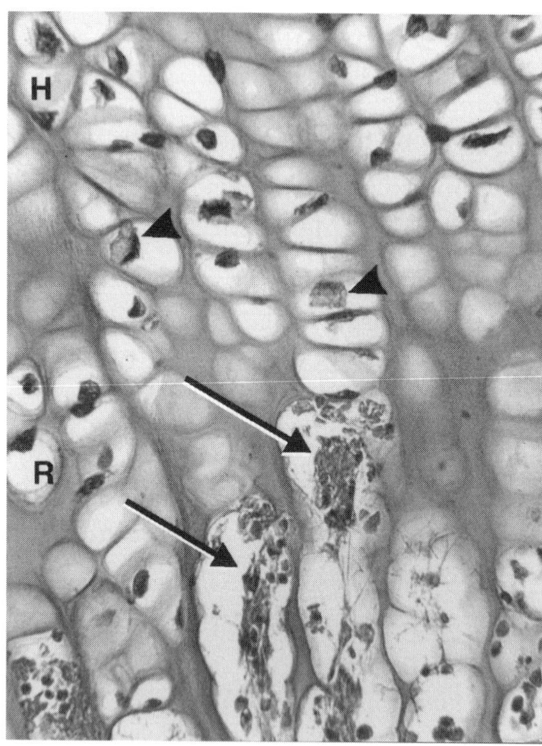

Figure 3.38. *Hypertrophic chondrocytes (arrowheads) degenerate in the zone of hypertrophy (H) just above the zone of resorption (R). Metaphyseal blood vessels (long arrows) invade the lacunae of the degenerating chondrocytes. Hematoxylin and eosin (×300).*

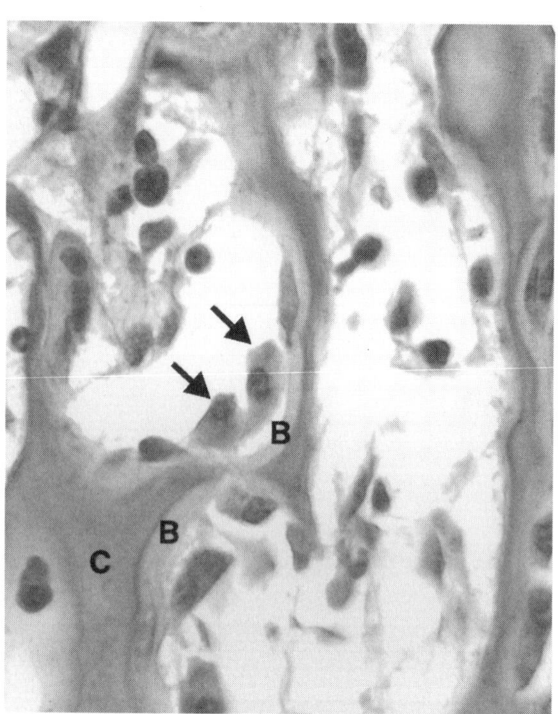

Figure 3.39. *Osteoblasts (arrows) form bone (B) on darker staining calcified cartilage (C) in the zone of ossification. Hematoxylin and eosin (×475).*

cent tubes filled with osteogenic cells and capillaries (Fig. 3.37).

Deeper in the metaphysis, trabeculae of the primary spongiosa decrease and trabeculae composed of lamellar bone predominate. Trabeculae without cartilage cores are known collectively as the **secondary spongiosa**.

Growth in width and circumference

The trabecular bone that formed in the original bony collar is converted to compact bone composed of primary osteons. Concurrent periosteal growth and endosteal resorption enlarge the marrow cavity and increase the width of the diaphysis. Because endosteal resorption lags behind periosteal production, the thickness of the shaft wall slowly enlarges and the circumference increases.

The outer surface of an actively growing bone is uneven, owing to numerous longitudinal ridges and grooves. Within these grooves, osteoblasts from the adherent periosteum deposit bone around the vessels. Eventually, the edges of the groove meet, forming a tube lined with osteogenic cells and enclosing the blood vessel derived from the periosteum. The osteogenic cells produce concentric layers of bone around the blood vessel within the new central canal. In this way, new primary osteons are added to the periphery of an actively growing young bone. These primary osteons are gradually replaced with more orderly secondary osteons.

Finally, the surface growth slows, and appositional growth in the subperiosteal and endosteal regions adds more layers, which smooth the surface. These layers are the inner and outer circumferential lamellae.

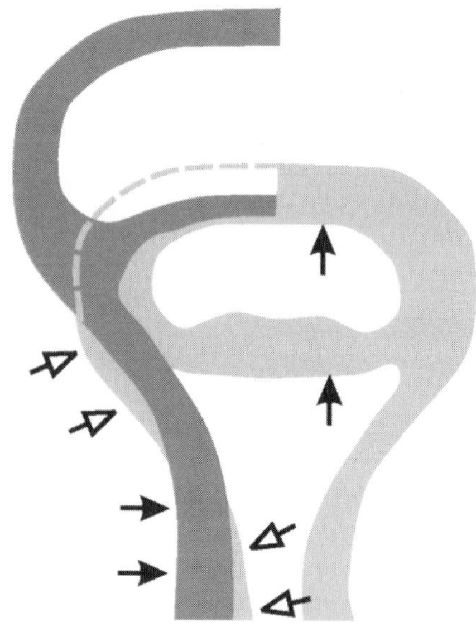

Figure 3.40. *During growth, modeling occurs as new bone is added on the outer periosteal surface of the diaphysis and within the metaphysis and epiphysis (solid arrows). Bone is concurrently resorbed on both the endosteal and periosteal surfaces to shape the adult bone (open arrows).*

The important principle to note is that growth in length is the result of endochondral ossification, whereas growth in width is the result of intramembranous ossification. Each type of growth responds to different rules, and each can be affected separately without necessarily influencing the other.

Bone modeling

The changes in size and shape of bones during the growth process are called **modeling**. The concurrent action of bone resorption and formation on different surfaces of a bone alters the overall shape. The process of modeling continues over most of the skeleton until the adult shape of the bones is reached. Modeling is rapid and results in a net gain of bone in the body. Examples of modeling include the drifting of the diaphysis during growth, shaping of the metaphyseal funnel, and enlargement of the cranial vault.

In the diaphyseal region, bone formation occurs on the periosteal surface while bone is resorbed on the endosteal surface, resulting in a wider diaphysis and larger marrow cavity (Fig. 3.40). If the modeling process occurs in an eccentric fashion, the entire diaphysis may drift in a specific direction.

In contrast, the shaping of the metaphyseal region is accomplished by periosteal resorption on the external surface to narrow the funnel shape in the direction of the diaphysis. Concurrent endosteal bone formation creates a thickened metaphyseal cortex.

Bone remodeling

Throughout life, bone is constantly being turned over. Early woven bone is of poorer quality than mature lamellar bone. In addition, as bone ages, the quality also diminishes. **Bone remodeling** is the process by which bone is constantly replaced.

In contrast to modeling, bone remodeling occurs in a cyclical fashion at a slower rate. The process generally does not alter the shape or size of the bone. Remodeling is coupled; it initiates and proceeds in only one way. First, activation of remodeling occurs, perhaps caused by a change in biomechanics. Osteoclastic resorption is then followed by osteogenic formation. The sequence is the hallmark of remodeling, and its balance is imperative for healthy bone.

Cortical bone is remodeled by **cortical remodeling units**. The unit, when viewed longitudinally, consists of a leading **cutting cone** composed of osteoclasts, which resorb bone without respect to osteonal barriers (Fig. 3.41). The cutting cone is followed by a **reversal zone**, in which resorption switches to osteoblastic formation. The structure terminates as a **closing cone**, in which osteoblasts close the newly excavated osteon by adding centripetal layers of lamellar bone inward from the cement line boundary. The osteoclasts of the cutting cone

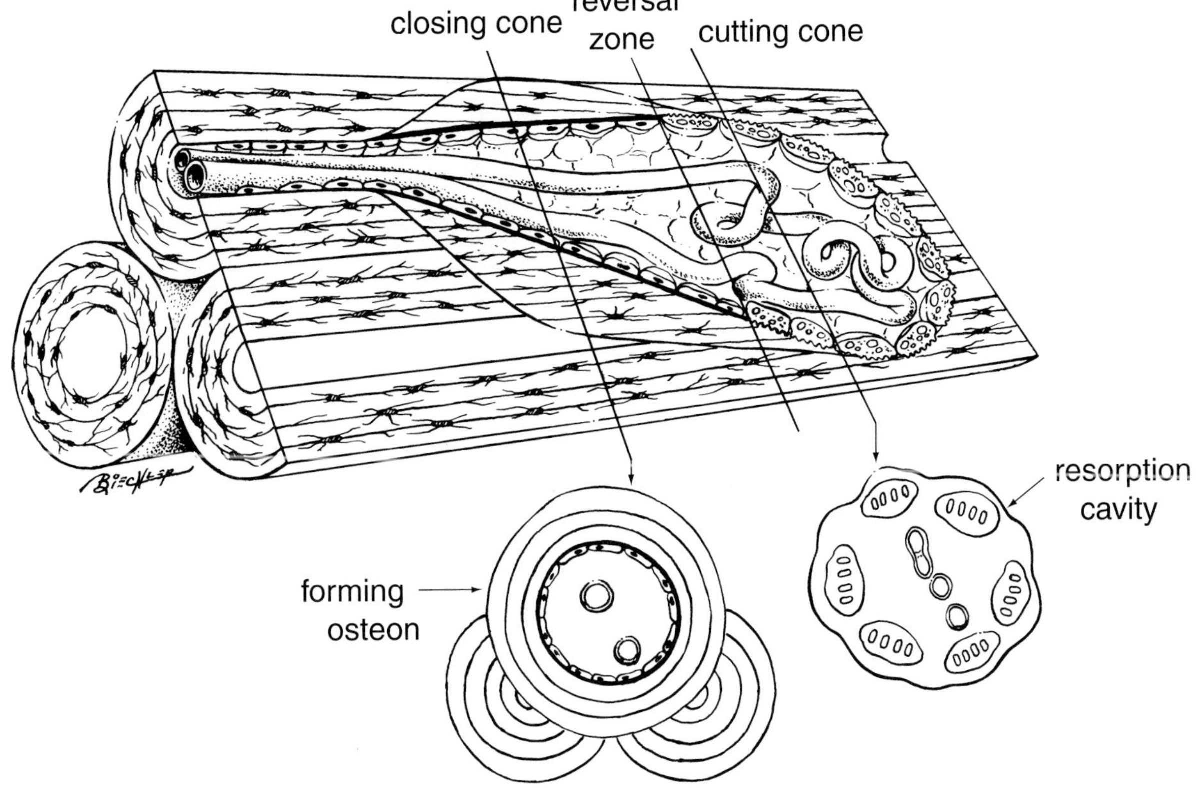

Figure 3.41. *The remodeling unit of cortical bone is composed of a cutting cone of osteoclasts, which resorbs bone. Osteoclasts change to osteoblasts at the reversal zone and the bone-forming cells of the closing cone fill in the resorption cavity to create a new osteon.*

are supported metabolically by a glomerulus, whereas the osteoblasts of the closing cone are within close diffusion distance from the central capillary.

In spongy bone, remodeling is accomplished on the endosteal surface of the trabecula. Osteoclasts resorb bone from the surface of the trabecula. Osteoblasts then form new bone in either the same location as the resorption or on the opposing surface of the trabecula. If bone is formed on the opposing surface, the alignment of the trabecula is changed in the direction of the bone formation.

Fracture repair

After a midshaft fracture of a bone, a certain sequence of events occurs during the healing process. Fracture repair involves changes in blood supply that affect cellular proliferation and differentiation as well as bone resorption.

The trauma that causes the bone to break also tears the adjacent soft tissues and blood vessels. The blood clot that forms at the fracture site stops circulation and results in necrosis or death of the surrounding tissue. Likewise, the interruption of the blood vessels within the osteons causes cessation of blood supply and death of the osteocytes on each side of the fracture site.

New tissue developing at the fracture site forms a bridge between the fragments. This formation is termed a **callus** and is composed of two parts. The **internal callus** develops between the opposing ends of the bone, and the **external callus** surrounds the outermost surface of the broken bone. The cells involved in the repair process are osteogenic cells of the periosteum and endosteum.

Early in the healing process, the cells of the periosteum proliferate to such an extent that the fibrous layer of the periosteum is lifted away from the bone. In addition, the endosteal cells proliferate, resulting in a thickened endosteum. The undifferentiated marrow cells increase in number in the same area. Differentiation of these cells takes place in one of two ways and depends on the vascular supply available. Those nearest the bone fragments differentiate in the presence of blood vessels; consequently, they become osteoblasts and form bony trabeculae. Those farther away from the bone proliferate in an area relatively devoid of capillaries; consequently, they form chondroblasts, which produce cartilage in the external callus. The cartilage is a temporary splint that eventually is replaced by bone, following the same sequence of events that occurs in endochondral ossification. Gradually, the callus is remodeled by resorption of the trabeculae at the periphery, until the original outline of the bone is restored.

No external callus develops when a bone fracture has smooth, even, opposing surfaces that are perfectly aligned without any space between the fragments, and the fragments are held rigidly throughout the healing period. Dead bone extends for some distance on both sides of the fracture line. Osteogenic cells and capillaries in the living bone proliferate and grow into the adjacent dead bone. Simultaneously, osteoclasts invade the area and form resorption tunnels, such as those described in bone remodeling. This results in new osteons that cross the fracture line and extend into the bone on the other side (primary osteosynthesis).

Fractures that are realigned in direct apposition but have a small space between the two fragments heal similarly, as long as rigid fixation is maintained. The only difference is that the two ends are joined initially by woven bone rather than by new osteons. Remodeling occurs as a secondary event.

Apparently, rigid fixation prevents osteogenic activity in the periosteum so that external callus formation does not occur. Any slight movement between the two ends of the fracture, however, stimulates callus formation.

JOINTS

Joints connect two or more bones. The various types of joints are classified according to the type of tissue that makes up the structure and the degree of movement permitted.

Synarthroses

Synarthroses range from slightly movable to highly immovable. The four types of synarthroses are classified according to the type of tissue involved in the connection between bones. Those held together by either col-

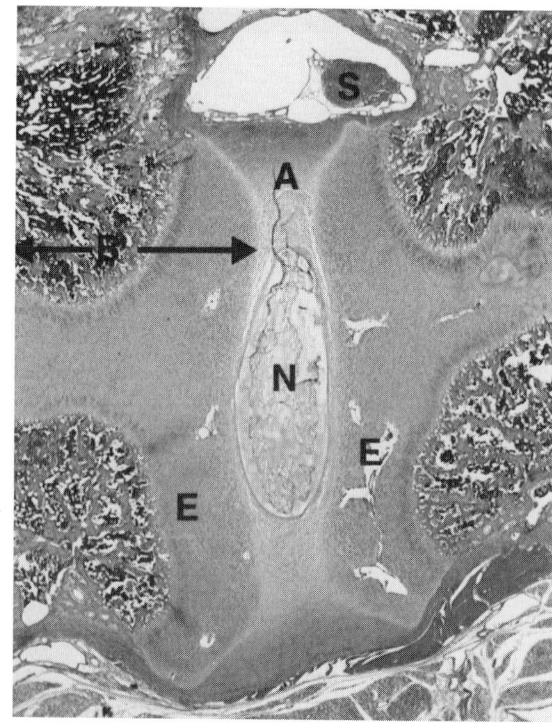

Figure 3.42. *Vertebral column, longitudinal section (puppy). The central nucleus pulposus (N) of the intervertebral disc is surrounded by the annulus fibrosus (A). The disc attaches to the cartilaginous end plates (E) of the vertebral bodies (B). A spinal nerve (S) exits from the spinal cord through the foramen above the disc. Hematoxylin and eosin (×8).*

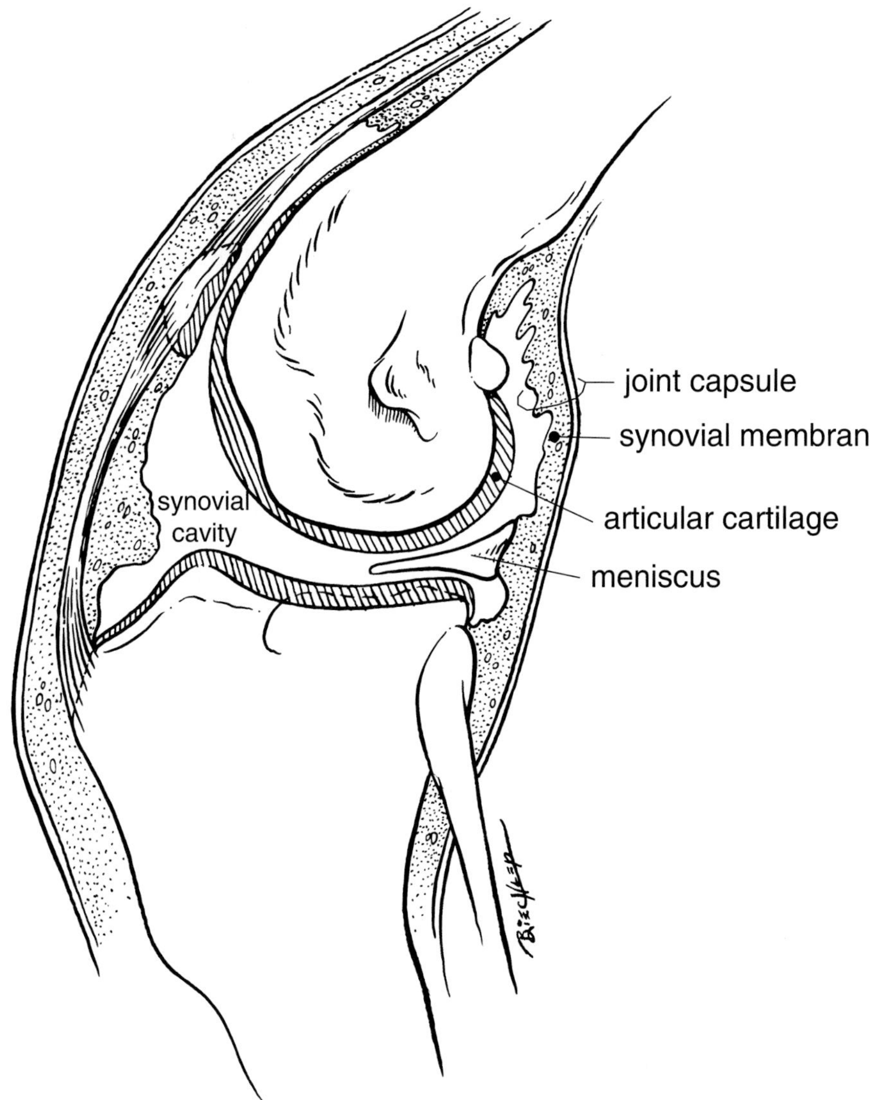

Figure 3.43. *Articular cartilage covers the opposing bony surfaces of a synovial joint as shown in this diagram of a stifle. The joint space is filled with synovial fluid from the synovial membrane of the surrounding joint capsule. A meniscus composed of fibrocartilage extends into the joint cavity.*

lagenous or elastic dense connective tissue are **syndesmoses**. Skull sutures are typical syndesmoses. Joints in which the two bones are connected by cartilage are **synchondroses**, such as those between epiphyseal plates and sternebrae. As the result of aging, syndesmoses and synchondroses become **synostoses**, because the respective connective tissues are eventually replaced by bone. In the **symphysis** joint, the hyaline cartilage caps of adjacent bones are joined by thick fibrous bands. Between the hyaline cartilage and the collagen fibers is a transition zone of fibrocartilage. The pubic symphysis is a good example of this type of joint.

The intervertebral disk is a symphysis that consists of an outer lamellated **annulus fibrosus** and an inner dorsally eccentric cavity, which is filled with a gelatinous **nucleus pulposus** in young animals (Fig. 3.42). The annulus is thicker ventrally than dorsally, and its fibers insert into a thin layer of hyaline cartilage covering the ends of adjacent vertebrae. The cells in the peripheral laminae of the annulus resemble fibrocytes, whereas the cells of the deeper lamellae resemble chondrocytes that are surrounded by a small area of metachromatic matrix. The nucleus pulposus in some breeds of dogs calcifies at approximately 5 years of age. The annulus is avascular and hence is sustained by diffusion from the vessels in the medullary cavity of the vertebrae and those of the periosteum.

Synovial Joints

Synovial joints are characterized by articular cartilage on the opposing bony surfaces, a lubricating synovial fluid within the closed joint cavity, and a joint capsule enclosing the entire joint (Fig. 3.43).

The articulating surfaces of synovial joints are covered by a specialized complex, the **articular cartilage**, which consists of hyaline cartilage, tidemark, and calcified cartilage (Fig. 3.44). The articular cartilage is devoid of perichondrium and can be divided into three zones by the arrangement of the type II collagen fibrils: *(a)* the **superficial zone** has flat cells that lie among collagen

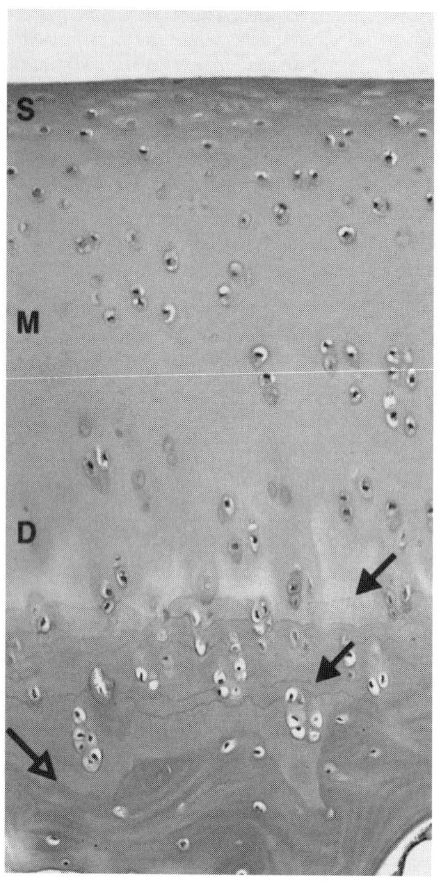

Figure 3.44. *Articular cartilage zones: superficial (S), middle (M) and deep (D). Multiple tidemarks (closed arrows) are present in the calcified cartilage region. The junction of the articular cartilage with the subchondral bone is indicated by the open arrow. Hematoxylin and eosin (×290).*

fibers oriented parallel to the surface; *(b)* the **middle zone** has larger, more spherical cells, displays a random arrangement of collagen fibers, and stains the most intensely of all zones for GAGs; *(c)* the **deep zone** has cells that are arranged perpendicular to the articular surface between columns of collagen fibers. These fibers are anchored into the calcified cartilage, which forms the deepest layer of this zone. The calcified cartilage is joined to underlying subchondral bone by simple adherence without traversing collagen fibers. Although uncalcified articular cartilage (superficial, middle, and upper deep zone) may vary in thickness during life, the thickness of the calcified cartilage layer remains constant.

The **tidemark** is a thin layer of clusters of mineral, glycoproteins, and lipids located between the calcified and uncalcified layers of articular cartilage. In decalcified sections, the tidemark stains with hematoxylin. Multiple tidemarks may be present in older animals and indicate that mineralization of the cartilage was interrupted and then resumed several times. This contrasting interface between calcified and uncalcified tissues is prone to fracture.

The highly anionic GAGs (e.g., chondroitin sulfate and keratan sulfate to a lesser degree) of articular cartilage normally bind water, which is released upon compression of the cartilage. Conversely, when the compression is released, the water is absorbed into the matrix and rebinds with the GAGs. This process provides a weeping lubrication of the articular surfaces, as well as a circulation of nutrients to and waste products from the articular chondrocyte. This circulation is important because the articular cartilage is avascular and alymphatic.

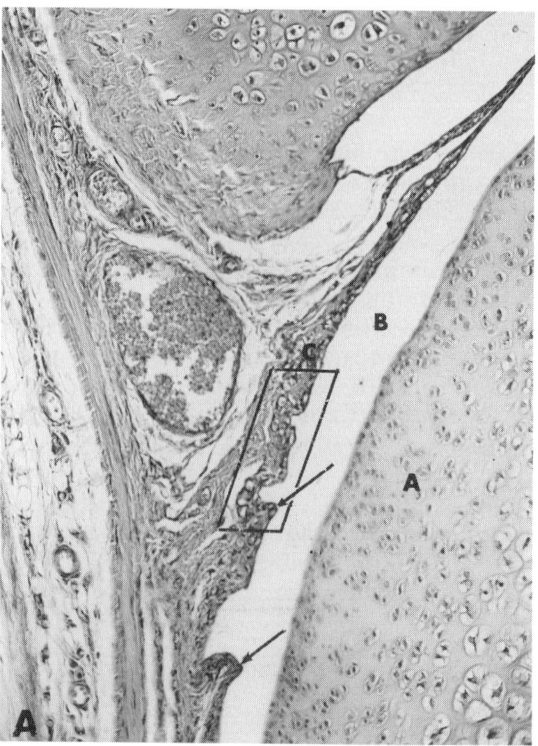

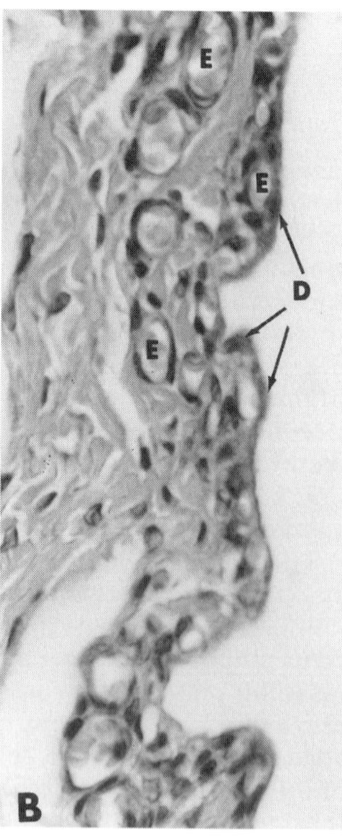

Figure 3.45. *Stifle joint (rat).* ***A.***, *The articular cartilage (A) is adjacent to the joint cavity (B). The synovial membrane (C) has synovial villi (arrows) (×160).* ***B.***, *Area outlined in* ***A.*** *Synovial cells (D) rest on loose connective tissue containing numerous capillaries (E). Hematoxylin and eosin (×750). (Reprinted by permission from Smith EM, Calhoun ML. The microscopic anatomy of the white rat. Ames, IA: The Iowa State University Press, 1968.)*

The joint capsule encloses the entire joint and comprises an inner **synovial membrane** and outer **fibrous layer** (Fig. 3.45A). The synovial membrane, in turn, is composed of synovial cells and subcellular connective tissue, which may be loose (Fig. 3.45B), fibrous, or adipose. The predominating type of connective tissue in the synovial membrane varies with the location in the joint and classifies the type of synovial membrane. The outer fibrous layer is composed of dense irregular connective tissue and is continuous with the periosteum of adjacent bones.

The synovial cavity is filled with **synovial fluid**, which has a composition similar to plasma. This fluid is derived as an ultrafiltrate of the blood with the addition of a substantial amount of polymerized hyaluronic acid from synovial cells. Synovial fluid provides the lubrication for the articulating surfaces of joints.

Some synovial joints (stifle) have intra-articular **menisci** composed of fibrocartilage (Fig. 3.43). Usually, menisci are anchored on one side to the fibrous layer of the joint capsule. If the cartilages are removed after traumatic injury, a new structure develops from the fibrous layer of the capsule; however, it is composed of dense collagen rather than fibrocartilage. These structures are important biomechanically in the joint, and the ends (horns) are heavily innervated with proprioceptive nerves.

REFERENCES

Alberts B, Bray D, Lewis J, et al. Molecular biology of the cell. 3rd ed. New York: Garland Publishing, 1994.

Anderson C. Manual for the examination of bone. Boca Raton, FL: CRC Press, 1982.

Cheville NF. Cell pathology. 2nd ed. Ames, IA: Iowa State University Press, 1983.

Everts V, Van der Zee E, Creemers L, et al. Phagocytosis and intracellular digestion of collagen, its role in turnover and remodeling. Histochem J 1996;28(4):229.

Freeman MAR, ed. Adult articular cartilage. New York: Grune and Stratton, 1972.

Frost HM. Intermediary organization of the skeleton. Boca Raton, FL: CRC Press, 1986;I, II.

Frost HM. The physiology of cartilaginous, fibrous, and bony tissue. Springfield, IL: Charles C. Thomas, 1972.

Ghosh P, ed. The biology of the intervertebral disc. Boca Raton, FL: CRC Press, 1988;I, II.

G thlin G, Ericsson JLE. The osteoclast. Clin Orthop 1976;120:201.

Hall BK, ed. Cartilage. San Diego: Academic Press, 1983;I, II.

Ibbotson KJ, D Souza SM, Kanis JA, et al. Physiological and pharmacological regulation of bone resorption. Metab Bone Dis Relat Res 1981;2(3):177.

Jee WSS. The skeletal tissues. In: Weiss L, ed. Histology, cell and tissue biology. 6th ed. New York: Elsevier Biomedical, 1988:213.

Jee WSS, Parfitt AM, eds. Bone histomorphometry. Paris: Societe Nouvelle de Publications Medicales et Dentaires, 1981.

Kimmel DB, Jee WSS. Bone cell kinetics during longitudinal bone growth in the rat. Calcif Tissue Int 1980;32:123.

Kincaid SA, Van Sickle DC. Bone morphology and postnatal osteogenesis potential for disease. In: Alexander JW, Roberts RE, eds. Symposium on orthopedic diseases. Philadelphia: WB Saunders, 1983;13(1):3.

Kuettner KE, Schleyerbach R, Hascall VC, eds. Articular cartilage biochemistry. New York: Raven Press, 1986.

Malluche HH, Faugere M-C. Atlas of mineralized bone histology. New York: S. Karger, 1986.

Piez KA, Reddi AH, eds. Extracellular matrix biochemistry. New York: Elsevier Biomedical, 1984.

Reddi AH, ed. Extracellular matrix: structure and function. In: UCLA symposia on molecular and cellular biology. New York, Alan R. Liss, 1985;25:1.

Ruggeri A, Motta PM, eds. Ultrastructure of the connective tissue matrix. Boston: M. Nijhoff, 1984.

Simon SR, ed. Orthopaedic basic science. Chicago: American Academy of Orthopaedic Surgeons, 1994.

Stockwell RA. Biology of cartilage cells. Cambridge: Cambridge University Press, 1979.

Talmage RV. Morphological and physiological consideration in a new concept of calcium transport of bone. Am J Anat 1970;129:467.

Tizard IR. Veterinary immunology. 5th ed. Philadelphia: WB Saunders, 1996.

Urist MR, ed. Fundamental and clinical bone physiology. Philadelphia: JB Lippincott, 1980.

Van Sickle DC, Kincaid SA. Comparative arthrology. In: Sokoloff L, ed. The joints and synovial fluid. New York: Academic Press, 1979;I:1.

Weiss L, Sakai H. The hemopoietic stroma. Am J Anat 1984;170:447.

Wilsman NJ, Van Sickle DC. Cartilage canals, their morphology and distribution. Anat Rec 1972;173:79.

Woo SL-Y, Buckwalter JA, eds. Injury and repair of the musculoskeletal soft tissues. Park Ridge: AAOS, 1988.

4

Blood and Bone Marrow

AHMED DELDAR

BLOOD CELLS

Blood is a fluid tissue that circulates through vascular channels to carry nutrients to cells and waste products to excretory organs. The total volume of circulating blood is kept remarkably constant and is expressed relative to body weight (% or ml/kg). In general, blood volume of large domestic animals is approximately 8 to 11% and that of common laboratory animals, from mice to monkeys, is approximately 6 to 7% of body weight.

Blood consists of a cellular component, blood cells, and a protein-rich fluid component, plasma. Cellular component contains erythrocytes (red blood cells), thrombocytes (platelets), and leukocytes (white blood cells). The five leukocyte types in the blood of most vertebrates are neutrophils, eosinophils, basophils, monocytes, and lymphocytes. Plasma contains 91 to 92% water and 8 to 9% solutes (e.g., proteins, lipids, electrolytes).

Freshly drawn blood rapidly clots into a jellylike mass. If clotting is prevented, however, the blood cells settle. Settled or centrifuged blood consists of three distinct layers. The lowest layer, approximately 45% of the blood volume, is red, consists of erythrocytes, and is called packed-cell volume (PCV) or hematocrit. A thin gray-white middle layer, the buffy coat, lies above the erythrocytes and accounts for approximately 1% of the blood volume. The buffy coat is composed of platelets above and leukocytes below. The uppermost layer of centrifuged blood is plasma (Fig. 4.1). On average, approximately 7×10^6 to 10×10^6 erythrocytes, 8×10^3 to 12×10^3 leukocytes, and 2×10^5 to 4×10^5 platelets per mm^3 are in most common large domestic animals. Variation

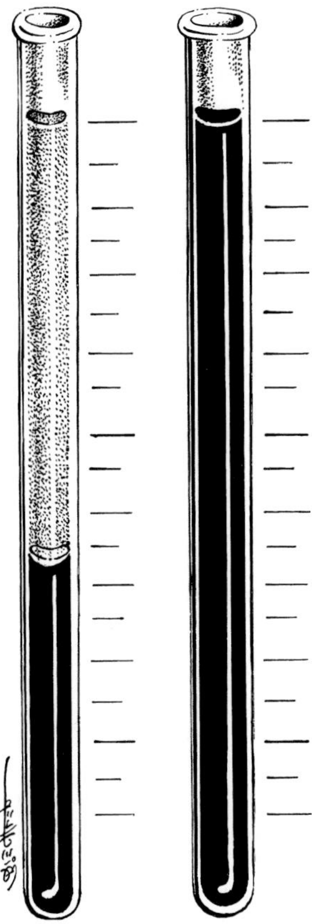

Figure 4.1. *Blood before and after sedimentation. The volume of packed erythrocytes is almost 45% of the total blood volume. The leukocytes and platelets form a buffy coat, accounting for approximately 1% of the blood volume. The remainder of the blood is the supernatant plasma.*

in erythrocyte numbers among animal species is generally related to the size of erythrocytes in various species.

Evaluation of Blood Cells

An evaluation of blood cells is performed routinely to assess general health, diagnose hematologic diseases, assess the body s ability to respond to a hematologic insult, and monitor the course of certain diseases.

Blood samples should be collected from animals at rest to minimize artifactual (physiologic) changes in blood cell counts. Blood is routinely drawn from large vessels (e.g., jugular vein) into a vial containing an anticoagulant. Other veins that are used less frequently in large animals for collecting the blood sample include femoral, brachial, and saphenous. Ethylenediaminetetraacetic acid (EDTA) is a preferred anticoagulant for evaluation of blood cell structure. Erythrocyte, leukocyte, and platelet counts are routinely performed using an electronic particle-counting analyzer.

Blood films are made by spreading a small drop of blood across a slide or a coverslip, immediately after blood collection. The film is then air dried, fixed in methanol, and stained with one of the modified Romanovsky s stains. The commonly used Romanovsky s stains are Wright s and Giemsa stains. Morphologic descriptions of various blood cells that follow are based on appearance of these cells in Wright s-stained blood films. Wright s stain is a mixture of a basic dye (methylene blue), which is attracted to acidic nuclei, and an acidic dye (eosin), which is attracted to alkaline cytoplasmic constituents. Blood films are initially screened with a low-power objective to assess the relative distribution of different blood cell types and to locate areas that are suitable for studying the cellular details. The oil-immersion objective (magnification) is used to examine erythrocyte, leukocyte, and platelet morphology, to perform a differential leukocyte count, and to estimate the adequacy of platelet number.

CHARACTERISTIC FEATURES OF BLOOD CELLS

Erythrocytes

The appearance of erythrocytes in stained blood films depends on the extent to which erythrocytes were flattened and shrunk during the smear preparation. Mature erythrocytes are non-nucleated biconcave discs; the degree of concavity varies among the domestic animals (Fig. 4.2). Typical biconcave erythrocytes are present in dogs, cows, and sheep; those in horses and cats have a shallow concavity; and most erythrocytes in goats and pigs are rather flat. Mature erythrocytes have a central pale area surrounded by orange (hemoglobinized) cytoplasm. The central pallor of erythrocytes is readily visible in dogs, less evident in cats and horses, and absent in cows, sheep, goats, and pigs.

The size and number of erythrocytes vary among animal species. The smaller the red cell, the greater the number per unit volume of blood. Dogs have the largest erythrocytes (7.0 μm) of all domestic animals, whereas goats have the smallest (4.1 μm). Slight **anisocytosis** (variation in size) of erythrocytes is common in most animal species, whereas **poikilocytosis** (variation in shape) is normally present in goats and deer (Fig. 4.3). Spindle, pear-, rod-, and triangle-shaped erythrocytes are normally seen in goats. Erythrocytes of the family *camellidae*

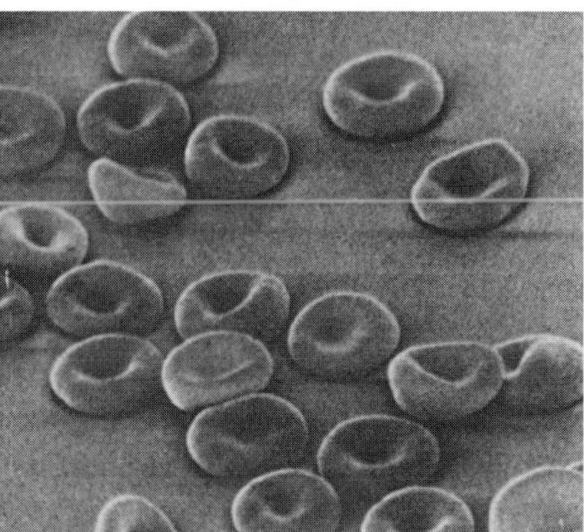

Figure 4.2. *Scanning electron micrograph of erythrocytes from a clinically normal dog. The erythrocytes are biconcave discs. (From Jain NC. Schalm s veterinary hematology. 4th ed. Philadelphia: Lea & Febiger, 1983.)*

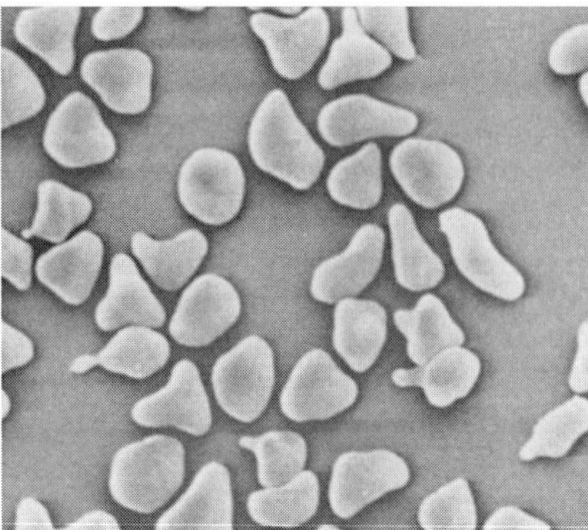

Figure 4.3. *Scanning electron micrograph of erythrocytes from a clinically normal goat shows a marked poikilocytosis. (From Jain NC. Schalm s veterinary hematology. 4th ed. Philadelphia: Lea & Febiger, 1983.)*

(e.g., camel, alpaca, llama) have a characteristic elliptical shape.

Erythrocytes tend to adhere to each other and form long chains resembling stacks of coins. This phenomenon, called **rouleau formation**, is prominent in blood of horses and cats, intermediate in blood of dogs and pigs, and rare in blood of ruminants. Reticulocytes and Howell—Jolly bodies are numerous when the marrow is responding to an increased demand for erythrocytes. Reticulocytes are immature anuclear erythrocytes that appear polychromatic (pinkish blue color) on Wright s-stained blood films. Reticulocytes contain residual ribonucleic acid (RNA) (ribosomes and polyribosomes) and mitochondria, which are aggregated into a reticular mesh when stained with vital stains (e.g., new methylene blue) but not with Wright s stain. Quantitation of reticulocytes in circulation is used as an index of bone marrow erythropoietic activity. **Howell—Jolly bodies** are DNA fragments that are derived from nuclear karyorrhexis. They appear as small, round, pyknotic, and deeply basophilic inclusions within erythrocytes. A few reticulocytes and Howell—Jolly bodies are seen normally in dogs and cats but are not seen in horses and ruminants. **Heinz bodies** (erythrocyte refractile bodies) appear as pale areas within the cytoplasm resulting from the oxidation of hemoglobin. These light-staining areas predominate in cats.

Lifespan of circulating erythrocytes varies among animal species: 110 to 120 days in dogs; 66 to 79 days in cats; 160 days in cows; 86 days in pigs; and 140 to 150 days in horses and sheep.

Leukocytes

Far fewer leukocytes than erythrocytes are present in the blood. Total blood leukocyte count refers to the total absolute counts of neutrophils, eosinophils, basophils, monocytes, and lymphocytes. The number of leukocytes varies among different animal species. Differential leukocyte count is the percentage of each population of leukocytes in peripheral blood and should be performed by counting and differentiating a minimum of 200 cells on stained blood films. Peripheral-blood leukocytes are also classified as **polymorphonuclear granulocytes**, consisting of neutrophils, eosinophils, and basophils, and **mononuclear agranulocytes**, consisting of lymphocytes and monocytes. Granulocytes are named according to the staining characteristics of their specific cytoplasmic granules. Eosinophils have pronounced acidophilic granules, basophils possess distinct basophilic granules, and neutrophils have neutral granules.

The proportion of different populations of leukocytes also varies among animal species. For example, neutrophils predominate in dogs and cats, whereas they slightly exceed lymphocytes in horses. In ruminants and laboratory animals (rats and mice), lymphocytes are predominant. The morphology of various populations of leukocytes are generally similar among animal species. These characteristics, as viewed on Wright s-stained blood films, are described below under each cell type.

NEUTROPHILS

The number of circulating neutrophils varies among animal species. Once released from the bone marrow, where they are produced, neutrophils circulate for 6 to 14 hours before migrating to tissues, where they function for an unknown period of time. Neutrophils account for approximately 40 to 70% of the total leukocyte count in most animal species. Mature neutrophils are approximately 12 to 15 μm in diameter and contain heterochromatic (clumped chromatin) segmented nuclei, with three to five lobes, joined by thin strands (Plate 4.I, Fig. 1). Occasionally, a nuclear appendage, an extra chromatin lobe resembling a drumstick, is present in neutrophils of female animals. This nuclear appendage is commonly known as a **Barr body** or sex body (Fig. 1.6). Fine-structural studies have shown that neutrophils contain occasional dense mitochondria, a few Golgi complexes, polyribosomes, glycogen, and granules. The neutrophil cytoplasm is pale grayish blue and contains a moderate number of fine pinkish or pale granules, depending on the animal species. Neutrophils contain two types of cytoplasmic granules: azurophilic (primary) and specific (Fig. 4.4). These granules contain different chemical substances that play a major role in regulating the neutrophil production and defending the body against bacterial infection. Cytoplasmic granules are large and reddish in rabbits, guinea pigs, and chicken; therefore, neutrophils are called **heterophils** in these species. In health, only mature neutrophils are present in circulation. Immature neutrophils are normally restricted to bone marrow, but they may be released into blood during granulocytic response to a disease process.

EOSINOPHILS

Eosinophils account for approximately 2 to 8% of the total leukocyte count. They are 10 to 15 μm in diameter and contain polymorphic nuclei that are less condensed and segmented than those of neutrophils. The cytoplasm contains eosinophilic granules that are loosely packed in the cell. Fine-structural studies have shown that Golgi complexes, mitochondria, ribosomes, and rough endoplasmic reticulum (rER) are more prominent in mature eosinophils than in mature neutrophils (Fig. 4.5). The cytoplasm contains only specific eosinophilic granules. As eosinophils mature in bone marrow, azurophilic granules disappear or transform into specific granules. Eosinophils play a role in allergic and anaphylactic reactions and in infestation caused by parasites. The size, shape, number, and staining characteristics of eosinophils vary among different animal species. Eosinophils in dogs often have pinkish or light orange vacuolated cytoplasm that contains granules. In dogs, eosinophil granules vary in size, shape, and number and rarely fill the cell. Eosinophils in cats have numerous uniform, rod-shaped granules that stain grayish orange. Eosinophils in sheep, goats, cows, and pigs have numerous uniform, spherical granules that stain bright orange and nearly fill the cell (Plate 4.I, Fig. 2). Eosinophils in horses have the largest granules of all, among different animal species. Granules stain bright orange, have mulberry-like appearances, and fill the cell completely (Plate 4.I, Fig. 3).

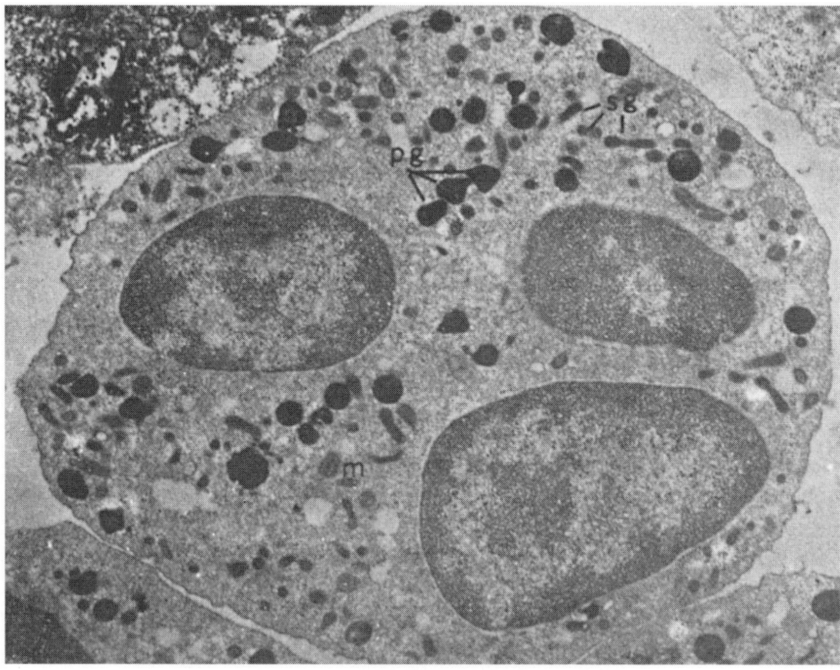

Figure 4.4. *Electron micrograph of a mature neutrophil from canine bone marrow stained for peroxidase. The neutrophil contains large, spherical, peroxidase-positive primary granules (pg) and small, pleomorphic, peroxidase-negative secondary granules (sg). Some mitochondria (m) are present. The nuclear lobes show chromatin condensation. (From Jain NC. Schalm s veterinary hematology. 4th ed. Philadelphia: Lea & Febiger, 1983.)*

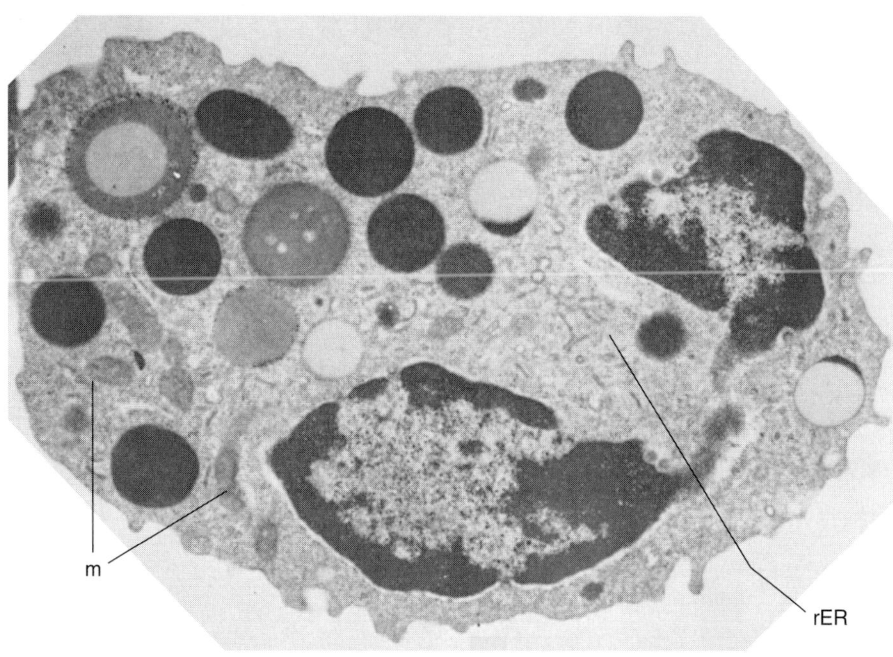

Figure 4.5. *Electron micrograph of a canine eosinophil. The cell contains pleomorphic granules. Dense and light homogeneous granules and clear vesicles are present. A few mitochondria (m) and remnants of rough endoplasmic reticulum (rER) are scattered throughout the cell. (From Jain NC. Schalm s veterinary hematology. 4th ed. Philadelphia: Lea & Febiger, 1983.)*

BASOPHILS

Basophils are rare in normal blood and account for 0 to 1.5% of the total leukocyte count. They measure 10 to 15 μm in diameter and have segmented or irregularly shaped heterochromatic nuclei. The nuclear segmentation, as in eosinophils, is less pronounced in basophils (two to three lobes) than in neutrophils. Fine-structural studies have shown that basophils contain homogeneous granules, rER, mitochondria, and Golgi complexes. Cytoplasmic granules are metachromatic and prominent, stain reddish violet, and invariably fill the cytoplasm, thereby masking the nucleus in some species. Basophilic granules are water soluble; therefore, some degranulation may occur during the staining of blood films. The size, number, and staining reaction of granules vary among animal species. Basophils of dogs have larger and fewer granules than those of cows and horses (Plate 4.I, Fig. 4). Granules of basophils in cats are rod-shaped and usually stain dull orange-gray. In other domestic species, granules are large, spherical, or oval, typically stain reddish violet, and usually fill the cell (Plate 4.I, Fig. 5).

Basophils have some morphologic resemblance to mast cells, which are widely distributed in connective tissues. Compared to mast cells, basophils are smaller with regular spherical or segmented nuclei and fewer granules that are evenly distributed in the cytoplasm. In contrast, tissue mast cells are large, have irregular or spherical nuclei, and contain numerous granules that are often eccentrically distributed. Basophils play a major role in mediating inflammatory reactions.

MONOCYTES

Monocytes are generally the largest blood leukocyte, 12 to 18 μm in diameter, and account for 3 to 8% of total leukocyte count. Monocytes are precursors of tissue macrophages and have highly pleomorphic nuclei (Fig. 4.6). The nucleus may appear elongated, irregularly contoured, folded, indented, horseshoe-shaped, and even slightly lobed. In contrast to that of lymphocytes, the nuclear chromatin of monocytes is lacy or reticular and may show some areas of condensation (Plate 4.I, Figs. 1 and 9). Nucleoli are present but not readily visible. The cytoplasm is abundant, grayish blue in color, and often appears foamy or vacuolated (Plate 4.I, Figs. 1 and 9). In cows, monocytes are difficult to differentiate from large lymphocytes, because nuclei of bovine lymphocytes may have different shapes and chromatin patterns. Prominent azurophilic granules are not a common feature of bovine monocytes. Activated monocytes often have a few large vacuoles and many fine or indistinct azurophilic granules in the cytoplasm.

LYMPHOCYTES

The number of circulating lymphocytes varies among animal species. Lymphocytes account for 20 to 40% of the total leukocyte count in dogs, cats, and horses; 60 to 70% in ruminants, mice, and rats; and 50 to 60% in pigs. Lymphocytes play a role in cell-mediated (T lymphocytes) and antibody-mediated (B lymphocytes) immunity. Morphologically, lymphocytes are classified as small

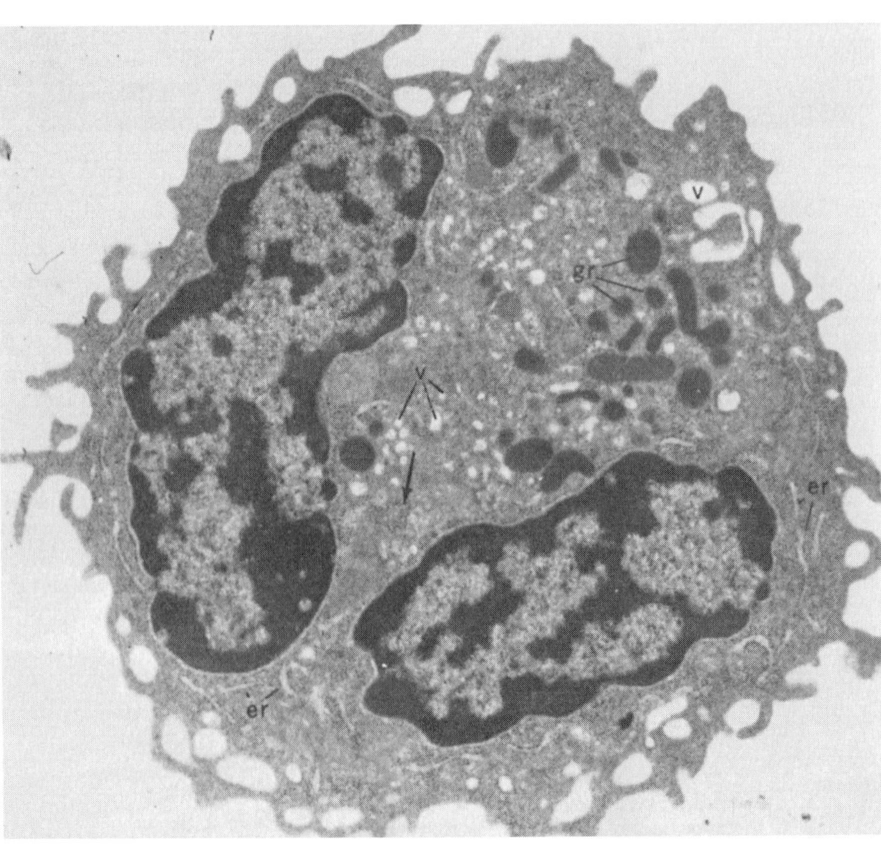

Figure 4.6. *Electron micrograph of a canine monocyte. The cell contains many lysosomal granules (gr), several small to large vesicles (v), abundant ribosomes (arrow), and prominent rough endoplasmic reticulum (er), especially along the cell periphery. This cell also has many microvillus-like projections along the cellular outline. The nucleus appears bilobed and shows areas of chromatin condensation. (From Jain NC. Schalm s veterinary hematology. 4th ed. Philadelphia: Lea & Febiger, 1983.)*

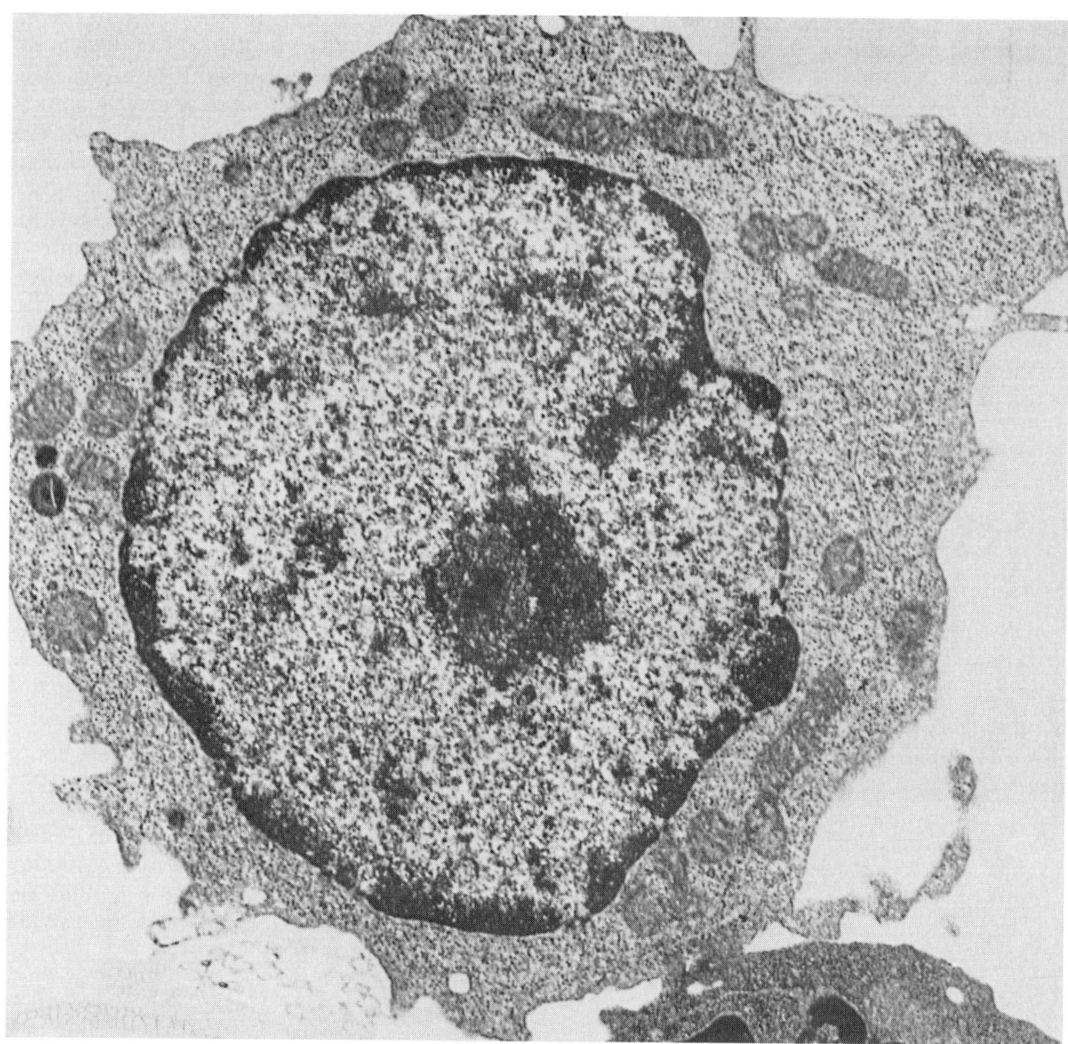

Figure 4.7. *Electron micrograph of a canine lymphocyte. The cell has a moderate amount of cytoplasm surrounding a large nucleus with nucleolus. The cytoplasm is rich in free ribosomes, has some profiles of rough endoplasmic reticulum and scattered mitochondria and contains dense granules (azurophilic granules). (From Jain NC. Schalm s veterinary hematology. 4th ed. Philadelphia: Lea & Febiger, 1983.)*

(6 to 9 μm) and large (9 to 15 μm) lymphocytes. Small lymphocytes have round, dense, or slightly indented heterochromatic nuclei and scant, pale blue cytoplasm with occasionally a few azurophilic granules (Fig. 4.7; Plate 4.I, Fig. 6). The nucleus of large lymphocytes contains a few nucleoli and is indented; the cytoplasm is more abundant and stains homogeneously blue, compared with dark-blue-staining cytoplasm of small lymphocytes.

The size, shape, and staining characteristics of lymphocytes vary among and within animal species. Small lymphocytes are prominent in dogs and cats. Both small and large lymphocytes are present in cows, sheep, and goats. Occasionally, in cows, large lymphocytes may have vacuolated cytoplasm with a few large azurophilic granules (Plate 4.I, Figs. 7 and 8). Large lymphocytes with vacuolated cytoplasm in cows should be distinguished from monocytes.

Platelets/Thrombocytes

The life span of circulating platelets is relatively short (approximately 9 to 12 days) and is generally comparable among all domestic animal species. Platelets generally vary in size and shape and are approximately 1.3 to 4.7 μm in diameter. In stained blood films, platelets are discoid, spherical, or elongated cells and may appear individually or in small to large clusters (Plate 4.I, Figs. 7 and 8). A slight platelet anisocytosis is present in most species. A direct platelet count is performed on blood samples, using a hematology analyzer. A subjective screening of platelet number (normal, increased, or decreased) can also be made from their relative distribution on stained blood films. The terms **platelet** and **thrombocyte** are used interchangeably; the term **thrombocyte** is used preferentially to describe nucleated platelets in fish, reptiles, and birds.

Fine-structural studies have shown that the platelet cytoplasm contains microfilaments, microtubules, mitochondria, lysosomes, a canalicular system, glycogen particles, and a heterogeneous population of granules (α granules, electron dense granules, and lysosomal granules) (Figs. 4.8 and 4.9). The external membrane of normal platelets is covered with amorphous material forming a thin **exterior coat**, which is responsible for platelet adhesive properties. Moreover, a number of plasma proteins (e.g., fibrinogen, immunoglobulins, and coagulation factors) are also adsorbed onto the exterior coat. Microfilaments and microtubules are present beneath the plasma membrane. They provide the cytoskeleton for maintenance of normal platelet shape and are responsible for platelet shape changes and pseudopod formation during activation and in subsequent secretion of cytoplasmic granules. Microfilaments are also involved in clot retraction. A spongelike system of channels, called the **open canalicular system** (OCS), is randomly distributed in the platelet cytoplasm. The OCS opens to the platelet surface and is used for externalization of platelet secretory products and for internalization of substances from plasma into the platelets. Another series of channels called the **dense tubular system** is also found beneath the cytoplasmic membrane and provides a site for sequestration of calcium and localization of enzymes needed for prostaglandin synthesis. The cytoplasmic α granules are membrane-bound and contain platelet factor 4 (antiheparin), coagulation factor V, fibrinogen, and several other proteins, including platelet-derived growth factor (PDGF). Electron dense granules contain adenosine diphosphate (ADP) and adenosine triphosphate (ATP), calcium, serotonin, histamine, and catecholamines. Lysosomal granules contain acid hydrolases such as phosphatase and β-glucuronidase.

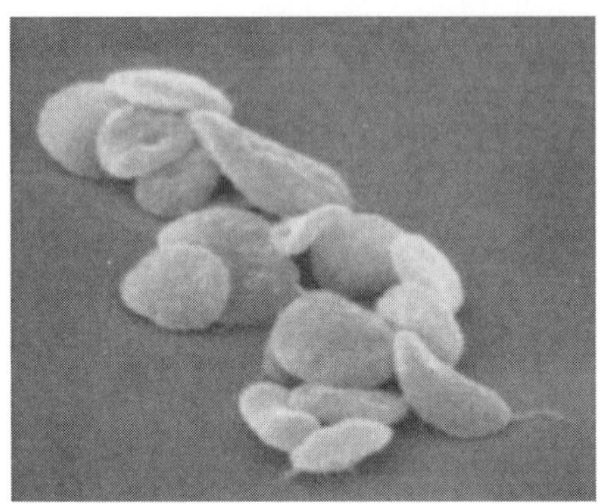

Figure 4.8. *Scanning electron micrograph of bovine platelets. Platelets vary in size and shape. (From Jain NC. Schalm s veterinary hematology. 4th ed. Philadelphia: Lea & Febiger, 1983.)*

FUNCTION OF BLOOD CELLS

Erythrocytes

Mature erythrocytes lack a nucleus, ribosomes, endoplasmic reticulum, and mitochondria. Therefore, they cannot synthesize proteins or new cell membrane. The biconcave shape of erythrocytes is maintained by spectrin, a contractile cytoskeletal protein that forms a net-

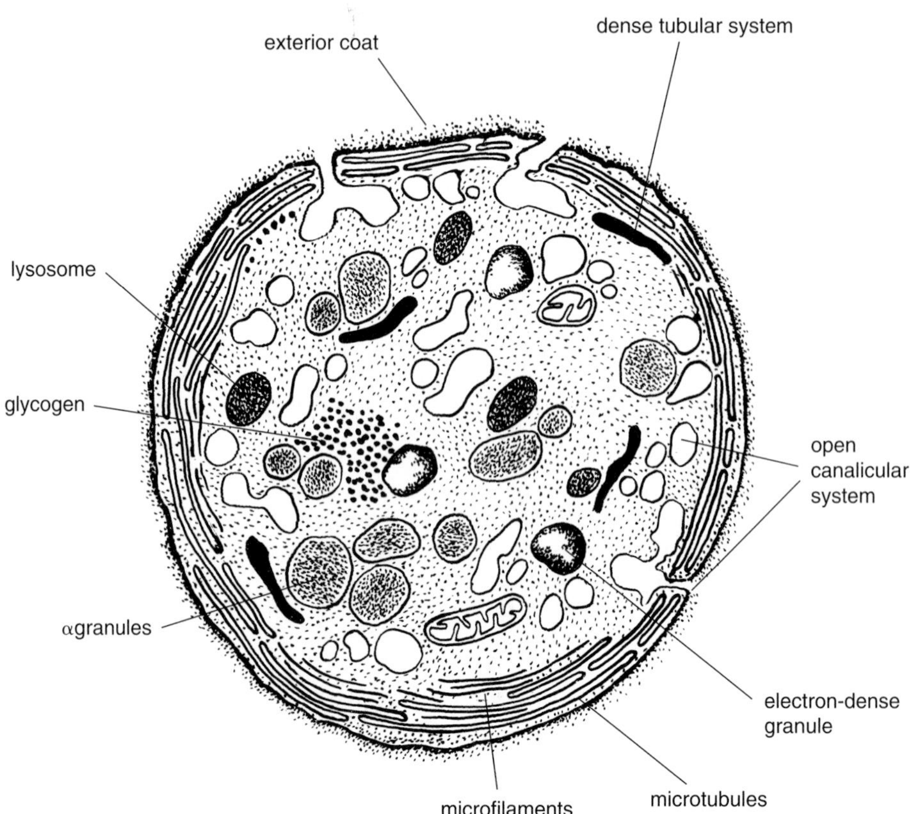

Figure 4.9. *A schematic drawing of the fine structure of a platelet.*

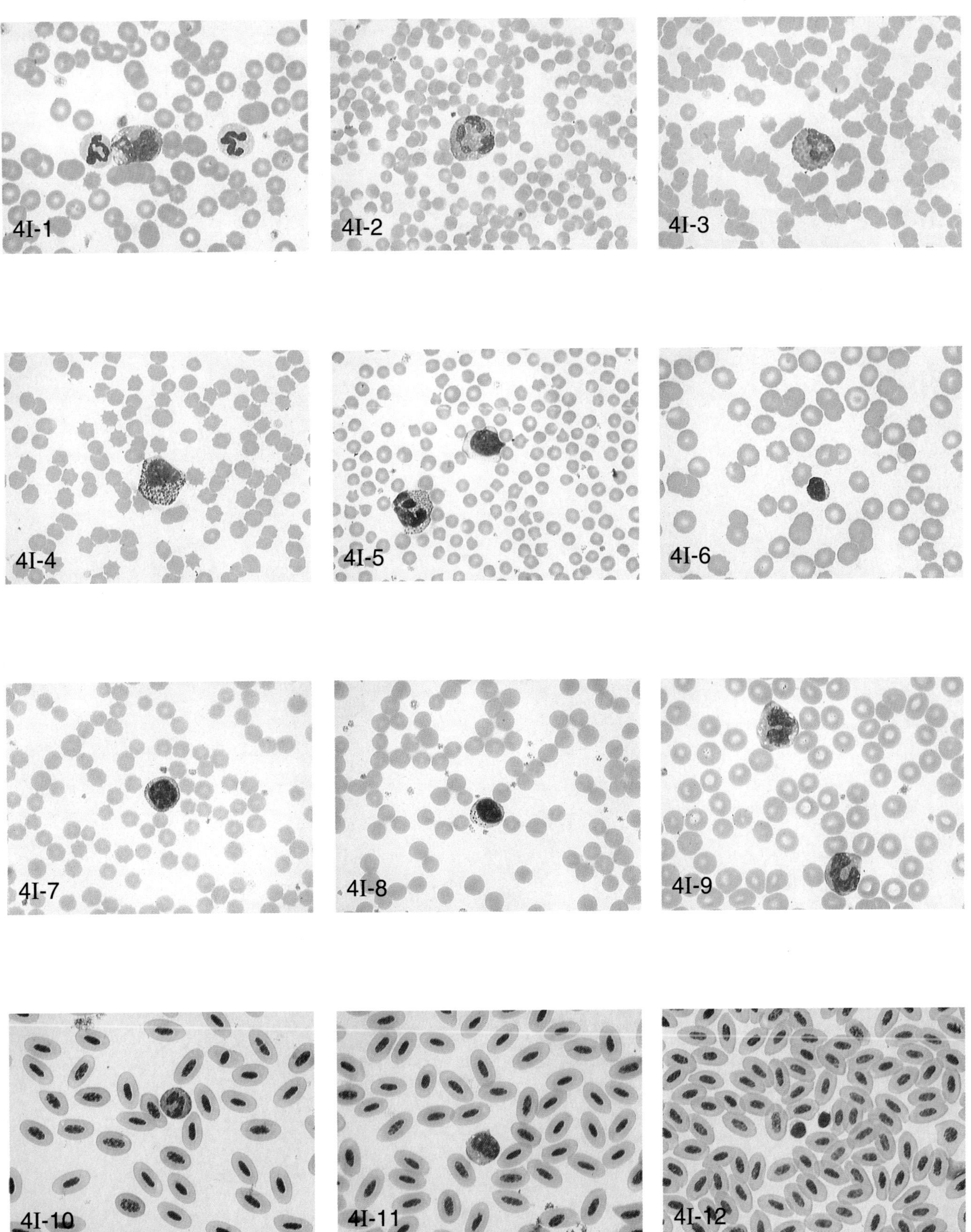

Plate I. *(Courtesy of Joanne B. Messick) 1. Two canine neutrophils and one monocyte. 2. Bovine eosinophil. 3. Equine eosinophil. The granules of the equine eosinophil are the largest of all the domestic species. 4. Equine basophil. 5. Ovine basophil and lymphocyte. 6. Small canine lymphocyte. 7 Large bovine lymphocyte and platelets. 8. Bovine lymphocyte with azurophilic granules and platelets. 9. Two canine monocytes. 10. Avian heterophil and nucleated erythrocytes. 11. Avian monocyte. 12. Two avian thrombocytes.*

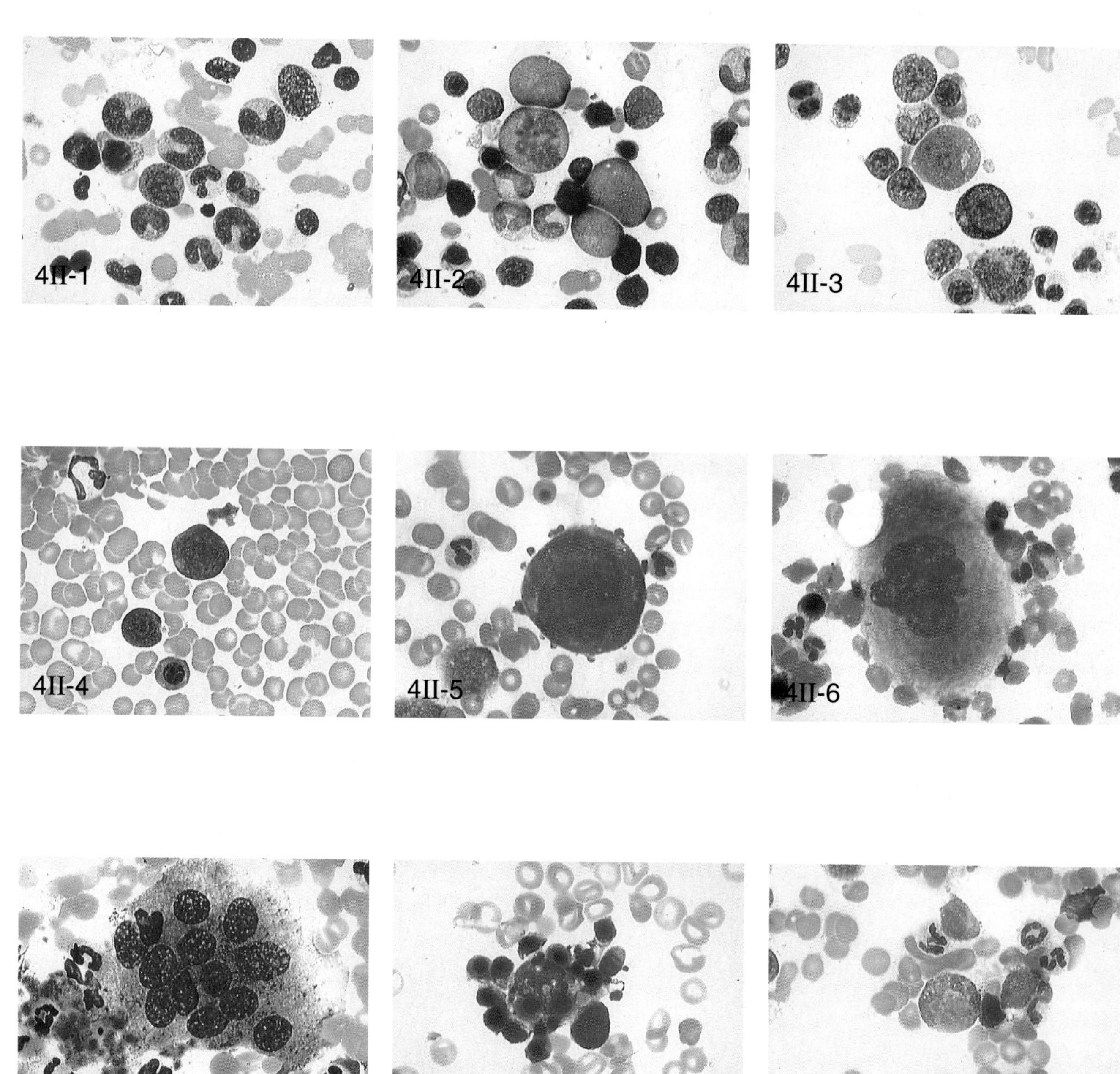

Plate II. *(Courtesy of Joanne B. Messick) 1. Bone marrow. Myeloid precursors; 1 = promyelocyte; 2 = myelocyte; 3 = metamyelocyte; 4 = band neutrophil; 5 = neutrophil. 2. Bone marrow. Myeloid precursors; 1 = promyelocyte; 2 = band neutrophil; 3 = mitotic figure. 3. Bone marrow. Myeloid and erythroid series; 1 = promyelocyte; 2 = rubriblast; 3 = basophilic rubricyte; 4 = polychromatic rubricyte. 4 = Bone marrow. Erythroid lineage. 1 = rubriblast; 2 = basophilic rubricyte; 3 = metarubricyte. 5. Bone marrow. Megakaryoblast. 6. Bone marrow. Megakaryocyte. Compare the multilobed nucleus with the multiple nuclei of the osteoclast in I-7. 7. Bone marrow. Osteoclast with multiple nuclei (compare with I-6). 8. Bone marrow. Erythroblastic island consisting of a central macrophage surrounded by erythroid cells in various stages of development. 9. Bone marrow. Myeloid and erythroid series; 1 = eosinophilic myelocyte; 2. = neutrophil; 3 = metarubricyte.*

work of filaments beneath the plasma membrane. Spectrin stabilizes the erythrocyte membrane against shear forces of blood flow and permits deformability during capillary blood flow. In spectrin-deficient animals, erythrocytes lose their biconcave shape and are short-lived. The plasticity of erythrocytes is also influenced by their colloidal contents. Approximately 60% of erythrocyte volume consists of water and the remainder is composed of hemoglobin (33 to 36%) and electrolytes.

The erythrocyte membrane is a bilayered structure composed of proteins (48%), lipids (44%) and carbohydrates (8%). The membrane surrounds the hemoglobin content of the cell and the two are bound together. Hemoglobin is essential to mammalian life, because it carries oxygen to tissues. It is a conjugated protein consisting of heme and globin and comprises approximately 33% of the weight of erythrocytes. The iron of heme must be maintained in ferrous form to transport oxygen. Erythrocytes contain an enzyme called methemoglobin reductase, which converts methemoglobin (having iron in ferric form) to a reduced functional hemoglobin (having iron in ferrous form), which is capable of transporting oxygen. Hemoglobin has a great affinity for oxygen and becomes readily saturated as blood passes through pulmonary alveolar capillaries. When hemoglobin is saturated with oxygen, it is called oxyhemoglobin; the oxidized form, methemoglobin, is functionally inactive.

Mature erythrocytes depend solely on anaerobic glycolysis for energy that is used to keep hemoglobin in its reduced state and maintain red-cell membrane integrity. With aging, a gradual decrease in the energy-producing capacity of erythrocytes occurs. Ultimately, senescent erythrocytes are removed from circulation. Mammalian erythrocytes contain 2,3-diphosphoglycerate (2,3-DPG), which regulates both the rate of energy metabolism through glycolysis and the release of oxygen from hemoglobin. The erythrocyte concentration of 2,3-DPG is inversely related to its hemoglobin concentration. An increase in concentration of 2,3-DPG decreases oxygen affinity of hemoglobin, causing the release of more oxygen to tissues. The latter phenomenon occurs during hypoxia, exercise, and anemia. Normal erythrocytic hemoglobin and 2,3-DPG concentrations vary among animal species and are related to muscular activity. Erythrocytes of humans, horses, and dogs have higher levels of hemoglobin and 2,3-DPG than those of cows, sheep, goats, and cats.

Leukocytes

NEUTROPHILS

Neutrophils form the first line of defense against microbial infection. They play an important role in bacterial phagocytosis and in modulating the inflammatory processes and subsequent tissue damage. The neutrophil granules (azurophilic and specific) work together to destroy phagocytized bacteria. Specific granules are prominent in mature neutrophils (Fig. 4.4).

Azurophilic granules contain substances that are involved in modulation of inflammatory processes, in generation and inactivation of chemotactic factors, and in migration of neutrophils to tissues. Specific granules contain factors that regulate neutrophil adhesiveness and aggregation, hydroxy radical (hydrogen peroxide) formation, complement-derived chemotactic factor generation, and myelopoiesis. Specific granules contain bactericidal lysozyme, lactoferrin, cationic proteins, and myeloperoxidase. Lysozyme is an enzyme that lyses certain bacteria by hydrolyzing the cell wall. Lactoferrin, which may act synergistically with lysozyme in bactericidal action, is an iron-binding protein that exerts its bacteriostatic and possibly bactericidal effects by chelating the iron needed by certain bacteria for growth. Lactoferrin also inhibits neutrophil production. Myeloperoxidase combines with hydroxy radical and halide (iodides and chlorides) to form a potent bactericidal complex. Azurophilic granules also contain acid hydrolytic enzymes and lysozyme.

Subsequent to bacterial infection, vascular permeability is increased and plasma escapes into surrounding tissues, thereby causing swelling. Neutrophils migrate to tissues in response to bacterial invasion. Tissue mast cells then respond, degranulate, and further intensify the inflammatory processes. Neutrophil migration occurs shortly after microbial infection and is mediated by chemotactic factors released from infected tissues and bacteria. The speed and magnitude of neutrophil migration vary with the degree, duration, and type of tissue injury.

Neutrophil chemotaxis and phagocytic activity require energy. Neutrophils derive energy primarily through anaerobic glycolysis. Different energy sources are used for chemotaxis and for phagocytosis. Chemotactic factors that cause neutrophils to sense and approach the site of inflammation accelerate uptake of extracellular glucose, whereas phagocytosis enhances glycogenolysis.

Complement component C5a is the most potent chemotactic factor for neutrophils. The serum complement system can be activated by several factors, including immune complexes and nonspecific proteases released from damaged tissues, neutrophils, and bacteria. Other complement components that induce the release of histamine from mast cells and basophils (see the following) also act as chemotactic factors for neutrophils. Bacterial phagocytosis is facilitated by opsonins, which are humoral factors (antibodies) that coat bacteria. Subsequent to phagocytosis, sequential degranulation and fusion of specific and azurophilic granules with phagosomes occur.

Neutrophils also play a role in coagulation, fibrinolysis, lymphocyte activation, and cytotoxicity. The extent of these activities, however, is beyond the scope of this chapter; interested readers should consult hematology textbooks.

EOSINOPHILS

Eosinophils are motile phagocytes. However, their phagocytic and bactericidal capacity is limited compared with that of neutrophils. The major source of energy in eosinophils, as in neutrophils, is anaerobic glycolysis.

Eosinophilic granules contain several cationic proteins, but they lack other bactericidal substances, such as lysozyme, lactoferrin, phagocytin, and neutral proteases. Cationic proteins also have little or no bactericidal activity, thus rendering eosinophils with limited bactericidal capacity. The lower density of immunoglobulin G (IgG) and complement receptors on eosinophils, compared with that on neutrophils, may account for low phagocytic activity of these cells.

Eosinophils play a major role in controlling parasitic infestation and regulating allergic and inflammatory processes. The latter function is mediated by phagocytizing the antigen—antibody complexes, inactivating histamine, and inhibiting the release and replenishment of histamine and other vasoactive mediators (serotonin). Histamine, a key chemotactic factor for eosinophils, is released from mast cells and basophils in response to tissue injury or allergic reactions. Other substances, such as antigen—antibody complexes, heterologous γ globulin, fibrin, fibrinogen, and substances released from stimulated T lymphocytes, also act as chemotactic factors for eosinophils. Eosinophils degranulate upon ingestion of inert particles, opsonized bacteria, antigen—antibody complexes, and after contact with metazoan parasites.

BASOPHILS

Basophils, like eosinophils, have limited phagocytic and bactericidal capacities. They respond chemotactically to bacterial products, complement components, and lymphokines. Although basophils and mast cells have evolved as separate systems, they are closely related and functionally complement one another. Basophil granules and those of mast cells are similar morphologically, cytochemically, and pharmacologically. Basophils play a major role in allergic and inflammatory reactions, lipid metabolism, and blood coagulation. Basophils and mast cells release their granule content through exocytosis and functionally are capable of resynthesizing their granules. Initial degranulation occurs within minutes of stimulation and may continue for several hours (6 to 72 hours); the degranulation is IgE mediated. Both basophils and mast cells have IgE surface receptors; on average, however, basophils have more receptors than do mast cells. Synthesized IgE quickly attaches to cell-surface receptors of basophils and mast cells. Upon contact with antigens, which stimulate IgE production, these IgE-loaded cells undergo acute degranulation, thereby releasing factors that affect blood vessels permeability and intensify the inflammatory reaction. After degranulation, new granules are synthesized and cytoplasmic substructures become normal within a few days.

The basophil and mast cell granules contain hydrolytic enzymes, heparin, histamine, hyaluronic acid, chondroitin sulfate, serotonin, and other vasoactive mediators. The content of granules, however, varies within and among animal species. Basophils of rats and mice contain serotonin, but basophils of humans and rabbits do not. Basophils of other species often contain both vasoactive amines. Heparin, a sulfated mucopolysaccharide responsible for metachromasia of granules, is an anticoagulant that also stimulates lipid metabolism by activating lipoprotein lipase released from vascular endothelium. Histamine, serotonin, and leukotrienes are vasodilators that increase vascular permeability. In contrast to the fast and transient action of histamine, the action of leukotrienes is delayed and more sustained. Therefore, depending on mediators and their release rates, the resulting reactions may occur quickly (immediate hypersensitivity) or may be delayed for several days (delayed hypersensitivity). In many instances, eosinophils and basophils are found together, because each releases chemotactic factors that attract the other.

MONOCYTES

Circulating monocytes rapidly migrate to tissues and body cavities and transform into tissue macrophages (Fig. 4.6). Once in tissues, monocytes generally do not reenter the bloodstream. Macrophages are long-lived phagocytic cells that are widely distributed throughout the body. Circulating monocytes and tissue macrophages are known as the **mononuclear phagocyte system** (MPS). Transformation of monocytes into macrophages is associated with increases in cell size, protein and lipid content, metabolism, surface receptor expression, phagocytic activity, and lysosomal/enzyme content and activity. The principal source of energy in monocytes and macrophages is anaerobic glycolysis. All macrophages have similar kinetics, structure, cytochemical properties, and functional activities, regardless of their locations. Macrophages are present in connective tissues (histiocytes), lymph nodes, spleen, bone marrow (osteoclasts), pleural and peritoneal cavities, liver (Kupffer cells), and lung (alveolar macrophages) and throughout the nervous system (microglial cells).

Monocytes and macrophages produce several substances of biologic importance, including colony stimulating factors (CSFs), cytokines (interleukin-1 [IL-1], interleukin-3 [IL-3]), tumor necrosis factor (TNF), endogenous pyrogens, lysosomal enzymes, and prostaglandins. The MPS plays an important role in phagocytizing and destroying intracellular organisms (fungi, protozoa, and viruses), transformed cells, and cell debris. The MPS is also involved in initiation and expression of immune response and in regulation of granulopoiesis and erythropoiesis. These cells also have surface receptors for all immunoglobulins. They take up and process antigens through their surface receptors. The processed antigens then are presented to T or B lymphocytes, which mount an appropriate immune response.

LYMPHOCYTES

Lymphocytes are the main cell type of the immune system. They circulate throughout the body and play an important role in immunologic defense for the host. Circulating lymphocytes are grouped into three functional types: T, B, and natural killer (NK) cells. These lymphocytes are morphologically similar, but each possesses a characteristic cytochemical surface marker. B lymphocytes have a primary role in humoral immunity and are precursors of plasma cells (antibody-producing cells). T lymphocytes comprise several subtypes and have a primary role in cellular immunity. They also regulate hematopoiesis and differentiation of B lymphocytes into plasma cells. NK cells lack B- or T-cell markers and are involved in cell-mediated cytotoxicity, including NK function and antibody-dependent cellular cytotoxicity. For more information on lymphocyte kinetics and functions, see Chapter 8.

Platelets

Platelets maintain the integrity of blood vessels and play a major role in blood coagulation and clot retraction. In response to vascular injury, platelets undergo profound morphologic, biochemical, and functional transformations. They adhere to injured endothelium and to one another, thereby forming an initial (primary) hemostatic plug at the site of vascular injury. Platelets are then stimulated and release their granular contents, resulting in the formation of a larger secondary hemostatic plug. Adequate number of functionally normal platelets is needed to stop bleeding effectively. Blood coagulation is simultaneously initiated by plasma factors and factors released from stimulated platelets and damaged endothelium. Blood coagulation results from sequential interaction of at least 13 plasma proteins. This interaction leads to the formation of a fibrinous jellylike clot, which along with platelet plugs, effectively stops bleeding. After its formation, the clot undergoes considerable retraction, which is mediated by contractile proteins released from activated platelets.

Platelets contain a variety of proteins that have procoagulant, antiheparin, inflammatory, and growth-promoting activities. Platelets play a role in formation of thrombi and emboli and in modulation of inflammatory processes through the release of their chemotactic factors and vasoactive amines.

BONE MARROW HEMATOPOIESIS

In adult animals, bone marrow is the primary production site for all blood-cell lines. Formation of blood cells is a complex process called hematopoiesis. Sustained hematopoietic activity depends on the ability of marrow to attract and hold a pool of stem cells that are capable of differentiating into a variety of blood-cell types. Marrow can be red or yellow. The red marrow is hematopoietically active, whereas the yellow marrow contains fat and is hematopoietically inactive. The red marrow can convert to yellow marrow and vice versa as demand for hematopoiesis changes.

Prenatal Hematopoiesis

Hematopoiesis begins in mammals in the wall of the yolk sac during intrauterine life. Primitive blood cells, originally derived by proliferation and differentiation of mesenchymal cells, are primarily erythroblastic and occur in small nests in the yolk sac. Later, during development of the embryo, hematopoietic cells migrate to the liver and form erythropoietic foci there. Subsequently, the bone marrow, spleen, lymph nodes, and thymus of the embryo are seeded with hematopoietic stem cells from the liver and become engaged in hematopoiesis.

Postnatal Hematopoiesis

Bone marrow is the major site of hematopoiesis during late gestation and at parturition. Extramedullary (outside the marrow) hematopoiesis persists in the liver and spleen for a few weeks after the birth and then gradually disappears. These organs, however, do retain their hematopoietic potential and become active hematopoietically in time of need. Early in life, marrow of all bones is red and hematopoietically active, producing all different blood-cell types. As the animal ages, demand for blood cells decreases; therefore, the red marrow is replaced gradually by yellow marrow. In adult animals, only the sternum, vertebrae, ribs, skull, pelvis, and epiphyses of long bones contain active marrow; the remainder of marrow is filled with fat cells.

BONE MARROW STRUCTURE

Blood supply to marrow is mainly provided by nutrient arteries that enter the midshaft in long bones. These arteries extend along the longitudinal axis of the bone and send off radial branches throughout the marrow. These branches terminate at the periphery of the marrow cavity and connect with venous vessels. Venous or vascular sinuses of marrow are thin-walled vessels that anastomose heavily and carry blood back to central veins. Marrow lacks lymphatic vessels. Nerves in marrow are vasomotor and found in association with vasculature. The hematopoietic compartment of marrow consists of irregular and anastomosing cords that lie between vascular sinuses (Fig. 4.10).

Blood cells are produced in the hematopoietic compartment of marrow and reach the circulation by crossing the wall of vascular sinuses. The sinus wall, in its fullest development, consists of an inner endothelial lining layer, discontinuous basal lamina, and an outer adventitial layer. Occasionally, the adventitial layer of vascular sinuses is incomplete, thus leaving the endothelial lining layer as the only layer of the sinus wall (Fig. 4.11). Adventitial cells are a type of reticular cell called adventitial reticular cells. These cells not only cover the outside surface of vascular sinuses but also branch out into surrounding hematopoietic compartments. These branches anastomose heavily and form a meshwork that supports hematopoietic cells and provides various hematopoietic microenvironments that influence early proliferation and differentiation of primitive stem cells (Fig. 4.11).

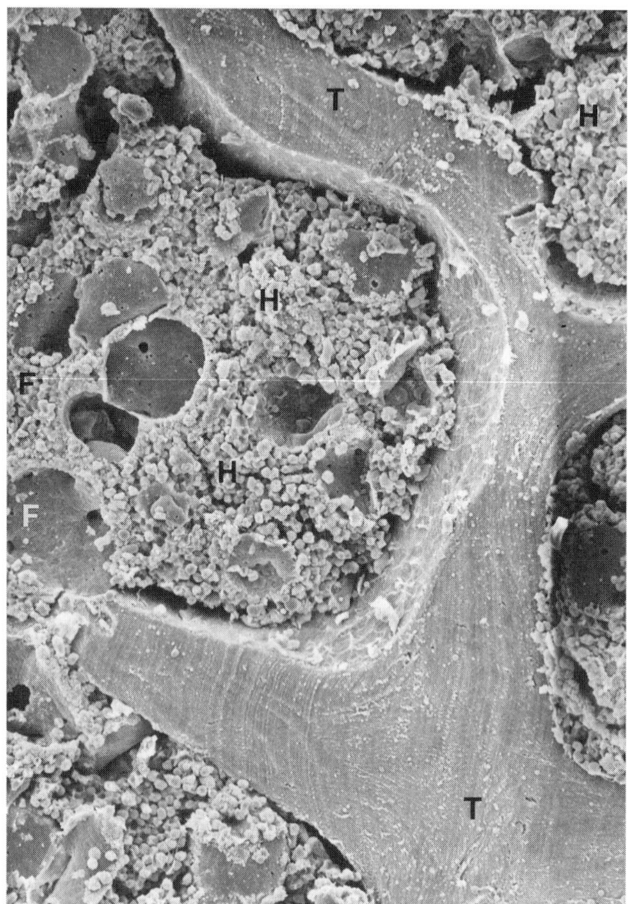

Figure 4.10. *Scanning electron micrograph of canine bone marrow. Marrow is compartmentalized by trabeculae (T). Hematopoietic spaces between the trabeculae are filled with hematopoietic (H) and fat (F) cells.*

Adventitial reticular cells are dynamic cells, i.e., they may fill with fat and become fat cells when demand for hematopoiesis is decreased. Marrow fat cells represent a mechanical buffer that occupies or releases space within the medullary cavity in response to changing demands for hematopoiesis. Moreover, fat cells may have an inductive influence on granulopoiesis. The extent of marrow fat and adventitial coverage of vascular sinuses varies inversely with the degree of hematopoiesis and the rate of cell delivery to the bloodstream. An increase in hematopoiesis with subsequent increased cell delivery to the bloodstream is associated with reduced marrow fat and adventitial coverage.

Marrow hematopoiesis is most active in areas close to bone. Fat cells are normally present in the center of marrow hematopoietic compartment, mainly around the large vessels. Hematopoietic cells held in reticular meshwork of reticular cells are arranged in particular patterns. Erythropoietic cells and megakaryocytes lie against vascular sinuses, whereas granulopoietic cells occur mostly deep within the marrow hematopoietic compartment away from vascular sinuses (Figs. 4.12 and 4.13).

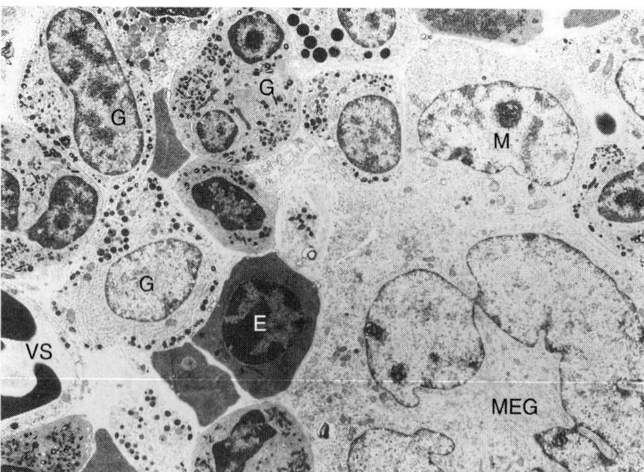

Figure 4.11. *Electron micrograph of canine bone marrow. Various hematopoietic cells, including erythrocytic, granulocytic (G), monocytic (M), and megakaryocytic (MEG) precursors, are present. A portion of a vascular sinus (VS), lined by the endothelial layer, is also shown.*

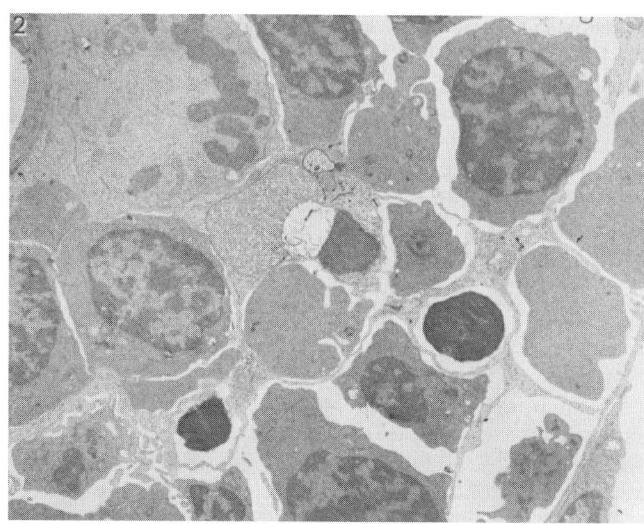

Figure 4.12. *Electron micrograph of the bone marrow of a rat shows an erythroblastic island. A macrophage lies amid a cluster of red cells. The cytoplasmic extensions of the macrophage enclose the surrounding red cells and reach the wall of a vascular sinus. (From Weiss L. The hematopoietic microenvironment of the bone marrow: an ultrastructural study of the stroma in rats. Anat Rec 1976;186:163.)*

Hematopoietic stem cells

In normal animals, production and utilization of blood cells are delicately balanced. Marrow contains several types of self-replicating stem cells with different proliferating and differentiating capacities. Stem cells of various lineages generally have similar structures, resembling lymphocytes. Stem cells are generally in a resting phase, but they proliferate in response to body demand for new blood cells. In vitro and in vivo studies have revealed the existence of **pluripotent**, **multipotent**,

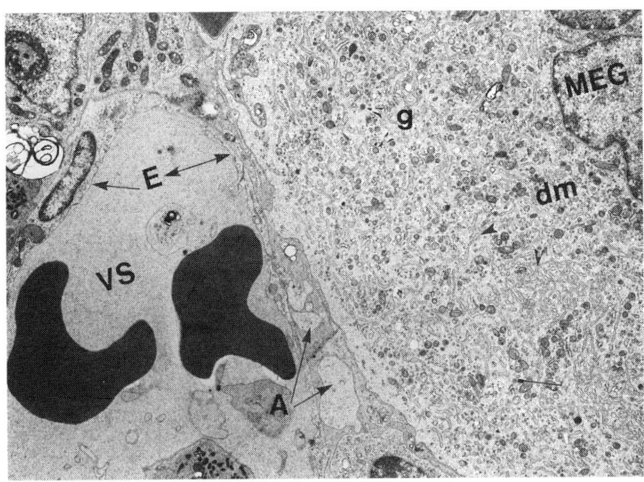

Figure 4.13. *Electron micrograph of canine bone marrow. A relatively mature megakaryocyte (MEG) lies next to a vascular sinus (VS). The megakaryocyte contains well-developed demarcation membranes (dm) and granules (g); its cytoplasmic process is extended toward the sinus (arrows). The vascular sinus is lined primarily by the endothelial layer (E) and partially by the adventitial reticular cell processes (A).*

and **unipotent** stem cells and have demonstrated their relationship to each other. Techniques such as radiation therapy, chromosomal and enzymatic markers, spleen colony assays, and bone marrow cell cultures have been used to identify the functional capacity of these different stem cells and their ability to repopulate the marrow after it has been damaged.

Primitive stem cells originally are supplied by embryonic yolk sac and later by fetal liver, spleen, and bone marrow. In most animal species, bone marrow is the primary source of these stem cells after the birth. Pluripotent stem cells proliferate and give rise to progenies that are capable of producing lymphocytes (lymphoid stem cells) and other blood cell types (myeloid stem cells). Progenies of lymphoid stem cells arise in the marrow but migrate in the bloodstream to the thymus, where T lymphocytes are formed, and to the spleen and lymph nodes, where B lymphocytes are produced. Progenies of myeloid stem cells, known as multipotent stem cells, are capable of differentiating into any of the blood-cell lines. Progenies of multipotent stem cells, in turn, differentiate into unipotent stem cells (progenitor cells), each committed irreversibly to a specific cell lineage, such as erythrocytic, granulocytic-monocytic, and megakaryocytic cell lines (Fig. 4.14).

Progenitor cells are morphologically similar but unrecognizable in conventional bone marrow preparations for cytologic and histologic evaluation. They can only be identified by their growth characteristics in various in vitro tissue cultures, in which they form colonies that contain morphologically recognizable precursors of a corresponding cell line. These progenitor cells are called colony-forming unit megakaryocyte (CFU-MK), colony-forming unit granulocyte/macrophage (CFU-GM), colony-forming unit eosinophil (CFU-EO), burst-forming unit erythroid (BFU-E), colony-forming unit erythroid (CFU-E), etc. Upon maturation, progenitor cells produce rubriblasts, myeloblasts, and megakaryoblasts, which undergo further maturation and give rise to mature erythrocytes, granulocytes, and platelets, respectively.

Local marrow microenvironment and systemic humoral factors influence hematopoiesis and stimulate or suppress the proliferation and differentiation of single or multiple cell lineages. In general, multispecific growth factors, such as IL-3, stimulate early progenitor cells, whereas monospecific factors, such as erythropoietin and CSFs, act on more differentiated progenitor cells, such as erythroid and granulocyte-monocyte progenitor cells, respectively. Factors furnished by marrow microenvironment regulate early differentiation and proliferation of hematopoietic stem cells.

Maturation and delivery of blood cells

Undifferentiated blood cells are generally larger than mature forms, and they have large euchromatic nuclei with high nuclear-to-cytoplasmic (N:C) ratios. As blood cells mature, the size and N:C ratio gradually decrease, nucleoli disappear, and nuclear chromatin becomes more heterochromatic. Megakaryocytes are the exceptions; they become larger upon maturation.

Mature blood cells pass from the bone marrow through apertures in the sinus wall to enter the circulation. As blood cells mature, they move to the adventitial surface of vascular sinuses. Adventitial cells then move away from the wall and the basal lamina subsequently depolymerizes, thereby leaving endothelium as the only barrier to the sinus lumen. The ability to pass through the sinus wall depends on a variety of factors, including deformability of migratory cells and surface characteristics of the endothelial layer. The adventitial layer regulates the rate of cell delivery to circulation by the extent to which it covers the sinus wall and by its dynamic contractile nature. Migration of blood cells into the bloodstream is a selective process in which, under normal conditions, only mature cells are allowed to cross the sinus wall. In response to an increased demand for cell delivery to the bloodstream, however, immature cells may also be released.

Maturation of erythrocytes occurs next to the sinus wall. As erythroid cells mature to reticulocytes, they press against the sinus wall, thereby creating an aperture in the endothelial layer through which reticulocytes squeeze into the sinus lumen. Alternatively, reticulocytes may enter the sinus through existing apertures, created by earlier passages of cells. Granulocytes and monocytes are produced in clusters away from the sinus wall. As these cells mature, they become motile, deformable, and move toward vascular sinuses. They enter the circulation by crossing the sinus wall through newly formed apertures. Megakaryocytes lie against the sinus wall, where they either release their platelets directly into the bloodstream or send long cytoplasmic projections (proplatelets) through the sinus wall into the lumen; these proplatelets will subsequently break into platelets.

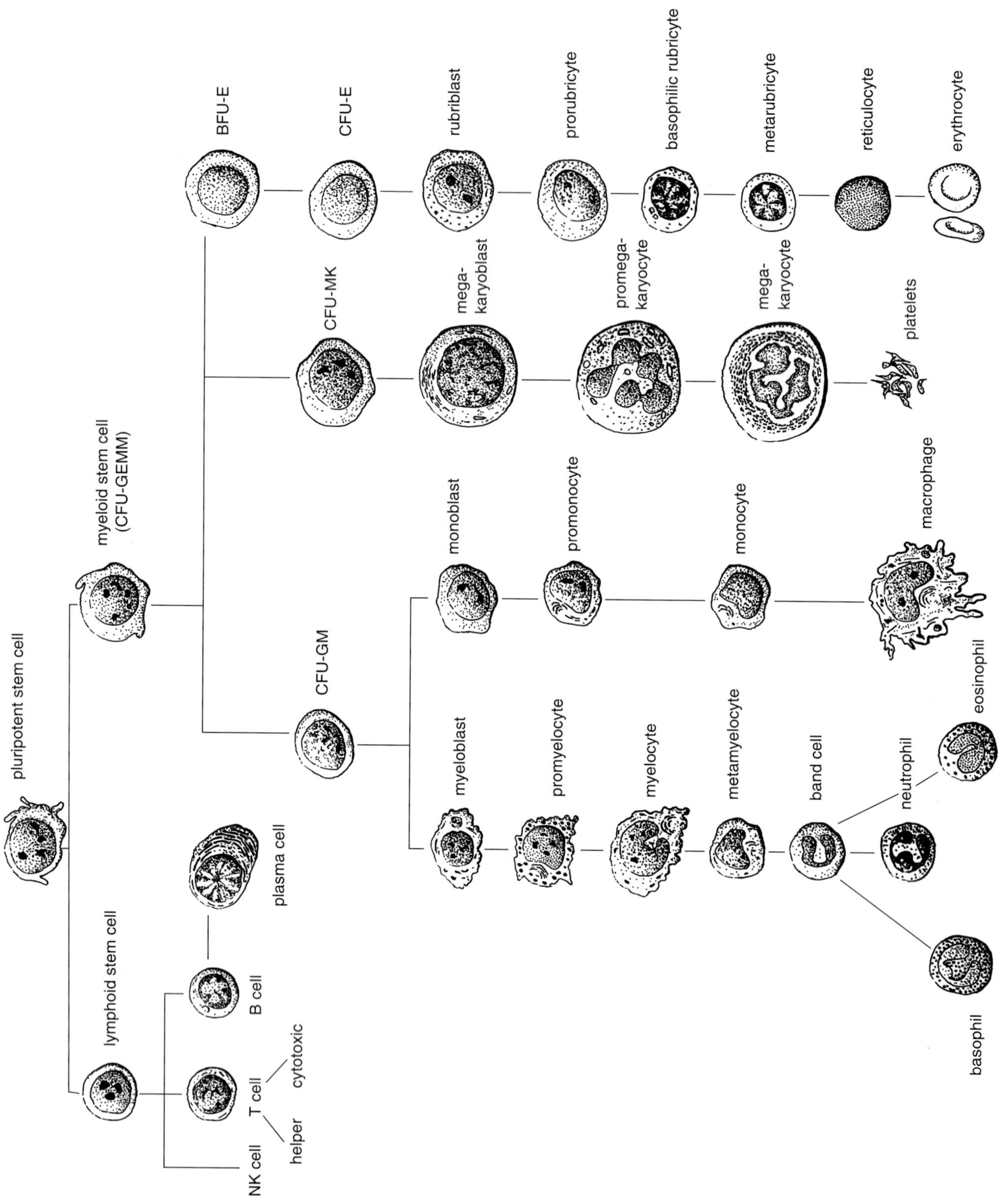

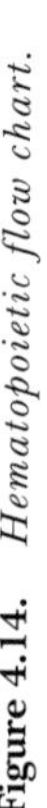

Figure 4.14. *Hematopoietic flow chart.*

ERYTHROPOIESIS

Erythropoiesis is defined as a developmental process that leads to the formation of mature erythrocytes. The mass of circulating erythrocytes and marrow erythropoietic tissue is called the **erythron**. In health, the erythron produces erythrocytes at a rate of about 1 million per second in a 15-kg dog. The daily production of erythrocytes equals the daily destruction of senescent erythrocytes. In response to an increased demand (e.g., anemia), erythrocyte production can be increased by sixfold to eightfold. In mammals, erythropoiesis begins with differentiation of multipotent stem cells (CFU-GEMM; colony-forming units granulocytic, erythrocytic, monocytic and megakaryocytic) into two morphologically unrecognizable erythroid progenitors: BFU-E (burst-forming unit erythroid) and its progeny, CFU-E (colony-forming unit erythroid). The CFU-E progenies produce morphologically identifiable erythroid precursors called rubriblasts (erythroblasts), which in turn differentiate to produce mature erythrocytes. Erythrocytic cells in marrow are organized into small anatomic units called **erythroblastic islands**. These islands occur next to vascular sinuses, and each consists of a central macrophage surrounded by one or two tiers of erythroid cells in various stages of maturation (Plate 4.II, Fig. 8). Cells of outer tiers are generally more mature than those of inner tiers. The cytoplasmic processes of the central macrophage extend between the surrounding erythroid cells (Fig. 4.12). As erythroid cells mature, they move along the macrophage processes toward the sinus wall.

Development of erythrocytic lineage

Maturation of rubriblasts to mature erythrocytes involves the following sequential stages: rubriblasts (erythroblasts), prorubricytes (proerythroblasts), basophilic rubricytes (basophilic erythroblasts), polychromatic rubricytes (polychromatic erythroblasts), normochromatic rubricytes, metarubricytes (orthochromatic erythroblasts), reticulocytes (polychromatophilic erythrocytes), and mature erythrocytes (Plate 4.II, Figs. 3, 4, and 9). Upon maturation, the cytoplasmic basophilia becomes progressively reduced as RNA is replaced by hemoglobin, the nucleus becomes smaller and loses its nucleoli, and the nuclear chromatin becomes progressively condensed.

The **rubriblast** is the largest cell of the erythrocytic series. It has a deep-blue cytoplasm and a spherical euchromatic nucleus (i.e., the nuclear chromatin is dispersed) with one to three nucleoli (Plate 4.II, Figs. 3 and 4). Rubriblasts are differentiated from myeloblasts by their spherical nuclei and deep cytoplasmic and nuclear staining, thus reflecting their higher RNA and deoxyribonucleic acid (DNA) content. The next maturation stage is **prorubricyte**, which is similar to the rubriblast, except for the absence of nucleoli. Condensation of nuclear chromatin begins at this stage. Mitotic division and progressive maturation of the prorubricyte lead to the formation of the **basophilic rubricyte**, which has a nucleus with clumped chromatin in a radial pattern and deep-blue cytoplasm (Plate 4.II, Figs. 3 and 4). Further division of the latter cell produces the **polychromatic rubricyte**, which has a dark condensed nucleus with prominent clumped chromatin and a grayish orange cytoplasm (Plate 4.II, Fig. 3). Usually at this stage of maturation, cytoplasmic hemoglobin level reaches a critical concentration (33 to 36% of the cell volume) and mitotic division stops. The next maturation stage is the **normochromatic rubricyte**, which has a dense nucleus and cytoplasm that is more reddish orange than the grayish orange of the **polychromatic rubricyte**. Further maturation produces the **metarubricyte**, the smallest nucleated erythrocyte (Plate 4.II, Figs. 4 and 9). The metarubricyte has a pyknotic nucleus and a slightly polychromatic to normochromatic cytoplasm, depending on the amount of hemoglobin present. Upon active extrusion of nucleus, the metarubricyte gives rise to the polychromatic erythrocyte (**reticulocyte**), which later matures to the erythrocyte.

Erythrocyte kinetics

Erythroid cells are divided into two main compartments: marrow erythroid precursors and reticulocytes, and circulating reticulocytes and erythrocytes. Development of rubriblasts to mature erythrocytes usually requires 5 to 7 days; however, in response to an increased demand for erythrocytes, the maturation time can be shortened to 3 to 5 days.

Newly formed reticulocytes normally undergo further maturation in the bone marrow for an additional 1 to 2 days before being released into the circulation. The released reticulocytes continue to mature further for 1 to 2 days in the spleen before becoming mature erythrocytes. Reticulocytes constitute up to 2% of circulating erythrocytes in most species. In health, horses and ruminants do not have circulating reticulocytes.

The life span of erythrocytes varies among animal species: 110 to 120 days in dogs, 66 to 79 days in cats, 160 days in cows, 86 days in pigs, and 140 to 150 days in horses and sheep. As erythrocytes age, changes in their surface membranes make them less deformable and mechanically more fragile. Senescent erythrocytes are sequestered and removed from the bloodstream by macrophages of the mononuclear phagocyte system, primarily in the spleen.

Regulation of erythropoiesis

Cellular and humoral growth factors are involved in the regulation of erythropoiesis. Macrophages and lymphocytes play an important role by stimulating the growth of both BFU-E and CFU-E progenitors. Differentiation of multipotent stem cells into BFU-E occurs under the influence of local diffusible growth factors, furnished by marrow microenvironment and a humoral growth factor known as burst-promoting activity (BPA). Erythropoietin is a fundamental growth factor for erythropoiesis. This glycoprotein is produced primarily by kidneys and has a molecular weight of 27,000 to 60,000. Erythropoietin plays a major role in differentiation of BFU-E to CFU-E, differentiation of CFU-E to rubriblasts, and all subsequent maturation stages.

GRANULOPOIESIS

Pluripotent stem cells differentiate and give rise to bipotent committed stem cells called CFU-GM. Progenies of CFU-GM undergo further differentiation and give rise to granulocytic and monocytic progenitor cells. Granulopoiesis usually occurs in clusters away from vascular sinuses in the midportion of the marrow hematopoietic compartment.

Development of neutrophils in marrow involves the following sequential stages: myeloblast, promyelocyte (progranulocyte), myelocyte, metamyelocyte, band neutrophil, and segmented neutrophil (granulocyte). As myeloblasts differentiate to form mature granulocytes, the cytoplasm becomes progressively granular and nuclei become condensed, flattened, indented, and segmented (Plate 4.II, Figs. 1, 2, and 9).

Development of granulocytic lineage

Morphologic changes associated with formation of all three granulocyte types (neutrophils, eosinophils, and basophils) are similar; therefore, the stages of development for these granulocytes are described together.

Myeloblasts are the earliest recognizable precursors of the granulocytic series and are derived from CFU-GM. Myeloblasts are ovoid or spherical cells, with spherical euchromatic nuclei containing three to five nucleoli. The cytoplasm is abundant and stains light blue, in contrast to the deeply basophilic cytoplasm of rubriblasts.

Promyelocytes are somewhat larger than myeloblasts but have similar nuclear features. The cytoplasm of promyelocytes is more abundant and stains lighter blue than that of myeloblasts (Plate 4.II, Figs. 1, 2, and 3). Promyelocytes also contain a variable number of large distinct azurophilic (peroxidase-positive) granules. Further maturation of promyelocytes produces **myelocytes**, which have spherical to slightly indented nuclei with some chromatin condensation and no nucleoli (Plate 4.II, Fig. 1). The cytoplasm of myelocytes stains pale blue and contains numerous specific (peroxidase-negative) (Plate 4.II, Fig. 9) and some azurophilic granules. Formation of azurophilic granules stops with the formation of specific granules; therefore, the number of azurophilic granules is reduced by half with each subsequent cell division. Production of specific granules, however, continues until **metamyelocyte** stage, during which division is no longer possible. The type of specific granules determines the type of granulocyte to be developed. Marrow myelocytes can be distinguished from lymphocytes by their abundant cytoplasm and lack of marked condensation of nuclear chromatin.

Myelocytes undergo nuclear transformation to form **metamyelocytes**, which have indented, kidney-shaped heterochromatic nuclei (Plate 4.II, Fig. 1). Specific granules of various granulocytes at the metamyelocyte stage have their characteristic colors. The next maturation stage is **band forms**, which result from further nuclear indentation, thereby forming C-, S-, or V-shaped nuclei with no definite constrictions (Plate 4.II, Figs. 1 and 2). The cytoplasm of band neutrophils is pale blue with pale (neutral) granules, as seen in mature neutrophils. **Mature granulocytes** have marked segmented heterochromatic lobular nuclei. Nuclei of mature eosinophils and basophils generally are less segmented (two to three lobes) than those of neutrophils (three to five lobes).

Granulocyte kinetics

Marrow granulocytic cells are divided into three compartments with no clear anatomic separation between them. These include **proliferative (mitotic)** compartment, consisting of myeloblasts, promyelocytes, and myelocytes; **maturative (postmitotic)** compartment, consisting of metamyelocytes and band neutrophils; and **reserve (storage)** compartment, consisting of predominantly mature neutrophils. The production time for granulocytes is approximately 5 to 7 days in most species. The size of the marrow neutrophil reserve is quite large, several times that of circulating neutrophils. The marrow reserve compartment provides neutrophils to blood and tissues during times of sudden demand. Mature neutrophils apparently leave the marrow randomly. Mechanisms controlling the release of neutrophils, however, are not well understood.

Blood neutrophils are divided into two pools: **circulating** and **marginating**. The marginating pool contains neutrophils marginating along capillary walls primarily in the lung and, to a lesser extent, in the liver and spleen. In most animal species, the two neutrophil pools are in dynamic equilibrium and together form the **total neutrophil** pool. In cats, the size of the marginating pool is approximately twice that of the circulating pool.

The two major sources of mature neutrophils that the body uses to meet the demand on short notice are the marrow reserve compartment and the blood marginating pool. Unlike erythrocytes, which normally stay in circulation throughout their life span, granulocytes are considered tissue cells. Once released from bone marrow, granulocytes circulate for 6 to 14 hours, then marginate along a blood-vessel wall, and subsequently migrate to tissues, where they function for an unknown period of time. The blood total neutrophil pool is replaced at least twice a day in most species.

Regulation of granulopoiesis

Under steady-state conditions, the rate of neutrophil production and release equals the rate of neutrophil removal from circulation. Early differentiation of pluripotent stem cells to committed (CFU-GM) progenitors is influenced by local growth factors furnished by the marrow microenvironment. Humoral growth factors known as CSFs play a major role in regulating the development of granulocytic precursors and in the formation of mature neutrophils. CSFs are produced by a variety of cells and tissues, including monocytes, macrophages, lymphocytes, fibroblasts, endothelial cells, placenta, and embryonic kidneys, spleen, and lung. Three major types of CSFs have been identified, each with a different molecular weight and functional specificity. CSFs stimulate granulopoiesis, whereas substances such as prostaglandins, produced by macrophages, and lactoferrin and chalones, produced by neutrophils, inhibit granulopoiesis.

The production and kinetics of eosinophils, basophils, and monocytes are similar to those of neutrophils. Basophils are rare in peripheral blood and bone marrow; they are more common in blood of ruminants and horses than in that of dogs and cats.

MONOCYTOPOIESIS

Monocytes, unlike granulocytes, retain their nucleoli as they mature, thus suggesting that mature monocytes are capable of synthesizing new granules. They enter the circulation as relatively immature cells and reach their full functional capacity only when they migrate into tissues and differentiate into macrophages.

LYMPHOPOIESIS

Lymphopoiesis is described in Chapter 8.

THROMBOPOIESIS

Development of megakaryocytic lineage

Progenies of pluripotent stem cells differentiate and give rise to unipotent stem cells called colony-forming units megakaryocyte (CFU-MK). CFU-MK give rise to **megakaryoblasts**, the earliest recognizable precursors of thrombocytes. Megakaryoblasts have relatively scant basophilic cytoplasm and large spherical or indented euchromatic nuclei with several distinct nucleoli (Plate 4.II, Fig. 5). Megakaryoblasts, in contrast to blasts of other blood cell lines, undergo endomitosis, i.e., the nucleus divides with no concurrent cytoplasmic division Endomitosis leads to production of a polyploid nucleus (nucleus with multiple connected lobes), an increase in size of the cell, and formation of abundant cytoplasmic demarcation membrane, which outlines platelet zones. The next maturation stage, the **promegakaryocyte**, has a multilobed nucleus, which often contains more than four lobes and a greater amount of cytoplasm. The cytoplasm is less basophilic and has a few azurophilic granules. Further maturation of promegakaryocytes leads to the formation of **megakaryocytes**. Megakaryocytes are not only the largest cell of the megakaryocytic series but are also the largest hematopoietic cells in marrow, measuring 40 to 100 μm in diameter (Plate 4.II, Fig. 6). The pleomorphic nucleus of megakaryocytes has two or more heterochromatic lobules and a few nucleoli, which are not readily visible. The abundant blue cytoplasm of megakaryocytes is rich in ribosomes and has numerous large azurophilic granules. The platelet demarcation membrane system is quite extensive at this stage.

Platelet kinetics

Platelets are produced by fragmentation of megakaryocytic cytoplasm along the demarcation membrane. Megakaryocytes usually lie against the sinus wall, where they either release their platelets directly into the bloodstream or extend their cytoplasmic projections (proplatelets) through the endothelial layer into the sinus lumen. Proplatelets have regular regional constrictions along their length that subsequently break, thereby releasing individual platelets into the circulation (Fig. 4.15).

The life span of circulating platelets is relatively short, 9 to 12 days, and is comparable among all domestic animal species. A large portion of circulating platelets is normally sequestered in the spleen. These stored platelets are in dynamic exchange with circulating platelets and can be rapidly mobilized and released into the bloodstream upon splenic contraction. Aged platelets are removed from the circulation by macrophages of the mononuclear phagocyte system primarily in the spleen and, to some extent, in the liver and bone marrow.

Regulation of thrombopoiesis

Differentiation of pluripotent stem cells to CFU-MK is influenced by local regulatory growth factors furnished by the marrow microenvironment and through cell-to-cell interaction. Differentiation of CFU-MK to megakaryoblasts is regulated by a specific growth factor called colony-stimulating factor megakaryocyte (CSF-Meg). A

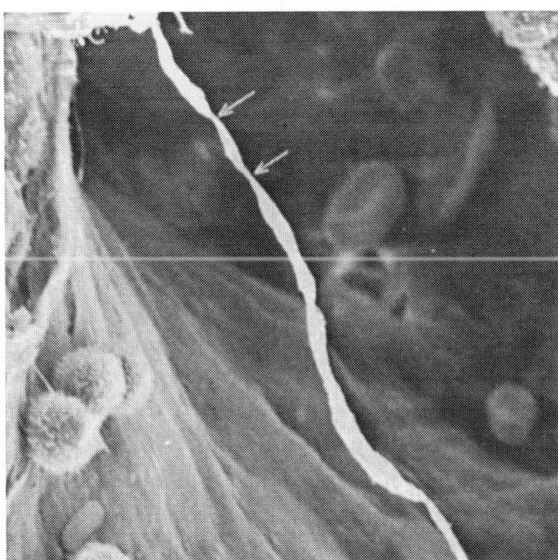

Figure 4.15. *Scanning electron micrograph of canine bone marrow. A long, slender proplatelet within the sinus lumen is shown. Individual platelets are shed by fragmentation of a proplatelet at the areas of intermittent constrictions (arrows).*

humoral factor known as thrombopoietin stimulates the maturation of megakaryocytes and influences the rate of platelet production and release. Megakaryocytopoiesis is regulated by the number of circulating platelets, which in health, is kept remarkably constant. The stimulatory influence of platelet number on megakaryocytopoiesis is mediated through thrombopoietin, which is produced primarily by the kidneys.

EVALUATION OF BONE MARROW

Evaluation of bone marrow is an adjunct to routine hematologic examination (complete blood-cell count) and is performed on a selective basis. It provides valuable information about the hematopoietic status of an individual animal and is recommended whenever a marrow disorder is suspected, e.g., lack of appropriate marrow response, nonregenerative anemia, persistent neutropenia, and/or production of abnormal cells. Bone marrow findings should be interpreted in the context of peripheral-blood findings. Therefore, both bone marrow and peripheral-blood evaluations should be performed simultaneously. Evaluation of bone marrow is performed on specimens collected by either aspiration or biopsy procedures. Although marrow aspiration is a more routine procedure and is widely used, the biopsy procedure is indicated whenever marrow topography, cellularity, and relative distribution of various blood-cell lines, particularly megakaryocytes, are to be evaluated.

Touch preparation should be made from all biopsy material, by gently rolling the specimen across a glass slide, before processing the specimen for histologic examination. Touch preparations are essential to determine cytologic details that are not visible in the usual histologic preparations. Decreased marrow cellularity is most easily recognized histologically, but the cell types affected are more easily determined in cytologic preparations. Aspirated marrow is discharged onto a glass slide for preparation of a film. Marrow films or touch preparations from a biopsy specimen are stained by one of the polychrome techniques, usually Wright s stain or Wright s stain followed by Giemsa stain. Paraffin-embedded bone marrow biopsy specimens are not ideal for assessment of various hematopoietic elements, especially the immature stages, because of processing artifacts such as tissue shrinkage. Techniques of embedding bone marrow in various plastics provide a superior means of evaluating 1- to 2-μm-thin sections for overall cellularity and cell types with high resolution and minimum artifacts. After the fixation and decalcification, marrow sections are stained with Giemsa, hematoxylin and eosin, or other histochemical and immunohistochemical procedures.

In evaluating the bone marrow, one should pay attention to the cellularity, cellular composition and distribution of various blood cell lines, and the myeloid:erythroid (M:E) ratio. Determination of M:E ratio is usually performed on bone marrow aspirate preparations. A positive identification of marrow precursor cells of various blood-cell lines, and of their characteristic maturation features, is challenging and requires experience. The M:E ratio is calculated by identifying 500 marrow nucleated cells and then by dividing the number of granulocytic cells by the number of erythrocytic cells. Although the term **myeloid** refers to all hematopoietic cells produced in marrow, in the context of the M:E ratio, myeloid refers only to cells of granulocytic series. The M:E ratio represents a relative value and should be interpreted in the context of peripheral-blood findings and bone-marrow cellularity. An M:E ratio of 1.0 indicates that erythrocytic and granulocytic precursors are present in equal numbers; a ratio of less than 1.0 indicates either that erythrocytic production exceeds granulopoiesis or that granulocytic series is hypoplastic. Conversely, an elevated M:E ratio of greater than 1.0 reflects granulocytic hyperplasia, erythroid hypoplasia, or a combination of the two.

AVIAN BLOOD AND BONE MARROW

Peripheral Blood

Birds, in contrast to mammals, have mature erythrocytes and thrombocytes (platelets) that are nucleated. Avian **erythrocytes** are typically elliptic and about 12 μm in length. They have elliptic central heterochromatic nuclei and orange—pink cytoplasm (Plate 4.I, Fig. 10). A few large young erythrocytes, which appear polychromatic in a Wright s-stained blood film, are often found in blood. The nuclei of these cells are less heterochromatic than those of mature erythrocytes. These polychromatic cells are reticulocytes, which can be identified positively with new methylene blue stain.

The cytologic/morphologic identification of various avian blood-cell types, particularly leukocytes, is challenging and requires practice. Avian **heterophils**, which are analogous to mammalian neutrophils, have segmented heterochromatic nuclei and red—orange cytoplasm with distinctive granules, which give them their name (Plate 4.I, Fig. 10). In birds, heterophils resemble eosinophils, as both cells have lobulated nuclei and granular cytoplasm. Although nuclear segmentation is more prominent in heterophils than in eosinophils, the nuclei are often masked by cytoplasmic granules. In normal birds, the most numerous segmented leukocytes with reddish granules are likely to be heterophils. **Basophils** have distinctive dark-blue granules and are readily distinguished from other leukocytes.

Identification of lymphocytes, monocytes, and thrombocytes in birds is also sometimes difficult. Both **small** and **large lymphocytes** are present in avian blood. Small lymphocytes have scant basophilic cytoplasm around their ovoid nuclei, whereas large lymphocytes have more cytoplasm that is less basophilic. Large lymphocytes resemble monocytes. A few large azurophilic granules are occasionally present within the cytoplasm of large lymphocytes. **Monocytes** are the largest of all leukocytes present in avian blood. They have pleomorphic nuclei, which may appear spherical, ovoid, elongated, or indented. Their cytoplasm is relatively abundant, foamy, and occasionally vacuolated with no visible granules (Plate 4.I, Fig. 11). **Thrombocytes** frequently have clear cytoplasm and few small reddish purple granules, which are more numerous than azurophilic granules present in large lymphocytes (Plate 4.I, Fig. 12).

Avian blood cells have functions similar to those of their mammalian counterparts. Erythrocytes transport oxygen and carbon dioxide to and from tissues; heterophils and monocytes are phagocytic and are important as a defense system against microbial infections; lymphocytes play a role in various immune functions; and thrombocytes play a role in hemostasis. Avian thrombocytes are also phagocytic, a feature that has not been observed in mammalian platelets.

Bone Marrow

Bone marrow erythropoiesis and thrombopoiesis in birds occur primarily inside the vascular sinuses, whereas granulopoiesis, as in mammals, takes place outside the vascular sinus. Fine-structural studies show that the sinus wall consists of elongated endothelial cells with discontinuous basement membranes. Intravascular erythrocytic precursors adhere to the sinus wall. As these cells mature and synthesize hemoglobin, they move away from the sinus wall toward the central area of the sinus lumen, where they are released into the bloodstream. The various maturation stages of erythrocytic and granulocytic cells are similar to those in mammals; however, the progressive condensation of nuclear chromatin is not as marked as that in mammals. The origin of thrombocytes in birds is unknown, as megakaryocytes are not found in avian bone marrow. Thrombocytes apparently develop intravascularly from cells that resemble erythrocytic precursors. Lymphocytic progenitors in birds, as in mammals, originate in bone marrow, from which they migrate to either the cloacal bursa or thymus, where they differentiate into B or T lymphocytes, respectively.

REFERENCES

Archer RK. Regulatory mechanisms in eosinophil leukocyte production, release, and distribution. In: Gordon AS, ed. Regulation of hematopoiesis. New York: Appleton Century-Crofts, 1970;2.

Arnalich F, Lahoz C, Zamorano AF, et al. Incidence and clinical significance of peripheral and bone marrow basophilia. J Med 1987;1:293.

Awadhiya RP, Vegad JL, Kolte GN. Demonstration of the phagocytic activity of chicken thrombocytes using colloidal carbon. Res Vet Sci 1980;29:120.

Bagby GC, Gigas VD, Bennett RM, et al. Interaction of lactoferrin, monocytes and T-lymphocyte subsets in the regulation of steady-state granulopoiesis in vitro. J Clin Invest 1981;68:56.

Baggionlini M. The enzymes of the granules of polymorphonuclear leukocytes and their functions. Enzyme 1972;13:132.

Bainton DF. Sequential degranulation of the two types of polymorphonuclear leukocyte granules during phagocytosis of microorganisms. J Cell Biol 1973;58:249.

Bass DA. The function of eosinophils. Ann Intern Med 1979;91:120.

Becker RP, De Bruyn PPH. The transmural passage of blood cells into myeloid sinusoids and the entry of platelets into the sinusoidal circulation; a scanning electron microscopic investigation. Am J Anat 1976;145:183.

Campbell F. Fine structure of the bone marrow of the chicken and pigeon. J Morphol 1967;123:405.

Chang CF, Hamilton PB. The thrombocyte as a primary phagocyte in chickens. J Reticuloendothelial Soc 1979;25:585.

Dein FJ. Avian clinical hematology. Proc Assoc Avian Vet 1982:5.

Deldar A, Lewis H, Bloom J. Electron microscopic study of the unique features and structural-morphologic relationship of canine bone marrow. Am J Vet Res 1989;50:136.

Denburg JA, Davison M, Bienenstock J. Basophil production. J Clin Invest 1980;65:390.

Deubelbeiss KA, Dancey JT, Harker LA, et al. Neutrophil kinetics in the dog. J Clin Invest 1975;55:833.

Dexter TM. Hematopoietic growth factors. Br Med Bull 1987;45:319.

Dvorak AM, Dvorak HF. The basophil: its morphology, biochemistry, motility, release reactions, recovery, and role in the inflammatory responses of IgE-mediated and cell-mediated origin. Arch Pathol Lab Med 1979;103:551.

Finch CA. Review: erythropoiesis, erythropoietin, and iron. Blood 1982;60:1241.

Gulati GL, Ashton JK, Hyun BH. Structure and function of the bone marrow and hematopoiesis. Hematol Oncol Clin North Am 1988;2:495.

Henry RL. Platelet function. Semin Thromb Hemostasis 1977;4:93.

Hodges RD. Normal avian (poultry) haematology. In: Archer RK, Jeffcott LB, eds. Comparative clinical haematology. Oxford: Blackwell Scientific Publications, 1977.

Huntley JF. Mast cells and basophils. A review of their heterogeneity and function. J Comp Pathol 1992;107:349.

Jain NC. Schalm s veterinary hematology. 4th ed. Philadelphia: Lea & Febiger, 1983.

Jones DG. The eosinophil: review article. J Comp Pathol 1993;108:317.

Lasser A. The mononuclear phagocytic system: a review. Hum Pathol 1983;14:108.

Lichtman MA. The ultrastructure of hemopoietic environment of the marrow: a review. Exp Hematol 1981;9:391.

Smith JE. Review: erythrocyte membrane; structure, function, and pathophysiology. Vet Pathol 1987;24:471.

Sorrel JM, Weiss L. Cell interactions between hematopoietic and stromal cells in the embryonic chick bone marrow. Anat Rec 1980;197:1.

Sun FF, Crittenen NJ, Czuk CI, et al. Biochemical and functional differences between eosinophils form animal species and man. J Leukocyte Biol 1991;50:140.

Tavassoli M. Marrow adipose cell, histochemical identification of labile and stable components. Arch Pathol Lab Med 1976;100:16.

Tavassoli M. Red cell delivery and the function of the marrow blood barrier: a review. Exp Hematol 1978;6:257.

Weisdorf DJ, Craddock PR, Jacob HS. Granulocytes utilizing different energy sources for movement and phagocytosis. Inflammation 1982;6:245.

Weiss L. The role of the spleen in the removal of normally aged red cells. Am J Anat 1962;111:175.

Weiss L. The structure of bone marrow. Functional interrelationships of vascular and hematopoietic compartments in experimental hemolytic anemia: an electron microscopic study. J Morphol 1965;117:467.

Weiss L, Chen LT. The organization of hematopoietic cords and vascular sinuses in bone marrow. Blood Cells 1975;1:617.

Williams N, Levine RF. The origin, development, and regulation of megakaryocytes. Br J Haematol 1982;52:173.

5

Muscular Tissue

JO ANN EURELL

MUSCULAR TISSUE

Muscular tissues contract to produce directed, organized movement. Cells of other tissue types are also capable of movement, but little integrated motion occurs. Only specialized collections of cells producing strong, concerted contraction, primarily in one direction, are categorized as muscle.

The specialized cells of muscular tissues have distinct morphologic characteristics directly related to their contractile activity. **Myocytes** are elongated cells with spindle-shaped, fiberlike profiles. Because of their shape, muscle cells are also referred to as **muscle fibers** or **myofibers**. The term **fiber** has a different meaning for muscle compared to connective tissue fibers, which are condensed extracellular substances rather than cells.

The myocytes are arranged in bundles with their long axes aligned parallel to the direction of their contractions. Within the cytoplasm of all myocytes are abundant fibrous proteins that stain intensely eosinophilic. The shape of the profiles of myocytes is dependent on the angle of sectioning. Myocytes sectioned parallel to their long axes appear as long rods or spindles, whereas those sectioned at right angles are polygonal. Oblique sectioning results in various elliptic profiles.

Muscular tissues are present in three principal areas of the vertebrate body: the walls of hollow organs (e.g., viscera of the gastrointestinal tract, urogenital tract, blood vessels), the skeletal muscles, and the heart. Microscopically, longitudinal sections of skeletal and cardiac muscular tissue have characteristic cross-striations, whereas the muscular tissue of hollow organs is composed of myocytes without cross-striations and hence has a smooth appearance. Therefore, three basic types of muscle fibers are recognized: *(a)* nonstriated **smooth muscle**, which forms the contractile portion of the walls of most viscera; *(b)* striated **skeletal muscle**, which comprises the skeletal muscles that originate and insert on the bones of the skeleton; and *(c)* striated **cardiac muscle**, which comprises the muscle of the walls of the heart. Skeletal muscle is considered to be voluntary in control, whereas cardiac and smooth muscle are involuntary.

SMOOTH MUSCLE

Light Microscopic Structure

Smooth muscle cells are elongated, spindle-shaped cells (Fig. 5.1A). Each cell contains a single, centrally located nucleus. The cells range from 5 to 20 μm in diameter and from 20 μm to 1 mm or more in length. The cytoplasm of smooth myocytes is acidophilic.

Within a tissue section, the cross-sectional size of cells is highly variable due to the tapered shape of the cells. Many cross sections of the cell lack nuclear profiles because of the extent of the cell beyond the central nuclear region (Fig. 5.1B).

Individual myocytes are surrounded by a fine network of reticular fibers, blood vessels, and nerves. In smooth muscle, reticular fibers are produced by myocytes rather than fibroblasts. Although the connective tissue is analogous to the endomysium of skeletal muscle described below, it is not termed as such.

Fine Structure

The cytoplasm of the smooth muscle myocyte contains numerous myofilaments in various orientations (Figs. 5.2 and 5.3). **Thin myofilaments** of smooth muscle contain **actin** and tropomyosin but lack troponin, which is present in skeletal muscle. **Thick myofilaments**, composed of **myosin-II**, are sparse. The thick and thin myofilaments are not arranged in a highly ordered pattern as in skeletal muscle, and various patterns have been proposed (Fig. 5.2). **Dense bodies** in the cytoplasm and the cell membrane serve as anchor sites for the myofilaments. **Intermediate filaments** further link the dense bodies into a meshwork array. The myofilament attachment sites on the cell membrane also form junctions that connect adjacent cells.

Numerous caveolae and vesicles are present along the cell membrane and are believed to play a role in calcium transport (Figs. 5.2 and 5.3). Transverse T tubules found in striated muscle are lacking and smooth endoplasmic reticulum is sparse. Gap junctions, which allow for cell coupling, occur at frequent periodic sites in the cell membrane. Other cell organelles, including mitochondria, Golgi apparatus, rough endoplasmic reticulum (rER), and free ribosomes, are located near the nucleus. Each myocyte is surrounded by a basal lamina, except at intercellular junctions.

Contraction

The contractile apparatus of smooth muscle is capable of greater shortening in length and more sustained contractions than that of striated muscle. Contraction is governed by the phosphorylation of the myosin-II molecule in contrast to striated muscle, which is regulated by a troponin–tropomyosin complex described below. A rise in cytosolic calcium leads to subsequent binding of the calcium to calmodulin. The calcium–calmodulin complex then interacts with myosin light-chain kinase, which initiates phosphorylation of myosin-II and interaction between the actin and myosin-II myofilaments. The overall process leading to actin–myosin interaction is slow, which results in slow contraction of smooth muscle compared with other muscle types.

The contraction of smooth muscle is involuntary in control. Innervation is both parasympathetic and sympathetic, and the effects of neural input on smooth muscle are variable. Unitary smooth muscle, found in the wall of visceral organs, behaves as a syncytium with cells that are extensively connected by gap junctions but sparsely innervated. In contrast, multiunit smooth muscle, found in the iris of the eye, is capable of precise contractions due to innervation of each individual myocyte. The multiunit myocytes lack gap junctions, therefore preventing networked communication between cells.

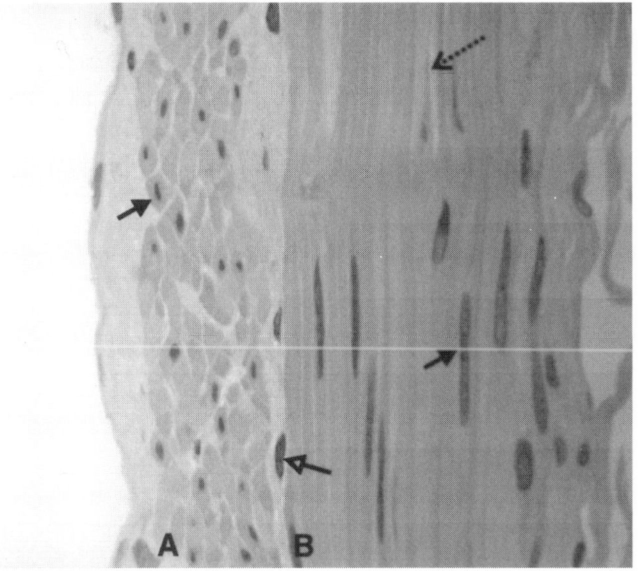

Figure 5.1. *Smooth muscle.* ***A****, Cross section.* ***B****, Longitudinal section. The central myocyte nuclei (solid arrows) are absent in several cross sections due to sectional geometry. The tip of a spindle-shaped cell is visible at the dotted arrow. Fibroblast nuclei (open arrow) are dark and smaller than smooth muscle nuclei. Hematoxylin and eosin (×490).*

Myogenesis, Hypertrophy, and Regeneration

Smooth muscle tissue increases in size by both hypertrophy (increase in size) and hyperplasia (increase in number) of myocytes. New smooth muscle cells can form through mitosis or by derivation from pericapillary mesenchymal cells. Formation of new myocytes is limited, so healing of smooth muscle primarily is through connective tissue scar formation.

SKELETAL MUSCLE

Light Microscopic Structure

Skeletal muscle myocytes are elongated cells that range from 10 to 110 μm in diameter and can reach up to 50 cm in length. These fibers are derived from the prenatal fusion of many individual mononuclear myoblasts. As a result of the fusion, a single myocyte contains multiple oval nuclei, which are peripherally located within the cell (Fig. 5.4). When viewed in longitudinal section, transverse striations are present as alternating light and dark bands. In transverse section, the myocyte has an angular outline and a stippled cytoplasm (Fig. 5.5). Peripheral nuclei may be absent in some planes of the cross section of the myocyte. The surrounding cell membrane is visible at higher magnification.

Each muscle cell contains **myofibrils**, which form the dots in cross sections of the fiber at the light microscopic level (Fig. 5.6). The myofibrils are cylindrical and 1 to 2 μm in diameter. Individual myofibrils are composed of thick and thin myofilaments, which are responsible for contraction. The myofibrils align in a longitudinal direction to create the light and dark banding pattern of the myocyte. Thick and thin myofilaments overlap in the darker **A band** (anisotropic), whereas

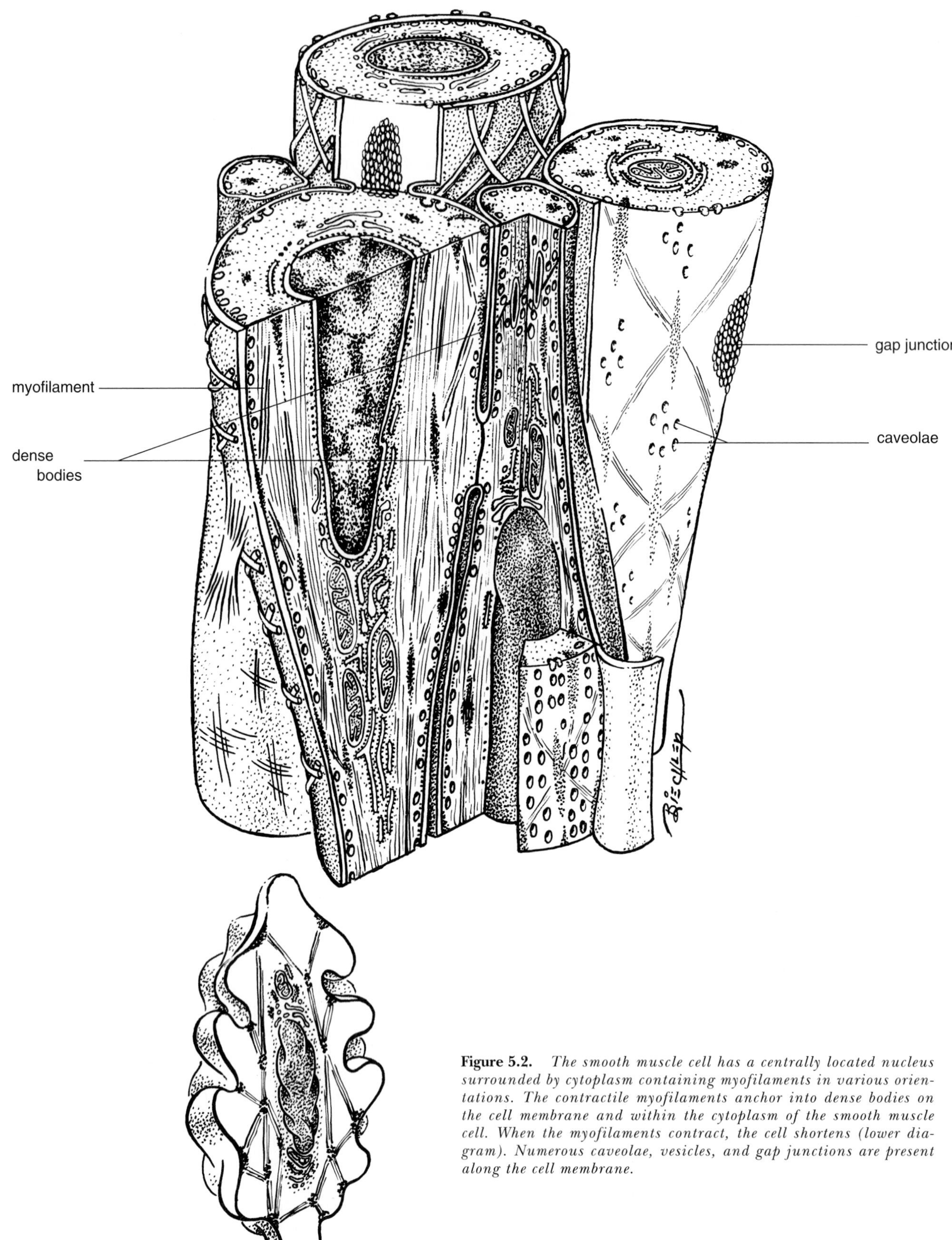

Figure 5.2. *The smooth muscle cell has a centrally located nucleus surrounded by cytoplasm containing myofilaments in various orientations. The contractile myofilaments anchor into dense bodies on the cell membrane and within the cytoplasm of the smooth muscle cell. When the myofilaments contract, the cell shortens (lower diagram). Numerous caveolae, vesicles, and gap junctions are present along the cell membrane.*

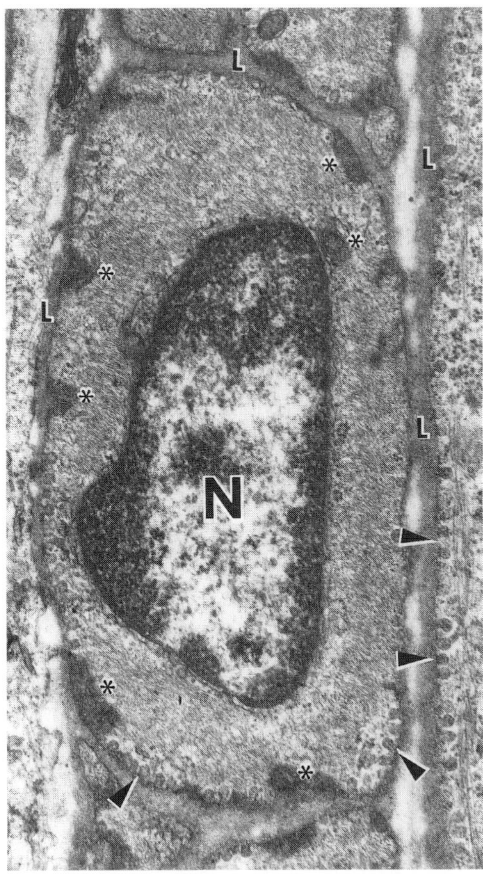

Figure 5.3. *Electron micrograph of a cross-sectioned smooth muscle cell. The nucleus (N) is centrally located, and the cytoplasm contains numerous myofilaments in various orientations. Electron dense bodies (*) serve as attachment sites for the myofilaments. Numerous caveolae (arrowheads) are present along the sarcolemma of an adjacent cell. The basal laminae (L) are visible between the two cells and appear fused at points (×23,900). (Courtesy of W.S. Tyler).*

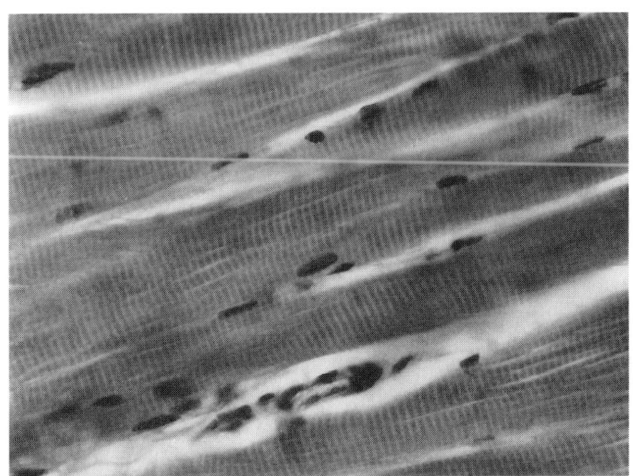

Figure 5.4. *Skeletal muscle, longitudinal section. Notice the cross-striations and the nuclei located in the periphery of the myocytes. Hematoxylin and eosin (×435).*

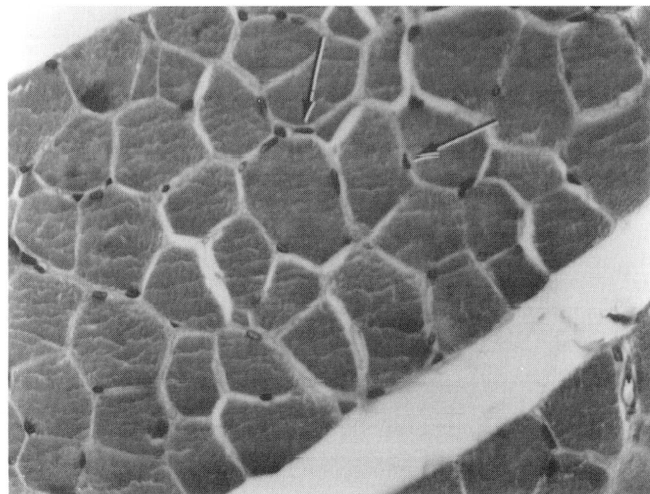

Figure 5.5. *Skeletal muscle, cross section. The nuclei in the sparse endomysium (arrows) belong to either fibroblasts or satellite cells. Hematoxylin and eosin (×435).*

only thin myofilaments are present in the lighter **I band** (isotropic).

Satellite cells are spindle-shaped cells located adjacent to the cell membrane of the myocyte and within its basement membrane. Their nuclei are heterochromatic in contrast to the lighter staining nuclei of the myocyte. Satellite cells may represent a population of inactive myoblasts, which can be activated upon injury to initiate regeneration of muscle fibers.

Individual myocytes are bound together into primary bundles or fascicles (Fig. 5.7). Within a fascicle, an individual myocyte is surrounded by a network of reticular fibers, the **endomysium**. An extensive capillary network and terminal nerve fibers are also present in the endomysium. Each fascicle is surrounded by dense irregular connective tissue, termed the **perimysium**. Supplying blood vessels and nerves plus muscle stretch receptors (muscle spindles) are also located in the perimysium. The muscle at the gross anatomic level is surrounded by a dense irregular connective tissue capsule, the **epimysium**. The connective tissues of skeletal muscle are interconnected and provide a means by which contractile forces are transmitted to other tissues.

Fine Structure

Contractile myofilaments of skeletal muscle cells are primarily actin or myosin-II. In addition, the myofilaments contain other proteins involved in either binding the primary filaments together (e.g., actinins, M-line proteins) or regulating the actin and myosin-II interaction (e.g., tropomyosin, troponin).

Thin myofilaments of skeletal muscle are composed of actin, troponin, and tropomyosin (Fig. 5.8). Globular molecules (G-actin) within the myoblast polymerize to form filamentous strands (F-actin). Two filamentous strands twist together to form a double helix, which contains binding sites for myosin-II. Filamentous

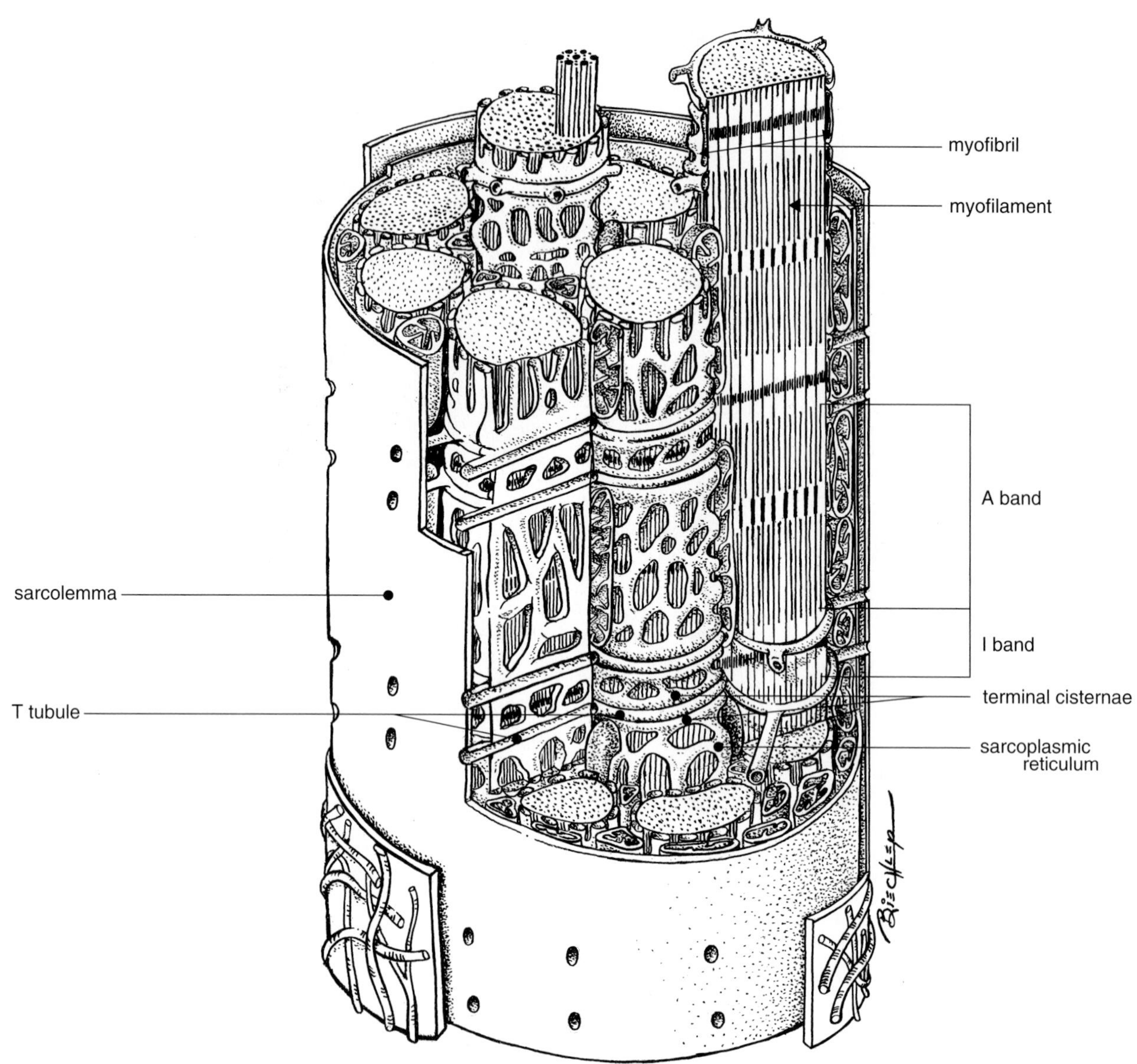

Figure 5.6. *The myofibrils of skeletal muscle are surrounded by sarcoplasmic reticulum. T tubules extend into the sarcoplasm from the sarcolemma and surround the myofibrils at the A–I junction.*

tropomyosin molecules lie in the groove between the two twisted strands of F-actin. The tropomyosin covers the myosin-II binding sites on the actin filament. In addition, triple globular units of **troponin** are spaced at regular intervals along the tropomyosin. Troponin binds to actin and inhibits actin–myosin interaction. When calcium increases, the troponin complex allows tropomyosin to move and myosin-II to bind to actin.

Thick myofilaments are composed of myosin-II, formed by two heavy chains and four light chains of amino acids. The two heavy chains twist together to form a rodlike tail with two protruding globular heads. Two light chains are associated with each head. The heads have binding sites for actin and for adenosine triphosphate (ATP). In addition, they have adenosine triphosphatase (ATPase) activity.

The myofilaments are arranged to form the light and dark banding pattern visible in a longitudinal section of the myofibril (Fig. 5.9). Adjacent thick myofilaments and overlapping thin myofilaments form the A band. Thin myofilaments do not extend to the center of the A band, leaving a more lucent region known as the **H band**. The thick myofilaments are interconnected down the center of the H band by an **M line**. The M line contains creatine kinase, which helps maintain levels of ATP for contraction. The **pseudo-H zone** is present on either side of the M line. In this region, thick myofilaments lack protruding cross-bridges and the area appears more electron lucent.

In a cross section of the myofibril within the A-band region, groups of six thin myofilaments surround one thick myofilament to form a hexagonal lattice. The myofilaments are linked to each other by myosin-II cross-

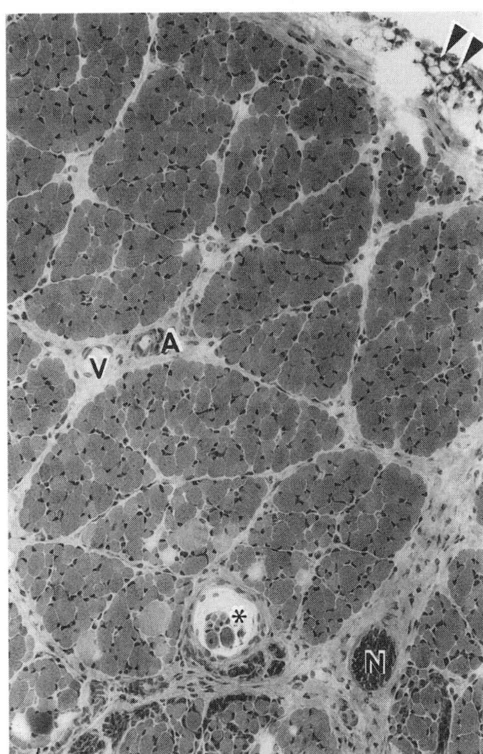

Figure 5.7. *The myofibers are organized into fascicles (bundles) and separated from other fascicles by perimysium. Within the larger divisions of the perimysium, notice the arteriole (A), venule (V), intramuscular nerve branch (N), and muscle spindle (*). At the margin of the section is a portion of the epimysium (arrowheads) (×125).*

bridges (side arms that protrude from the filaments) in the A band except in the pseudo-H zone, where cross-bridges are absent.

The I band is composed of the portion of the thin filaments that do not extend into the A band. These thin myofilaments are interconnected in the center of the I band by a **Z line** composed of α-actinin. A **sarcomere** extends from one Z line to the next and represents the repeating unit of myofilament arrangement within the myofibril.

Several structural proteins that link the contractile myofilaments are found within skeletal muscle. Spring-like **titin** anchors the end of myosin-II filaments to the Z line and helps maintain the A band width when muscle is stretched. **Nebulin** is associated with actin and may regulate the assembly and length of actin filaments. **Desmin** links adjacent myofilaments together side by side, whereas **spectrin** and **dystrophin** connect the myofilament system to the surface membrane of the myocyte.

The **sarcolemma**, another term for the cell membrane of the myocyte, invaginates to form a tubular network, the **T tubule** (Figs. 5.6 and 5.10). Within the sarcoplasm (cytoplasm of the myocyte), individual myofibrils are surrounded by **sarcoplasmic reticulum**, which is a highly specialized smooth endoplasmic reticulum. The sarcoplasmic reticulum forms an anastomosing network of tubules around the myofibrils and dilates to create **terminal cisternae** at the A–I band junction. The T tubule courses adjacent to the two terminal cisternae and the three structures collectively form a **triad**. Mitochondria and glycogen granules are located in the cytoplasm between the myofibrils and provide energy during muscle contraction.

Contraction

A **motor unit** is composed of a nerve fiber and the muscle cells it innervates. One nerve fiber may innervate multiple myocytes. The axon contacts the skeletal muscle fiber and branches to form a **motor end plate** on the surface of the myocyte. When stimulated, an action potential travels down the axon and causes release of

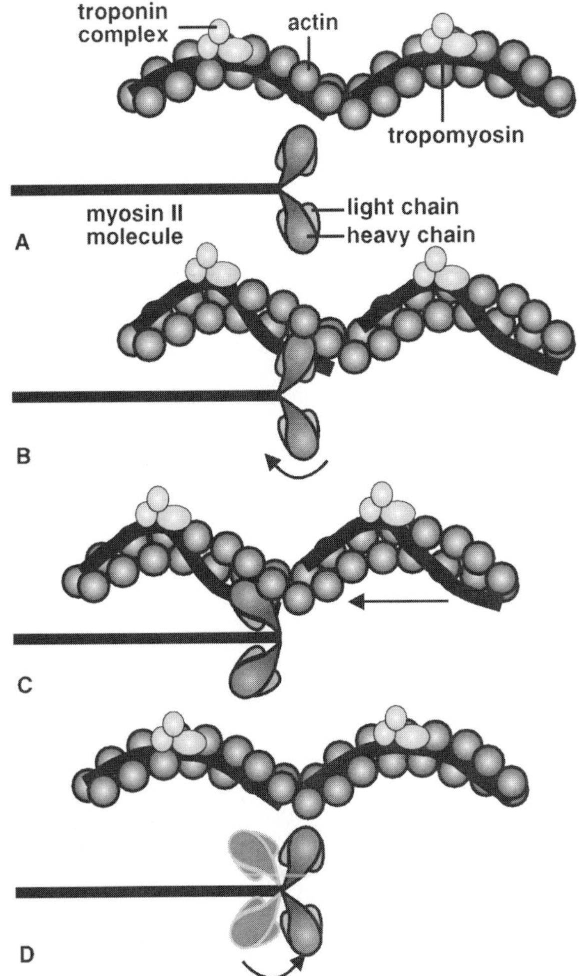

Figure 5.8. *Schematic representation of a thin myofilament (actin, troponin, tropomyosin) and a myosin-II molecule. Several myosin-II molecules aggregate to form a thick myofilament.* ***A.****, The muscle is relaxed; actin and myosin-II are not linked.* ***B.****, As contraction begins, the troponin–tropomyosin complex moves off the actin binding site and allows myosin-II to bind. The myosin-II head then bends.* ***C.****, The thin myofilament is pulled toward the center of the sarcomere (to the left in this drawing).* ***D.****, The actin–myosin complex then dissociates, troponin–tropomyosin covers the actin binding site, and the myosin head swings forward to repeat the cycle.*

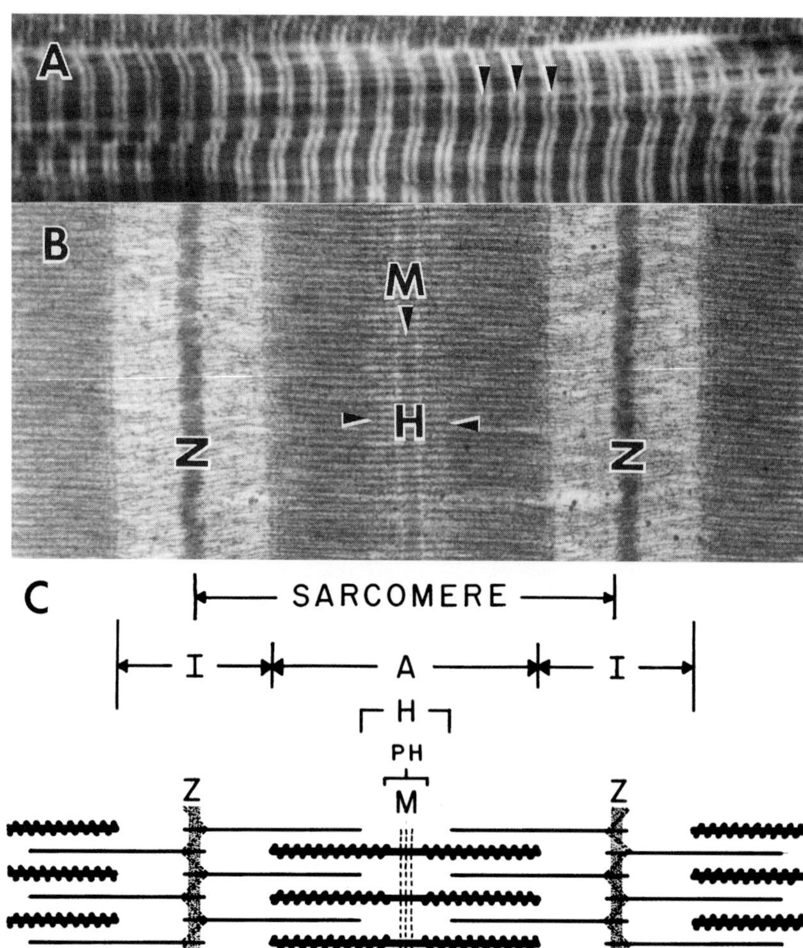

Figure 5.9. *Light micrograph (**A**) and electron micrograph (**B**) of longitudinally oriented skeletal muscle and schematic representation (**C**) of a sarcomere. In **A**, transverse striations consisting of alternating light bands (I bands) and dark bands (A bands) are present. Each I band is bisected by a Z line (arrowheads) (×1150). In **B**, the transverse striations can be further resolved into Z lines (Z) that define a sarcomere and bisect the light I band (not labeled). The A band is electron dense and is bisected by the M line (M, arrowhead), which connects adjacent thick myofilaments. On either side of the M line, an electron-lucent area represents the H band (H) where there is no overlap of thick and thin myofilaments (×22,500). In **C**, the arrangement of myofilaments is shown in relation to the electron micrograph. PH is the pseudo-H zone, a more electron-lucent region in which thick myofilaments lack cross-bridges. The bottom diagram represents a cross section of the region indicated by the arrows. Large dots represent thick myofilaments and small dots represent thin myofilaments.*

acetylcholine from the axon terminal into the synaptic cleft adjacent to the muscle fiber. Acetylcholine binds to receptors on the cell membrane and opens receptor-gated sodium channels into the myocyte. Sodium influxes into the muscle fiber and initiates a wave of depolarization that spreads across the cell membrane.

In the resting state before depolarization of the cell membrane, the tropomyosin–troponin complex covers the myosin-II binding sites on the actin filament. Myosin-II heads are bound to ATP. As depolarization begins, an action potential spreads across the cell membrane and extends into the T tubules. The depolarization causes the adjacent sarcoplasmic reticulum to release its stored calcium into the cytoplasm around the myofibrils. The calcium binds to troponin on the thin myofilaments, causing the troponin to undergo a conformation change. The change in troponin results in the movement of tropomyosin to expose the myosin-II binding sites. Actin and myosin-II interact, allowing the increased hydrolysis of ATP. Energy from the ATP hydrolysis is used to bend the head of the myosin-II complex. The movement of the head pulls the attached actin toward the center of the sarcomere, thus shortening the sarcomere and contracting the myocyte overall. The myosin-II head binds to a new ATP and then detaches from the actin filament and the cycle repeats. If ATP is depleted, the filaments cannot detach and rigor mortis sets in. After depolarization ends, the sarcoplasmic reticulum actively transports calcium back into the terminal cisternae and contraction ceases.

Classification of Skeletal Muscle Fibers

Skeletal muscle fibers can be classified as **red**, **white**, or **intermediate** based on gross anatomic appearance and physiologic principles of contraction. Red muscle fibers are smaller than white fibers and have a more extensive blood supply. The red fibers contain large amounts of myoglobin, which contributes to their red color. The fibers have extensive mitochondria, which are densely packed under the sarcolemma and between myofibrils. This type of skeletal muscle fiber depends on the oxidative pathway for energy production. Most red muscle fibers contract and fatigue slowly and are termed slow-twitch fibers; however, some fast-twitch red fibers do exist. In contrast to red muscle fibers, white muscle fibers are larger and have a less extensive blood supply. Fewer mitochondria are present, often clustering as pairs between myofibrils near the I bands. The sarcoplasmic reticulum is more extensive, allowing for rapid release of calcium to initiate contraction. The energy for white muscle fiber contraction is primarily from anaerobic glycolysis. White muscle fibers contract and fatigue more rapidly compared with red muscle fibers and are known as fast-twitch fibers. Intermediate muscle fibers have characteristics of both red and white fibers.

Within individual muscles, variable distribution of fiber types occurs. The fiber types are identified by using antibodies against either fast- or slow-twitch myosin isotypes.

Myogenesis, Hypertrophy, Atrophy, and Regeneration

During development, mesenchymal cells differentiate into skeletal muscle myoblasts. Myoblasts may migrate to remote locations from their original site of development. As development progresses, multiple myoblasts fuse and form elongated myotubes. Within the myotube, contractile myofibrils are formed. As additional myoblasts fuse to the developing myocyte and myofibrils increase in number, the nuclei peripheralize within the cell. Satellite cells remain as potential myogenic cells within the basal lamina next to the mature myocyte.

Hypertrophy of mature muscle cells occurs through the activity of satellite cells. One satellite cell divides into two daughter cells. One daughter cell remains as a satellite cell, whereas the other fuses with the muscle cell and adds additional nuclei. The new nuclei direct the synthesis of additional myofibrils and other cytoplasmic elements. Neither the myocyte nor its nuclei divide during the process of hypertrophy. In contrast, during atrophy of skeletal muscle, myofibrils and nuclei are lost.

Regeneration of muscle is dependent on the extent of injury. Small areas of muscle can be regenerated through fusion of satellite cells with each other to form new muscle cells or fusion with existing muscle cells. If damage is extensive, muscle is replaced by connective tissue instead.

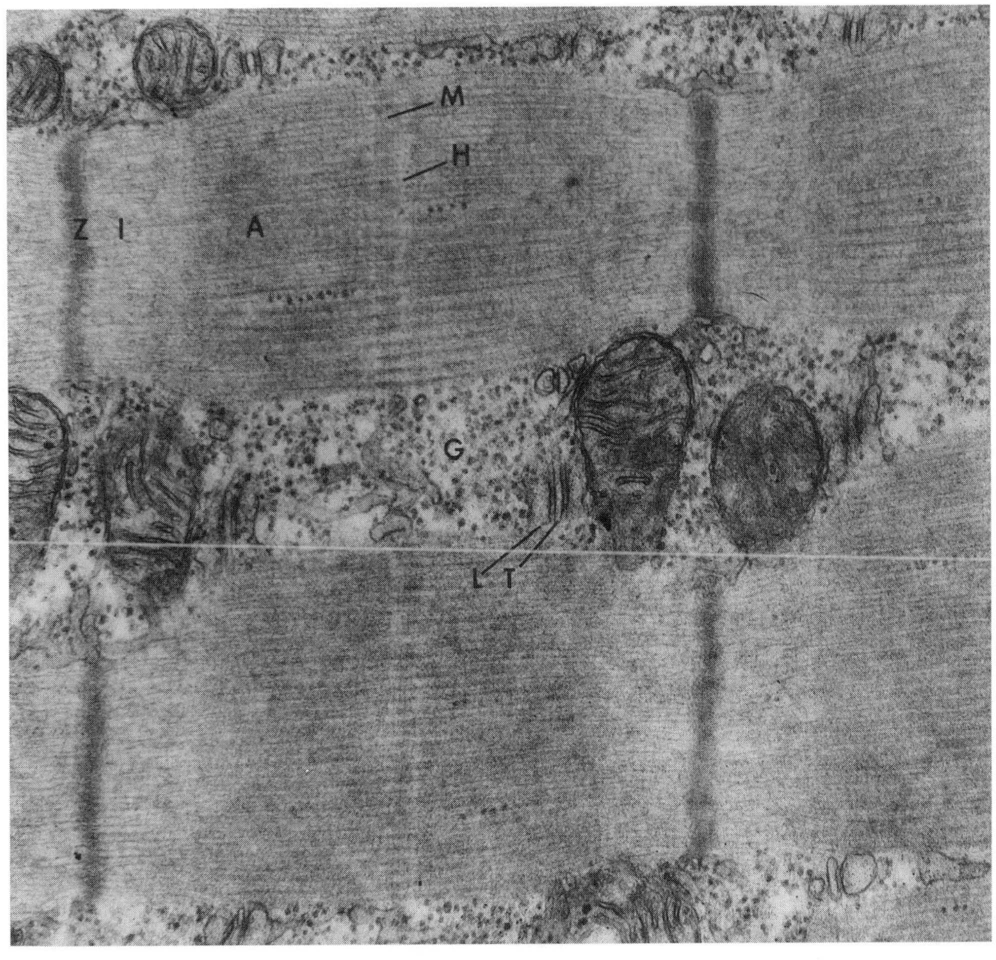

Figure 5.10. *Electron micrograph of a longitudinal section through a skeletal muscle cell. Structures identified include: A band (A); I band (I); Z line (Z); M line (M); pseudo-H band (H); glycogen (G) within the cytoplasm adjacent to mitochondria; terminal cisternae of sarcoplasmic reticulum (L); T tubule (T); and other triads (*) located at the A–I junction (×34,000).*

CARDIAC MUSCLE

Light Microscopic Structure

The striated myocytes of cardiac muscle branch and anastomose (Fig. 5.11). At the end-to-end junction of adjacent cells, dense **intercalated disks** are present. Cardiac myocytes are approximately 15 μm in diameter and 85 to 100 μm in length. The single nuclei of cardiac muscle cells are located in the center of the cell and the cytoplasm is acidophilic.

A network of fine reticular and collagenous fibers surrounds each cardiac muscle fiber. The network corresponds to endomysium of skeletal muscle but is more irregular. In the heart, cardiac myocytes are subdivided into groups by more dense connective tissue analogous to the perimysium of skeletal muscle. No tissue that corresponds to skeletal muscle epimysium is present. Individual cardiac myocytes are surrounded by a dense capillary network.

Fine Structure

Cardiac myocytes have myofibrils similar to skeletal muscle (Fig. 5.12). The same banding pattern of myofilaments is present. T tubules, located at the Z line, are larger than in skeletal muscle (Fig. 5.13). The sarcoplasmic reticulum is usually present on one side of the T tubule, forming a diad instead of a triad as found in skeletal muscle.

The mitochondria of cardiac myocytes are larger and more numerous than in skeletal muscle, indicating the degree of aerobic metabolism that occurs in this tissue (Fig. 5.13). The cytoplasm also contains lipid droplets and glycogen.

The intercalated disk is the means by which cells are mechanically and electrically linked (Figs. 5.12 and 5.14). The disk is formed by junctions between laterally adjacent cells (lateral region) and continues between cells that are in contact end to end (transverse region). The lateral region of the disk contains gap junctions, which allow transfer of chemical signals between adjacent cells. Desmosomes and fasciae adherentes are present in the transverse region of the disk. The desmosomes have intermediate filaments that extend into the cytoplasm and result in strong attachment between cells. Actin filaments of the myofibrils anchor into the fasciae adherentes, which in turn provide a junction between adjacent cells.

Atrial myocytes are smaller and have fewer T tubules than myocytes of the ventricle. In addition, atrial cardiac muscle has membrane-bounded dense granules in the cytoplasm that contain **atrial natriuretic peptides** (ANPs). ANPs stimulate the inner medullary collecting ducts of the kidney to excrete sodium (natriuresis) and water (diuresis). The peptides also cause smooth muscle in blood vessels' walls to relax.

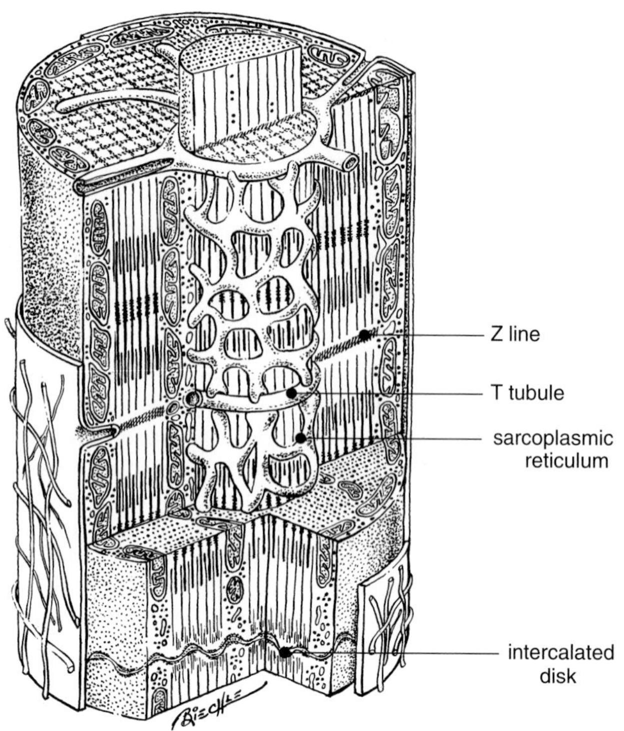

Figure 5.12. *The T tubules of cardiac muscle are located at the Z line. Sarcoplasmic reticulum surrounds the myofibrils and contacts the T tubules. The ends of the adjacent muscle fibers are joined by an intercalated disk.*

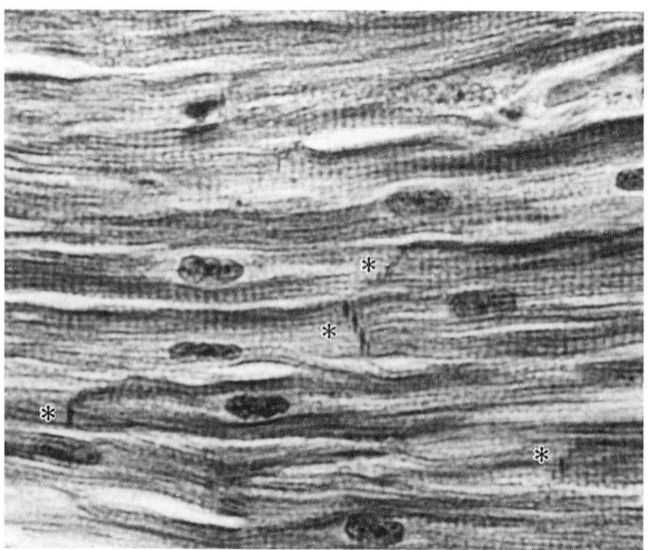

Figure 5.11. *Cardiac myocytes in longitudinal section. Notice the transverse striations and branching of the myocytes, the central location of their nuclei, and the dark-stained intercalated disks (*) (×690).*

Cardiac Impulse Conduction Fibers

Cardiac muscle contains specialized **impulse conduction fibers** (Purkinje fibers), which are modified cardiac myocytes (Fig. 5.15). The largest cells form the atrioventricular bundle. The conduction fibers have more cytoplasm and fewer myofibrils than cardiac myocytes, accounting for their large size and light staining cytoplasm.

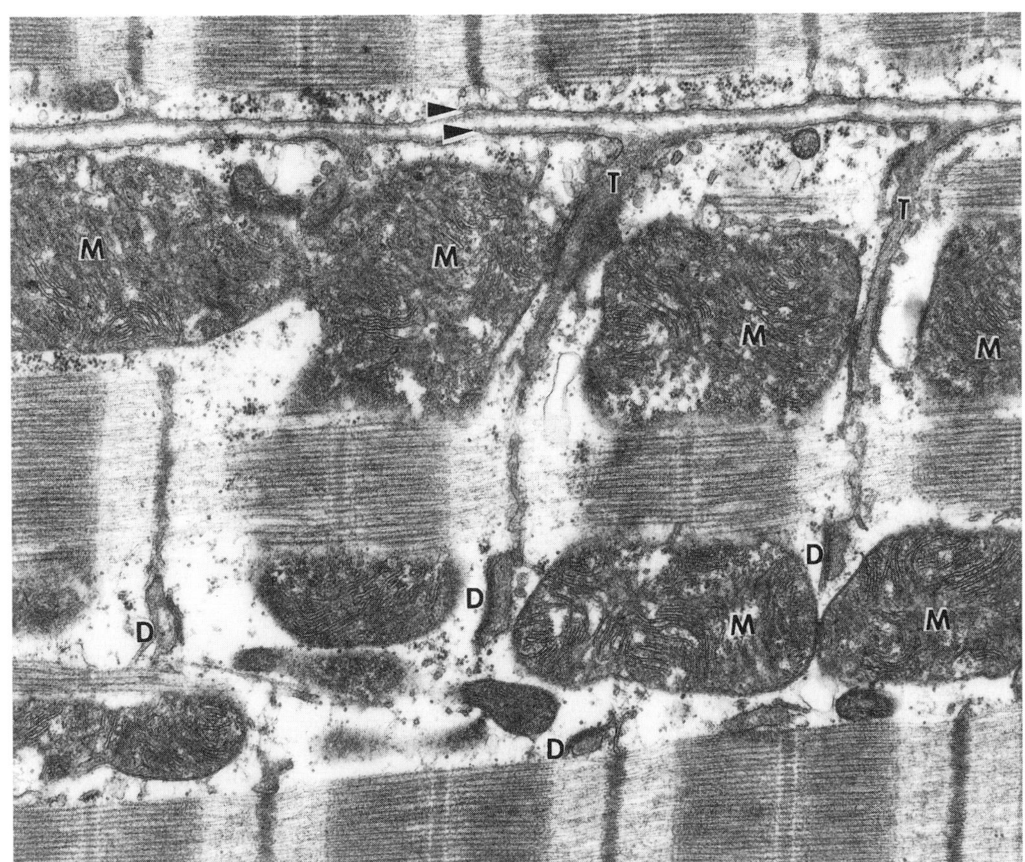

Figure 5.13. *Electron micrograph of a longitudinal section of cardiac muscle. The sarcolemma and basement membrane of each myocyte are indicated with arrowheads. Large mitochondria (M) with densely packed cristae are located just below the sarcolemma. Notice the two large T tubules (T) entering the lower myocyte at the Z lines. Diads (D) composed of a T tubule and sarcoplasmic reticulum are present deeper in the cell between the myofibrils (×22,500). (Courtesy of W.S. Tyler.)*

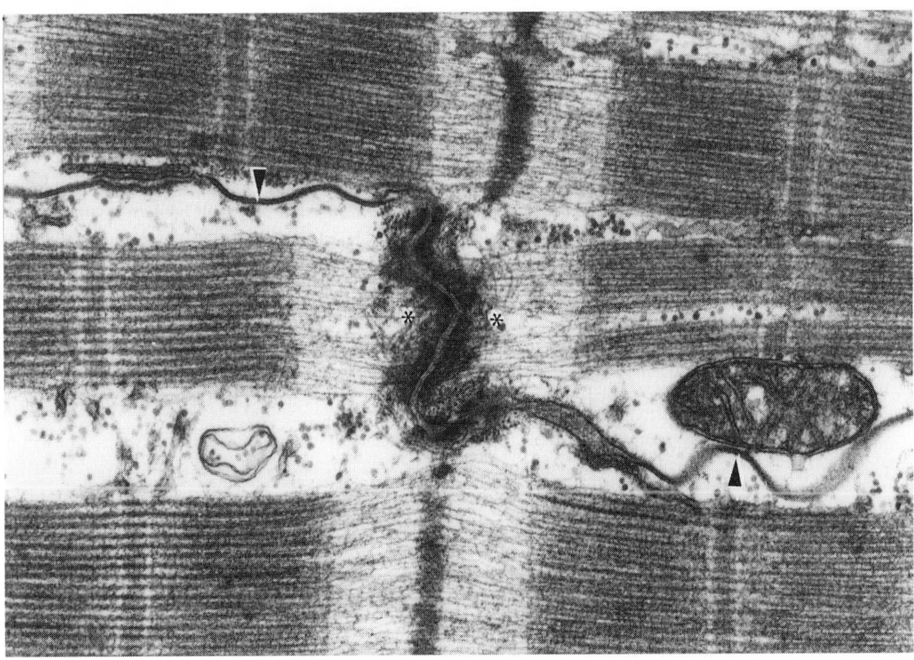

Figure 5.14. *Electron micrograph of an intercalated disk from cardiac muscle. The fascia adherens junction (*) is oriented transversely to the long axis of the myofibril. Gap junctions (arrowheads) are oriented parallel to the long axis (×42,100). (Courtesy of W.S. Tyler.)*

A large, pale area near the nucleus represents the storage site of glycogen, which is removed during tissue processing. The cells stain positively for acetylcholinesterase, which relates to their conductive function. At the ultrastructural level, the cells have mitochondria and sarcoplasmic reticulum but lack T tubules.

Contraction

Cardiac muscle is stimulated to contract by a mechanism similar to skeletal muscle. An action potential triggers the release of calcium from the sarcoplasmic reticulum. Contraction is activated through the interaction

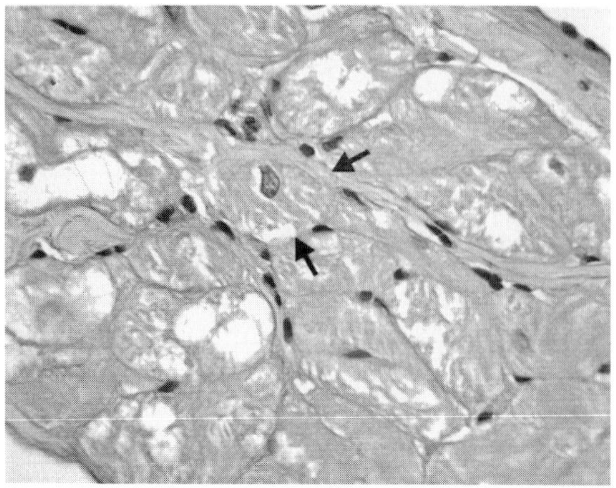

Figure 5.15. *Cardiac impulse-conducting fibers (one is outlined by arrows) are larger than myocytes. They have a centrally located nucleus and sparse myofibrils in their cytoplasm. Hematoxylin and eosin (×335).*

of actin and myosin myofilaments. Sequential contraction of heart chambers is stimulated by the orderly spread of the action potentials via gap junctions in the intercalated disks. The number, size, and distribution of the gap junctions plus the type of connexin (the structural protein of the gap junctions) influences the rate of impulse conduction.

Myogenesis, Hypertrophy, and Regeneration

Cardiac muscle develops from splanchnic mesoderm surrounding the endocardial heart tube. The fibers arise by differentiation and growth of single cells. As the cells grow, new myofilaments form. The ability of cardiac muscle to divide is lost soon after birth. Enlargement of the heart wall during exercise or cardiac insufficiencies is primarily through hypertrophy rather than hyperplasia. Damage to a section of the heart wall, with the resulting death of that section, is repaired primarily by proliferation of connective tissue rather than by regeneration of any significant number of new cardiac myocytes. However, the potential for cell proliferation does exist because cardiac muscle cells grown in tissue culture do grow and proliferate.

REFERENCES

Alberts B, Bray D, Lewis J, et al. Molecular biology of the cell. 3rd ed. New York: Garland Publishing, 1994.

Cardinet GH III, Leong DL, Means PS. Myocyte differentiation in normal and hypotrophied canine pectineal muscles. Muscle Nerve 1982;5:665.

Cardinet GH III, Orvis JA. Skeletal muscle function. In: Kaneko J, ed. Clinical biochemistry of domestic animals. New York: Academic Press, 1980.

Dellmann H-D, Carithers JR. Cytology and microscopic anatomy. Baltimore: Williams & Wilkins, 1996.

Ebashi S. Excitation-contraction coupling. Ann Rev Physiol 1976;36:293.

Guyton AC, Hall JE. Textbook of medical physiology. Philadelphia: WB Saunders, 1996.

Horowitz A, Menice CB, Laporte R, et al. Mechanisms of smooth muscle contraction. Physiol Rev 1996;76:967.

Huxley HE. Electron microscopy studies of the structure of natural and synthetic protein filaments from striated muscle. J Mol Biol 1963;7:281.

Huxley HE. The structural basis of contraction and regulation in skeletal muscle. In: Heilmeyer LMG, Rüegg JC, Wieland T, ed. Molecular basis of motility. New York: Springer-Verlag, 1976.

Jones DA, Round JM. Skeletal muscle in health and disease. New York: Manchester University Press, 1990.

Pardo JV, D'Angelo Siliciano J, Craig SW. A vinculin-containing cortical lattice in skeletal muscle: transverse lattice elements ("costameres") mark sites of attachment between myofibrils and sarcolemma. Proc Natl Acad Sci U S A 1983;80:1008.

Peachey LD, ed. Handbook of physiology. Section 10: skeletal muscle. Bethesda, MD: American Physiological Society, 1983.

Severs NJ. Cardiac muscle cell interaction: from microanatomy to the molecular make-up of the gap junction. Histol Histopathol 1995;10:481.

Tokuyasu KT, Dutton AH, Singer SJ. Immunoelectron microscopic studies of desmin (skeleton) localization and intermediate filament organization in chicken cardiac muscle. J Cell Biol 1983;96:1736.

Wang K, Ramirez-Mitchell R. A network of transverse and longitudinal intermediate filaments is associated with sarcomeres of adult vertebrate skeletal muscle. J Cell Biol 1983;96:562.

6

Nervous Tissue

THOMAS F. FLETCHER

Nervous tissue parenchyma consists of **neurons** and supportive cells called **neuroglia**. Nervous tissue forms the nervous system, which may be divided into the central nervous system and the peripheral nervous system.

The **central nervous system** (CNS) includes the brain and spinal cord. The **peripheral nervous system** (PNS) consists of cranial and spinal nerves, including associated nerve roots and ganglia. Nerves and ganglia that innervate viscera are designated the **autonomic nervous system**.

Meninges are tissue layers that surround the CNS and the roots of peripheral nerves. Cerebrospinal fluid is present in a space within meninges and inside cavities within the brain and spinal cord.

NEURONS

Neurons are the structural and functional units of the nervous system. They are also trophic units because often they transform and sustain what they innervate. With the exception of olfactory receptor cells, neurons are typically incapable of mitosis. Each neuron must last a lifetime.

Morphologically, neurons feature elongated processes that extend variable distances from the cell body (perikaryon). Neuronal processes usually consist of one axon and multiple dendrites per neuron (Fig. 6.1). Metabolically, neurons are actively involved in maintaining their structural integrity and in synthesizing, packaging, transporting, and releasing secretory products.

Neurons specialize in excitability and they communicate by releasing chemical agents (neurotransmitters, neuromodulators, or neurohormones). Excitation involves ions passing through protein channels embedded in neuronal plasma membrane that otherwise acts as a hydrophobic barrier to ion flow. Via chemical secretion, neurons transmit excitation to other neurons or to muscle or gland.

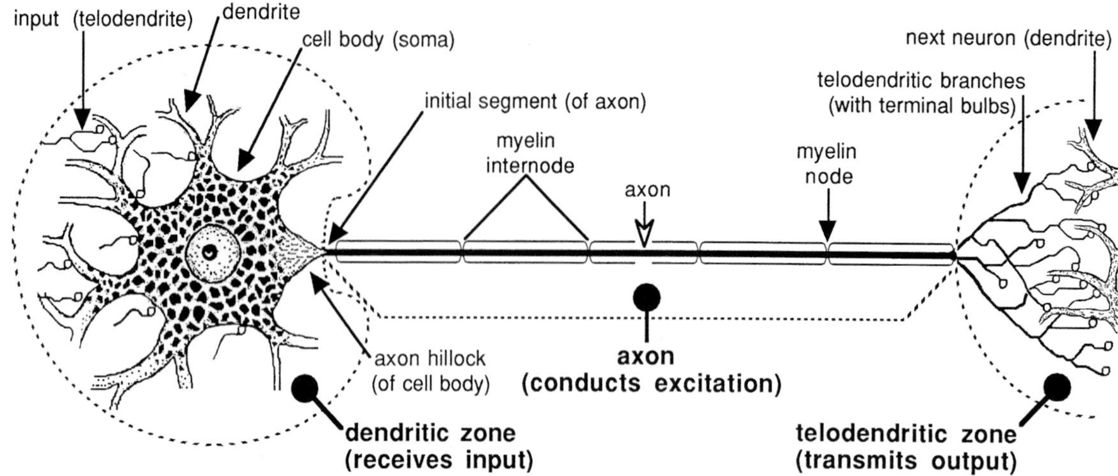

Figure 6.1. *Schematic illustration of a typical (multipolar) neuron, showing multiple dendrites and one axon emanating from the cell body. Functional regions include the dendritic zone (cell body and dendrites), which receives synaptic input; the telodendritic zone, which makes synaptic contact with other neurons; and the axon, which conducts excitation between the two zones. The axon is myelinated. The myelin insulation is interrupted by nodes (gaps). The myelin of each internode is formed by an individual gliocyte (not shown).*

Classification

Neurons are anatomically classified as unipolar, bipolar, or multipolar according to the number of processes that emanate from the cell body (Fig. 6.2).

In a **unipolar** neuron, the cell body gives off a single axon that soon bifurcates into central and peripheral branches. The peripheral branch terminates in receptors that are sensitive to environmental energy. The central branch conveys the environmentally induced excitation into the CNS. Unipolar cell bodies are found in sensory ganglia located in roots of cranial and spinal nerves. Mammalian unipolar neurons are often referred to as pseudounipolar, because they originate as bipolar cells and only become unipolar during development.

In a **bipolar** neuron, two processes emanate from the cell body, which is situated within the axon (vestibulocochlear afferent neurons; bipolar cells of the retina) or situated at the juncture of the axon and a solitary dendrite (olfactory afferent neurons). Like unipolar neurons, bipolar neurons are afferent neurons that convey sensory information to the CNS.

In a **multipolar** neuron, the cell body gives rise to multiple branches, several dendrites, and an axon. Nearly all of the billions of neurons comprising the CNS are multipolar, as are the neurons contained in autonomic ganglia of the PNS. Multipolar neurons can be classified further into those with long axons (type I neurons) and those with short axons (type II neurons).

Regions of a Neuron

A typical neuron becomes excited at its input region, conducts excitation to its output region, and transmits excitation via chemical secretion at synapses (Fig. 6.1). Reception, conduction, and transmission of excitation require functionally different ion channels and cellular features. Thus, an individual neuron has distinct regions: *(a)* an input region or **dendritic zone**, where excitation is initially received; *(b)* an output region or **telodendritic zone**, where excitation is transmitted to other cells; *(c)* an **axon**, which conducts excitation between the dendritic and telodendritic zones; and *(d)* a **cell body**, which nurtures the cell. The cell body may be found within the dendritic zone (multipolar neurons) or associated with the axon (unipolar and bipolar neurons).

In a typical multipolar neuron (Fig. 6.1), the receptive dendritic zone features a large surface area encompassing the cell body and highly branched processes called **dendrites**. An elongated, cylindrical axon originates from the cell body. The telodendritic zone is a highly branched region located at the distal end of the axon. The terminal branches feature localized expansions (bulbs) where neurotransmitter molecules are stored and released at synapses.

In the case of a unipolar afferent neuron, the cell body is situated along the axon and the dendritic zone consists of receptors that change environmental energy into neural excitation. Dendritic zones of bipolar afferent neurons may involve receptors (olfaction) or synaptic contact with receptor cells (in the retina and inner ear). From dendritic zones, excitation is conveyed along the axon to terminal branches within the CNS.

The protein composition of plasma membrane is necessarily different at each functional region of a neuron. For example, dendritic zone membrane has ligand-reactive receptors that open ion channels, either directly or through second messengers. Axon membrane has voltage-gated Na^+ channels that enable membrane polarity reversal and regenerative conduction. Terminal

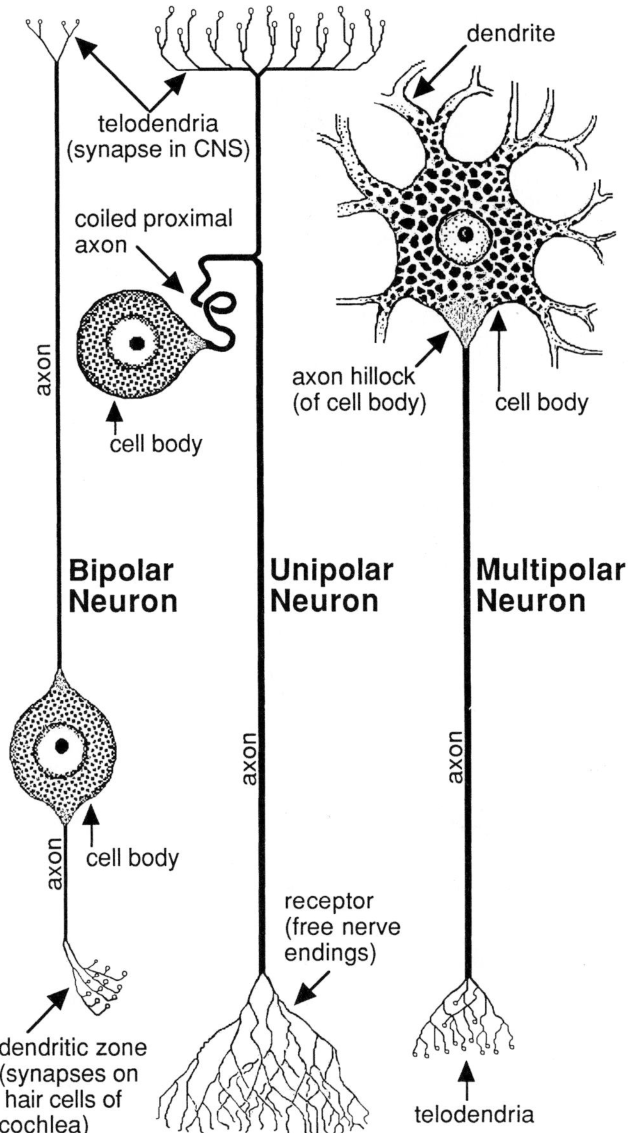

Figure 6.2. *Schematic illustration of a bipolar neuron (left), a unipolar neuron (center), and a multipolar neuron (right). Neurons are anatomically classified according to the number of processes emanating from the cell body. Unipolar and bipolar neurons are sensory. Most neurons are multipolar; however, their shapes vary considerably. The cytoplasm of the cell bodies features clumps of chromatophilic substance (Nissl substance).*

branches and bulbs have voltage-gated Ca^{++} channels (Ca^{++} is involved in the release of neurotransmitter molecules) and receptors for reuptake of released neurotransmitter.

Neuronal Structure

Neurons assume a variety of shapes and sizes, related to their functional roles. Neuronal processes are configured according to the connections that must be made. Neurons with processes that extend long distances must necessarily be larger than less extensive neurons. Also, because larger axons conduct more rapidly than smaller ones, neurons that convey urgent information are large.

CELL BODY

The cell body (perikaryon; soma) of a neuron consists of the nucleus plus the cytoplasm and plasma membrane surrounding the nucleus. In routine histologic stains, the cell body is the most identifiable feature of a neuron. The axon arises from a distinct, conical portion of the cell body called the **axon hillock**. Cellular constituents are synthesized within the cell body. They flow distally into the axon and dendrites.

Cell bodies range from less than 10 μm to more than 100 μm in diameter. Cell body size is proportional to neuronal total volume, although the cell body itself represents a minor portion of the total volume (and an even smaller fraction of total surface area). In multipolar neurons, where the cell body plasma membrane integrates synaptic input, smaller cell bodies are more easily excited to threshold than larger ones, i.e., less synaptic activity is required to trigger action potentials in small neurons (which have high input impedance, by virtue of their size).

Nucleus

Typically, the nucleus of a neuron is centrally positioned, spherical or ovoid, and relatively euchromatic. Small neurons have rather heterochromatic nuclei. Neurons in autonomic ganglia have eccentric nuclei. Nuclear size is proportional to neuron size. The nucleus appears relatively large in a neuron because the cell body cytoplasm surrounding it represents only a minor fraction of total cell volume.

A prominent nucleolus is evident within the nucleus. In females of some species, **sex chromatin** (Barr body) may be evident in the vicinity of the nucleolus (cats, rodents) or nuclear membrane (primates).

Cell body cytoplasm

Many proteins are synthesized in cell body cytoplasm, including cytoskeletal proteins (e.g., for neurofilaments and microtubules), membrane proteins (e.g., for ion channels and active transport), enzymatic proteins (e.g., for glucose metabolism and neurotransmitter synthesis), and secretory peptides (e.g., neuromodulators and neurohormones).

The cell body cytoplasm of large neurons stained with aniline dyes and examined by light microscopy features clumps of **chromatophilic substance** (Nissl substance), which represents aggregations of rough endoplasmic reticulum (rER), free ribosomes, and polyribosomes. Nissl substance extends into the trunks of dendritic trees, but it is absent from the axon hillock, which instead features neurofilaments and grouped microtubules. In small neurons, cytoplasmic chromatophilia appears relatively pale and diffuse.

When a neuron is injured (e.g., by transection of its axon), the cell body swells, the nucleus shifts to an eccentric position, and ribosomes disperse so that Nissl substance disappears centrally in the cell body (**chromatolysis**). This response to injury, called the **axonal reaction** (Fig. 6.3), begins within days and may persist several weeks. It is one of the features that a pathologist looks for as evidence of nervous system damage in the CNS.

A Golgi complex is usually prominent in cell body cytoplasm. **Secretory vesicles** originate from the complex and are transported through the axon to terminal bulbs. Secretory vesicles commonly contain neuroactive peptides that influence the excitability or growth of target cells. In the case of certain hypothalamic neurons, secretory vesicles contain neurohormones. Although **synaptic vesicles** may be evident in the cell body, they are primarily formed and stored in telodendritic bulbs.

Microtubules (25 nm in diameter) and **neurofilaments** (10 nm in diameter) are numerous in the cell body. Microtubules are involved in the rapid transport of membrane-bound organelles within the neuron. Neurofilaments are the cytoskeletal elements that form the neurofibrils of light microscopy. Neurons are aerobic and thus dependent on mitochondria, which are plentiful. Neurons are long-lived and may accumulate lipofuscin granules as a residue of lysosomal activity.

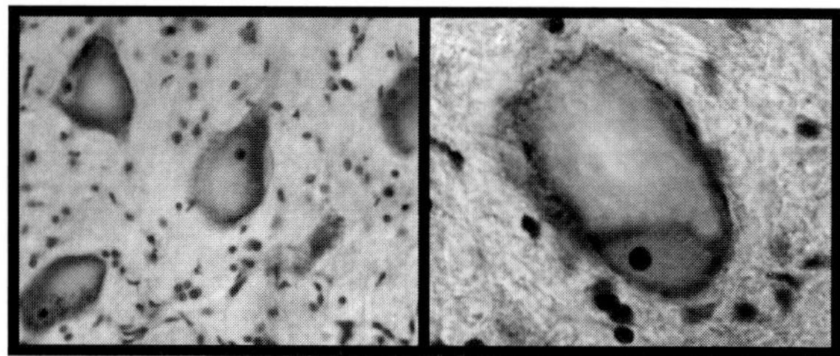

Figure 6.3. *Two light micrographs at different magnifications of chromatolytic cell bodies from the spinal cord of a dog that had spinal nerves transected. The cell bodies are swollen, nuclei are shifted to an eccentric position, and chromatophilic substance is lost except for small amounts accumulated marginally. Nissl's stain (left, ×200; right, ×400).*

NEURON PROCESSES

A typical neuron has a single axon and multiple dendrites originating as processes from its cell body. The axon ends in terminal branches that synapse with dendrites and cell bodies of other neurons or innervate muscle or gland. Each type of neuronal process has a distinct functional role within the neuron. Thus, the processes feature different populations of plasma membrane proteins (channels, receptors, transporters, pumps).

Dendrites

Dendrites are highly branched processes designed to receive numerous synaptic contacts from other neurons. Treelike, each dendrite emerges as a main trunk that branches repeatedly into smaller and smaller twigs. The trunk has an organelle content similar to that of the cell body. Small dendritic branches feature predominantly microtubules, augmented by neurofilaments, mitochondria, and smooth endoplasmic reticulum (sER).

Synaptic sites on dendrites are distinguished by a variably thick band of electron-dense cytoplasm lining a region of postsynaptic membrane that faces a presynaptic element across a synaptic cleft (Fig. 6.4). The dense material represents proteins (receptors, channels, enzymes, etc.) responsible for postsynaptic activity.

Some neurons display numerous **dendritic spines** (gemmules). A spine is a short expanded process at-

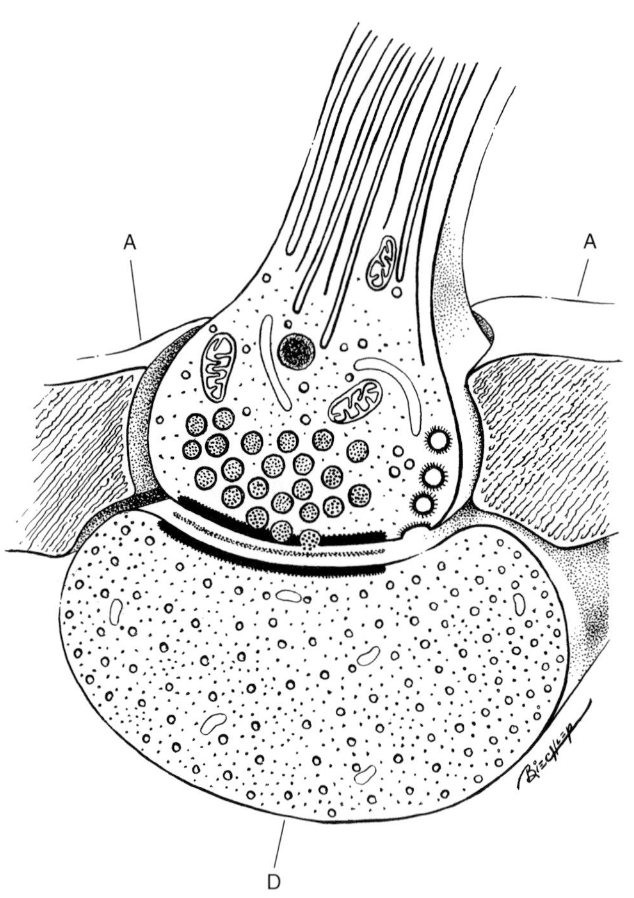

Figure 6.4. *Schematic illustration of a symmetric axodendritic synapse. A terminal bulb containing synaptic vesicles is separated from a dendrite (D) by a synaptic cleft containing glycoprotein material. Astrocyte processes (A) border the synaptic cleft bilaterally. Within the terminal bulb, synaptic vesicles are clustered around an active zone in which an electron-dense band lines the plasma membrane. As a consequence of Ca^{++} influx, synaptic vesicles are able to dock with the plasma membrane and release neurotransmitter molecules by exocytosis. Vesicle membrane is recovered from the plasma membrane and conveyed, as coated vesicles, to sER for re-cycling. A solitary, large, dense-core secretory vesicle containing a peptide neuromodulator is also shown, along with mitochondria, microtubules, and neurofilaments. The transverse section of the dendrite features an electron-dense band along the postsynaptic membrane. Numerous microtubules and neurofilaments and a few sER profiles are evident in the dendrite.*

tached to the dendritic branch by a narrow stalk, like a bud on a twig (Fig. 6.5). A spine apparatus, consisting of alternating membrane sacs and dense material, may be found within the spine. Spines increase dendritic surface area and act to restrict the spread of postsynaptic excitation.

Axon

The **axon** is a relatively long, cylindrical process that originates from the axon hillock of the cell body and ends in terminal branches and bulbs. Except at its termination, axonal branches are sparse. When branches are present along the course of the axon, they emerge at right angles (from nodes in the case of myelinated axons) and are called **collateral branches**. Axoplasm contains microtubules, neurofilaments, mitochondria, and sER. Being devoid of rER, axoplasm is not well stained by hematoxylin and eosin and other routine histologic stains.

The **initial segment** of the axon is a site just distal to the axon hillock, where action potentials normally originate. It is narrower than the rest of the axon. Ultrastructurally, bundled microtubules are present and electron-dense material is evident along the inner surface of the plasma membrane of the initial segment. The density represents protein accumulation associated with ion channels and pumps. Similar electron-dense protein accumulations are also found at nodes of myelinated axons.

A slow flow of cytoplasm (1 mm/day) and a slow transport of cytoskeletal elements (10 mm/day) progress along the axon, from axon hillock to terminal branches. In addition, axons have a fast transport capability (up to 400 mm/day) involving microtubule-linked movement of mitochondria and constituents packaged in vesicles. There is also a retrograde transport mechanism that rapidly conveys remnants of organelles from terminal branches to lysosomes in the cell body. Viruses (e.g., rabies) and neurotoxins (e.g., tetanus toxin) can also be carried to the cell body by this route.

Axons are capable of regenerative conduction, i.e., they convey an excitation signal that arrives at the end of the axon with the same magnitude as it had when it began at the initial segment. Large axons conduct more rapidly than small ones, but to further increase conduction velocity, large axons are myelinated (coated with a myelin sheath formed by glial cells). Small nonmyelinated axons are ensheathed by glial cells in peripheral nerves, but they are not ensheathed at all in the CNS.

Terminal branches (telodendrites)

Axons terminate by successively branching (Fig. 6.1). The collective terminal branches constitute the telodendritic zone of a neuron. Each terminal branch ends in an expansion called a **terminal bulb** (synaptic bouton). In some neurons, terminal branches have a series of expansions proximal to the terminal bulb, called **preterminal bulbs** (varicosities). Both preterminal and terminal bulbs are sites where neurotransmitter molecules are packaged and stored within synaptic vesicles.

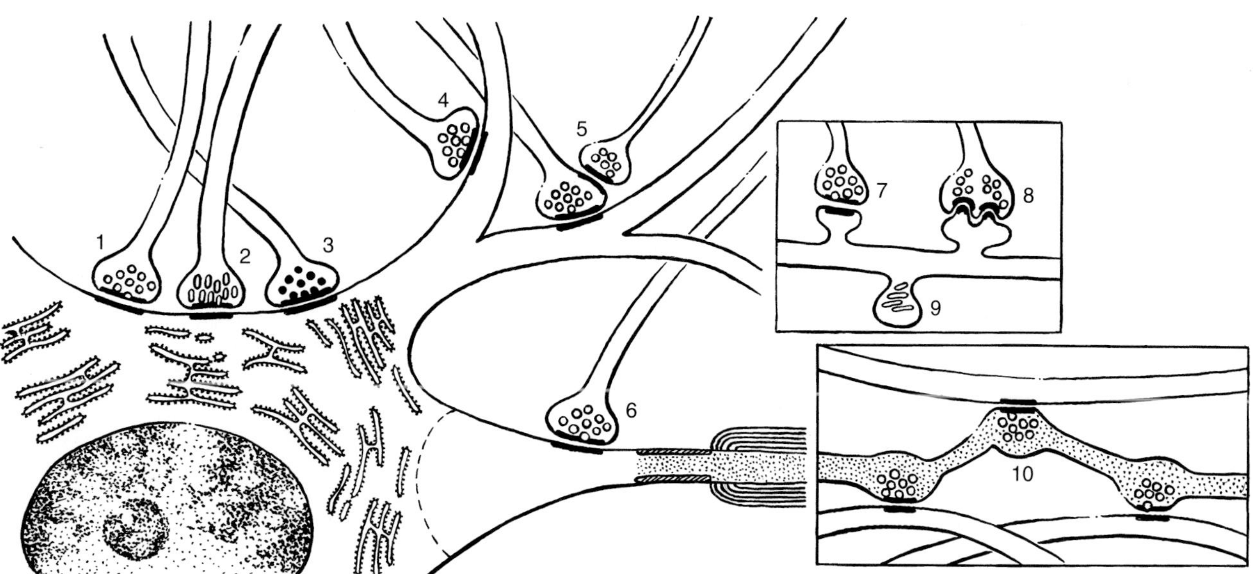

Figure 6.5. *Schematic illustrations of types of CNS synapses. 1) Axosomatic synapse with electron-lucent, spherical, synaptic vesicles. 2) Axosomatic synapse with synaptic vesicles that are flattened (an artifact associated with inhibitory synapses). 3) Axosomatic synapse with electron-dense synaptic vesicles. 4) Axodendritic synapse. 5) Axoaxonic synapse in which one terminal bulb synapses on another (associated with presynaptic inhibition). 6) Synapse on an axon hillock, close to the initial segment of the axon. 7) Axodendritic synapse on a dendritic spine. 8) Relatively elaborate synapse on a dendritic spine. 9) Dendritic spine exhibiting a spine apparatus (sER plus electron dense material). 10) Three axonal varicosities making synapses in passing (en passant).*

The most common **synaptic vesicle** is spherical (40 to 50 nm in diameter) with an electron-lucent (agranular) core. Such vesicles may contain any one of a number of neurotransmitters. Electron-lucent synaptic vesicles that appear flattened when exposed to solutions of high osmolarity are associated with inhibitory synapses. Some neurons have spherical vesicles (40 to 60 nm in diameter) with an electron-dense (granular) core. The electron-dense synaptic vesicles usually contain dopamine or norepinephrine molecules.

Synaptic vesicle proteins are synthesized in the cell body and transported rapidly to telodendritic sER, where they supplement local production of synaptic vesicles from recycled vesicular membrane. Transporter proteins in vesicle membrane load newly formed synaptic vesicles with neurotransmitter molecules that were also recycled. Linked by cytoskeletal actin filaments, synaptic vesicles are clustered together, in ready reserve for plasma membrane docking and exocytosis during synaptic activity (Fig. 6.4).

In addition to synaptic vesicles, terminal branches may contain **secretory vesicles** that store neuroactive peptides (several dozen have been identified). Peptides are found in spherical, electron-dense vesicles that are relatively large (100 to 200 nm in diameter). The secretory vesicles are synthesized in the cell body and transported to preterminal and terminal bulbs for storage and release. The peptides generally act as neuromodulators (agents that augment neurotransmitter effects). Secretory vesicles of certain hypothalamic neurons contain peptide hormones (e.g., vasopressin and oxytocin are stored and released in the neurohypophysis).

Neuronal Communication

Neurons communicate with one another and with the muscles and glands they innervate. Alterations in excitation communicated from neuron to neuron (neural circuits) constitute the basis of nervous system function.

A few neurons communicate through gap junctions (electrotonic synapses), especially in invertebrates and fish. In mammals, gap junction communication is common among neuroblasts during embryonic development, but it is relatively rare among mature neurons.

Some neurons communicate by producing a gas that passes freely through neuronal membranes (e.g., nitric oxide, which can inhibit neurotransmitter release in target neurons by gas activation of an enzyme that produces cyclic guanosine 5′-monophosphate (cGMP) second messenger molecules).

Among the billions of neurons that comprise the nervous system, the primary means of communication is localized release of neurotransmitter molecules at interneuronal chemical synapses. Also, chemical synaptic arrangements are encountered between efferent neurons and the muscles and glands they innervate (see Peripheral Nervous Tissue section).

INTERNEURONAL CHEMICAL SYNAPSES

An interneuronal chemical synapse is a site of morphologic specialization where one neuron influences the excitability of another by releasing neurotransmitter molecules from synaptic vesicles. Neurotransmitters are biogenic amines (e.g., glutamate, glycine, dopamine, norepinephrine, serotonin, acetylcholine, etc.). Generally, each neurotransmitter can interact with more than one variety of receptors. Sometimes, one receptor type is excitatory, whereas another receptor type activated by the same neurotransmitter has an inhibitory effect. Thus, it is the nature of the receptor type, rather than the neurotransmitter itself, that determines the function of a synapse (e.g., excitatory or inhibitory, short or long acting, etc.). Nonetheless, some neurotransmitters (e.g., glutamate) are consistently associated with excitatory synapses, and others (e.g., glycine) are associated with inhibitory synapses.

Most synapses between neurons involve terminal bulbs of one neuron contacting the input region of another neuron, forming axodendritic or axosomatic synapses (Fig. 6.5). However, among the trillions of synapses in the nervous system, every synaptic combination has been observed, including axoaxonic, dendrodendritic, dendrosomatic, somatodendritic, and somatosomatic synapses.

The input region of a typical multipolar neuron receives thousands of synaptic contacts. Excitatory and inhibitory synaptic effects are collectively summated and integrated at the spherical cell body of the target neuron, so that the cell body membrane potential continually registers the net effect of total synaptic input to the neuron. In turn, the massive cell body affects the membrane potential at the nearby initial segment of the axon. At any moment, the collective synaptic input to a neuron will be sufficient to trigger an action potential at the initial segment of the axon or be insufficient to do so.

The influence that one neuron has on another depends on the number of synaptic contacts it makes with the target neuron and where the synapses are positioned. Synapses close to the initial segment will have much greater influence triggering an action potential than will synapses on distal dendrites.

SYNAPTIC ULTRASTRUCTURE AND FUNCTION

Ultrastructurally, an interneuronal chemical synapse may be identified by the juxtaposition of a presynaptic element, a synaptic cleft, and a postsynaptic membrane (Fig. 6.4). The presynaptic element contains multiple synaptic vesicles clustered around an active zone indicated by electron density (protein accumulation) just inside the plasma membrane. The synaptic cleft (in the CNS, approximately the same width as the general intercellular space, 20 to 30 nm wide) contains a protein that holds presynaptic and postsynaptic membranes together. The postsynaptic plasma membrane features an electron density that is similar to the presynaptic density (symmetrical synapse) or is thicker (asymmetrical synapse). The densities reflect the high-protein content of synaptic membranes.

When an action potential arrives at the end of an axon, it passively depolarizes the presynaptic element (e.g., terminal bulb). Voltage-sensitive channels in the presynaptic membrane open to allow Ca^{++} influx. Elevated cytoplasmic Ca^{++} activates enzymes that phosphorylate synaptic vesicle proteins responsible for reversibly linking vesicles to cytoskeletal actin filaments and merging vesicles with plasma membrane. This mobilizes synaptic vesicles, enabling them to dock with the plasma membrane and then release several thousand neurotransmitter molecules by exocytosis. The molecules diffuse into the synaptic cleft and bind with various receptors and transporters.

A receptor is a site on a membrane protein to which a neurotransmitter binds briefly. The receptor protein may be a channel that undergoes reconfiguration to allow passage of selective ions. Or, the receptor may be coupled to a G-protein cascade that opens ion channels either directly or indirectly by activating second messengers (such as cyclic adenosine monophosphate [cAMP]). Second messengers provide a means of amplifying the scope and impact of a neurotransmitter signal as well as prolonging its time course. Autoreceptors (receptors in presynaptic plasma membrane that influence neurotransmitter synthesis and release) and neuromodulators (peptides released from secretory vesicles) typically act via second messengers.

Synaptic activity ceases when neurotransmitter molecules are removed from the synaptic cleft (or degraded in the case of acetylcholine). Molecules are actively transported intracellularly by transporters (protein pumps) located in the presynaptic membrane or in membranes of adjacent glial cells. Thus, neurotransmitter molecules are recycled to minimize the need for synthesis within presynaptic cytoplasm. As well, synaptic vesicle membrane is recycled. Vesicle membrane is extracted from the presynaptic plasma membrane and transported as coated vesicles to sER within the presynaptic cytoplasm (Fig. 6.4).

NEUROGLIA

Neuroglia comprise well more than 90 percent of the cells that make up the nervous system. Neuroglial cells (gliocytes) are relatively small. With routine stains, only their nuclei and perikarya are evident. Collectively, they provide structural and functional support. Unlike mature neurons, gliocytes remain capable of mitosis, and they can give rise to tumors of the nervous system.

The gliocytes found in the CNS are astrocytes, oligodendrocytes, microglial cells, and ependymal cells. Except for microglial cells, which migrate into the CNS from mesoderm, CNS gliocytes are derived from the cells that form the embryonic neural tube. The PNS gliocyte is the neurolemmocyte, which ensheathes or myelinates axons and becomes a satellite cell in ganglia. Neurolemmocytes are derived from the embryonic neural crest (as are neurons that have cell bodies in ganglia).

Astrocytes

With routine stains, astrocytes are identified by their pale, ovoid nuclei, which are largest among glial nuclei. With silver stains, astrocytes exhibit numerous processes that contain glial fibrils. In white matter, the processes are long, slender, and moderately branched; in gray matter, the processes appear shorter and highly branched. Thus, white matter is said to contain **fibrous astrocytes**, whereas gray matter contains **protoplasmic astrocytes** (Fig. 6.6).

Under the electron microscope, astrocytes feature packed bundles of intermediate filaments (8-nm diameter) and pale cytoplasm. The glial filaments, which are composed of glial fibrillar acidic protein, are unique to astrocytes and form the glial fibrils seen with light microscopy. The filaments are denser in fibrous astrocytes than in protoplasmic ones.

Adjacent astrocytes are joined by gap junctions. In response to local stimulation, a widening excitatory wave of elevated cytoplasmic Ca^{++} can spread outward from cell to cell. The adjacent astrocytes are also linked by small, buttonlike adhering junctions (spot desmosomes).

Astrocyte processes terminate in expansions called **end feet**. Collections of end feet form a **glial-limiting membrane** to which pia mater is attached at the CNS surface. End feet are prominent in the subependymal glial layer, and they form septa in the spinal cord. End feet cover vessels within the brain and spinal cord, and they are believed to be responsible for inducing formation of tight junctions between capillary endothelial cells (a basis for the blood–brain barrier).

Astrocytes, through their glial fibrils, provide structural support. By storing glycogen and releasing glucose, they represent a source of reserve energy. Astrocyte plasma membranes have ionic pumps that regulate K^{+} throughout the narrow extracellular space of the CNS. Astrocyte processes insulate synapses and take up neurotransmitter molecules to stop ongoing synaptic activity. Astrocytes are capable of phagocytosis, and they can proliferate to form glial scars in the event of CNS injury. Finally, astrocytes seem to have an immune function; they can present antigens to T lymphocytes.

Oligodendrocytes

Oligodendrocytes have relatively few branches (Fig. 6.6). In routine stains, they are recognized by their small, spherical, densely stained nuclei. Ultrastructurally, oligodendrocyte cytoplasm is electron dense and rich in microtubules and organelles, especially rER

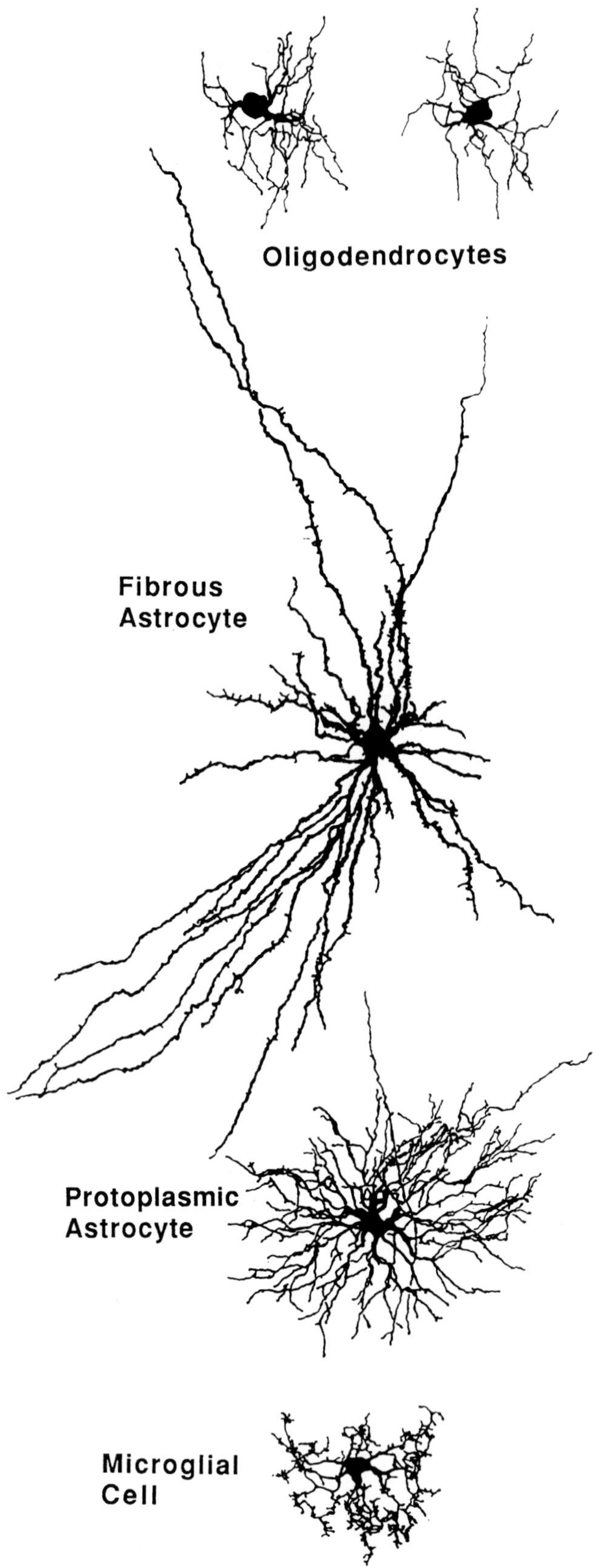

Figure 6.6. *CNS gliocytes are drawn as they appeared following Golgi silver impregnation of monkey cerebral cortex (×700). (Adapted from Weiss L. Histology. 6th ed. New York: Elsevier Biomedical, 1988.)*

and mitochondria. Oligodendrocytes lack gap junctions.

In gray matter, oligodendrocytes serve as perineuronal satellites. Their specific function is unclear. In white matter, oligodendrocytes form myelin sheath internodes around axons of the CNS.

Microglia

Microglia are cells of mesodermal origin that invade the CNS when it is vascularized embryologically. They are sparse and difficult to find in normal tissue. In routine stains, microglia are identified by their small, elongated, chromophilic nuclei. With silver impregnation, they are seen as small, elongated cells with polar processes (Fig. 6.6). In the event of CNS damage, microglia can transform into macrophages with antigen-presenting and phagocytic capabilities.

In addition to microglia, other cell types also respond to CNS damage. Hematogenous macrophages can invade the CNS. Astrocytes can become phagocytic. Pericytes, cells associated with CNS capillaries and believed to have contractile capability, are believed to have the capacity to become phagocytic.

Ependymal Cells

Ependymal cells line ventricular cavities within the brain and the central canal within the spinal cord. The cells are typically cuboidal or columnar with numerous motile cilia (Fig. 6.7). Ependymal cells are linked by zonulae adherentes and gap junctions near their luminal borders. Large molecules from the CNS extracellular space can pass between ependymal cells to reach cerebrospinal fluid (which functions like a lymphatic drainage system for the CNS).

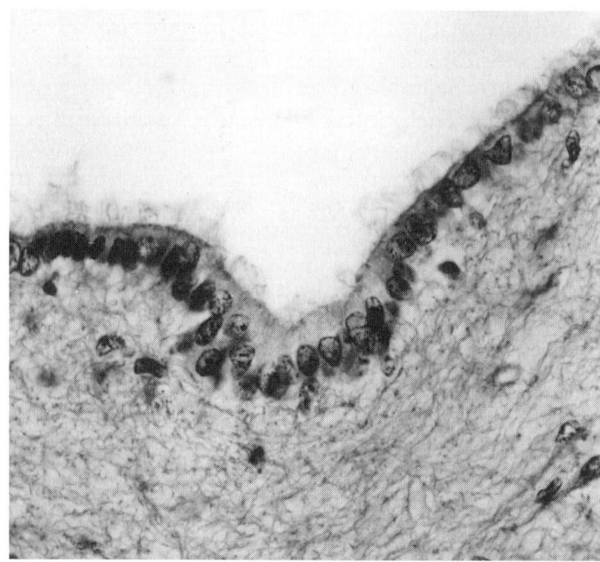

Figure 6.7. *Light micrograph of ependymal cells lining the fourth ventricle (camel). The cells have motile cilia (×400). (From Dellmann H-D. Veterinary histology: an outline text–atlas. Philadelphia: Lea & Febiger, 1971.)*

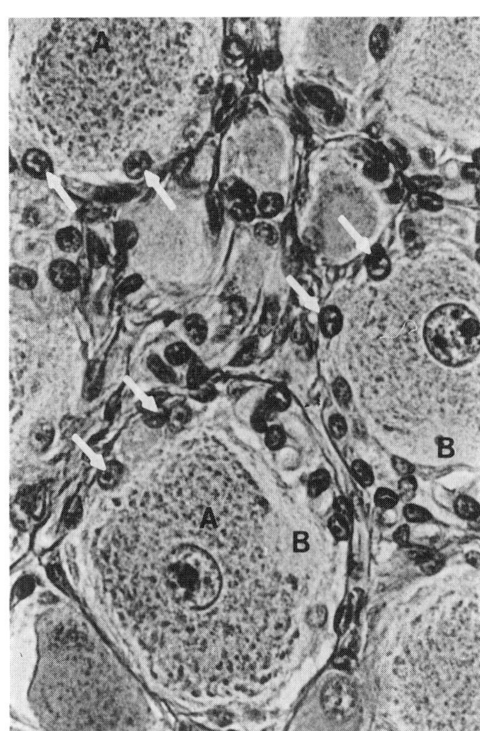

Figure 6.8. *Light micrograph of a sectioned spinal ganglion (dog). The arrows indicate nuclei of ganglionic gliocytes (satellite cells), which completely encapsulate unipolar neuron cell bodies (A). An axon hillock (B) is evident where chromatophilic substance is absent (×625). (Courtesy of E.M. Brown.)*

Modified ependymal cells, called **choroid plexus epithelium**, cover the surfaces of choroid plexus villi and produce cerebrospinal fluid by a mechanism that involves active secretion of Na^+. Modified ependymal cells are also present at certain sites (circumventricular organs) within brain ventricles. In both cases, the modified ependymal cells are cuboidal and have microvilli instead of cilia extending into cerebrospinal fluid. Adjacent cells are linked by relatively impermeable junctions (zonulae occludentes), establishing a localized ependymal barrier in association with a locally reduced blood–brain barrier due to the presence of fenestrated capillaries.

Tanycytes are modified ependymal cells found in the hypothalamic wall of the third ventricle. The luminal border of a tanycyte has microvilli; the basal border features an elongated process that makes contact with capillaries and neurons. It is speculated that tanycytes convey substances from cerebrospinal fluid to blood and/or neurosecretory neurons.

At certain sites, neuronal processes extend between ependymal cells to contact cerebrospinal fluid. The processes, which end in bulbs with stereocilia, are presumed to serve a receptive function. Also, neurons containing secretory vesicles can be found among ependymal cells. They are believed to release catecholamines.

Neurolemmocytes

Neurolemmocytes are gliocytes of the PNS that either ensheathe and myelinate axons (Schwann cells) or encapsulate neuron cell bodies as ganglionic gliocytes (satellite cells). Neurolemmocytes provide a protected immediate environment for PNS neurons. Each neurolemmocyte is enclosed within a basal lamina. Neurolemmocytes can proliferate and become phagocytic in the event of nerve damage.

In craniospinal (sensory) ganglia, satellite cells form a complete, tight capsule around each neuron cell body (Fig. 6.8). In autonomic ganglia (Fig. 6.9), capsules formed by satellite cells may have gaps and may enclose more than one postganglionic cell body. Away from the cell body, satellite cells are replaced by neurolemmocytes that ensheathe or myelinate axons.

Every axon in the PNS is ensheathed or myelinated along its entire length by neurolemmocytes (except for the most terminal branches in some cases). Because an individual neurolemmocyte is less than 1 mm in length, a tandem series of many neurolemmocytes is required to enclose the entire length of a long axon.

In the case of small, nonmyelinated axons, each neurolemmocyte ensheathes a number of axons simultaneously (Fig. 6.10). Each axon resides in a furrow, protected by a pair of neurolemmocyte processes so that the space surrounding the axon communicates with the

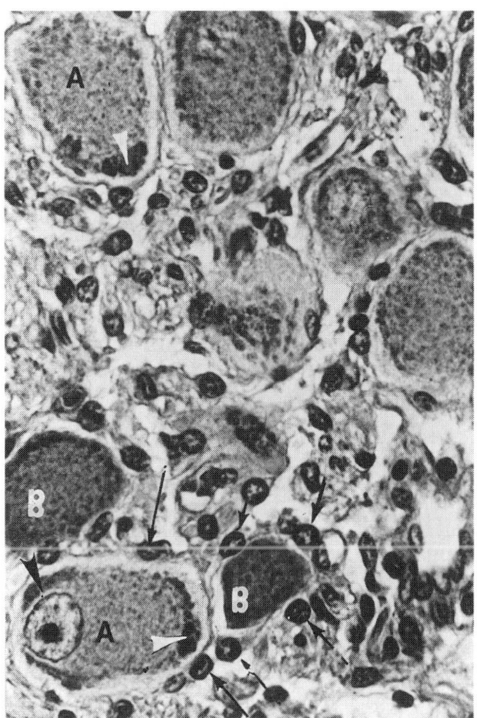

Figure 6.9. *Light micrograph of a sectioned autonomic ganglion (dog). The thin arrows indicate nuclei of ganglionic gliocytes, which form an incomplete capsule around multipolar neuron cell bodies. Cell bodies of postganglionic autonomic neurons normally exhibit eccentrically positioned nuclei, marginal accumulations of chromatophilic substance (A, arrowheads), or generalized chromatophilia (B) (×625). (Courtesy of E.M. Brown.)*

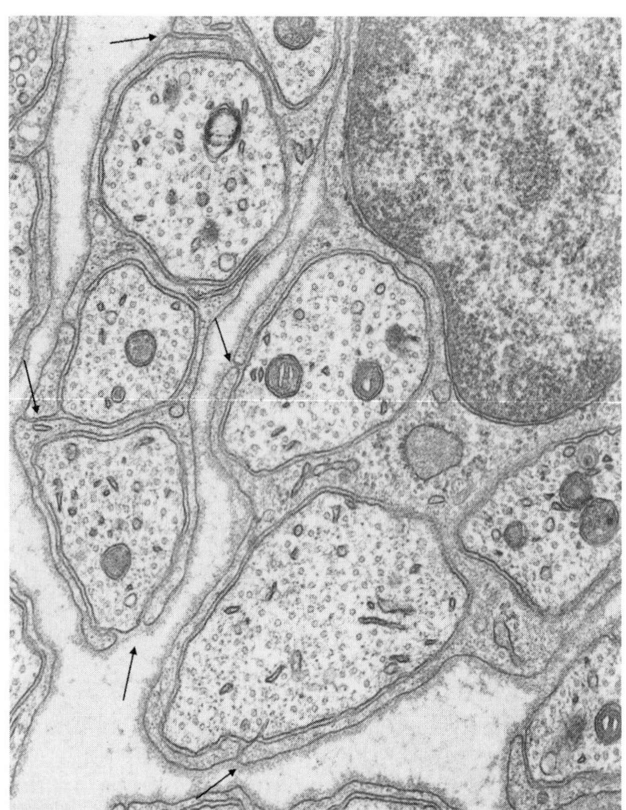

Figure 6.10. *Electron micrograph of a neurolemmocyte ensheathing nonmyelinated axons of the peripheral nervous system. Each axon is enclosed by neurolemmocyte processes. Mesaxons (arrows) are formed where the processes meet (×33,600). (Courtesy of H.-D. Dellmann.)*

general interstitial space only by means of a narrow gap (referred to as a mesaxon because of a resemblance to mesentery). For axons larger than 1 μm in diameter, each neurolemmocyte encloses a single axon and its processes wrap around the axon to form a myelin sheath (Fig. 6.11).

Myelin Sheath

The term **myelin sheath** refers to wrappings of gliocyte plasma membrane that surround an axon and insulate it. The myelin sheath is necessarily interrupted at the juncture of adjacent gliocytes, forming uninsulated sites called nodes. Because action potentials jump from node to node and skip over the long insulated internodes, myelin greatly increases excitation conduction velocity. Myelin is formed by oligodendrocytes in the CNS and neurolemmocytes in the PNS.

In the PNS, a transverse section of a myelinated fiber viewed by light microscopy reveals an axon enclosed in a myelin sheath surrounded by neurolemmocyte cytoplasm (Fig. 6.12). With electron microscopy, one can see that the myelin sheath is composed of multiple layers of neurolemmocyte plasma membrane and the neurolemmocyte is within a basal lamina (Fig. 6. 11).

Myelin formation in the PNS begins with a neurolemmocyte draped around a solitary axon, establishing a simple mesaxon (Fig. 6.13). Induced by the axon itself, neurolemmocyte processes elongate, slide past one another, and proceed to produce multilayered neurolemmocyte wrappings around the axon. Cytoplasm is extruded from the wrappings, thereby leaving the concentric lamellae of plasma membrane that constitute the myelin sheath.

At high magnification, the myelin sheath exhibits a periodicity of concentric **major dense lines** separated by intraperiod lines. Each major dense line is formed by fusion of inner surfaces of plasma membrane as cytoplasm is extruded during myelin sheath formation. An **intraperiod line** is formed where the outer surfaces of adjacent plasma membranes are separated by a small gap. The gap is continuous with the **inner mesaxon** and the **outer mesaxon**, all of which are derived from the original simple mesaxon. Occasionally, a major dense line appears to split and contain a pocket of cytoplasm. Adjacent pockets of cytoplasm may extend throughout the thickness of the myelin sheath, thereby establishing a **myelin incisure** in the sheath.

A longitudinal view of a myelinated nerve fiber shows myelin sheath gaps. Each gap is referred to as a **node** (of Ranvier), and the myelin sheath between nodes is called an **internode**. The internodal transition region adjacent to a node is referred to as a **paranode** (Fig. 6.14). At the paranode, major dense lines split and cytoplasm is re-

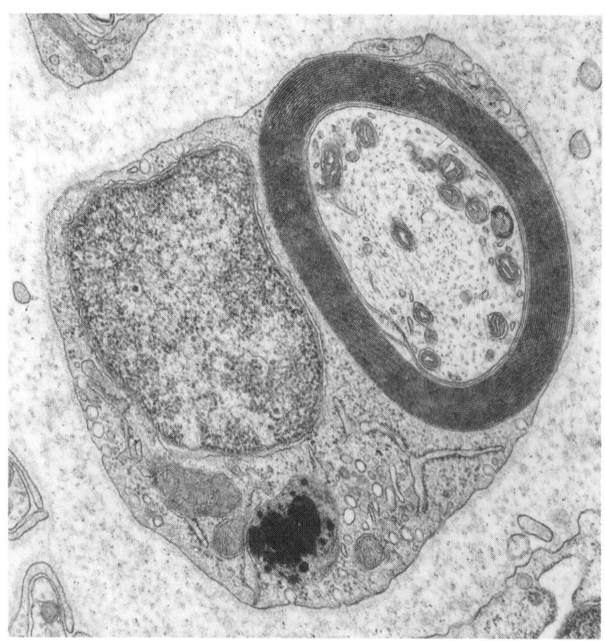

Figure 6.11. *Electron micrograph of a myelinated fiber of the peripheral nervous system. A neurolemmocyte has produced a myelin sheath around a single axon. The neurolemmocyte is enclosed by basal lamina, and external to this, collagen fibrils of the endoneurium are evident. (The electron-dense mass in the neurolemmocyte cytoplasm is a lipofuscin inclusion.) The myelin consists of multiple wrappings of neurolemmocyte membrane. An external mesaxon is evident above the myelin sheath, and an internal mesaxon can be seen at the lower left of the axon. The axoplasm features neurofilaments, microtubules, and mitochondria (×29,325). (From Dellmann H-D. Veterinary histology: an outline text–atlas. Philadelphia: Lea & Febiger, 1971.)*

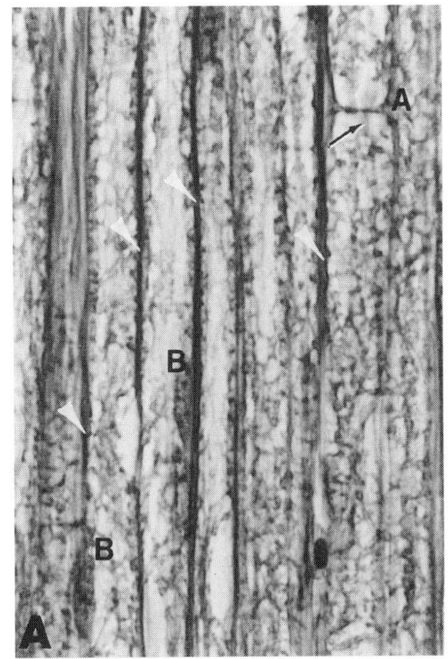

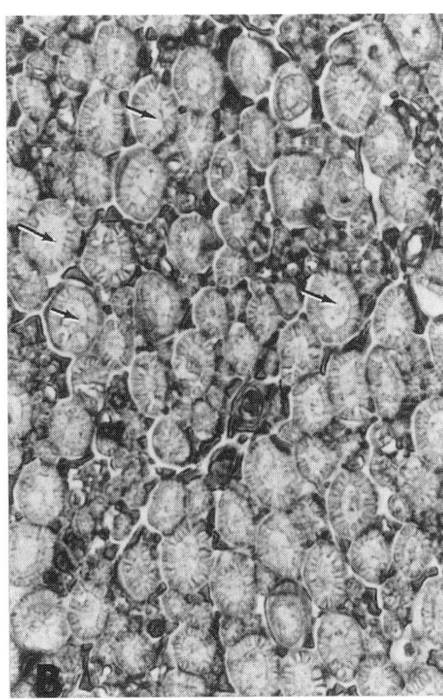

Figure 6.12. *Light micrographs of longitudinal (**A**) and transverse (**B**) sections of a canine peripheral nerve. Lipid extraction during tissue preparation disintegrates the myelin sheath, leaving a protein residue (neurokeratin). In **A**, endoneurium (white arrowheads) surrounds each myelinated nerve fiber; a myelin sheath is interrupted at a node (A); an axon (black arrow) is evident in the center of a fiber; neurolemmocyte nuclei (B) and cytoplasm are present at the surface of each fiber. In **B**, each myelinated fiber consists of an axon (arrow) surrounded by a myelin sheath (neurokeratin) within a cytoplasmic rim. Nonmyelinated axons are not visible at this magnification, but they are more numerous than the myelinated fibers in the field (×625). (Courtesy of E.M. Brown.)*

tained in processes that overlap one another as each contacts the axon plasma membrane. Outermost cytoplasmic processes of adjacent neurolemmocytes make contact, thus enclosing the node in the PNS. A continuous basal lamina is present external to the neurolemmocytes. At the node, the axon bulges slightly and exhibits subplasmalemmal electron-dense material.

In the CNS, where myelin sheaths are formed by oligodendrocytes, nodes are not covered by cytoplasmic processes and they are exposed to the extracellular space (Fig. 6.15). Internodes are thinner and nodes are wider in the CNS compared to the PNS. A single oligodendrocyte is known to contribute internodes to as many as 50 myelinated fibers and the outer cytoplasm of the internode is restricted to a single ridge that is connected to the oligodendrocyte perikaryon by a thin process.

Myelin sheaths provide electrical insulation so that action potentials jump from node to node instead of progressing continually, as in nonmyelinated axons. The jumping process, called **saltatory conduction**, is much faster than nonmyelinated conduction and the longer the internode, the faster the conduction. Internode length is proportional to myelin sheath thickness, and both are proportional to axon diameter. However, because neurolemmocytes develop an association with axons early in development, axons that subsequently grow farther (e.g., in the limbs) have longer internodes than axons (e.g., in the head) that do not grow as far.

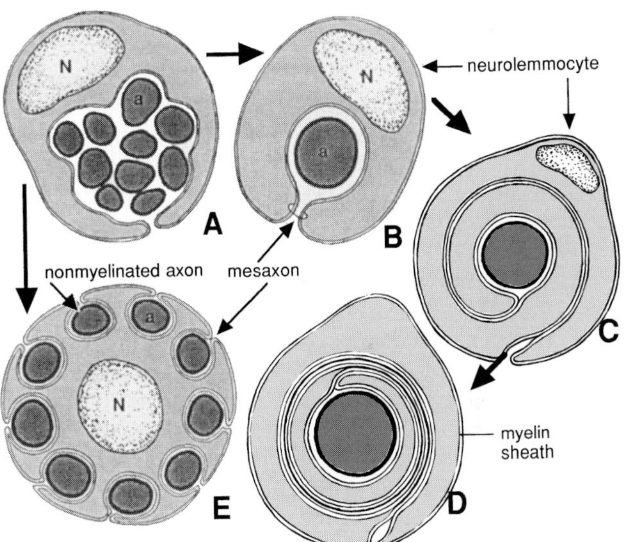

Figure 6.13. *Schematic illustration of myelinated and nonmyelinated developmental relationships between axons (a) and neurolemmocytes in cross-section perspective. **A.**, Early in development, several axons are ensheathed in common by a neurolemmocyte. **B.**, After neurolemmocyte proliferation, a solitary large axon that is destined to be myelinated is ensheathed by a neurolemmocyte; a mesaxon is formed where neurolemmocyte processes meet. **C.**, Neurolemmocyte processes elongate and encircle the axon, thereby lengthening the original mesaxon. **D.**, A myelin sheath is formed when cytoplasm is extruded from encircling neurolemmocyte processes, thereby leaving layers of plasmalemma. The sheath features major dense lines, where plasmalemmal cytoplasmic surfaces make contact, alternated with intraperiod lines formed by the elongated mesaxon. Cytoplasm is generally retained internal and external to the myelin sheath, where an inner mesaxon and outer mesaxon are evident. **E.**, In the case of nonmyelinated axons, neurolemmocyte invaginations provide a separate compartment and mesaxon for each ensheathed axon. N = neurolemmocyte nucleus. (Adapted from Copenhaver WM, Bunge RP, Bunge MB. Bailey's textbook of histology. 16th ed. Baltimore: Williams & Wilkins, 1971.)*

PERIPHERAL NERVOUS TISSUE

Tissue of the PNS consists of cranial and spinal nerves, including their roots, distal branches, and ganglia. **Cranial nerves** originate from the brain and exit from the cranial cavity. **Spinal nerves** originate from the spinal cord and exit from the vertebral canal. A **nerve**

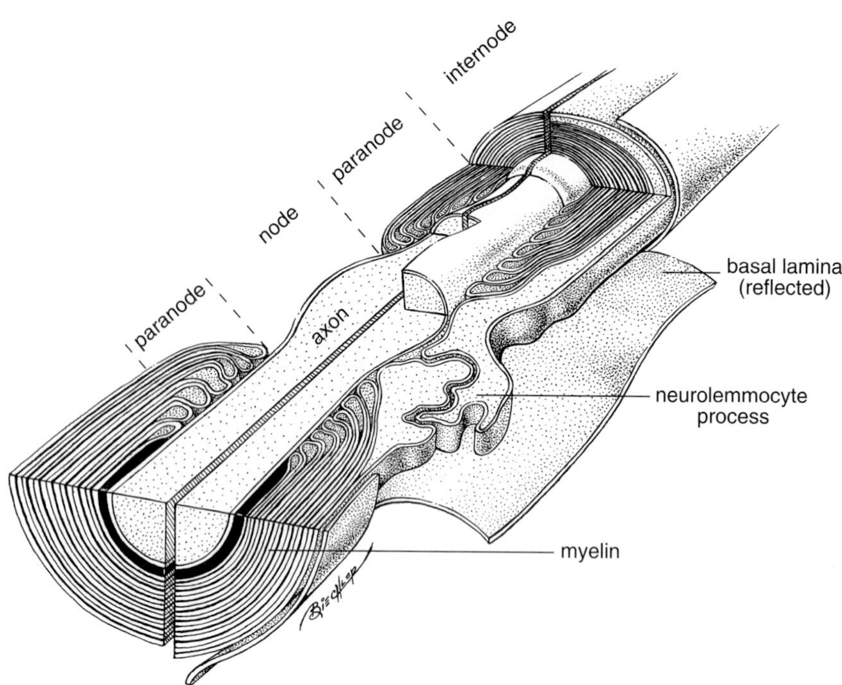

Figure 6.14. *Schematic illustration of nodal and paranodal regions of myelinated fibers from the central nervous system (CNS) (left) and the peripheral nervous system (PNS) (right). In the CNS, myelin is formed by oligodendrocytes and nodes are broadly exposed to the extracellular space. In the PNS, outer cytoplasmic processes of adjacent neurolemmocytes (Schwann cells) overlap to restrict node exposure to the extracellular space. Also, neurolemmocytes are surrounded by a continuous basal lamina. Myelin consists of compressed membranes of glial cells, distinguished by a series of major dense lines separated by intraperiod lines. At each paranode, major dense lines split to contain terminal cytoplasmic "loops" that contact the axon plasma membrane and impede ionic flow beyond the node.*

root is the proximal region of a cranial or spinal nerve that is enveloped by meninges within the cranial cavity or vertebral canal. The term **nerve fiber** refers to one axon within a nerve. In the case of a myelinated axon, the term **nerve fiber** (myelinated nerve fiber) includes the axon plus the myelin sheath and surrounding neurolemmocyte.

Individual nerve fibers may be classified as either **afferent** or **efferent**. Afferent fibers are sensory because they conduct excitation to the CNS. Typical afferent neurons have unipolar cell bodies located in craniospinal (sensory) ganglia. The dendritic zone of an afferent neuron consists of receptors or postsynaptic endings on sensory epithelial cells in the case of sense organs. Efferent axons arise from multipolar cell bodies located in the brain or spinal cord or in autonomic ganglia. They activate muscle or gland or neurons in autonomic ganglia.

Individual nerve fibers are classified also as **somatic** or **visceral**. The somatic fibers innervate skin, skeletal muscles, and joints, whereas visceral fibers innervate cardiac and smooth muscles and glands. Visceral efferent fibers, in particular, (and often visceral fibers in general) are designated the **autonomic nervous system**. The visceral efferent pathway involves two neurons. The first (preganglionic) neuron has its cell body in the CNS. The cell body of the second (postganglionic) neuron is located in an autonomic ganglion.

Nerves

A **nerve** typically consists of thousands of axons, each ensheathed or myelinated by neurolemmocytes and all organized into fascicles enveloped by connective tissue (Fig. 6.16). A **nerve fascicle** is delimited by **perineurium**, which consists of fibrous tissue surrounding epithelioid cells. The **perineural epithelioid cells** are squamous and arranged in concentric sheets. The **fibrous perineurium** is collagenous connective tissue. The multiple fascicles of a nerve are bound together by connective tissue called **epineurium**. Within a nerve fascicle, the fibrocytes and collagen fibers surrounding individual neurolemmocytes constitute **endoneurium**. Blood vessels supplying a nerve are designated **vasa nervorum**.

Individual perineural epithelioid cells are joined by zonulae occludentes and enveloped by basal laminae. Multiple concentric sheets of the squamous cells, along with interposed collagen fibrils, form a continuous tube enclosing nerve fibers and endoneurium within a fascicle (Fig. 6.17). A perineural epithelioid tube may have a dozen concentric layers at its origin, at the juncture of the nerve with its meningeal-covered root. The number of layers gradually decreases as a nerve branches. A single layer surrounds terminal branches, but epithelioid cells proliferate to encapsulate certain receptors. Because it is a diffusion barrier, the perineural epithelioid tube affords nerve fibers a protected environment. However, the enclosed intrafascicular space may also serve as a channel for infectious or toxic agents once they invade the epithelioid cell barrier.

The morphologic distinction between fibrous perineurium, which surrounds individual fascicles, and epineurium, which binds fascicles together, varies with species. In the dog, for example, nerves are composed of a few relatively large fascicles and fibrous perineurium is dense compared to epineurium, which is a flimsy, fatty connective tissue. In contrast, fibrous perineurium and endoneurium tend to be indistinguishable in bovine nerves, which feature multiple small fascicles.

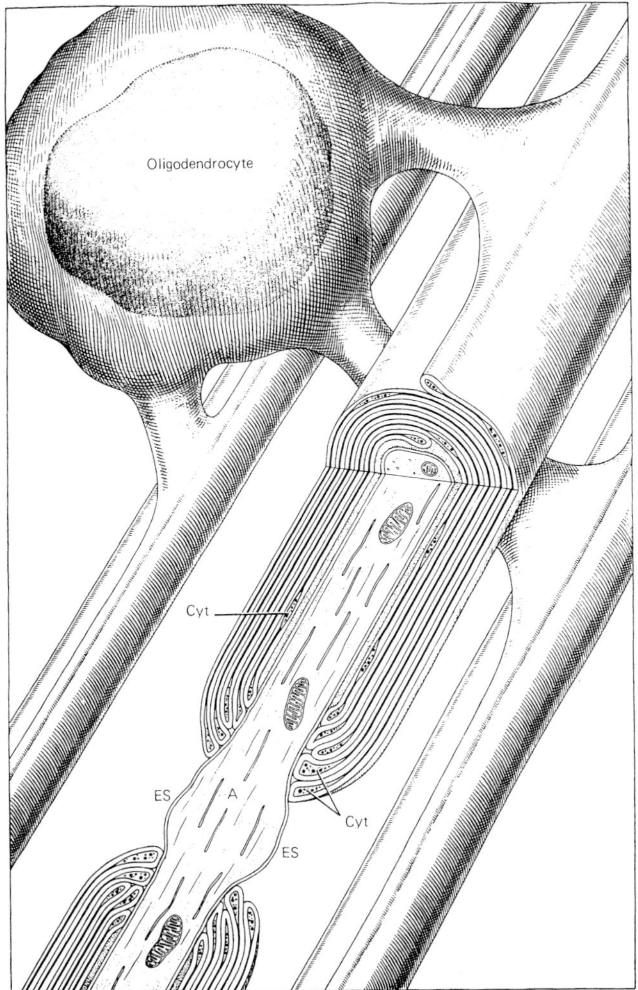

Figure 6.15. *Illustration of an oligodendrocyte providing myelin internodes to three axons. A bisected view of a node, adjacent paranode regions, and part of an internode is shown in the foreground. The axon (A) bulges at the node and is exposed to extracellular space (ES). Loop profiles containing cytoplasm (Cyt) contact the axon at the paranodal regions. Cytoplasm is retained along the ridges associated with inner and outer mesaxons, and small cytoplasmic pockets may be seen interrupting major dense lines. (Adapted from Bunge MB, Bunge RP, Ris H. Ultrastructural study of remyelination in an experimental lesion in adult cat spinal cord. J Biophys Biochem Cytol 1961;10:67.)*

Ganglia

A **ganglion** is a localized enlargement of a nerve produced by the accumulation of neuron cell bodies. Spinal ganglia located in dorsal spinal roots and ganglia in cranial nerve roots are referred to as **sensory ganglia**, because they contain cell bodies of primary afferent neurons (see Fig. 6.8). Afferent neurons are unipolar, except in the case of sense organs (vestibular apparatus, cochlea, retina, and olfactory epithelium), in which afferent neurons are bipolar.

Within a sensory ganglion, unipolar cell bodies are distributed superficially and nerve fibers course through the center of the ganglion. Each unipolar cell body gives rise to a single axon that may coil initially before bifurcating into central and peripheral branches; the peripheral branch is usually thicker than the central branch. Large cell bodies give rise to myelinated axons that bifurcate at a node. Each cell body is tightly encapsulated by ganglionic gliocytes.

Autonomic ganglia are accumulations of multipolar cell bodies within autonomic nerves (Fig. 6.9). The cell bodies, which have eccentric nuclei and marginally distributed Nissl substance as normal features, are loosely encapsulated by ganglionic gliocytes. Synapses occur in autonomic ganglia, where terminals of cholinergic preganglionic neurons synapse on dendritic zones of postganglionic neurons. Microscopic accumulations of postganglionic cell bodies within nerve plexuses of visceral organs (especially the gut) constitute terminal autonomic ganglia.

Postganglionic neurons are classified as **cholinergic** if they synthesize and release acetylcholine and are classified as **adrenergic** if their neurotransmitter is noradrenaline (norepinephrine). Adrenergic neurons feature dense-core synaptic vesicles. Some autonomic ganglia contain a few small intensely fluorescent (SIF) cells. These SIF cells feature numerous large, dense-core vesicles containing dopamine, which is released under neural control. The significance of SIF cells is unknown, but they form somatodendritic synapses and thus appear to function as interneurons.

Efferent Neurons

Somatic efferent neurons innervate skeletal muscle. One such neuron, together with all the muscle fibers it

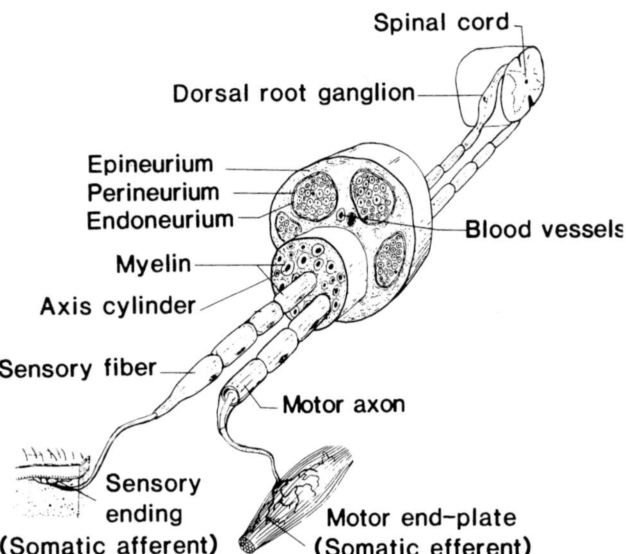

Figure 6.16. *Diagram of peripheral nerve constituents: Five fascicles are joined by epineurium. Each fascicle is encircled by perineurium, which consists of epithelioid-cell layers surrounded by fibrous connective tissue. Within a fascicle, endoneurium surrounds individual myelinated fibers. A myelinated fiber consists of an axon (axis cylinder) surrounded by a myelin sheath formed by neurolemmocytes and interrupted by nodes. Somatic afferent and efferent myelinated fibers are diagrammed. (From Jenkins TW. Functional mammalian neuroanatomy. 2nd ed. Philadelphia: Lea & Febiger, 1978.)*

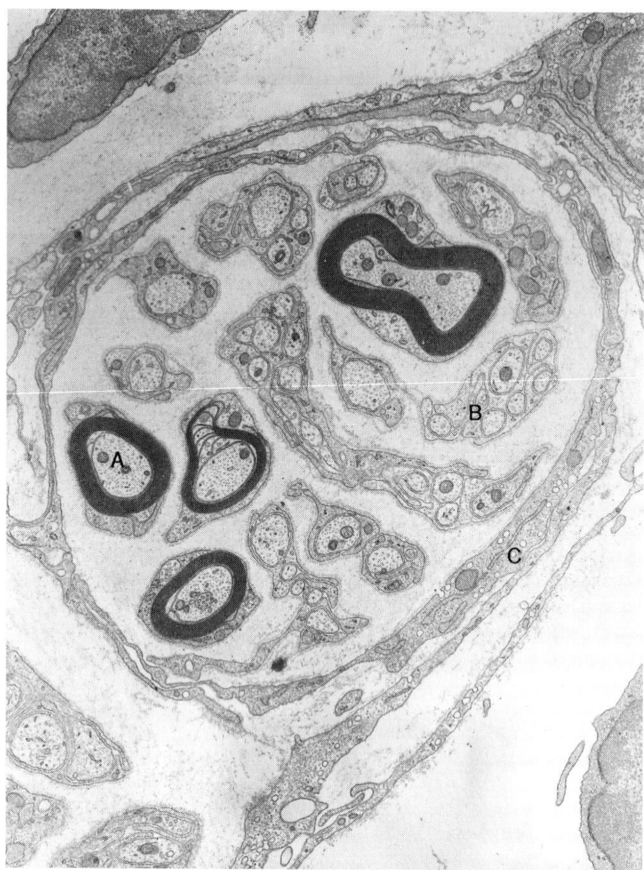

Figure 6.17. *Electron micrograph of a small nerve (within an organ) consisting of a single fascicle. Four myelinated fibers (A) are present; in one (to right of A), a myelin incisure is evident where major dense lines have split to contain pockets of cytoplasm. Several bundles of ensheathed non myelinated axons (B) are seen. Layers of perineural epithelioid cells (C) border the fascicle (×10,400). (Courtesy of H.-D. Dellmann.)*

innervates, is regarded as a **motor unit**, because the muscle fibers contract as a unit when the neuron is excited. A motor unit may have several or several hundred muscle fibers, depending on muscle size. Typical muscles have a range of large and small motor units. Small motor units have fatigue-resistant muscle fibers innervated by small neurons that are the first to begin firing and the last to cease firing during muscular contraction. Large motor units have hundreds of muscle fibers innervated by large neurons. The muscle fibers are readily fatigued and, because large neurons require additional synaptic input to reach threshold, they fire only when strong muscle contractions are needed.

A neuromuscular synapse consists of a presynaptic neuronal end plate overlaying a postsynaptic muscle sole plate at the midregion of a muscle fiber (Fig. 6.18). A **motor end plate** is formed by very short branches within a circumscribed zone (plate) at the end of one terminal branch of a somatic efferent neuron. Each branch of the end plate lies in a corresponding trough of the sole plate. The width of the neuromuscular gap is 40 to 50 nm; however, the gap is increased by junctional folds, where sarcolemma of the trough undergoes transverse enfolding. Neurolemmocytes cover the end plate, and associated basal lamina extends into the neuromuscular gap and junctional folds (Fig. 6.19).

End-plate cytoplasm contains many mitochondria and numerous agranular synaptic vesicles (40 nm in diameter). The vesicles contain acetylcholine, which is released at active sites opposite the junctional folds. Acetylcholine molecules diffuse across the neuromuscular gap and bind to postsynaptic receptor sites that open cation channels, leading to muscle fiber depolarization. Some binding sites are cholinesterase enzymes that degrade acetylcholine and thereby stop synaptic activity. Transporter protein molecules are present in the presynaptic membrane to recapture choline and recycle it.

Figure 6.18. *Drawing of three motor end plates synapsing on skeletal muscle fibers. Each of three terminal branches ends in a perfusion of short branches collectively designated an end plate. The bottom end plate is viewed from its edge. Neurolemmocytes that ensheathe the terminal branches proceed to overlay the end-plates. N. nuc. = neurolemmocyte nucleus; M. nuc. = muscle fiber nucleus. (Adapted from Krstic RV. General histology of the mammal. New York: Springer-Verlag, 1985.)*

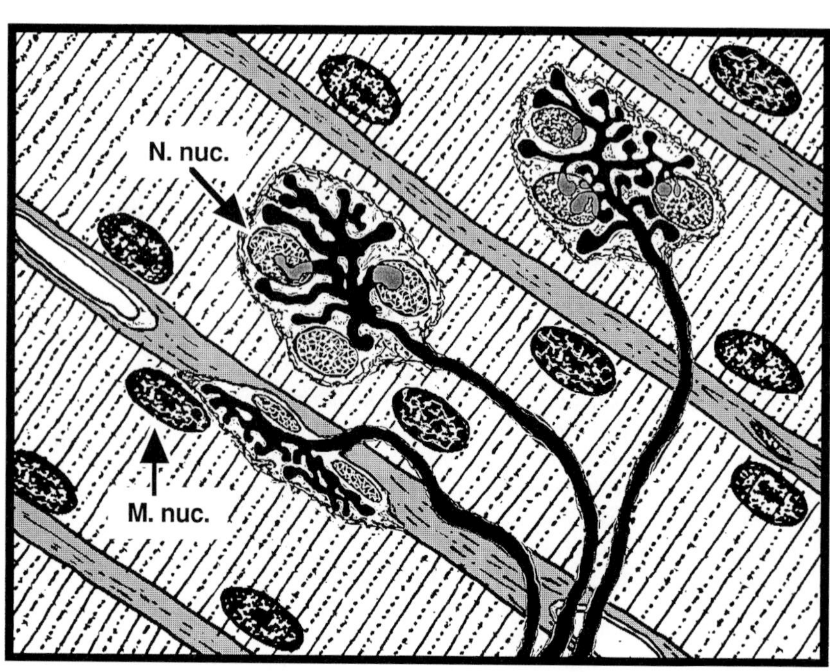

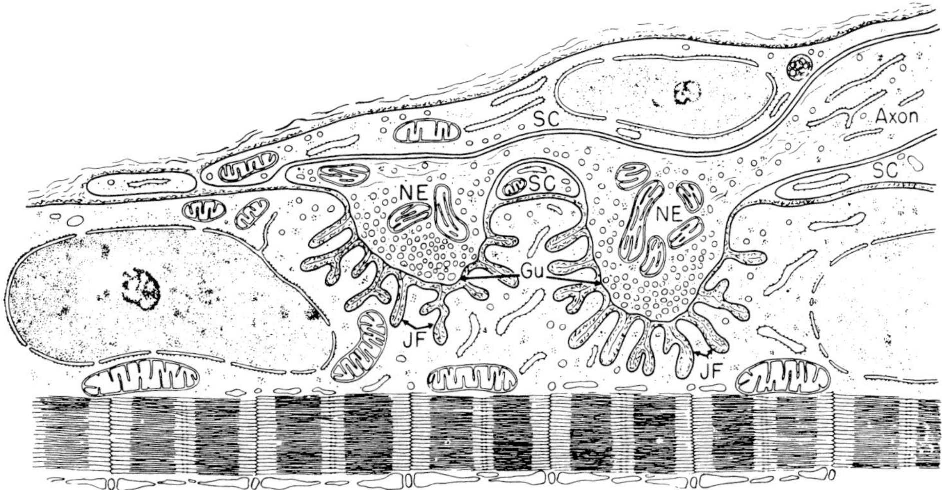

Figure 6.19. *Schematic ultrastructural illustration of a segment of motor end plate synapsing on the sole plate of a muscle fiber. Terminal branches (NE) featuring synaptic vesicles are in sole plate troughs (Gu). The synaptic cleft is elaborated further by junctional folds (JF). The cleft contains basal lamina continuous with that covering the muscle fiber and neurolemmocytes (Sc) overlaying the end plate. (From Porter KR, Bonneville MA. Fine structure of cells and tissues. 4th ed. Philadelphia: Lea & Febiger, 1973.)*

The **fusimotor** or **gamma motor neuron** is another type of somatic efferent neuron. It innervates intrafusal muscle fibers within muscle spindles. These relatively small neurons have myelinated axons that terminate as end plates or trail endings (multiple synaptic contacts along the muscle fiber surface).

Preganglionic autonomic neurons originate in the CNS and synapse on postganglionic neurons in autonomic ganglia, making typical interneuronal synapses. **Postganglionic autonomic neurons** have nonmyelinated axons that innervate cardiac muscle or smooth muscle or gland. The postganglionic axons terminate in branches that individually wander long distances without evidence of specialized contact with muscle or gland cells.

Ultrastructurally, terminal autonomic nerves consist of isolated neurolemmocytes ensheathing one or more terminal branches. The terminal branches present numerous preterminal bulbs along their course. Each preterminal bulb (varicosity) bulges beyond the confines of the ensheathing neurolemmocyte and contains a concentration of synaptic vesicles. Thus, neurotransmitter is released from multiple sites and diffuses variable distances to bind with receptors on target cells. Postsynaptic specializations are not evident.

Receptors

Afferent axons convey information to the CNS from receptors or from sense organs. Sense organs are organized collections of sensory epithelial cells, neurons, and supporting cells that detect visual, auditory, olfactory, or taste stimuli. In contrast, receptors are individual, isolated stimulus detectors widely distributed in the body (Fig. 6.20). Generally, the peripheral branch of an afferent axon branches repeatedly, and a receptor is located at the termination of each branch. All receptors of a single neuron have the same structure and function.

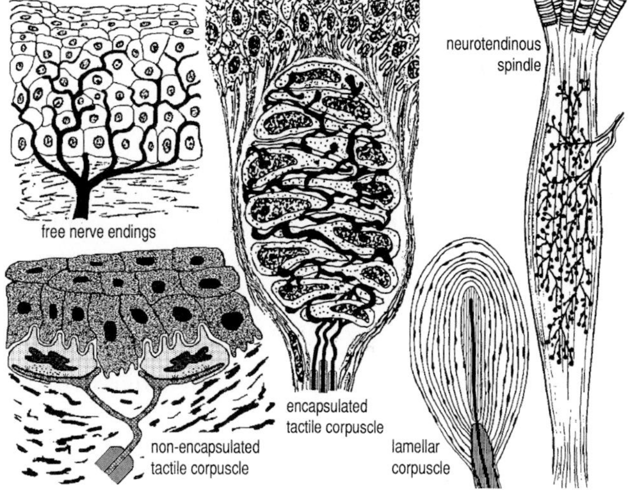

Figure 6.20. *Schematic drawings of five receptors at various magnifications. Free nerve endings branch among cells of the epidermis. Two nonencapsulated tactile corpuscles embrace a specialized tactile cell (Merkel's cell) at the base of the epidermis. An encapsulated tactile corpuscle (Meissner's corpuscle) is located in the dermis; dendritic branches from multiple myelinated axons weave among flattened neurolemmocytes within a capsule of perineural epithelioid cells. A lamellar corpuscle (Pacini's corpuscle) features the dendritic branch of a myelinated axon encased in a core of flattened neurolemmocytes within a laminated capsule composed of perineural epithelioid cells. A neurotendinous spindle splays among the collagen bundles of a small tendon; the receptor has a thin capsule and is associated with a myelinated axon (not shown). (Encapsulated tactile corpuscle and neurotendinous spindle from Krstic RV. General histology of the mammal. New York: Springer-Verlag, 1985.)*

Receptors are classified in several ways. By location, **exteroceptors**, **proprioceptors**, and **enteroceptors** are found at the body surfaces, in musculoskeletal structures, and in viscera, respectively. Receptors are classified according to the type of stimulus they are sensitive to as mechanoreceptors, chemoreceptors, and thermoreceptors. Morphologically, receptors may be classified as encapsulated and nonencapsulated. The following is a list of common receptors.

NONENCAPSULATED RECEPTORS

Free nerve endings are found throughout the body. They detect stimulation described as pain (noxious), warmth, cold, or touch. Simultaneously, the same stimulus information is used for subconscious reflex activity. The receptors are associated with nonmyelinated or thinly myelinated axons that branch extensively to innervate a wide area (receptive field). The actual receptors are simply unsheathed terminal branches enveloped by basal lamina (Fig. 6.20).

Hair follicle terminals, which detect body hairs being displaced, are derived from myelinated axons that branch extensively to innervate hundreds of follicles. Each follicle is encircled by a nonmyelinated plexus that disperses free nerve endings among follicle epithelial cells. (A different situation prevails for tactile hair follicles [vibrissae], each of which receives several myelinated axons, giving rise to several kinds of receptors.)

Nonencapsulated tactile corpuscles are often collected at the base of a slight skin elevation called a tactile pad (Fig. 6.20). Each receptor consists of a neural expansion embraced by processes of an epithelioid tactile cell (Merkel's cell) that develops under the trophic influence of the nerve ending. Tactile corpuscles are derived from a myelinated axon that distributes to a restricted receptive field. The receptors are capable of persistent firing (tonic receptors).

ENCAPSULATED RECEPTORS

Encapsulated tactile corpuscles (Meissner's corpuscles) are phasic touch receptors found in the dermis of glabrous skin (Fig. 6.20). Several myelinated axons give rise to nonmyelinated dendritic branches that permeate a stack of flattened neurolemmocytes encapsulated by perineural epithelioid cells.

Lamellar corpuscles (Vater's corpuscles, Pacini's corpuscles) are widely distributed throughout the body. A terminal branch of a myelinated axon is encased in several layers of flattened neurolemmocytes that are surrounded by a fluid space and multiple concentric layers derived from perineural epithelioid cells (Fig. 6.20). The ellipsoid receptor is large enough to be seen without magnification (0.5 × 1.0 mm). These receptors are sensitive to transient pressure, such as in vibratory stimuli.

Bulbous corpuscles (Krause's corpuscles, Golgi–Mazzoni corpuscles, genital corpuscles) vary in location, size, and shape. They are mechanoreceptors derived from myelinated axons that have highly coiled terminal branches enclosed in a relatively thin capsule derived from perineural epithelioid cells.

Neurotendinous spindles (Golgi tendon organs) are located at muscle–tendon junctions and are activated by tension. Derived from a large myelinated axon, the receptor consists of terminal branches traveling on bundles of collagen fibers within a fluid-filled, thin capsule derived from perineural epithelioid cells (Fig. 6.20).

Ruffini's corpuscle, found in dermis, fascia, and ligaments, is structurally similar to the neurotendinous spindle. It is a tonic mechanoreceptor.

Neuromuscular spindles (muscle spindles) are so elaborate, they could qualify as sense organs. Located in most muscles, the spindle features an elongated (1.5 mm) capsule derived from perineural epithelioid cells. The capsule encloses afferent and efferent innervation and two kinds of intrafusal muscle fibers, designated nuclear bag and nuclear chain fibers (Fig. 6.21).

A typical spindle has one or two **nuclear bag** fibers. Each has a dilated middle zone filled with nuclei and polar ends that project beyond the spindle capsule. A spindle has several **nuclear chain** fibers. These are smaller than nuclear bag fibers, contained entirely within the spindle capsule, and characterized by a chain of nuclei at the middle of the fiber. The middle nuclear region of both types of intrafusal muscle fibers lacks myofilaments and is stretched when the striated polar regions contract. The striated regions are innervated by fusimotor (gamma) motor neurons that establish either end-plate or trail-type neuromuscular synapses. Trail endings form multiple synaptic contacts as terminal branches ramify on a surface of the muscle fiber.

Two types of receptors are found on intrafusal muscle fibers (Fig. 6.21). A **primary ending**, also called an **annulospiral ending**, is derived from a single, large myelinated axon that has terminal branches that spiral around the nuclear regions of intrafusal muscle fibers. A **secondary ending** is derived from a myelinated axon with dendritic branches arranged in a flower-spray configuration, situated on nuclear chain fibers adjacent to the annulospiral endings. Collectively, the receptors are activated by the rate and degree of stretch that occurs when either the polar ends of intrafusal muscle fibers contract or the whole muscle is stretched. Information from spindle receptors is primarily subconscious and important for regulating muscle tone, adjusting posture, and coordinating movements.

CENTRAL NERVOUS TISSUE

The CNS consists of the brain and spinal cord (plus the optic nerve and retina, which originate embryologically as an extension of the brain). The brain may be divided into brainstem, cerebellum, and cerebrum. When the CNS is sliced, one can identify white-matter regions, gray-matter regions, and regions where white and gray matter are mixed together.

White matter is formed by dense accumulations of myelinated axons (myelin is rich in lipid and has a white appearance). Individual myelin sheaths are relatively thin in the CNS compared to the PNS. Nonmyelinated axons of the CNS are not ensheathed; they are totally exposed to the CNS extracellular space. White matter is composed of collections of tracts (called fasciculi or lemnisci in particular cases). A tract consists of functionally related nerve fibers having a similar origin and destination.

An absence or scarcity of myelin results in CNS tissue having a gray appearance. **Gray matter** is rich in neuronal cell bodies, glial cells, and neuropil. **Neuropil** refers to the axons, terminal branches, dendrites, and glial processes that collectively form a background matrix for the cell bodies seen with light microscopy. Most synapses occur in the neuropil. Neuropil appears dense because the CNS extracellular space is uniformly narrow (approximately 20 nm wide).

Gray matter on the surface of the cerebellum and cerebrum is called **cortex**. Distinctive gray matter masses within the CNS are usually designated **nuclei**. Generally, a nucleus receives input from some tract(s) and projects output to another tract or tracts, which, in turn, are input to a different nucleus or to cortex. For a given nucleus, incoming terminals typically synapse on small neurons with short axons, called **interneurons** because they are interposed between the input and output of the nucleus. The interneurons in a nucleus determine the appropriate output for a particular input.

Nervous tissue exhibits a variety of configurations among the different regions of the CNS. Gray- and white-matter features of three major CNS regions will be presented: cerebral cortex, cerebellum, and spinal cord.

Cerebral Cortex

The cerebrum of the brain is composed of paired cerebral hemispheres (Fig. 6.22). The surface of each hemisphere presents **gyri** (ridges) demarcated by **sulci** (grooves). The surface is coated by gray matter called cerebral cortex. The characteristic neuron of the cerebral cortex has a pyramid-shaped cell body, oriented with its apex directed toward the surface. Dendrites emerge from the apex and basal edges of the pyramidal cell; the axon leaves the center of the base and enters the white matter.

In mammals, all but the ventral cerebral cortex is designated neocortex, because it is phylogenetically recent. Cerebral **neocortex** is divisible into six layers, although the layering is evident only in thick sections and the prominence of individual layers varies from region to region. From superficial to deep, the six layers are as follows (Fig. 6.23):

1. **Molecular layer** — predominantly neuropil-oriented tangentially; composed of apical dendrites from pyramidal cells and terminal branches of superficial cortical afferent fibers.
2. **External granular layer** — predominantly small neurons that serve as interneurons.
3. **External pyramidal layer** — small and medium pyramidal neurons that send axons to adjacent cerebral cortex.
4. **Internal granular layer** — small stellate neurons that receive specific sensory input, a thick layer in sensory areas of cortex (e.g., primary visual area).

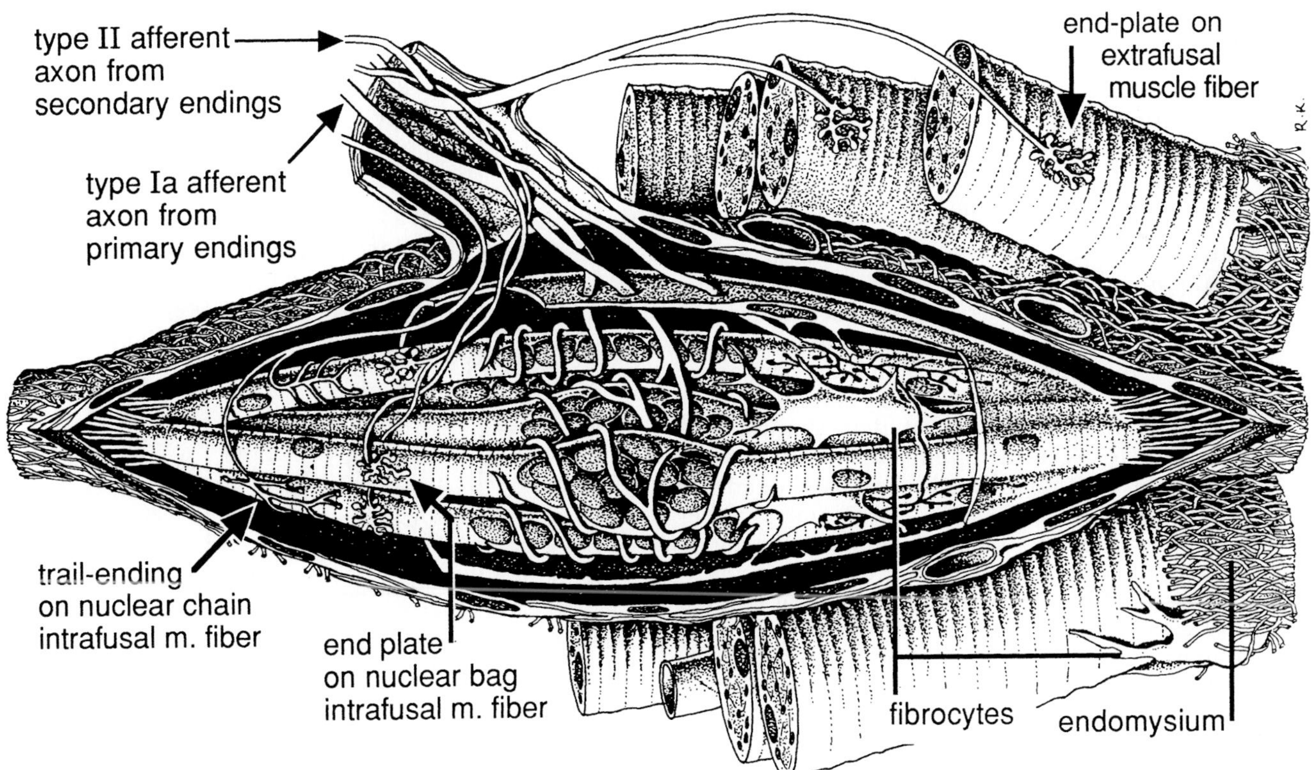

Figure 6.21. *Schematic drawing of a muscle spindle and several extrafusal muscle fibers linked by collagen fibrils of the endomysium. Perineural epithelioid cells that surround nerve fibers continue to form the spindle capsule (cut open). The contents of the spindle include nuclear bag and nuclear chain intrafusal muscle fibers, primary and secondary receptors, two types of neuromuscular synapses, and fibrocytes and collagen fibrils. Primary or annulospiral endings, which spiral around nuclear bag, and chain regions of intrafusal muscle fibers arise from a large (myelinated) axon. Secondary or flower-spray endings, which contact nuclear chain fibers adjacent to the primary ending, arise from a medium-sized (myelinated) axon. Small (myelinated) axons of fusimotor (gamma) neurons synapse on the polar regions of intrafusal muscle fibers. They form small end-plates and trail endings. The trail-endings are on nuclear chain fibers. Terminal branches of an alpha motor neuron form end-plates on extrafusal muscle fibers. (From Krstic RV. General Histology of the Mammal. New York: Springer-Verlag, 1985.)*

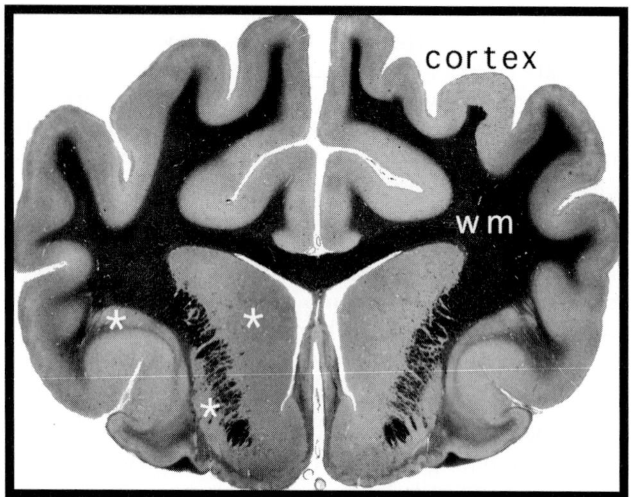

Figure 6.22. *Transverse section through the cerebrum of a canine brain; white matter is stained dark. The cerebrum is composed of two cerebral hemispheres joined across the midline by white matter (corpus callosum). The cerebral surface features gyri (elevations) separated by sulci (grooves). Gray matter at the surface of the cerebrum is cerebral cortex. Cerebral white matter (wm) is deep to the cortex. Internal masses of gray matter at the base of the cerebrum constitutes basal nuclei (*).*

5. **Internal pyramidal layer** — medium to large pyramidal neurons that send axons into the white matter; a thick layer in the motor area of the cortex.
6. **Fusiform** (multiform) **layer** — many spindle-shaped neurons; deep to this layer, cerebral white matter is composed of nerve fibers going to and coming from the cortex.

The functional unit of the cerebral cortex is a vertical column (approximately 0.3 mm in diameter) extending from the white matter to the cortical surface. Individual cortical columns are not histologically distinct, but physiologically, all neurons within a column become active in response to a certain feature of a stimulus and become inactive in the absence of that feature. The anatomic basis for vertical column organization is the pyramidal neuron. Pyramidal cells have basal dendrites for making radial connections within a column and they establish vertical contact by means of superficially directed apical dendrites and deeply directed axons.

Two types of afferent fibers enter a cortical column from white matter. One, which lacks specific information content, ramifies in all cortical layers, but especially in superficial layers. This fiber produces background excitation and represents a means of alerting selected cortical columns. The other type of input fiber conveys the modality-specific information with which the column is functionally concerned. It synapses on the small neurons of the internal granular layer, which serve as interneurons to distribute excitation throughout the column.

Output from the cortical column is predominantly from pyramidal neurons, which send their axons into the white matter. Superficial neurons send axons to neighboring regions of cortex (short association fibers). Neurons in the deepest two layers of the cortex send long axons to the brainstem (projection fibers), to the contralateral cerebral hemisphere (commissural fibers), or to distant regions of the same hemisphere (long association fibers).

Cerebellum

The cerebellar surface features **folia** (narrow ridges) separated by **sulci** (grooves). The surface is coated by gray matter, called **cerebellar cortex**. White matter is located deep to the cortex, and three bilateral pairs of cerebellar nuclei are embedded within the white matter (Fig. 6.24).

The cerebellar cortex is divisible into three layers (Fig. 6.25). The **molecular layer**, composed predominantly of neuropil, is most superficial. The **granule cell layer**, situated adjacent to white matter, features densely packed granule cells (small neurons with chromatic nuclei). Finally, a single layer of large cell bodies is located at the interface of the molecular and granule cell layers. This is called the **piriform cell layer** (Purkinje cell layer)

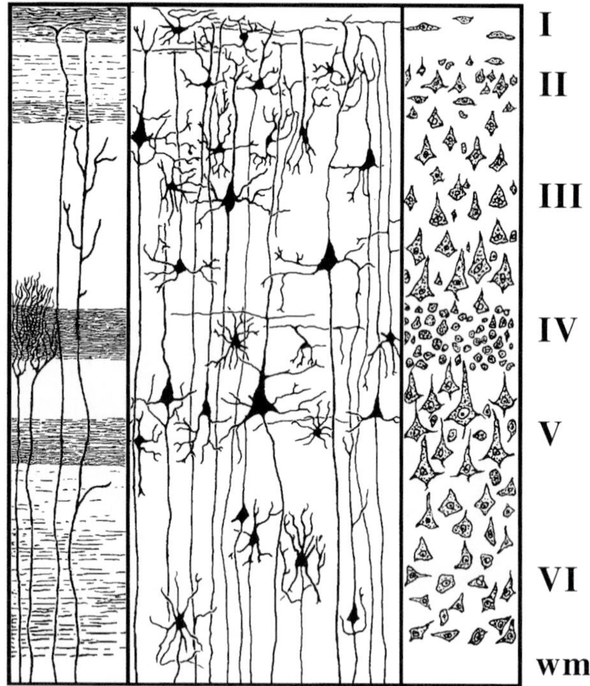

Figure 6.23. *Schematic illustration of the six layers (I to VI) of cerebral cortex (neocortex), shown in three perspectives. The left panel illustrates nerve fibers (axons, telodendria, and dendrites) in the cortex. From the white matter (wm), modality-specific input fibers terminate in layer IV; nonspecific input fibers terminate especially in the superficial layers. The middle panel displays individual neurons as they are seen with silver impregnation (Golgi stain). The characteristic neuron of the cerebral cortex has a pyramidal shape. Notice that pyramidal neurons have an apical dendrite that ascends to the surface, radially oriented basal dendrites, and a single axon that courses into the white matter. The right panel shows neuron cell bodies in the different layers of cerebral cortex as they appear in a Nissl stain. (Modified from Crosby EC, Humphrey T, Lauer EW. Correlative anatomy of the nervous system. New York: The Macmillan Co., 1962.)*

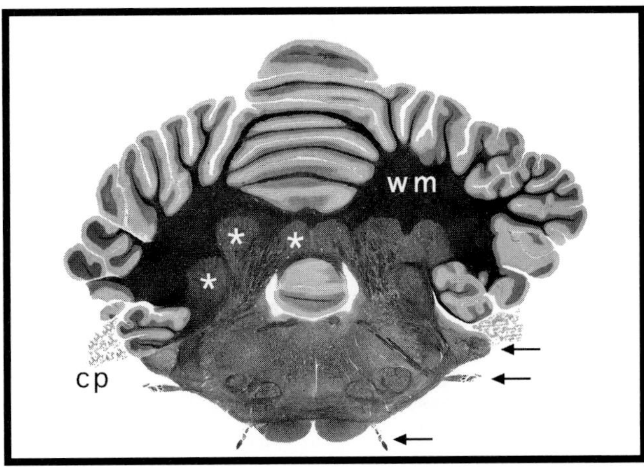

Figure 6.24. *Transverse sections of the canine hindbrain. The cerebellum (above) is joined to the brainstem (below). The cerebellar surface features folia (elevations) separated by sulci (grooves). Cerebellar cortex, the surface gray matter, appears two-toned because of a cell-sparse molecular layer covering a cell-dense granule layer. Three cerebellar nuclei (*) are located bilaterally deep to the white matter (wm). The brainstem exhibits white matter tracts, gray matter nuclei, regions in which white and gray matter are mixed, and emerging cranial nerve roots (arrows). On each side, the tip of a choroid plexus (cp) is seen in the surrounding subarachnoid space.*

The **piriform** (Purkinje) **cells** send axons into the white matter to synapse on neurons of cerebellar nuclei. Each **piriform cell** has an elaborate dendritic tree that projects into the molecular layer (Fig. 6.26) and makes more than 200,000 synaptic contacts with granule cell axons. Axons of **granule cells** enter the molecular layer, bifurcate, travel longitudinally within a folium, and synapse on numerous piriform cell dendritic trees. Another neuron of the cerebellar cortex is called a **basket cell** because its terminal branches form "baskets" surrounding cell bodies of adjacent piriform cells. The cell bodies of basket cells are found in the piriform cell layer; their axons course transversely in the folium and inhibit laterally positioned piriform cells.

Two types of input fibers enter the cerebellar cortex. One type (climbing fibers) has terminal branches that climb like vines on piriform dendritic trees, each fiber making numerous synapses-in-passing on one dendritic tree. The other type of input fiber has terminal expansions (mossy endings) within the granule cell layer. Neighboring granule cells send dendrites to synapse with each mossy ending, thereby creating a synaptic complex known as a glomerulus.

The cerebellum regulates muscle tone, posture, and movement so that these are expressed in an appropriate, coordinated pattern. It operates in the following manner: neurons of cerebellar nuclei are spontaneously active; they send their axons out of the cerebellum to excite brain neurons responsible for initiating posture and movement. Input to the cerebellum comes from these brain neurons and from muscle and joint proprioceptors. Input fibers excite cerebellar nuclei and specific regions of cerebellar cortex. Excitatory granule cells and inhibitory basket cells interact to produce a localized pattern of active piriform cells in the cerebellar cortex. Piriform axons, the only output from the cortex, inhibit neurons of cerebellar nuclei. Thus, the cerebellar cortex continuously compares movement initiation with movement performance and regulates movement execution by selectively inhibiting the generalized excitatory influence of cerebellar nuclei.

Spinal Cord

The cylindrical spinal cord is divisible into segments that are demarcated by the bilateral emergence of dorsal and ventral roots of spinal nerves. A transverse section of the spinal cord shows a **central canal** surrounded by an H-shaped profile of gray matter, which is in turn surrounded by white matter (Fig. 6.27). The spinal cord is sagittally divided by a **ventral median fissure** and a **dorsal median septum** (the septum is replaced by a fissure in the caudal half of the cord). Spinal cord and particularly spinal gray matter are enlarged at segments supplying limbs because limb innervation requires additional nervous tissue.

Spinal gray matter contains three categories of neurons: interneurons (contained within the gray matter, connecting afferent and efferent neurons), projection neurons (which project axons through white matter

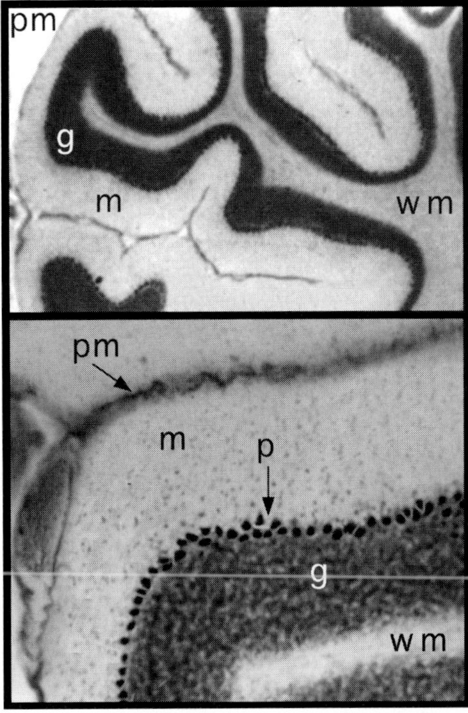

Figure 6.25. *Two light micrographs at different magnification of cerebellar cortex (pig). Nissl stain. Top: white matter (wm) extends into the center of a cerebellar folium. Cortex covering the white matter exhibits a cell dense layer (g) and a relatively acellular layer (m). Pia mater (pm) covers the cerebellar surface and extends into sulci separating folia (×15). Bottom: cerebellar cortex, situated between white matter (wm) and pia mater (pm), is composed of three layers. From deep to superficial: the granule cell layer (g); piriform (Purkinje) cell layer; and molecular layer (m) (×55).*

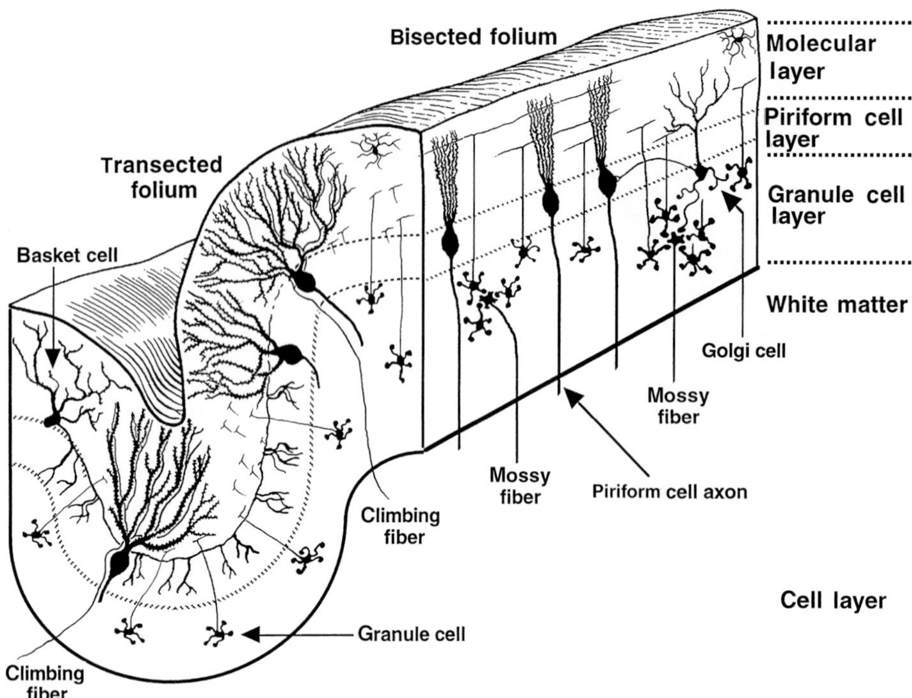

Figure 6.26. *Schematic diagram of cerebellar cortex. The three layers of cortex (labeled on the right) are shown in bisected (right side) and transected (left side) views of a folium. The molecular layer of cerebellar cortex is composed of neuronal processes plus a few small stellate neurons (upper right, unlabeled). The piriform (Purkinje) cell layer features cell bodies of Piriform (piriform) neurons, which send their axons into the white matter. The piriform cell dendritic tree is flattened and oriented perpendicular to the long axis of the folium. The granule cell layer is packed with small granule cell neurons that send axons into the molecular layer to synapse on Piriform dendrites. Two additional neurons include the Golgi cell (right) and the basket cell (left). The Golgi cell (great stellate cell) is an inhibitory interneuron located in the upper part of the granule cell layer. The basket cell, an inhibitory neuron located in the depths of the molecular layer, has axonal branches that form "baskets" around Piriform cell bodies. Cerebellar white matter is composed of Piriform cell axons leaving the cortex and two types of cortical afferents: mossy and climbing fibers. A mossy fiber makes synaptic contact with granule cell dendrites; the mossy ending forms the center of a synaptic glomerulus. Climbing fibers make many synaptic contacts on one Piriform dendritic tree. (Modified from Jenkins TW: Functional Mammalian Neuroanatomy. 2nd ed. Philadelphia: Lea & Febiger, 1978.)*

tracts to the brain), and efferent neurons (which send axons into ventral roots). A group of related neuron cell bodies is designated a nucleus (e.g., the intermediolateral nucleus is composed of sympathetic preganglionic neuron cell bodies). Spinal gray matter is sometimes subdivided into 10 defined laminae (boundaries of laminae are indistinct in ordinary tissue sections).

Bilaterally, spinal gray matter consists of dorsal and ventral gray columns connected by intermediate gray matter. In transverse sections, gray column profiles are usually called **horns**. The **ventral gray column** (horn) contains somatic efferent neurons that innervate skeletal muscle. The **dorsal gray column** (horn) contains interneurons and projection neurons on which primary afferent neurons synapse. Intermediate gray matter features visceral neurons. In thoracolumbar segments, a **lateral gray column** (horn) containing sympathetic preganglionic neurons (intermediolateral nucleus) is present.

Spinal white matter is composed of fibers that form ascending and descending tracts plus fibers entering from dorsal roots or exiting to ventral roots. Ascending tracts terminate in the brain. Axons of descending tracts originate in the brain and mainly synapse on interneurons within the gray matter. Afferent axons of dorsal roots enter white matter at a dorsolateral sulcus and terminate principally in the dorsal gray column. Axons of efferent neurons exit ventrolaterally as ventral root fibers.

Bilaterally, spinal white matter is divided into three anatomic regions. The **dorsal funiculus** is located between the midline and dorsal root attachments. The **ventral funiculus** is situated between the midline and ventral root attachments. The **lateral funiculus** is positioned between dorsal and ventral root attachments.

MENINGES, VESSELS, AND CEREBROSPINAL FLUID

Meninges

The brain and spinal cord and the roots of peripheral nerves are enveloped by meninges. Meninges also surround the entire optic nerve (which is CNS tissue). Meninges contain cerebrospinal fluid and constitute a protective barrier.

Traditionally, three meningeal layers are described, from superficial to deep: dura mater, arachnoid, and pia mater (Fig. 6.28). **Dura mater** is sometimes called **pachymeninx** because it is thick and strong. The **arachnoid** and **pia mater** are collectively termed **leptomeninges**, because they are delicate and connected embryologically and physically. A **subarachnoid space** containing cerebrospinal fluid separates arachnoid from pia mater.

Dura mater is composed of variably oriented planes of collagen fibers. Elastic fibers, fibrocytes, nerves, and

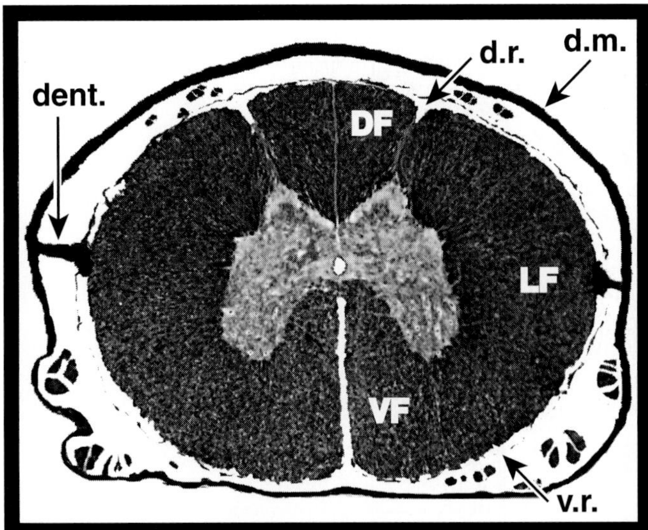

Figure 6.27. *Photomicrograph of a canine spinal cord at the midthoracic region. The central canal is surrounded by butterfly-shaped gray matter, which is surrounded by white matter (stained dark). In this thoracic segment, gray matter features a small dorsal horn, a subtle lateral horn, and a large ventral horn, bilaterally. Meninges and transected nerve roots are external to the white matter. Bilaterally, a denticulate ligament (dent.) connects pia mater to dura mater (d.m.). The spinal cord is divided into bilateral halves by a ventral median fissure and a dorsal median sulcus and septum. In each half, white matter is divided into three regions: dorsal funiculus (DF), lateral funiculus (LF), and ventral funiculus (VF). A prominent dorsolateral sulcus, where dorsal roots (d.r.) would enter, separates dorsal and lateral funiculi. The boundary between lateral and ventral funiculi is demarcated by the emergence of ventral roots (v.r.). Luxol blue and hematoxylin (×18).*

lymph and blood vessels are also present. The inner surface of dura mater is lined by multiple layers of flattened fibrocytes to which outer cells of arachnoid membrane adhere. Although there is no subdural space, hemorrhage can result in blood accumulation between fibrocyte layers (subdural hematoma), giving the false impression of a subdural space.

Spinal dura mater is surrounded by an epidural space that separates the dura mater from periosteum lining the vertebral canal. **Cranial dura mater** is composed of two laminae. The internal lamina is comparable to spinal dura mater; the external lamina serves as periosteum for the cranial cavity. The two laminae are distinct only where the inner lamina separates from the outer one to form partitions between parts of the brain (Fig. 6.28). Endothelium-lined spaces, called **dural venous sinuses** are present where the internal and external laminae separate. Venous blood drains into the sinuses, which resist collapse because of their rigid walls.

Arachnoid (arachnoid membrane) consists of outer layers of flattened fibrocytes and inner, loosely arranged, flattened fibrocytes associated with small bundles of collagen fibers. **Arachnoid trabeculae** are thin strands of inner arachnoid that traverse the subarachnoid space and establish continuity with pia mater. **Arachnoid villi** are microscopic projections of arachnoid that penetrate walls of dural venous sinuses and act as one-way valves for drainage of cerebrospinal fluid. When cerebrospinal fluid pressure exceeds sinus blood pressure, arachnoid villi expand to facilitate fluid transfer into the bloodstream. The villi collapse to preclude blood reflux when venous pressure exceeds cerebrospinal fluid pressure. Cerebrospinal fluid can also drain into lymphatics of peripheral nerves.

Pia mater is composed of variable amounts of loosely arranged collagen fibers covered superficially by flattened fibrocytes. A basal lamina separates pia mater collagen from the underlying glial limiting membrane (astrocyte processes). Pia mater coats the entire CNS surface, lining every sulcus and fissure. It is highly vascularized.

Together with arachnoid, pia mater bounds the subarachnoid space, which contains cerebrospinal fluid. The entire subarachnoid space, including the surfaces of nerves and vessels that traverse the space, is lined by flattened fibrocytes joined by zonulae adherentes. The fibrocytes are capable of phagocytosis, and macrophages are sporadically found on the lining of the subarachnoid space.

Along each midlateral surface of the spinal cord, an increase in the amount of pia mater collagen creates an elongated ligament called the **denticulate ligament**. A periodic series of projections extends laterally from the ligament and attaches to spinal dura mater (Fig. 6.17). Thus, bilateral denticulate ligaments act to suspend the spinal cord within the dura mater so the spinal cord is completely surrounded by the cerebrospinal fluid within the subarachnoid space.

As nerve roots enveloped by meninges become cranial and spinal nerves enveloped by connective tissue, there is a transition between meninges and neural connective tissue at cranial and intervertebral foramina. Flattened fibrocytes of the leptomeninges are continued by the epithelioid cells of the perineurium. Dura mater is continued by fibrous perineurium and epineurium. Pia mater collagen is continued by endoneurium.

Vessels

Vessels in the subarachnoid space are covered by leptomeningeal tissue derived from arachnoid trabeculae

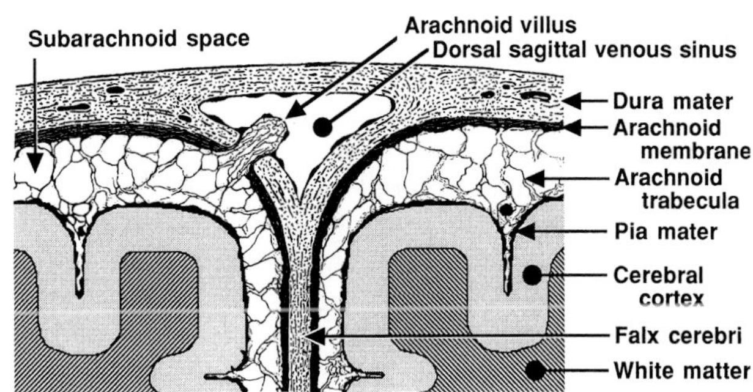

Figure 6.28. *Schematic illustration of meningeal relationships at the dorsal midline of the cranial cavity. The internal lamina of dura mater separates from the external (periosteal) lamina and forms a partition, the falx cerebri, between cerebral hemispheres. The separation also encloses a venous sinus lined by endothelial cells (into which veins drain). Arachnoid membrane merges with flattened fibrocytes lining the internal surface of dura mater. Arachnoid trabeculae connect to pia mater by traversing the subarachnoid space, which is filled with cerebrospinal fluid. The fluid drains into venous blood through an arachnoid villus that expands or collapses according to the pressure differential across it. (Adapted from Weed LH. The absorption of cerebrospinal fluid in to the venous system. Am J Anat 1923;31:191.)*

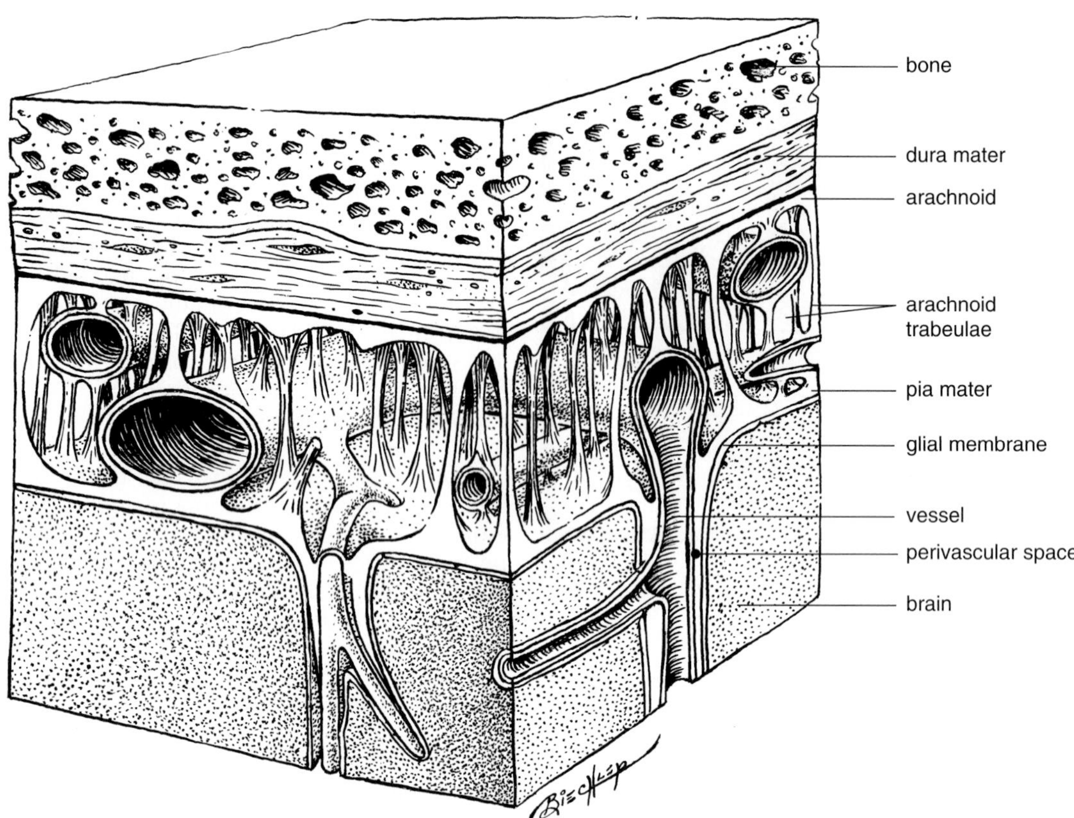

Figure 6.29. *Schematic illustration showing cranial meninges and perivascular space around vessels. The entire subarachnoid space, including surfaces of vessels, is coated by leptomeninges (arachnoid and pia mater). The perivascular space that is present between the glial limiting membrane and the vessel wall is filled with pia mater collagen fibers.*

or pia mater (Fig. 6.29). When a vessel penetrates the CNS, it is surrounded by a perivascular space, i.e., a space situated between the vessel wall and the glial limiting membrane The space persists to the level of small vessels, where the basal lamina associated with the glial limiting membrane merges with vascular basal lamina. Leptomeninges, particularly pia mater collagen fibers, fill the perivascular space so space is not obvious, except when it fills with inflammatory cells under pathologic conditions. Communication between perivascular spaces and the subarachnoid space is blocked by a continuous barrier of leptomeningeal cells, formed by cells on surfaces of vessels uniting with those on the pia mater surface.

In contrast to most endothelial cells in the body, endothelial cells of CNS capillaries are generally nonfenestrated and joined by tight junctions. These endothelial features are responsible for the **blood–brain barrier**, which impedes diffusion of hydrophilic molecules from the bloodstream to the CNS (polar molecules must be specifically transported into the CNS). The trophic influence of astrocyte end feet in contact with the basal lamina surrounding CNS capillaries induces CNS endothelial cells to become nonfenestrated and joined by tight junctions. A blood–brain barrier is not present either neonatally or at the few sites in the adult brain where modified ependymal cells are found (choroid plexuses and circumventricular organs).

A blood–brain barrier is also present in peripheral nerves. Capillaries within the endoneurium of peripheral nerves (but not ganglia) exhibit zonulae occludentes. Perineural epithelioid cells surrounding nerve fascicles also have zonulae occludentes. These tight junctions establish a blood–nerve barrier for hydrophilic molecules.

Cerebrospinal Fluid

Cerebrospinal fluid is produced by choroid plexuses in brain ventricles. A region of each ventricular wall is formed by **tela choroidea**, a term that refers to ependyma in contact with pia mater without intervening nervous tissue. A **choroid plexus** arises from tela choroidea as a mass of villi that collectively form a fuzzy tufted growth extending into the ventricle. Each villus consists of pial vasculature in loose connective tissue covered by modified ependymal cells, called choroid plexus epithelium. The epithelial cells are joined by zonulae occludentes near their luminal surfaces. Choroid plexus capillaries have fenestrated endothelial cells.

Cerebrospinal fluid is produced by choroid plexus epithelium through a process that involves active Na^+ secretion. Choroid plexus epithelial cells exhibit pinocytotic vesicles at the base of each cell and migration of the vesicles toward the luminal surface.

Cerebrospinal fluid flows through brain ventricles. By exiting through lateral apertures, the fluid leaves the ventricles and enters the subarachnoid space, where it surrounds the brain and spinal cord. Besides offering the physical protection of a fluid buffer, cerebrospinal fluid compensates for the absence of lymphatics in the CNS because large molecules from the CNS extracellular space are able to pass between ependymal cells and into the cerebrospinal fluid.

REFERENCES

Bergman RA, Afifi AK, Heidger PM Jr. Atlas of microscopic anatomy. 2nd ed. Philadelphia: WB Saunders, 1989.

Calakos N, Scheller RH. Synaptic vesicle biogenesis, docking, and fusion: a molecular description. Physiol Rev 1996;76:1.

Cooper JR, Bloom FE, Roth RH. The biochemical basis of neuropharmacology. 7th ed. New York: Oxford University Press, 1996.

Fawcett DW. A textbook of histology. 12th ed. Philadelphia: WB Saunders, 1994.

Jones EG. The nervous tissue. In: Weiss L, ed. Cell and tissue biology. 6th ed. Baltimore: Urban & Schwarzenberg, 1988.

Junqueira LC, Carneiro J, Kelly RO. Basic histology. 8th ed. Norwalk, CT: Appleton & Lange, 1995.

Krstic RV. General histology of the mammal. New York: Springer Verlag, 1985.

Orlin JR, Osen KK, Hovig T. Subdural compartment in pig. A morphologic study with blood and horseradish peroxidase infused subdurally. Anat Rec 1991;230:22.

Pannese E. Neurocytology. Fine structure of neurons, nerves processes, and neuroglial cells. New York: Thieme Medical Publishers, 1994.

Peters A, Palay SL, Webster HDeF. The fine structure of the nervous system, neurons and supporting cells. 3rd ed. New York: Oxford University Press, 1991.

Sternberg SS. Histology for pathologists. New York: Raven Press, 1992.

7

Cardiovascular System

H. DIETER DELLMANN

The connective tissues of domestic animals are permeated by a network of tubular passages through which the more fluid components of the intercellular milieu flow. Two types of fluids circulate within these tubes of the vascular system: the highly cellular and viscous **blood**, and the relatively acellular and watery **lymph**. The vascular systems conducting these different fluids are called blood and lymphatic vascular systems, respectively.

In domestic mammals, the blood vascular system forms circulatory arcs emanating from and returning to the heart, whereas the lymphatic vascular system forms drainage channels, which join the major veins at the thoracic inlet, and through which accumulating tissue fluid returns to the circulating blood.

Blood and lymph flow because of the pressure gradients within the lumina of their respective vascular networks. These pressure gradients arise from several forces: the pumping action of the heart, the movements of the muscular and skeletal parts, and gravity. The pressure inside the vascular tubes differs from the pressure outside, and the resulting pressure gradients, coupled with the shearing forces of fluid flow, probably determine the structure of the various tubular portions composing the vascular system.

BLOOD VESSELS

Structure–Function Relationships of Blood Vessels

The blood vascular system includes the heart and blood vessels. The blood vessels of the **macrovasculature** are visible with the naked eye and include elastic and muscular arteries and accompanying veins. Arteries of the macrovasculature carry the blood from the heart to the **microvasculature**, which comprises arterioles, metarterioles and thoroughfare channels, capillaries, venules, and arteriovenous anastomoses. Veins return the blood from the microvasculature to the heart.

Blood vessels are commonly defined by their position in the vascular circuit. They are characterized histologically by their individual structures, which reflect the particular forces withstood and the control over vascular function provided by each type.

Arteries control flow to the microvasculature, in which blood flows slowly and can stop intermittently because its pressures are only slightly above or below those of the surrounding tissues. In veins, the velocity of the blood is back again to at least half that in corresponding arteries, but the pressures are reduced.

Ventricular contractions are the greatest impelling force to blood circulation. The thick **elastic**, **conducting arteries**, such as the aorta, receive the first surge of blood from each contraction, during which both velocity of flow and pressure reach their peaks. The great pressure of the cardiac blood pumped out during contraction of the cardiac ventricles (systole) is absorbed largely by the stretch of the highly elastic arterial walls. At the time of ventricular dilation (diastole), release of the arterial wall tension partially maintains blood pressure, and the volume of flow is dissipated into the more numerous **muscular**, **distributive arteries**. These vessels lead to specific organs or body parts and eventually into the smallest branches of the arterial tree, the **arterioles**. The velocity of flow is gradually reduced in the distributive arteries because their increasing number of branches greatly expands the total volume accepting this flow. Pressure in muscular arteries remains high. Peripheral outflow is regulated by the sympathetic division of the autonomic nervous system, which determines contraction or relaxation of the smooth muscle cells of the walls of these arteries.

Frequently, the elastic, muscular, and arteriolar arteries are referred to as **large**, **medium- sized**, and **small**, respectively. On a comparative anatomic basis, the latter nomenclature is confusing, because an elastic artery of a cat may be of smaller caliber than a muscular artery of a large ruminant. But within one species, the assumption of a relationship between structure and relative size is valid.

From the arterial tree, the vessels open into voluminous networks of small, uniformly thin-walled tubules called **capillaries**. In the liver parenchyma, the capillaries are called **sinusoids**. The total blood volume in capillaries and sinusoids is so much greater than that in arterioles that the velocity of blood flow decreases from meters per second in the arterial tree to less than 1 mm per second in the capillary. The shearing forces generated by the viscous blood flowing within the narrow arterioles decrease the pressure of the blood until it exceeds that of the surrounding tissue fluid only by 10 mm Hg or less. Thus, capillaries oppose only small-scale forces and have thin walls structured from single cells. Blood-tissue exchanges take place within the capillary network, as well as within postcapillary venules, which have a comparable structure.

Blood from the capillaries and sinusoids returns to the heart via the **veins**. Veins of increasing size, usually classified simply as **small, medium-sized**, and **large**, form inverse trees, analogous to and in most instances parallel with the arterial trees. Consequently, arteries and their accompanying veins are seen together in most tissue sections. Usually, a nerve and sometimes a lymphatic vessel are seen along with the paired blood vessels. There are, however, specific exceptions, such as in the lung.

Because they receive blood from capillaries, veins oppose little residual pressure from the pumping action of the heart. They do withstand, however, pressures caused by gravity and surrounding tissues, particularly muscle. Flow of blood through the veins results from pressure of blood flowing from the capillaries into the veins and pressure differences between peripheral tissues and the thorax. This flow is augmented by a series of valves in the long veins of the extremities, whereby strong forces from adjacent skeletal muscles cause a flow that is directed toward the heart.

The small pressure gradients within the veins provide relatively low velocities of flow as compared to those within arteries. However, the venous channels are large in comparison to those of the satellite arteries; consequently, the rate of flow through the two is equal.

Because veins are larger than arteries, they hold nearly half of the total blood volume, and the contractile state of the walls of the larger veins is an important determinant of total vascular volume.

The blood vessels of the **macrovasculature** are visible with the naked eye and include elastic and muscular arteries and accompanying veins. The **microvasculature** comprises arterioles, metarterioles and thoroughfare channels, capillaries, venules, and arteriovenous anastomoses, and thus blood vessels that are only visible microscopically.

General Structural Organization of Blood Vessels

The walls of all blood vessels larger than capillaries are composed of three concentric layers or tunics that comprise an inner **tunica interna** (intima), a middle **tunica media**, and an external **tunica externa** (adventitia) (Fig. 7.1). The tissues that comprise these layers and their relative importance depend on the type of blood vessel and vary within wide limits.

The **tunica interna** is lined with **endothelium**, a simple squamous epithelium, and its underlying basal lamina. A **subendothelial layer** includes collagen and elastic fibers, fibrocytes, and smooth muscle cells. The outermost layer is the **internal elastic membrane**. This membrane is a sheet of elastin that has gaps, which permit diffusion of nutrients into the tunica media; it is usually absent in the smaller veins and thin or inconspicuous in the larger ones. The internal elastic membrane is often indistinct under the light microscope but can be identified readily by electron microscopy (see Fig. 7.4). The tunica interna is avascular and is nourished through transendothelial transport of substances from the circulating blood.

The **tunica media** consists of several layers of smooth muscle in helical arrangement, interspersed with varying numbers of elastic laminae and elastic and collagen fibers. Approximately the inner half of the tunica media receives nutrients from the tunica interna; the remainder is supplied by vasa vasorum. An **external elastic membrane**, similar in structure to the internal elastic membrane, is clearly distinguishable only in the largest muscular arteries.

In the outermost **tunica externa** (adventitia), collagen

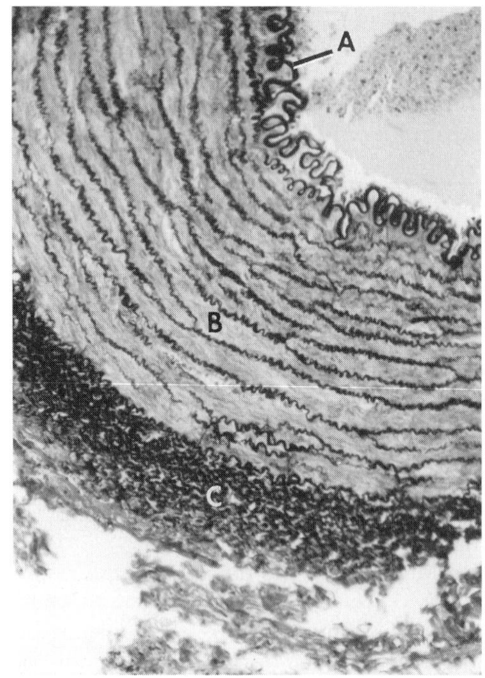

Figure 7.1. *Cross section through part of the wall of a canine muscular artery. The most prominent layer of the tunica interna is the internal elastic membrane (A); the tunica media consists of several alternating layers of smooth muscle cells and elastic lamellae or fibers (B). In the tunica externa, elastic fibers predominate (C); its innermost elastic layer is the external elastic membrane. Verhoeff's elastic stain (×130).*

and elastic fibers predominate, and smooth muscle cells may be present. This tunic contains small blood vessels (**vasa vasorum**), which penetrate the outer layers of the tunica media. Vasomotor nerves (**nervi vasorum**) form plexuses in most large blood vessels. A few axons penetrate the tunica media and terminate in proximity of smooth muscle cells.

Arteries

ELASTIC ARTERIES

The tunica interna of elastic arteries is often thicker than that of the other types of arteries (Fig. 7.2). The endothelial cells often have a bricklike shape. The subendothelial layer contains smooth muscle cells, fibroblasts, and primarily longitudinally oriented collagen and numerous fine elastic fibers. In the large domestic mammals, this layer is particularly thick. The internal elastic membrane is often split into lamellae that may merge with the elastic laminae of the tunica media.

The tunica media is the thickest of the three layers and consists primarily of concentrically arranged, fenestrated elastic laminae (Fig. 7.3). Smooth muscle cells lie between adjacent laminae to which they are attached by collagen and elastic fibers. In addition, fine elastic fibers and collagen fibers are present (Fig. 7.3). The amorphous ground substance is basophilic because it contains a great amount of sulfated glycosaminoglycans. All intercellular fibers and ground substances of the media are synthesized by the smooth muscle cells. With increasing distance from the heart, the number of smooth muscle cells increases and the amount of elastic tissue decreases. The external elastic membrane is either absent or indistinct.

In the tunica externa, longitudinally arranged bundles of collagen fibers predominate and are intermixed with a few elastic fibers and fibroblasts. The interlacing of the collagen fibers limits the elastic expansion of the vessel.

Transition from elastic to muscular arteries may be either gradual or abrupt. In the dog, typical muscular renal arteries arise abruptly at right angles from the elastic abdominal aorta. Carotid, femoral, vertebral, and brachial arteries commonly begin as elastic arteries but gradually transform peripherally into muscular types. The sites of transitional zones vary among species and individual animals.

MUSCULAR ARTERIES

The tunica interna of muscular arteries consists of the endothelium, followed by a thin subendothelial layer composed of collagen and elastic fibers. In large muscular arteries, a few fibroblasts and smooth muscle cells

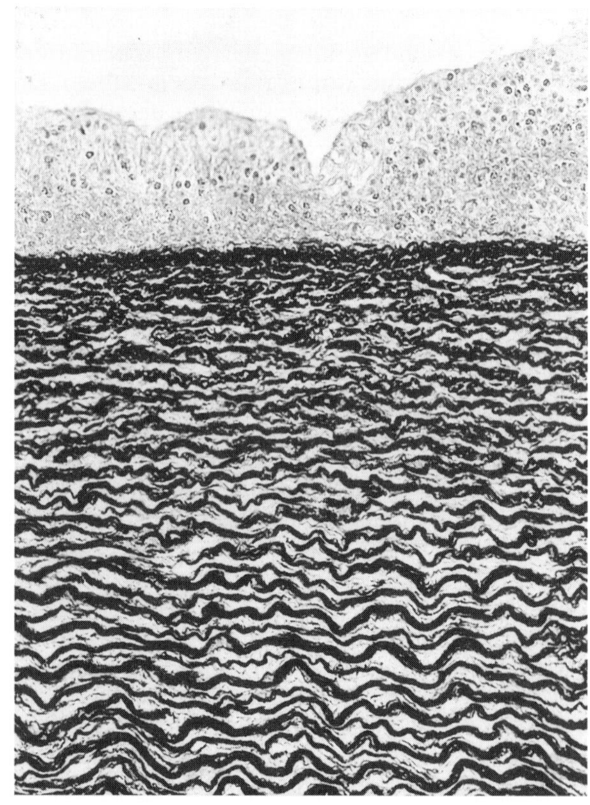

Figure 7.2. *Cross section through part of the wall of the equine thoracic aorta. A particularly thick subendothelial layer contains many longitudinally oriented elastic fibers. In the tunica media, elastic laminae predominate. Resorcin-fuchsin-van Gieson's stain (×50). (Courtesy of A. Hansen.)*

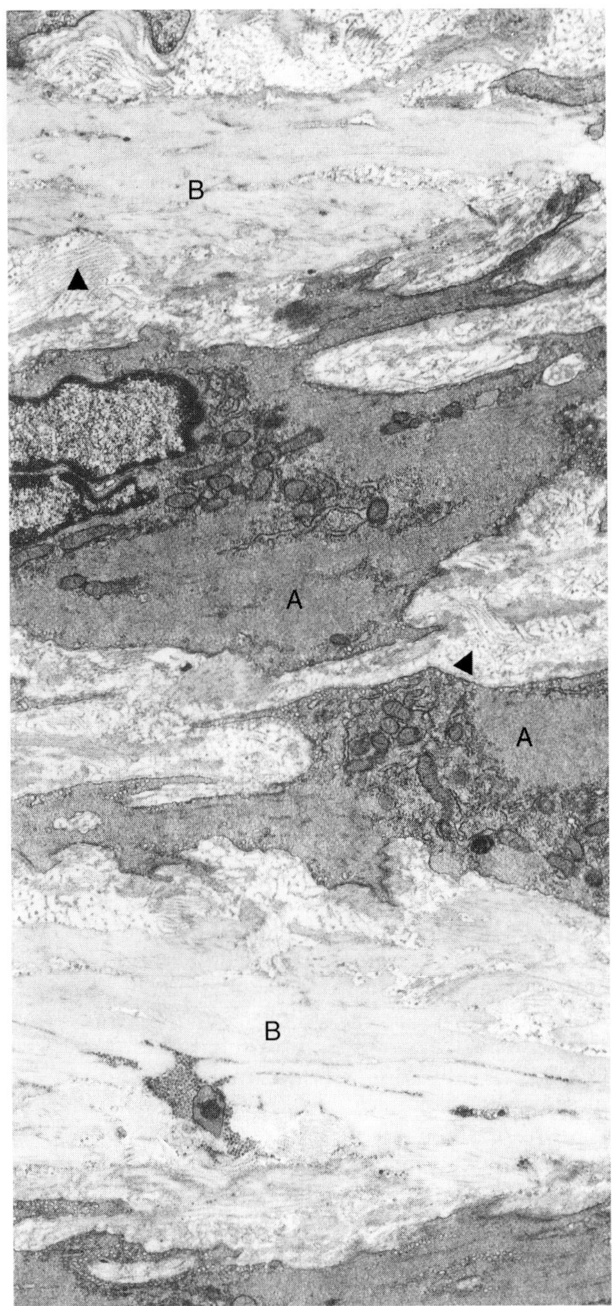

Figure 7.3. *Electron micrograph of part of the tunica media of the aorta (rat). Smooth muscle cells (A) surrounded by collagen fibrils (arrowheads) alternate with elastic laminae (B) (×9000).*

are present. With decreasing vessel size, the subendothelial layer gradually becomes thinner and eventually disappears. The thick internal elastic membrane (Figs. 7.1 and 7.4) possesses fenestrations through which cytoplasmic processes of endothelial cells contact the smooth muscle of the tunica media.

Muscular arteries are characterized by a thick tunica media, composed mainly of smooth muscle cells in the form of circular or helical wrappings from three to more than 40 cell layers in thickness. Interspersed between these smooth muscle cells are elastic fibers or lamellae, as well as collagen fibers (Figs. 7.1, 7.3, and 7.4). The external elastic membrane is often discontinuous and not always clearly defined. It consists of a dense feltwork of elastic fibers adjacent to the tunica externa (see Fig. 7.1).

The tunica externa consists of collagen fibers, fibroblasts, and elastic fibers, the number of which decreases in parallel with the size of the vessel.

When living tissues are prepared for fixation or when an animal dies, the muscular arteries contract considerably and blood is forced out of the lumina. Consequently, the tunica interna, the underlying internal elastic membrane, and the external elastic membrane are thrown into longitudinal folds. Thus, the cross-sectional profiles of muscular arteries in most histologic preparations possess relatively small lumina containing little blood, and the internal elastic membranes appear scalloped (see Fig. 7.1).

Microvasculature

ARTERIOLES

In its simplest form, the microvasculature comprises afferent arterioles that break up into capillary networks

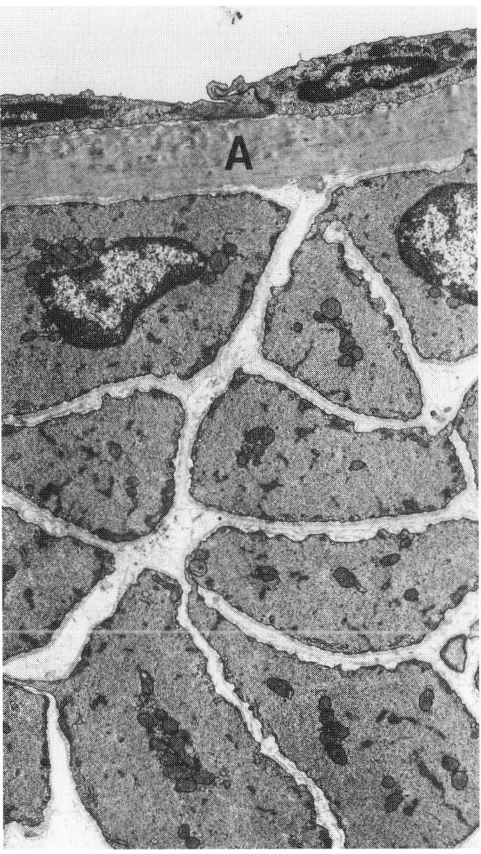

Figure 7.4. *Electron micrograph of part of the wall of a muscular artery (rat). The endothelium rests on a thick internal elastic membrane (A). The smooth muscle cells of the tunica media are surrounded by a basal lamina and collagen fibrils are present in the intercellular spaces (×7800).*

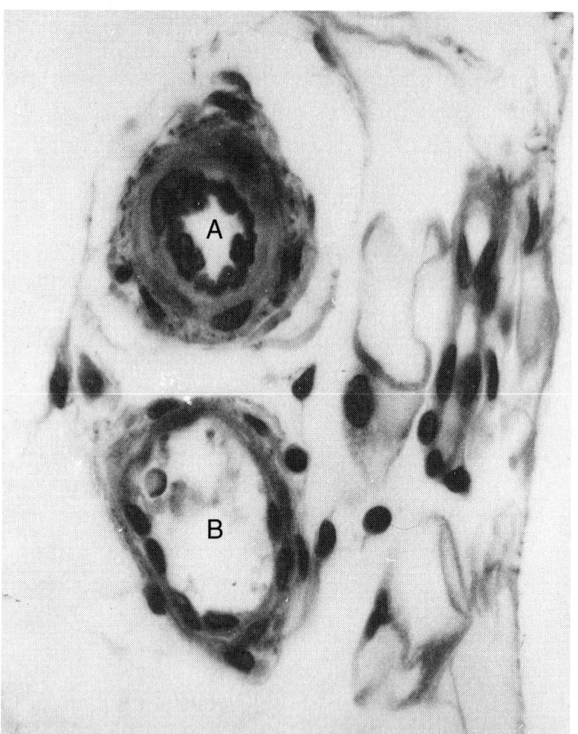

Figure 7.5. *Cross sections through an arteriole (A), with two layers of smooth muscle in the tunica media, and a venule (B), classified as intermediate between pericytic and muscular because of the presence of one incomplete layer of smooth muscle. Hematoxylin and eosin (×400). (From Dellmann H-D, Carithers JR. Cytology and microscopic anatomy. Philadelphia: Williams & Wilkins, 1996.)*

drained by efferent venules. Shunts may exist between arterioles and venules in the form of arteriovenous anastomoses and thoroughfare channels. In many organs, the microvasculature possesses unique architectural and structural characteristics that are described with these organs.

The tunica interna of arterioles consists of endothelium, a thin subendothelial layer of collagen and elastic fibers (which is absent in the smallest arterioles), and an internal elastic membrane. This membrane is fenestrated and eventually disappears in the smallest arterioles. Basal processes of the endothelial cells may establish direct contact with smooth muscle cells. In addition to one to three layers of smooth muscle cells, the tunica media may contain collagen fibers (Fig. 7.5). An external elastic membrane is absent. The tunica externa is loose connective tissue.

Arterioles continue directly into either capillaries or metarterioles (Fig. 7.6). Capillary openings are surrounded by a few smooth muscle cells forming a precapillary sphincter that regulates the blood flow through the capillary bed. **Metarterioles** are narrow vessels surrounded by isolated bundles of smooth muscle. They give rise to capillaries, again provided with precapillary sphincters, and continue into **thoroughfare channels** (preferential channels) that have the same structure as capillaries but a wider lumen. Thoroughfare channels connect directly with venules. Blood circulating through these channels bypasses the capillary bed, especially when precapillary sphincter contraction limits blood flow into capillaries.

CAPILLARIES

Capillaries are tubules of uniform diameter, approximately 8 μm wide (ranging from 5 to 10 μm), the walls of which are composed of endothelial cells, an associated basal lamina, pericytes, and a thin adventitial connective-tissue layer that is lacking around brain capillaries. A tunica media is absent (Figs. 7.7 and 7.8).

Pericytes of capillaries and postcapillary venules are basal lamina-enclosed cells with numerous processes. They are considered to be undifferentiated mesenchymal cells, readily stimulated to divide mitotically and to migrate around or away from the vessels. Pericytes are believed to transform into other cell types, especially fibroblasts and smooth muscle cells. A capillary apparently can transform by this means into the other types of vascular tubes if the internal flow characteristics change. Indeed, this description is compatible with the method by which arteries and veins develop from simple endothelial tubes during embryogenesis.

Capillaries form networks, called **capillary beds**, the density of which is a reflection of the metabolic requirements of different organs. For example, capillary beds are most dense in cardiac and skeletal muscle and relatively less dense in tendons. Within the capillaries beds, exchange takes place between the circulating blood and interstitial fluid, with water and water-soluble substances leaving the arterial end of the capillaries and reentering at the venous end and in postcapillary venules. Plasma molecules may leave the capillary lumen via transcytosis, through temporary transendothelial channels, across monolayered diaphragms, and by free diffusion (e.g., lipid-soluble substances).

On the basis of fine-structural characteristics of the capillary wall, continuous capillaries, fenestrated capillaries, porous capillaries, and sinusoids are distinguished. The structural differences correspond to measurable differences in capillary permeability. Fenestrated and porous capillaries have the highest permeability, continuous neural capillaries have the least permeability, and the permeability of continuous muscular capillaries lies between these limits.

Continuous capillaries are virtually ubiquitous in the organism. Individual endothelial cells are held together by tight junctions (Fig. 7.8). Usually, these cells contain only a few mitochondria and ribosomes, little endoplasmic reticulum, and small Golgi complexes. Transcytotic vesicles are a common finding. They may be either numerous, as in muscular capillaries (Fig. 7.8), or scarce or nonexistent, as in neural capillaries (Fig. 7.9).

Fenestrated capillaries (visceral capillaries) commonly occur in the gastrointestinal tract (Fig. 7.10) and in endocrine glands, where they are referred to as sinusoidal capillaries. They have a large diameter and their shape is adapted to the surrounding parenchymal cells from which they are separated by only a basal lamina

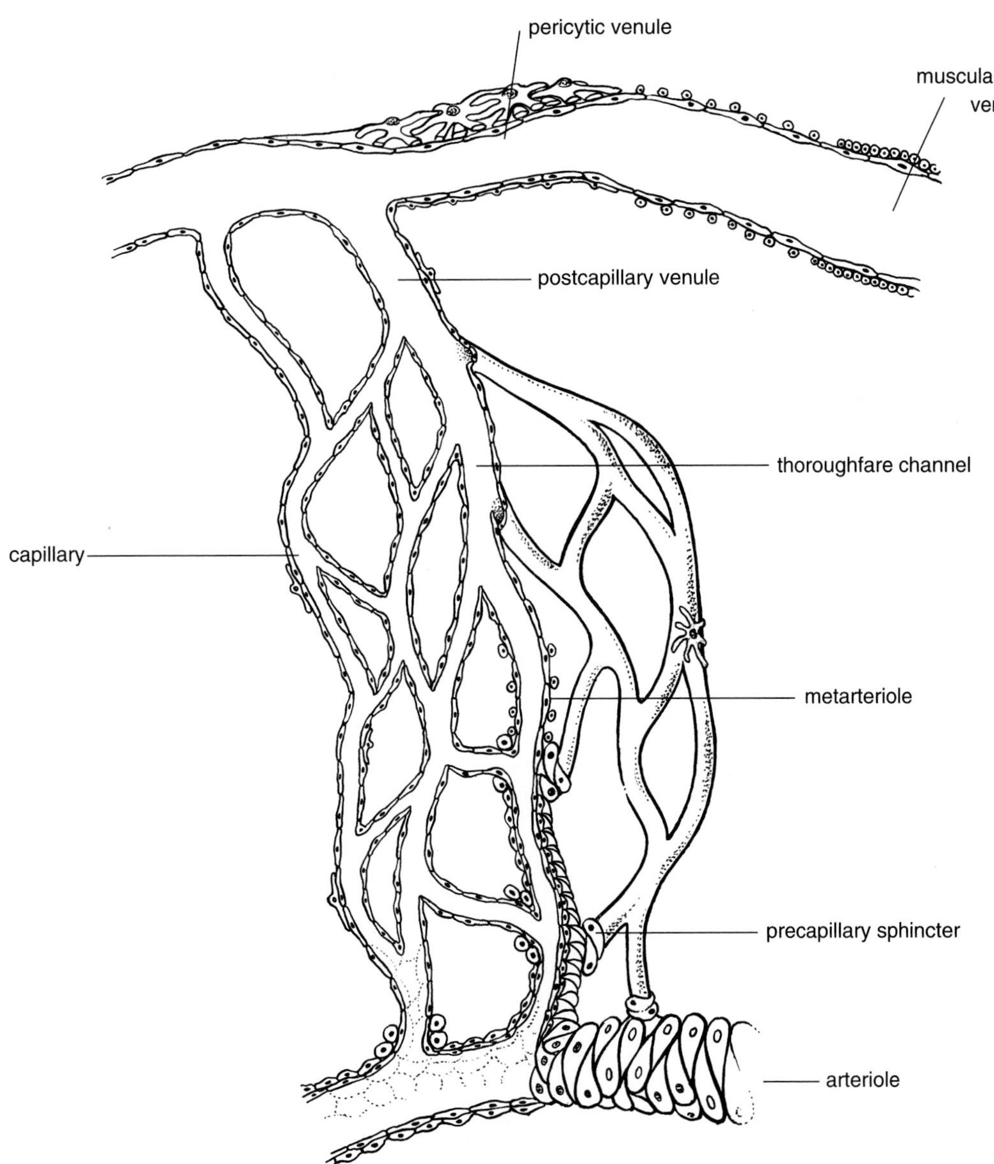

Figure 7.6. *Schematic drawing of the microvasculature. Capillaries arise from both an arteriole and a metarteriole; precapillary sphincters are present. The metarteriole continues into a thoroughfare channel, followed by a postcapillary venule, pericytic venule, and muscular venule, linked by a venule with an incomplete layer of smooth muscle.*

and small amount of adventitial connective tissue. In these capillaries, portions of the endothelial cells are attenuated and possess circular fenestrae, 60 to 80 nm in diameter, that are closed by monolayered diaphragms that are thinner than a cell membrane (Fig. 7.10). Fenestrations facilitate the passage of substances across the endothelium.

Porous capillaries are characteristic of the kidney glomerulus. In these capillaries, endothelial diaphragms are absent, and consequently, the endothelial cells are pierced by pores (Fig. 7.11).

Sinusoids are present in the liver parenchyma. They are larger than other capillaries, lack uniformity in diameter, the shape themselves to fill the space within the confines of the surrounding parenchyma. Large openings between and pores in the endothelial cells, with a concomitant discontinuity or absence of the surrounding basal lamina, provide for a maximum exchange between blood and surrounding parenchyma.

VENULES

Immediate **postcapillary venules** are similar in structure to capillaries but are larger in diameter (10 to 30 μm) (Fig. 7.6). The tunica interna is formed by continuous and occasionally fenestrated endothelial cells connected by incomplete tight junctions, a basal lamina, and a thin subendothelial layer of longitudinal collagen fibers. Occasional pericytes are present. Postcapillary venules have a functional significance not made evident by simple morphologic studies. The junctions between the endothelial cells are more permeable than those in capillaries and are more sensitive to leakage induced by such agents as serotonin and histamine. These compounds play a role in the inflammatory reaction, with the resultant accumulation of excessive extravascular fluid, soluble substances, and blood cells. Pericytic venules are a definite site for large molecular exchange between the vascular and connective-tissue spaces. Immediate postcapillary venules in many lym-

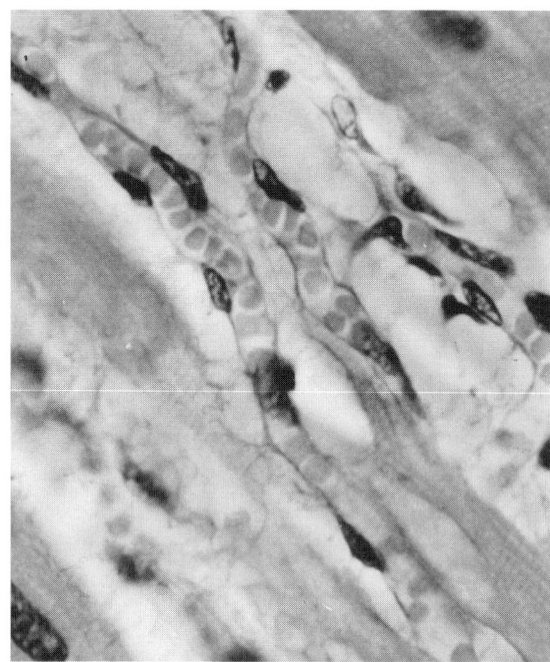

Figure 7.7. *Capillaries in the canine myocardium. Note that the variable widths of the capillaries may be barely greater than or slightly smaller than the diameter of an erythrocyte. It is not always possible to distinguish clearly between the nuclei of endothelial cells and pericytes. Hematoxylin and eosin (×750).*

phatic organs have a special structure and significance (see Chapter 8).

As the venules increase in diameter (30 to 50 μm), they are called **pericytic venules** or **collecting venules**, in which pericytes form a continuous layer (Fig. 7.6). Fibrocytes and collagen fibers form a thin tunica externa. As venules increase further in diameter (50 to 100 μm), the pericytes are gradually replaced by circularly disposed muscle cells (Fig. 7.6). When these form one to two complete layers, the venule is referred to as a **muscular venule** (Fig. 7.6). The tunica externa, containing elastic and collagen fibers and scattered fibrocytes, becomes more prominent.

ARTERIOVENOUS ANASTOMOSES

Direct connections between arterioles and venules without an intervening capillary bed are called **arteriovenous anastomoses**. These anastomoses are short, usually nonbranched, and often coiled vessels. They possess a thick smooth muscle layer that receives a dense vasomotor nerve supply. Often, longitudinally oriented smooth muscle fibers form cushions or sleeves. When arteriovenous anastomoses are open, the blood essentially bypasses capillary beds and is shunted directly into the venous system; when they are closed, the blood flow to capillary areas is increased. Arteriovenous anastomoses are particularly numerous in the skin, lips, intestine, salivary glands, nasal mucosa, and male and female reproductive tracts. They function in the regulation of blood pressure and blood flow into capillary beds, thermoregulation, and erection.

Several convoluted arteriovenous anastomoses surrounded by venules and enclosed by a thick connective-tissue capsule are called a **glomus**. Arteriovenous anastomoses in glomera are characterized by numerous longitudinal, subendothelial epithelioid muscle cells surrounded by circularly arranged muscle cells in the media. An internal elastic membrane is absent. Glomera are particularly numerous in digital pads and the external ear and have a thermoregulatory function.

Veins

The structure of veins varies within wide limits and is apparently determined by varying local mechanical conditions. Consequently, a classification of veins is difficult, especially because layers in their walls are often absent or difficult to distinguish.

The terms **small**, **medium-sized**, and **large** used to classify veins have only relative meaning in any one animal. The large veins of a cat may be smaller than the medium-sized veins of a cow. Small veins are the continuation of muscular venules. The medium-sized veins correspond in function and location to the distributive arteries. They are actually collecting veins, because blood courses through venous trees in a direction opposite to that in arterial trees. Veins corresponding to the aorta are referred to as the great veins or large veins, or simply by their gross anatomic names, such as vena cava.

All types of veins that carry blood against gravity, including venules, and especially the small and medium-sized veins of the extremities, are equipped with flap-like, usually paired, semilunar **valves**. Their free margins are oriented toward the heart. When closed, they prevent the backflow of blood. **Venous valves** are folds of interna with a core of collagen fibers. Proximal to the attachment of valves, the vein wall is slightly distended to form a valve sinus.

SMALL VEINS

As venules increase further in diameter, they become **small veins**. Endothelium and associated basal lamina are surrounded by a distinct media of two to four continuous layers of circularly oriented smooth muscle cells, interspersed with a varying amount of connective tissue that blends with that of the surrounding tunica externa.

MEDIUM-SIZED VEINS

The wall structure of veins of the **medium-sized** range reflects that they must withstand the physical stresses of gravity and the centrifugal forces of locomotion. Because the variation in position and orientation of smooth muscle components is considerable in different veins within the various species, attempts to provide inclusive descriptions are difficult.

The tunica interna consists of an endothelial lining and a thin subendothelial layer of collagen and elastic fibers. An internal elastic membrane may be present in the larger vessels. Usually, the tunica media consists of several layers of smooth muscle with associated collagen and elastic networks, commonly arranged circularly or spirally. In the outer tunica media, smooth muscle cells may be longitudinally oriented. The tunica externa is composed predominantly of collagen networks anchored to both the tunica media and the surrounding connective tissue and of longitudinally oriented elastic fibers.

LARGE VEINS

The tunica interna of **large veins** has essentially the same structure as that of medium-sized veins. The endothelium is, however, often slightly thicker and blocklike; occasionally, smooth muscle cells are present, and the internal elastic membrane is more prominent.

The tunica media is thin, compared to the size of the vessel or to the diameter of the lumen. It consists of collagen, elastic fibers, and smooth muscle cells in varying

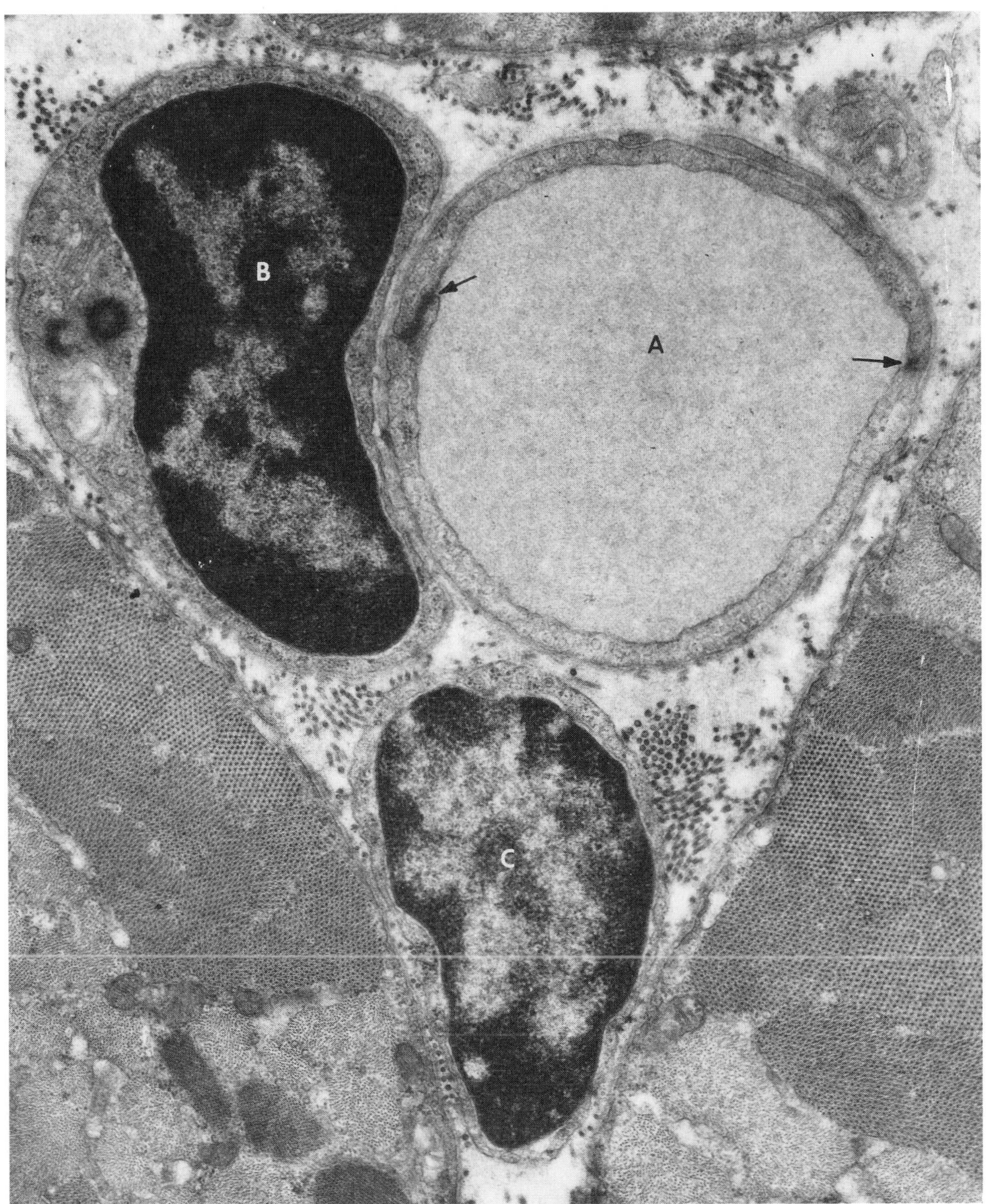

Figure 7.8. *Electron micrograph of a continuous (muscular) capillary (A). Tight junctions are present between the endothelial cells (arrows). The basal lamina of the endothelium continues around the adjacent pericyte (B). The black dots are cross sections of collagen fibrils (×16,000).*

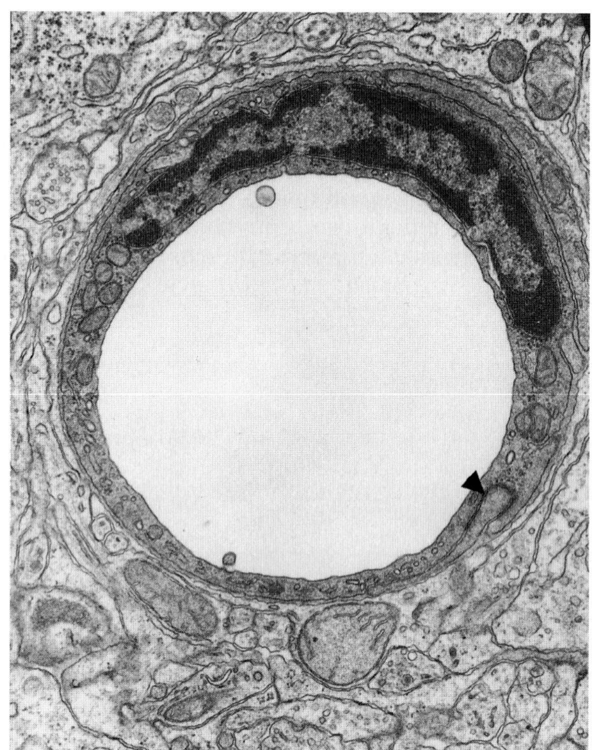

Figure 7.9. *Electron micrograph of a continuous (neural) capillary. Tight junctions (arrowhead) are present between adjacent endothelial cells (×21,000).*

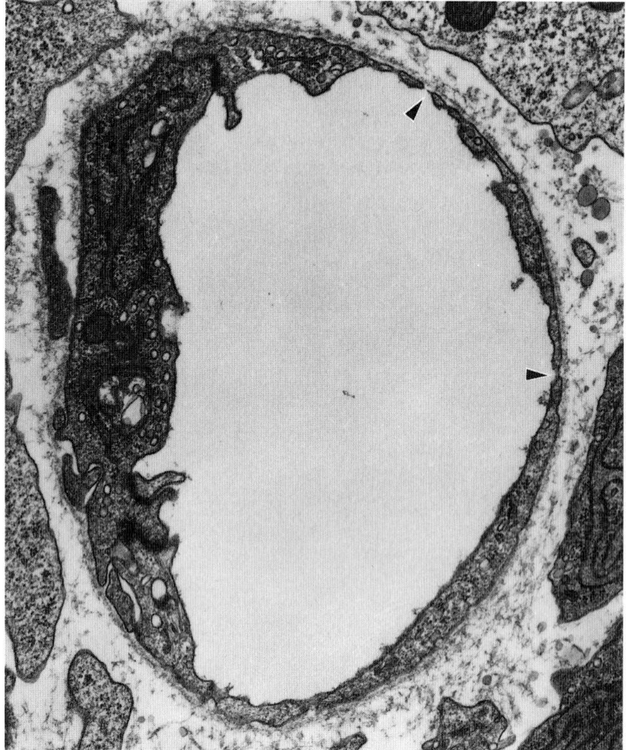

Figure 7.10. *Electron micrograph of a fenestrated capillary in the propria of the small intestine (rat). The fenestrations (arrowheads) are closed by a monolayered diaphragm (×15,600).*

proportions (Fig. 7.13). In most large veins, the smooth muscle layer is insignificant.

The tunica externa, on the contrary, is prominent and composed of longitudinally or spirally oriented bundles of smooth muscle cells, together with collagen and elastic fibers that maintain the proper tension of the wall. The thickness of this muscular layer depends on the location of the vein and is more pronounced in veins on which greater pressure is exerted by the environment (e.g., in the thoracic and abdominal cavities) (Fig. 7.13).

Specialized Blood Vessels

Many blood vessels have special structural features that fulfill specific functions in the regulation of the

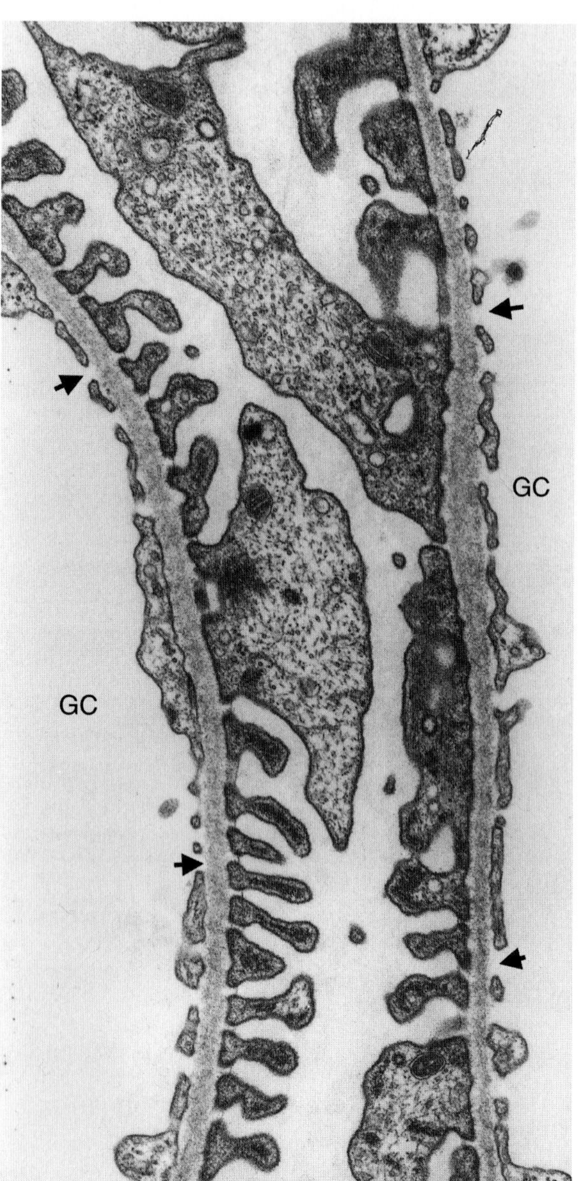

Figure 7.11. *Electron micrograph of part of the walls of two glomerular capillaries (GC) of the kidney. The endothelial cells have pores (arrowheads) (×27,600).*

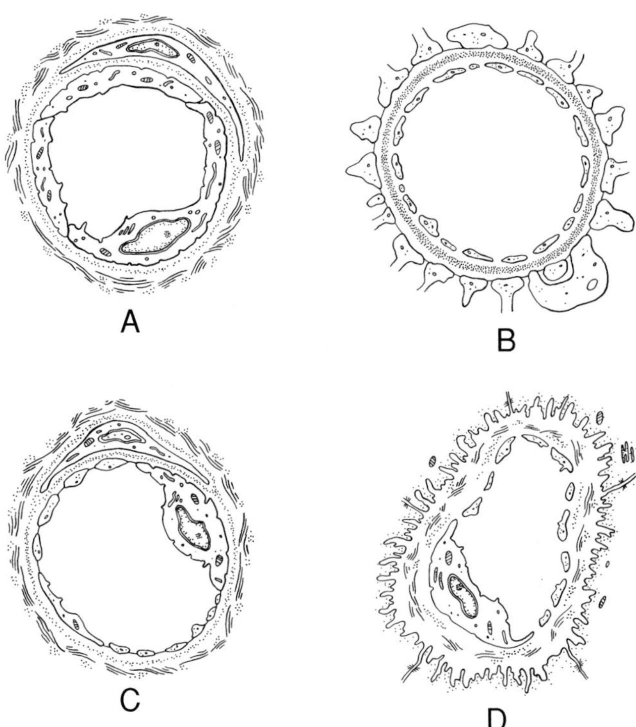

Figure 7.12. *Drawing of the fine structural characteristics of the four types of capillaries: continuous capillary (**A**), porous capillary (**B**), fenestrated capillary (**C**), and sinusoid (**D**). The fine dots around the endothelial cells and pericytes (in **A** and **C** only) indicate the basal lamina, which is particularly thick in porous capillaries and discontinuous in sinusoids.*

blood flow. An increase in the thickness of the wall is observed in vessels subjected to unusual blood pressures, such as arteries and veins of the teat (Fig. 7.14), veins of the glans penis, and coronary arteries. Conversely, a decrease in the thickness occurs in protected, low-pressure areas, such as the skull (e.g., arteries of the brain, dural venous sinuses), bones, and lungs. Longitudinal muscle bundles that can stop the blood flow occur in the tunica interna in both arteries and veins of the penis, ovary, and uterus. Circular, sphincterlike thickenings of the tunica media of veins perform similar functions in the large intestine, liver, and skin.

Sensory Receptors

Sensory receptors are present in the area of the bifurcation of the carotid artery. They comprise the carotid body and the carotid sinus, which monitor changes in blood chemical composition (chemoreceptors) and blood pressure (baroreceptors), respectively.

CAROTID BODY

The carotid body is enclosed by a connective-tissue capsule and consists of a dense sinusoidal capillary network surrounding clusters of cells. Two cell types are present within these clusters: **type I cells** or **chemoreceptor cells**, which contain many granules rich in catecholamines and serotonin, and **type II cells** or **sustentacular cells**, which have few or no granules. The type II cells incompletely invest several type I cells (Fig. 7.15). Nonmyelinated afferent and efferent nerve terminals are present on type I cells. Changes in the concentrations of blood pH and oxygen and carbon dioxide tension generate action potentials in afferent nerve fibers to the central nervous system, triggering responses primarily in the respiratory and cardiovascular systems.

CAROTID SINUS

The baroreceptor area of the **carotid sinus** is a dilatation of the internal carotid artery where it originates from the common carotid artery. At this point, the tunica media is thin and surrounded by a thick tunica ex-

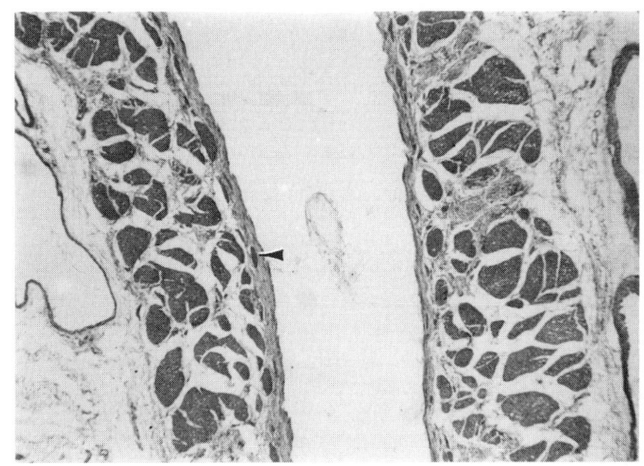

Figure 7.13. *Cross section through part of the ovine vena cava. The thin tunica media consists of a few bundles of smooth muscle cells (arrowhead). The tunica externa is the most prominent layer and contains many bundles of longitudinally oriented smooth muscle. Hematoxylin and eosin (×40).*

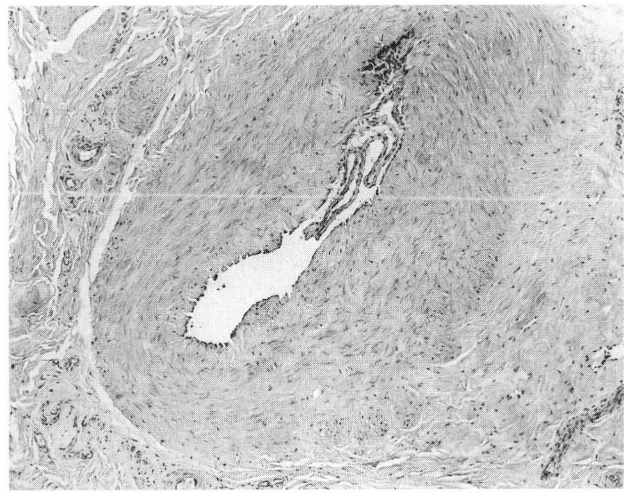

Figure 7.14. *Cross section through a vein with a thick muscular media in the ovine teat. Hematoxylin and eosin (×200).*

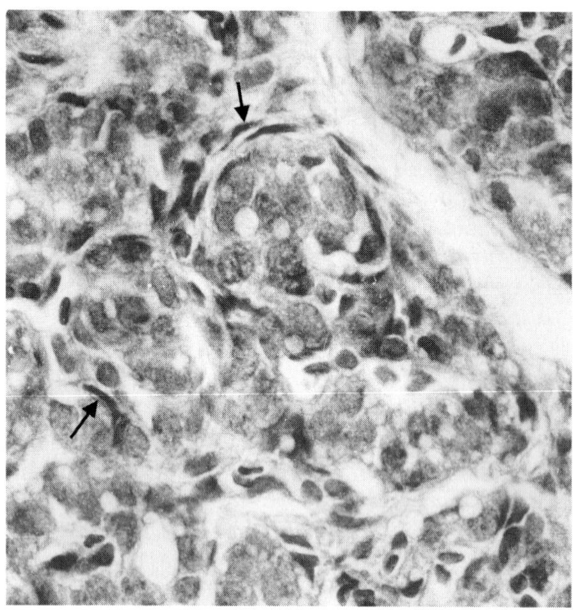

Figure 7.15. *Ovine carotid body. Groups of large type I cells are invested by flatter type II cells (arrows) Hematoxylin and eosin (×350). (Preparation courtesy of J.H. Riley.)*

terna that contains many terminals from the sinus branch of the glossopharyngeal nerve. The terminals are mechanoreceptors that, when stimulated by increased blood pressure, cause reflex bradycardia, a fall in blood pressure, and dilatation of the splanchnic blood vessels.

HEART

The thick wall of the heart is mainly composed of cardiac muscle cells capable of spontaneous rhythmic contraction, which pumps the blood into the vascular system. The inner layer of the heart is referred to as **endocardium** and is continuous with the tunica interna of the large blood vessels leaving and entering the heart. The contractile middle muscular layer is called the **myocardium** and is by far the thickest layer of the organ. The outermost layer is the **epicardium**.

Endocardium

The **endocardium** completely lines the ventricles and atria, including the cardiac valves and associated structures. The endocardium usually consists of three layers (Fig. 7.16). A continuous **endothelium** composes the innermost layer. Underneath the endothelium are an inner and outer subendothelial layer. The **inner subendothelial layer** is composed of dense irregular connective tissue with collagen and elastic fibers and occasional smooth muscle cells. The elastic fibers are particularly abundant in the atrial walls and are usually arranged parallel to the endocardial surface. The **outer subendothelial layer** is also referred to as the subendocardial layer and is predominantly composed of loosely arranged collagen and elastic fibers. Adipose cells may be present, along with a rich supply of blood and lymph vessels, and in some locations, the impulse-conducting cardiac muscle fibers (Purkinje fibers) (Fig. 7.16). The connective tissue is continuous with that of the myocardium.

The **cardiac valves** are endocardial folds that consist of a central layer of dense irregular connective tissue covered by endothelium. In the central layer of the **atrioventricular valves**, collagen fibers predominate, which connect with the fibrous rings surrounding the atrioventricular openings. They also continue with the collagen fibers of the fibrous cords (chordae tendineae) that arise from the endomysium of the papillary muscles. The central layer is covered on both surfaces by thin layers of elastic fibers. In the **semilunar valves** of the aorta and the pulmonary artery, the central connective-tissue fibers have a predominantly circular arrangement and are reinforced by a thin layer of elastic fibers nearest the vessel and a thick layer of elastic fibers on the ventricular side. The thickening of the free edge of the cardiac valves is caused by the presence of loose connective tissue and cartilaginous tissue.

Myocardium

The middle and thickest layer of the heart is the **myocardium**, which is composed of bundles and groups of bundles of cardiac muscle cells, the impulse-generating and conducting system, and the cardiac skeleton.

Bundles of cardiac muscle cells are embedded in loose connective tissue that contains a dense capillary network, lymph vessels, and autonomic nerve fibers; the amount of interstitial connective tissue is subject to local variations and is greater in the myocardium of the right than of the left ventricle. The atrial cardiac muscle cells are usually smaller than the ventricular cardiac muscle

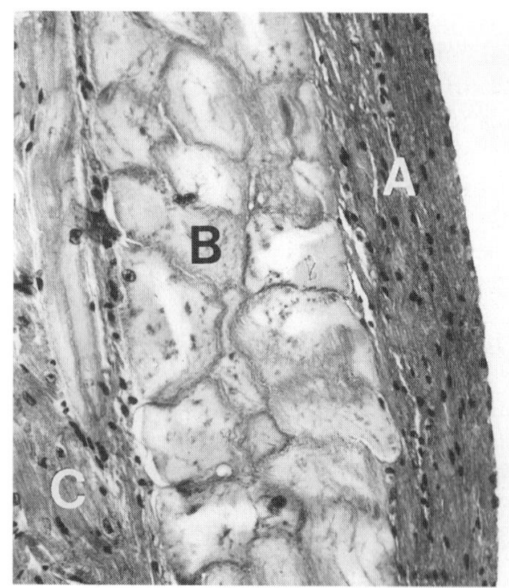

Figure 7.16. *Horizontal section through part of the bovine heart wall. Peripheral to the inner subendothelial layer (A) is the outer subendothelial layer, with large impulse-conducting muscle fibers (B), and the myocardium (C). Trichrome (×200).*

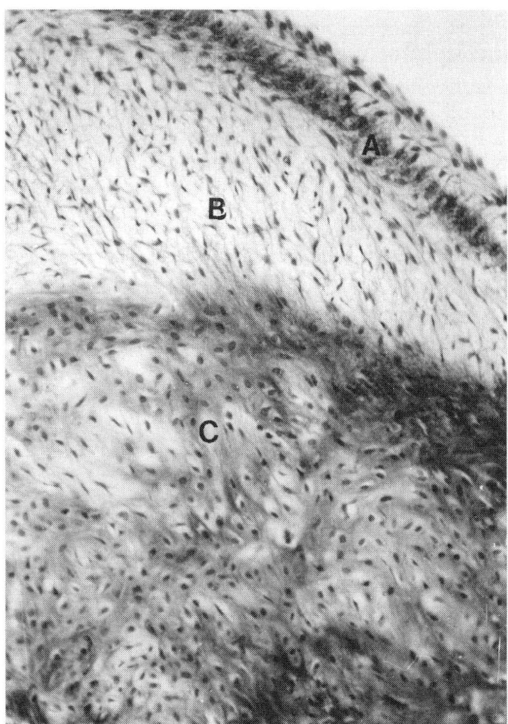

Figure 7.17. *Horizontal section through the canine trigonum fibrosum. The innermost endothelial layer is followed by an inner subendothelial layer of dense irregular connective tissue (A) and an outer one of loose connective tissue (B). The trigonum (C) is a highly cellular fibrocartilage. Hematoxylin and eosin (×130).*

cells. In atrial cardiac muscle cells, numerous specific atrial granules containing atrial natriuretic peptide (ANP) are present; ANP plays an important role in fluid homeostasis (e.g., diuresis, natriuresis, vasodilation).

The impulse for cardiac contraction is generated in the sinoatrial node, subsequently spreads to the atrioventricular node, and continues in the atrioventricular bundle. The **sinoatrial node** is composed of a network of thin, branching nodal muscle cells that contain scarce myofibrils and lack intercalated disks. They are continuous with ordinary cardiac muscle fibers of the atrial myocardium. Nodal muscle fibers are separated by a relatively large amount of highly vascularized connective tissue, containing many autonomic nerve fibers and occasional ganglion cells (vagus nerve).

The **atrioventricular node** is composed of irregularly arranged, small, branching nodal muscle fibers, the morphology of which is similar to that of the sinoatrial node. Nodal muscle fibers are continuous with the atrial myocardial fibers and the impulse-conducting cardiac fibers. These impulse-conducting fibers form the **atrioventricular bundle**. They are readily identified by their large diameter, centrally located large spherical nuclei, scarce and usually peripherally located myofibrils, and a central area that is rich in glycogen (Fig. 7.16). In longitudinal sections, characteristic cross-striations and intercalated disks are visible. The conducting fibers connect with smaller transitional cells that lack intercalated disks and in turn connect with ordinary myocardial cells.

The musculature of the atrial and ventricular walls is inserted into the **cardiac skeleton**, which is made of three parts: *(a)* the fibrous rings (annuli fibrosi), *(b)* the fibrous triangle (trigonum fibrosum), and *(c)* the fibrous (or membranous) part of the interventricular septum. The **fibrous rings** are composed of intermingling bundles of collagen and a few elastic fibers that surround the atrioventricular openings and those of the aorta and the pulmonary artery. The **fibrous triangle** is the connective tissue that fills the space between the atrioventricular openings and the base of the aorta. The nature of this connective tissue is species- and age-dependent. It may be predominantly dense and irregular connective tissue (in pigs and cats), fibrocartilage (in dogs) (Fig. 7.17), hyaline cartilage (in horses), or bone (in large ruminants). The fibrous part of the **interventricular septum** consists of collagen fiber bundles.

Epicardium and Pericardium

The myocardium is covered peripherally by the **epicardium.** It is covered externally by the mesothelial cells of the visceral pericardium. Under this epithelium is a loose connective-tissue layer rich in elastic fibers that forms protective sheaths around blood vessels and nerves. It is particularly abundant around the large subepicardial (e.g., coronary) blood vessels.

The epicardium becomes continuous with the parietal pericardium at the orifices of the large blood vessels entering or leaving the heart. The **pericardium** consists of an innermost mesothelial layer, the parietal pericardium, resting on a thin layer of loose connective tissue, followed by a thick, resistant layer of collagen fiber bundles and elastic fibers. The pericardial cavity, located between the visceral and parietal pericardium, contains serous fluid lubricating the surfaces for frictionless cardiac movement. Like the epicardium, the pericardium can readily adapt to the normal continual changes in the size of the heart but provides a limit to overfilling of the heart and will cause cardiac tamponade if the pericardial sac fills with excess fluid.

Cardiac Blood Vessels, Lymph Vessels, and Nerves

The coronary arteries are thick muscular arteries and often contain bundles of longitudinal smooth muscle cells and epithelioid muscle cells in the interna that regulate the blood flow within these vessels. From the coronary arteries, a dense capillary network supplies the myocardium, epicardium, cardiac skeleton, and peripheral portions of cardiac valves. Blood is collected by venules and veins that open into the right atrium either through the coronary sinus or through direct openings (venae cordis minimae).

Lymph capillaries form a network in the cardiac connective tissue. They are continuous with larger lymph vessels, especially in the outer subendothelial layer of the endocardium and the subepithelial connective tissue of the epicardium.

Both sympathetic and parasympathetic nerves inner-

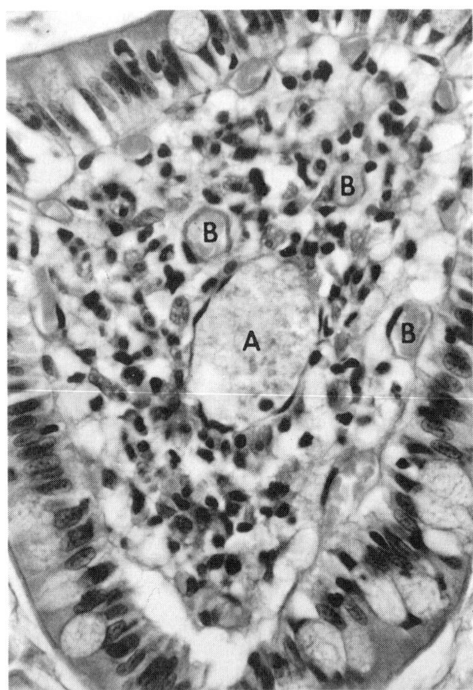

Figure 7.18. *Cross section through a canine intestinal villus. Lymph capillary (A); blood capillaries (B). Hematoxylin and eosin (×435).*

vate the heart. They are numerous in the atria but scarce in the ventricles, where mainly sympathetic fibers are represented. They form extensive plexuses that are particularly dense around the sinoatrial and atrioventricular nodes. The parasympathetic (vagus) fibers terminate on ganglion cells, which in turn contribute fibers to the aforementioned plexuses. Both the myocardium and epicardium receive sensory fibers that terminate with club-shaped or platelike enlargements.

LYMPH VESSELS

The lymph vascular system is an integral part of both the circulatory and the defense systems. It originates as a network of anastomosing lymph capillaries in the connective tissue of the organism. It continues with larger lymph vessels that pass through at least one lymph node and even larger collecting ducts that drain the lymph into the venous system.

Lymph Capillaries

Lymph capillaries are endothelium-lined tubes that are usually larger than blood capillaries (Fig. 7.18). Their shape is variable, and the endothelial lining is usually thin. Adjacent endothelial cells are joined by intimate interdigitations, simple overlapping, or adhering junctions. Frequently, variably sized gaps are observed between adjacent cells. These gaps probably are temporary, i.e., they appear and disappear continuously, presumably depending on local circumstances.

A basal lamina is either absent or discontinuous around lymph capillaries (Fig. 7.19). Fine anchoring extracellular matrix filaments link the outer surface of the endothelial cells to pericapillary collagen fibrils and elastic fibers. These filaments are responsible for keeping the lumina of the capillaries open, especially when the tissues are edematous.

As a general rule, lymph capillaries are found in conjunction with loose connective tissue from which they drain excess interstitial fluid, including fat, proteins, cells, and particulate matter. They are absent in the central nervous system, structures within the eye bulb, bone marrow, cartilage, red pulp of the spleen, liver lobules, and tonsils.

Small and Medium-Sized Lymph Vessels

The structure of the walls of these vessels is subject to great variability according to location and the species involved.

Postcapillary lymph vessels differ from lymph capillaries by their larger diameter and a continuous basal lamina. With increasing diameter, first a thin subendothelial connective tissue layer is present; then one or two layers of smooth muscle and elastic fibers are added. A tunica externa is not distinguishable from the surrounding connective tissue.

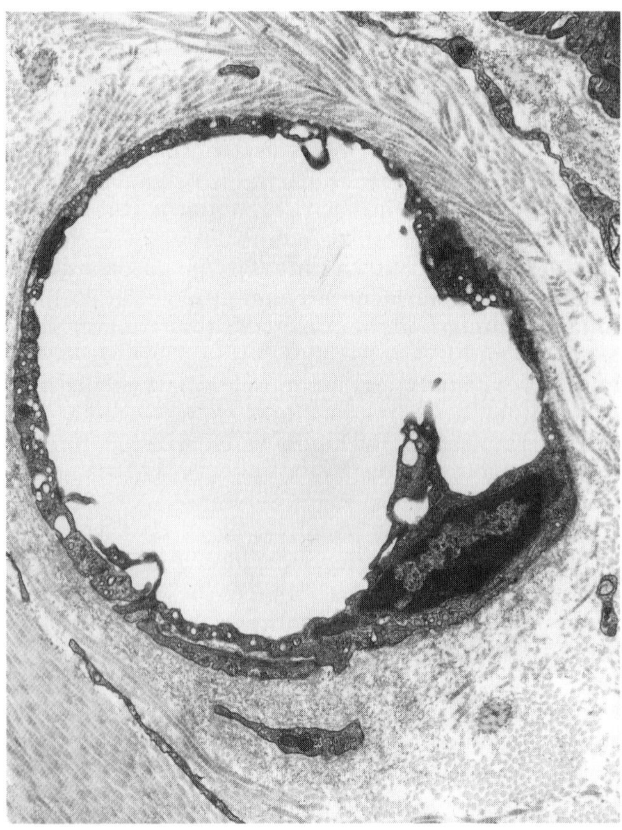

Figure 7.19. *Electron micrograph of a lymph capillary. The thin endothelium contains numerous pinocytotic vesicles and lacks a basal lamina (×16,000).*

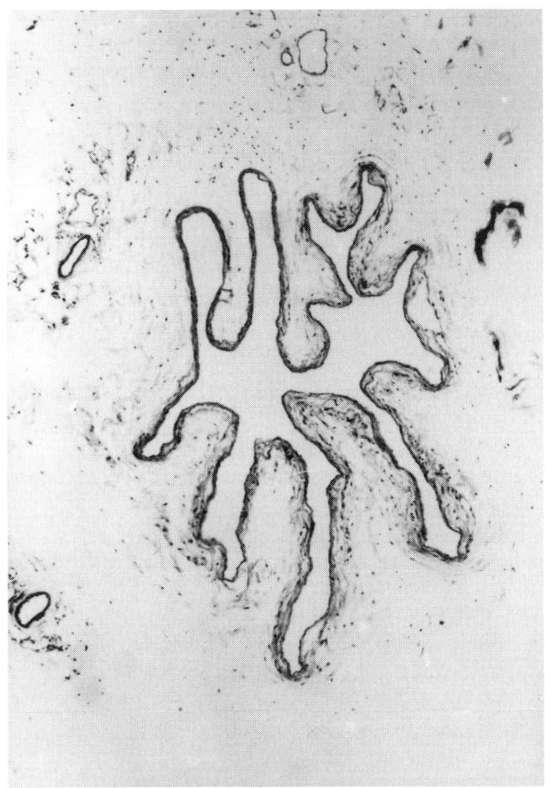

Figure 7.20. *Cross section through the canine thoracic duct. The wall consists of an endothelium and a thin tunica media with sparse muscle cells; a distinct tunica externa is absent. Hematoxylin and eosin (×110). (From Dellmann H-D, Carithers JR. Cytology and microscopic anatomy. Philadelphia: Williams & Wilkins, 1996.)*

Large Lymph Vessels and Collecting Ducts

As in blood vessels, the walls of these lymph vessels (ducts) comprise three layers that are not always well delineated (Fig. 7.20). The tunica interna consists of the endothelium and a layer of longitudinal, interlacing collagen and elastic fibers. An internal elastic membrane is usually absent. The tunica media contains smooth muscle cells, surrounded by many elastic and collagen fibers, the number and orientation of which vary with the location and species. The tunica externa is composed of collagen and elastic fibers and may contain muscle cells.

Valves may be present occasionally in lymph capillaries and are a constant feature of all other lymph vessels. They are composed of an endothelial fold with little intervening connective tissue, except at the junction with the vessel wall, where it is more abundant. Occasional smooth muscle fibers are found in the valves of the larger lymph vessels.

REFERENCES

Bagshaw RJ, Fisher GM. Morphology of the carotid sinus in the dog. J Appl Physiol 1971;31:198.

Biscoe TJ. Carotid body: structure and function. Physiol Rev 1971;51:437.

Johansson BR. Size and distribution of endothelial plasmalemmal vesicles in consecutive segments of the microvasculature of cat skeletal muscle. Microvasc Res 1979;17:707.

Kaley G, Altura BM, eds. Microcirculation. Baltimore: University Park Press, 1977, 1978;1,2,3.

Leak LV. Lymphatic capillary ultrastructure and permeability. Eur J Physiol 1972;336:S46.

Majno G, Joris I. Endothelium 1977: a review. Adv Exp Med Biol 1978;104:169.

Marais J, Fossum TW. Ultrastructural morphology of the canine thoracic duct and cysterna chyli. Acta Anat 1988;133:309.

Maul GG. Structure and function of pores in fenestrated capillaries. J Ultrastruct Res 1971;36:768.

Opthof T, de Jonge B, Masson-Pevet M, et al. Functional and morphological organization of the cat sinoatrial node. J Mol Cell Cardiol 1986;18:1015.

Racker DK. Atrioventricular node and input pathways: a correlated gross anatomical and histological study of the canine atrioventricular junctional region. Anat Rec 1989;224:336.

Simionescu N, Simionescu M, Palade GE. Structural basis of permeability in sequential segments of the microvasculature. Microvasc Res 1978;15:1.

Stone EA, Stewart GJ. Architecture and structure of canine veins with special reference to confluences. Anat Rec 1988;222:154.

Thaemert JC. Atrioventricular node innervation in ultrastructural three dimensions. Am J Anat 1970;128:239.

Verna A. Ultrastructure of the carotid body in mammals. Int Rev Cytol 1979;60:271.

Viragh S, Challice CE. The impulse generation and conduction system of the heart. In: Dalton AJ, Challice CE, eds. Ultrastructure in biological systems. New York: Academic Press, 1973;6:43.

8

Immune System

THOR LANDSVERK
CHARLES MCL. PRESS

The immune system comprises organs and cells that work in a coordinated manner to maintain the integrity of the body. The immune system serves to identify and protect against pathogenic organisms and to ensure the body's response is appropriate. The system has innate components that act rapidly but nonspecifically and adaptive components that act specifically but need some time to respond. Threats to the integrity of the individual are not limited to extrinsic sources. The processes of wear and tear and pathologic changes in tissues result in alterations of cell surface molecules that are detected and responded to by components of the immune system with measures that restore the tissues.

The ability of the system to distinguish between "self" and "altered self" or "foreign" is therefore critical. This ability appears early in ontogeny, and initially, the ability is probably restricted to phagocytic cells but then, as the various components of the immune system develop, other cell types also acquire the capacity for discrimination. The recognition of a foreign substance or antigen is usually followed by a response, involving the concerted action of immune components. Diverse effector molecules present either at the cell surface or in secretions mediate the response and bind to the foreign molecule or to other interacting components of the immune system, often in the form of a ligand–receptor interaction.

CELLS OF THE IMMUNE SYSTEM

The cellular participants of the immune response can be categorized as either migratory or fixed cells. The

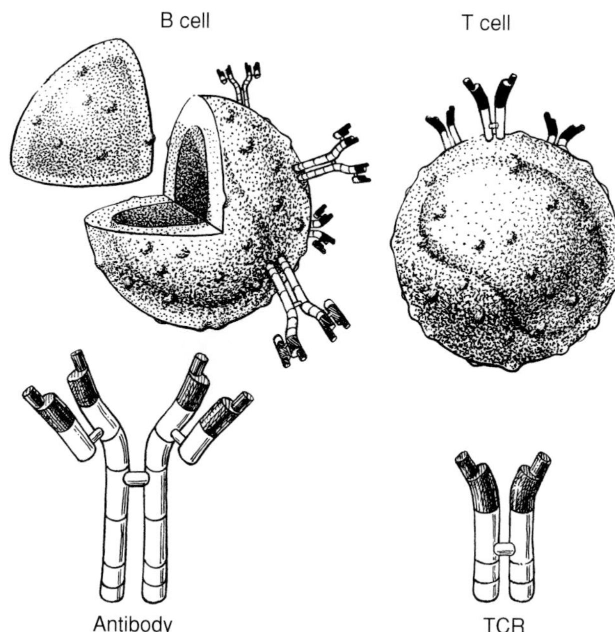

Figure 8.1. *Schematic drawing of lymphocyte surface antigen receptors. The B-cell receptor is an immunoglobulin (antibody) molecule that has two antigen-binding sites (dark segments), whereas the T-cell receptor (TCR) has a single antigen-binding site.*

leukocytes are **migratory cells** that are, in principle, free to move anywhere in the body. Recirculation through the lymph or blood is a prominent feature of the leukocytes ensuring effective surveillance of the tissues. The **fixed cells** are mesenchymal or epithelial cells that are restricted to a lymphatic organ forming its stroma. These cells create a microenvironment that provides support for the leukocytes during phases of development or function. The leukocytes are channeled into specific microenvironments by a set of directing receptors or addressins that reside on vascular endothelial cells. It is important to realize that in these microenvironments, the leukocytes may be less mobile, particularly during phases of interaction with the stroma, antigen, and other leukocytes.

The remarkable diversity of both migratory and fixed cells creates the character of each tissue. As the fetus develops, the immune system is molded into two principal types of tissues: the diffuse and the organized lymphatic tissues. The diffuse lymphatic tissues are found scattered throughout the loose connective tissues of the body and in extranodular areas of lymphatic organs. The contribution of the diffuse lymphatic tissue to the immune system is considerable, as exemplified by the diffuse lymphatic tissues of the gut, the respiratory tract and skin, and the leukocyte populations found in the epithelia of these organs. The organized lymphatic tissues include encapsulated organs such as the lymph nodes and spleen and contain focal accumulations of lymphatic tissue called lymphatic nodules.

Lymphocytes

The lymphocytes are responsible for the adaptive immune responses. The lymphocytic lineage gives rise to two major cell types: B cells and T cells. **B cells** undergo differentiation in the bone (B) marrow, or the cloacal bursa (B) in birds, and **T cells** differentiate in the thymus (T). B cells and T cells can be distinguished by the different structure of the surface molecule that recognizes antigen, called the antigen receptor (Fig. 8.1). Surface molecules involved in signal transduction and cell cooperation are also important in distinguishing between B cells and T cells. There is a fundamental difference in the way the B-cell and T-cell antigen receptors recognize antigen. The T-cell antigen receptor recognizes antigen in the form of short peptides presented on the surface of a cell, an antigen-presenting cell, by a particular class of molecule called a major histocompatibility complex (MHC) molecule. However, for B cells, the binding of antigen alone to the B-cell antigen receptor, called antibody or immunoglobulin, is sufficient to induce a response (Fig. 8.2).

B cells and T cells also differ in the way they put an immune response into effect. After antigen stimulation, both lymphocyte types undergo proliferation and differentiation to become either effector cells or memory cells. **Memory cells** are long-lived cells that have the ability to mount an enhanced response upon a re-encounter with antigen. The effector function of B cells is mediated by the secreted antigen receptor, and in their active secretory phase, B cells typically are manifest as **plasma cells**. Released to the extracellular fluids, the antibodies serve an important role in humoral immunity. Antigen with attached antibody is more easily recognized by phagocytes and eliminated. The antigen–antibody complex also triggers a collection of plasma proteins that form the complement system. This important component of innate defense has wide ranging effects that include the ability to kill microorganisms.

T cells, on the other hand, act more directly on adjacent cells within tissues. The two major subsets of T cells mediate their effects in different ways. The **T helper cells** act through the secretion of soluble short-range effector molecules, called cytokines, whereas the **T cytotoxic cells** need to attach to the target cells to kill them.

A third category of lymphocyte, the **natural killer cell** (NK), lacks an antigen receptor that is typical for either B or T cells. In some species, these cells appear as large granular lymphocytes. The NK cells seem to rely on a recognition system that is less specific than that used by B cells and T cells. The cell-mediated killing of NK cells is similar to the function of T cells and NK cells in the elimination of tumors and virus-infected cells or other cells that show altered expression of "self" molecules.

The threat posed to the individual by the large number of microbial antigens has been met by a prodigious diversity among lymphocytes. The strategy has been to develop lymphocytes that are individually different; the concept being — one cell, one specificity. Genetic mechanisms, including random sampling of germline gene segments, allelic exclusion, and hypermutation, have evolved that provide an enormous variation in the lymphocyte antigen receptors. In B cells, other gene events may be superimposed during final differentiation. Class switching of the constant region of the heavy

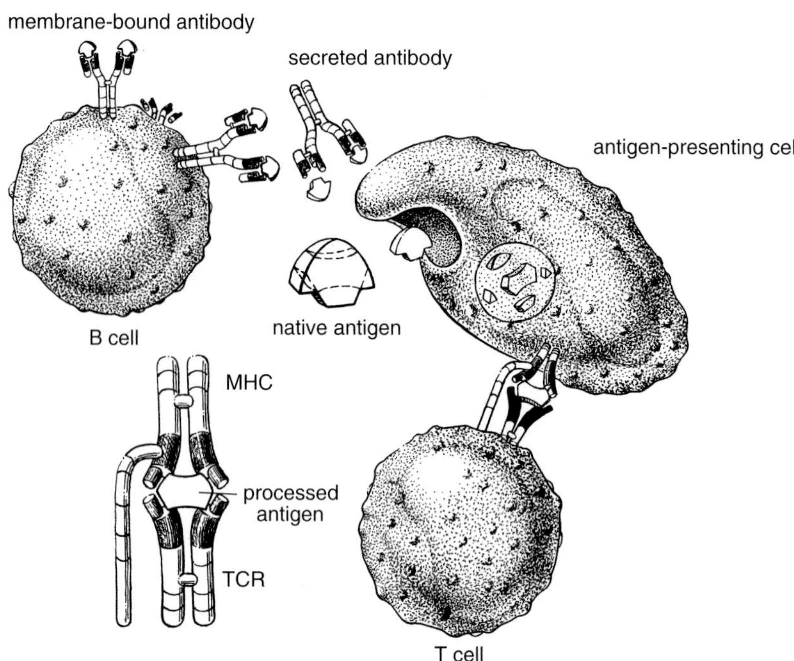

Figure 8.2. *Schematic drawing of antigen–antigen receptor interaction. The B-cell receptor can interact directly with native antigen either while bound to the plasma membrane of a B cell or as secreted antibody. The T-cell receptor recognizes processed antigen presented by a major histocompatibility complex (MHC) molecule on the surface of an antigen-presenting cell. Accessory molecules such as CD4 or CD8 contribute to the stability of this interaction.*

chain gene results in the production of B cells with different functional characteristics. Thus, the immunoglobulin (Ig) of M isotype, which is produced first, may be switched to one of the other major classes, i.e., IgA, IgG, or IgE.

In addition to a vast range of antigen specificities and subpopulations with diverse functional abilities, lymphocytes circulate continuously from blood through lymphatic and nonlymphatic tissues and return to the blood either directly or via the lymph. This process, called **lymphocyte recirculation**, facilitates the dissemination of an immune response throughout the body and enables effective immune surveillance for foreign invaders and alterations in the body's own cells. Most lymphocytes enter organs such as the lungs, liver, and bone marrow and return to the blood via venules, whereas a few lymphocytes leave these organs via the lymph and drain to lymph nodes via afferent lymph vessels. Tissue fluid from large peripheral areas also drains into lymph nodes, further enhancing the likelihood of an encounter between a lymphocyte and its antigen. A proportion of lymphocytes migrates from blood directly into lymphatic tissues through specialized postcapillary venules, called **high endothelial venules**. High endothelial venules have lining cells that are tall and rounded, in contrast to the flattened endothelial cells of other blood vessels. These specialized venules are abundant in the T-cell areas surrounding B-cell nodules and serve as the sites of entry for both T cells and B cells. The spleen is an exception, because it does not possess specialized postcapillary venules or afferent lymphatics, and lymphocytes migrate into the spleen via blood capillaries in the marginal zone. Normally, relatively few lymphocytes migrate into organs such as the skin, synovia, muscle, and brain; however, during acute and chronic inflammation, an influx of large numbers of lymphocytes can occur.

Stromal Cells

A three-dimensional network of stellate reticular cells with a fibroblastic structure forms a supportive mesh or stroma for lymphocyte and other leukocyte populations that constitute the parenchyma of lymphatic organs.

RETICULAR CELLS

Reticular cells, which are of fibroblastic origin and structure, form a reticulum in lymphatic tissues and synthesize reticular fibers that are closely associated with or invaginated in their cell surface. Because of their numerous long and branching processes, reticular cells have a stellate or fusiform appearance.

FOLLICULAR DENDRITIC CELLS

Follicular dendritic cells are specialized stromal cells localized within lymphatic nodules and are known to retain antigens on their surface for long periods of time. Whereas macrophages and dendritic cells originate from hemopoietic stem cells in the bone marrow, follicular dendritic cells are derived from fibroblastic cells.

Antigen-Presenting Cells

For antigen recognition and the induction of an immune response to occur, T cells require antigen to be presented on the surface of a cell by an MHC molecule and a complex to form between the MHC-bound antigen and the T-cell antigen receptor (Fig. 8.2). Most nucleated cells express a class of MHC molecule, MHC class I, and the presence of this molecule serves as the identifying password for self recognition. The MHC class I molecules also play a role in the presentation of antigen derived from the cytoplasm of cells, such as are present during virus infections or in neoplastic cells. The endogenous antigens presented by MHC class I molecules usually induce a T-cytotoxic-cell response. Exogenous antigens are usually presented by another class of MHC molecule, MHC class II, to T helper cells. The induction of a T-cell response is greatly facilitated by the presence of accessory molecules on the T-cell surface that bind the MHC molecule and enhance signal transduction to the cell. CD4 is an accessory molecule on the surface of T helper cells that binds to the MHC class II molecule, whereas the CD8 molecule performs a similar function for T cytotoxic cells, binding the MHC class I molecule. The CD, or cluster of differentiation, number is a classification system used to define cell surface molecules on leukocytes and platelets and is based on the specificities of monoclonal antibodies.

The range of cells expressing MHC class II is more restricted than for MHC class I, although many cell types may be induced to express MHC class II, particularly during an inflammatory reaction. A group of cells has specialized in the presentation of antigen to T helper cells. This diverse group includes dendritic cells, macrophages, and B cells.

DENDRITIC CELLS

Dendritic cells constitutively express high levels of MHC class II and are particularly important in the induction of an immune response in naive T helper cells. Dendritic cells have the capacity to bind antigens or cluster lymphocytes on their surface. When in lymph, dendritic cells possess prominent surface folds and have been called "veiled cells." When lodged in the extranodular domains of the lymph nodes, these cells become "interdigitating" cells, and dendritic cells can also be present in lymphatic nodules. In the stratified squamous epithelia, dendritic cells localize in the upper spinous layer and are termed "Langerhans cells" (see Chapter 16, Integument).

MACROPHAGES

Macrophages or mononuclear phagocytes exist in various types but have the common feature of being active in the phagocytosis and degradation of foreign substances. The degradation of foreign substances into short peptides is essential for presentation of antigen in the peptide-binding groove of the MHC class II molecule (Fig. 8.2). Macrophages express MHC class II and are able to present antigen to T helper cells, although antigen presentation is more typically performed by other cell types.

B CELLS

B cells also express MHC class II and are very efficient in the presentation of antigen to T helper cells. In contrast to macrophages, which will ingest any foreign substance, B cells bind only one antigen through surface immunoglobulin. The bound antigen is endocytosed, fragmented, and presented by MHC class II molecules. B cells are particularly important for antigen presentation in a secondary immune response.

ORGANS OF THE IMMUNE SYSTEM

Primary Lymphatic Organs

Hemopoietic stem cells give rise to erythroid, megakaryocytic, granulocytic-monocytic, and lymphoid cell lineages (see Chapter 4). In the chicken, these pluripotent stem cells are found in the embryonic yolk sac, in the periaortic mesenchyme, and later in the bone marrow. In rodents and man, hemopoietic stem cells are present in the paraaortic splanchnopleure and fetal liver, spleen, and bone marrow but throughout adult life are normally only found in the bone marrow. Lymphocytes develop from stem cells in the primary lymphatic organs. Other processes of lymphocyte development that occur in primary lymphatic organs include the generation of preimmune diversification, i.e., the rearrangement of antigen-receptor genes.

It is within the primary or central lymphatic organs during the development of the fetus that the identity of lymphocytes first becomes established. In primary lymphatic organs, stem cells are in an environment suitable for differentiation and development. Intense cell proliferation is accompanied by random rearrangement of the genes responsible for the antigen receptor and expression of accessory molecules, processes that allow interaction with other cells and confer effector functions. Scrutiny of the emerging cells is followed by elimination of more than 90% of the cells, which are identified as unsuitable, largely because of their reaction with the body's own molecules (autoreactivity). These lymphocytes are eliminated by apoptosis, a mechanism that involves activation of a gene protocol ensuring rapid disintegration of the selected cells with minimal harm to the surrounding tissues.

Even with the elimination of most of their cells, primary lymphatic organs produce vast numbers of B cells and T cells, which constitute a diverse repertoire of antigen specificities. The released cells are disseminated to the secondary or peripheral lymphatic organs distributed throughout the body, i.e., the mucosa-associated lymphatic tissues, lymph nodes, spleen, and hemal nodes.

BONE MARROW

The structure and major hematopoietic functions of the bone marrow are presented in Chapter 4. The bone marrow is the site of origin of pluripotent stem cells and B-cell precursors in some species. B-cell precursors are located adjacent to the endosteum of the bone lamellae and undergo differentiation and selection as they migrate toward the venous sinus at the center of each cav-

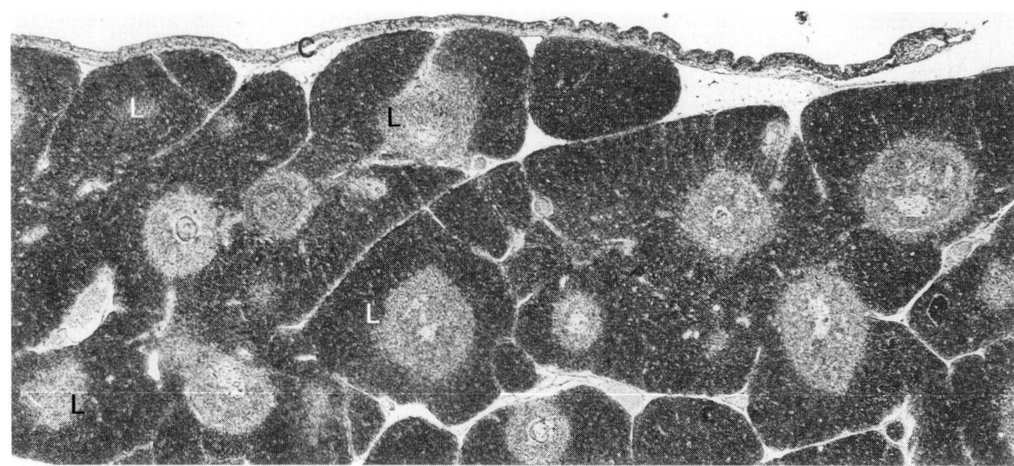

Figure 8.3. *Thymus (cat). The thymic lobules (L) are partially separated by thin septa of connective tissue. Capsule (C). Hematoxylin and eosin (×20).*

Figure 8.4. *Schematic drawing of a portion of a thymic lobule. The lobule consists of a cortex and medulla and has a border of flattened epithelial cells. The epithelial reticulum of the cortex is heavily infiltrated by lymphocytes undergoing cell division and differentiation. The epithelial cells of the medulla may form concentric arrangements called thymic corpuscles or Hassall's corpuscles. Blood vessels supply the lobule via the capsule and thin connective tissue septa to reach the corticomedullary junction.*

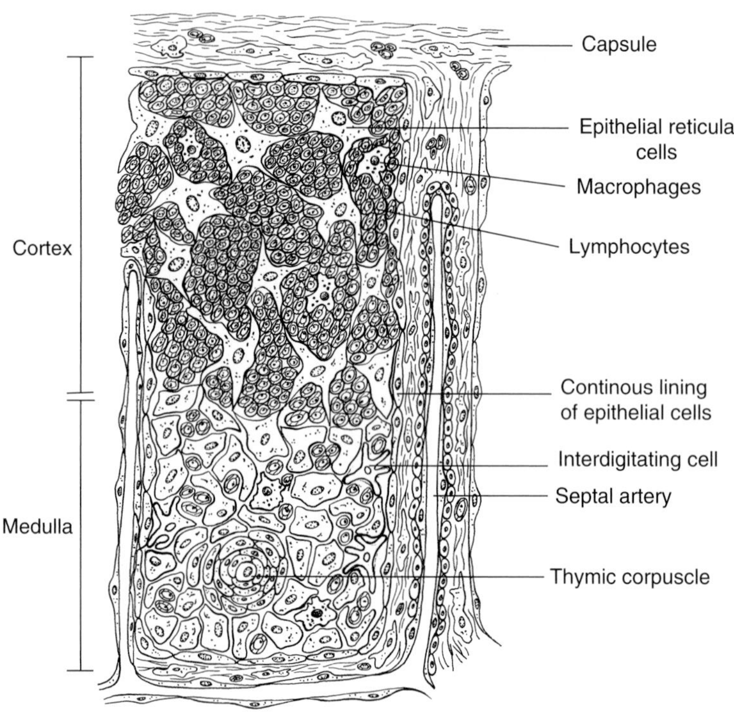

ity of the spongy bone. B-cell maturation occurs in close association with stromal reticular cells.

THYMUS

The thymus originates as a solid outgrowth from the epithelium of the third pharyngeal pouch. The spreading of epithelial cells gives rise to a thymic epithelial reticulum, which is invaded by blood vessels from the surrounding mesenchyme. Migration of lymphocytic stem cells into the thymus occurs from early in ontogeny and is probably associated with chemotactic signals produced by the thymic anlage. The lymphocytic stem cells invade the interstices, filling the spaces between the epithelial cells. The thymus is therefore often referred to as a "lymphoepithelial organ."

Structure

The thymus comprises **lobes**, each of which is surrounded by a capsule of connective tissue continuous with thin septa that subdivide the lobes into partially separated **lobules**. The central medulla of each lobule is a branch of tissue that arises from a central stalk in the lobe and is surrounded by a cortex (Fig. 8.3).

CORTEX. The thymic cortex consists mainly of an epithelial reticulum and lymphocytes (Fig. 8.4). The stellate **epithelial reticular cells** possess large, pale, ovoid nuclei and long, branching processes that contain numerous intermediate filaments and are connected to each other by desmosomes. Their organelles are inconspicuous. At the periphery of the lobules and around the perivascular spaces, a single layer of long and flattened epithelial cells forms a continuous lining.

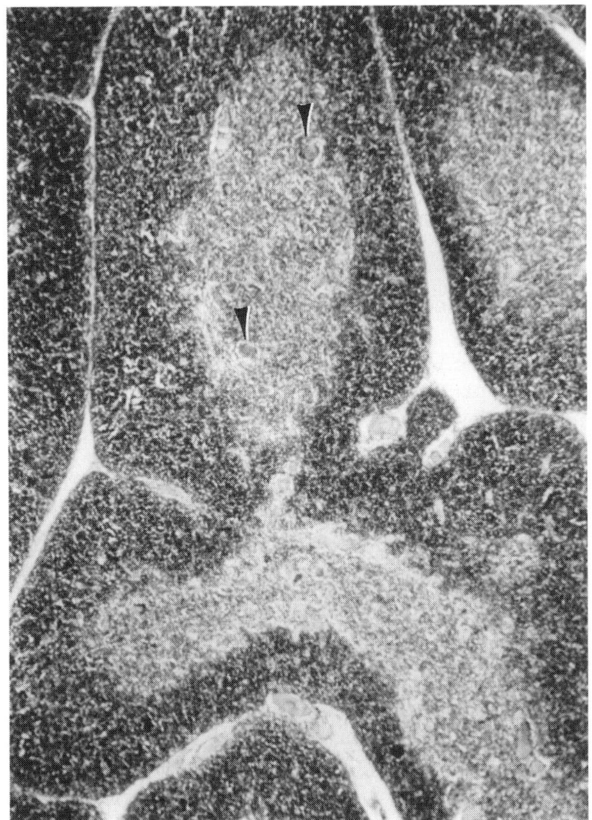

Figure 8.5. *Thymus (dog). The dark cortex is clearly distinguishable from the light medulla, in which thymic corpuscles (arrowheads) are readily identified. Hematoxylin and eosin (×40).*

Lymphoblasts and **medium-sized lymphocytes** predominate in the meshes of the peripheral epithelial reticulum, where they undergo mitotic divisions producing small lymphocytes that differentiate in the deep cortex. **Tingible body macrophages**, which are macrophages that phagocytose and eliminate dead lymphocytes and often contain remnants of lymphocytes, are present, especially in the vicinity of the medulla. Because it contains a greater number of lymphocytes than the medulla, the cortex always stains much darker (Fig. 8.5).

MEDULLA. Some of the epithelial reticular cells in the medulla have the same structure as those in the cortex; however, others are much larger and their epithelial nature is thus more obvious. They contain more mitochondria and have an extensive rough endoplasmic reticulum, Golgi complex, and granules. Medullary epithelial cells form **thymic corpuscles**, also called Hassall's corpuscles (Fig. 8.6). The corpuscles consist of one or several calcified or degenerated large central cells, which are surrounded by flat keratinized cells in a concentric arrangement. These cells contain many desmosomes and bundles of intermediate filaments. **Interdigitating cells** similar to those present in the T-cell areas of secondary lymphatic organs are also present. The cells in the meshes of the reticular network are predominantly small lymphocytes, along with a few macrophages.

BLOOD VESSELS, LYMPH VESSELS, AND NERVES. The blood supply of the thymus is derived from arteries that penetrate the parenchyma at the corticomedullary junction by way of the connective tissue septa. The arteries divide into arterioles that course along the junction and give rise to a capillary network that forms arcades in the cortex. These capillaries drain into postcapillary venules located in the medulla or at the junction between the cortex and medulla; the postcapillary venules join veins in the connective tissue septa. Cortical capillaries are characterized by a continuous endothelium, perivascular connective tissue, and a sheath of epithelial cell processes. Together, these lay-

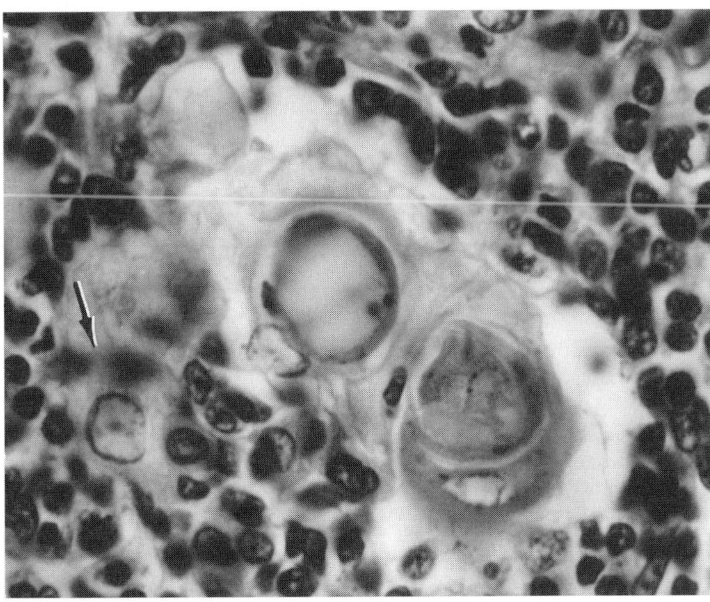

Figure 8.6. *Thymic corpuscles, thymus (dog). Notice the arrangement of the cells in concentric layers and an enlarged epithelial reticular cell (arrow), which is probably the point of origin of a new thymic corpuscle. Hematoxylin and eosin (×735).*

ers form the **blood–thymus barrier**. This barrier reduces the access of antigens to the cortical parenchyma, and it is also impermeable to tracers, such as horseradish peroxidase. However, some circulating antigens may filter into the cortical tissues via the capsule. The venules at the corticomedullary junction are permeable to blood-borne macromolecules and cells.

The parenchyma of the thymus is devoid of lymph vessels. Efferent lymph vessels drain the capsule and septa. A network of nerve fibers derived from the vagus and sympathetic nerves accompanies the blood vessels.

Immunologic function

The thymus is populated by bone-marrow-derived stem cells that commit to developing into T cells. The developing T cells or thymocytes initially populate the outer cortex and undergo population growth, rearrangement of their antigen-receptor genes, and surface expression of the antigen-receptor and accessory molecules such as CD4 and CD8. A high mitotic rate results in a rich supply of thymocytes, which is then subjected to rigorous selection processes. The aim of thymic selection is to produce T cells that have an antigen receptor capable of recognizing self- MHC molecules as well as foreign antigen. After the successful rearrangement of the antigen-receptor genes, also called T-cell receptor genes, the developing T cells are subjected to a process of **positive** and **negative selection**. First, T cells having a moderate affinity for self-MHC are selected, resulting in deletion of those lymphocytes with low or high affinity for MHC. The next step involves elimination of T cells that recognize a self antigen other than MHC. Thus, T cells capable of attacking the body's own cells are destroyed. It is believed that positive selection is mediated by the cortical epithelial cells and negative selection is mediated by interdigitating cells and macrophages that are prevalent in the medulla and at the corticomedullary junction. Through these processes, more than 90% of the newly formed lymphocytes are destroyed. Elimination of unsuitable cells is brought about by apoptosis, and tingible body macrophages are frequent in the thymus. The blood–thymus barrier reduces the access of circulating antigens, which could interfere with the processes of positive selection in the cortical tissue. The absence of such a barrier at the corticomedullary junction allows circulating antigens to contribute to the negative selection processes.

The T cells enter the blood by migrating through the endothelium of postcapillary venules at the corticomedullary junction. The T cells released from the thymus settle within the T-cell areas of secondary lymphatic organs.

The thymus is particularly active in young animals, and involution of the organ is a normal occurrence after puberty and aging. **Involution** is characterized by a gradual depletion of lymphocytes (especially from the cortex), enlargement of the epithelial reticular cells, and invasion of the parenchyma by adipocytes originating from the interlobular connective tissue. In adult animals, the thymus consists of narrow strands of parenchyma, in which enlarged epithelial reticular cells predominate, surrounded by adipose tissue (Fig. 8.7).

CLOACAL BURSA OF BIRDS

The dichotomy of lymphocyte lineages was first revealed in birds. The cloacal bursa of birds (bursa of Fabricius) is a lymphatic organ situated in the dorsal cloaca and, like the thymus, is a lymphoepithelial organ. From day 8 to day 15 of embryonic incubation in the chicken, precursor cells committed to the B-cell lineage migrate into the developing organ. The nodules develop as invaginations of the cloacal epithelium at approximately day 12 of incubation. Longitudinal plicae protruding inside the bursal lumen are then formed. Buttonlike epithelial formations penetrate the tunica propria from the plicae, and lymphopoiesis begins inside the epithelial buds. In the developed bursa, the supporting stroma of the nodular medulla is formed by long irregular reticular epithelial cells. Macrophages and lymphoid cells of various size occur between the cytoplasmic extensions of these cells. The nodular cortex also has a stroma of epithelial reticular cells. Small lymphocytes predominate in the cortex, and some macrophages are seen. The epithelium overlying the nodule has a remarkable capacity for transcytosis of macromolecules from the bursal lumen into the nodules. Transcytosed antigen could contribute to the high rate of proliferation of B cells in the bursa, an apparent prerequisite for the gene events occurring there. The lymphocytes undergo repetitive conversions of genes coding for the variable regions of immunoglobulin, using pseudogenes, which are genes that have structures homologous to other genes but are incapable of being expressed, as sequence donors. This process of gene conversion expands the B-cell antigen-receptor repertoire. Strict selection processes ensure that the antibodies of the emigrant lymphocytes have suitable specificities for their tasks in the secondary lymphatic tissues.

GUT-ASSOCIATED LYMPHATIC TISSUE

Most organized lymphatic tissue associated with the gut has been attributed with functions related to mucosal and systemic immunity (see below). In young ruminants, pigs, and carnivores, a single large aggregate of lymphatic nodules (the ileal Peyer's patch) is present in the distal jejunum/ileum. It is characteristic for this patch to show atrophy in young age and is, in this respect, different from the numerous discrete aggregates in the proximal jejunum and the scattered aggregated or solitary nodules of the colon and rectum. A role for the ileal Peyer's patch in the diversification of the preimmune antigen-receptor repertoire and expansion of B-cell populations has been defined in sheep. Thus, in sheep, removal of the ileal Peyer's patch before birth results in a drastic decline in the number of circulating B cells. At 2 months of age, the weight of the ileal Peyer's patch is more than twice that of the thymus. It has been shown that more than 90% of the cells in the nodules are eliminated by apoptosis. The intense cell division in the nodules is independent of foreign antigen. The antigen-receptor genes are subjected to a diversity-enhancing process that includes point muta-

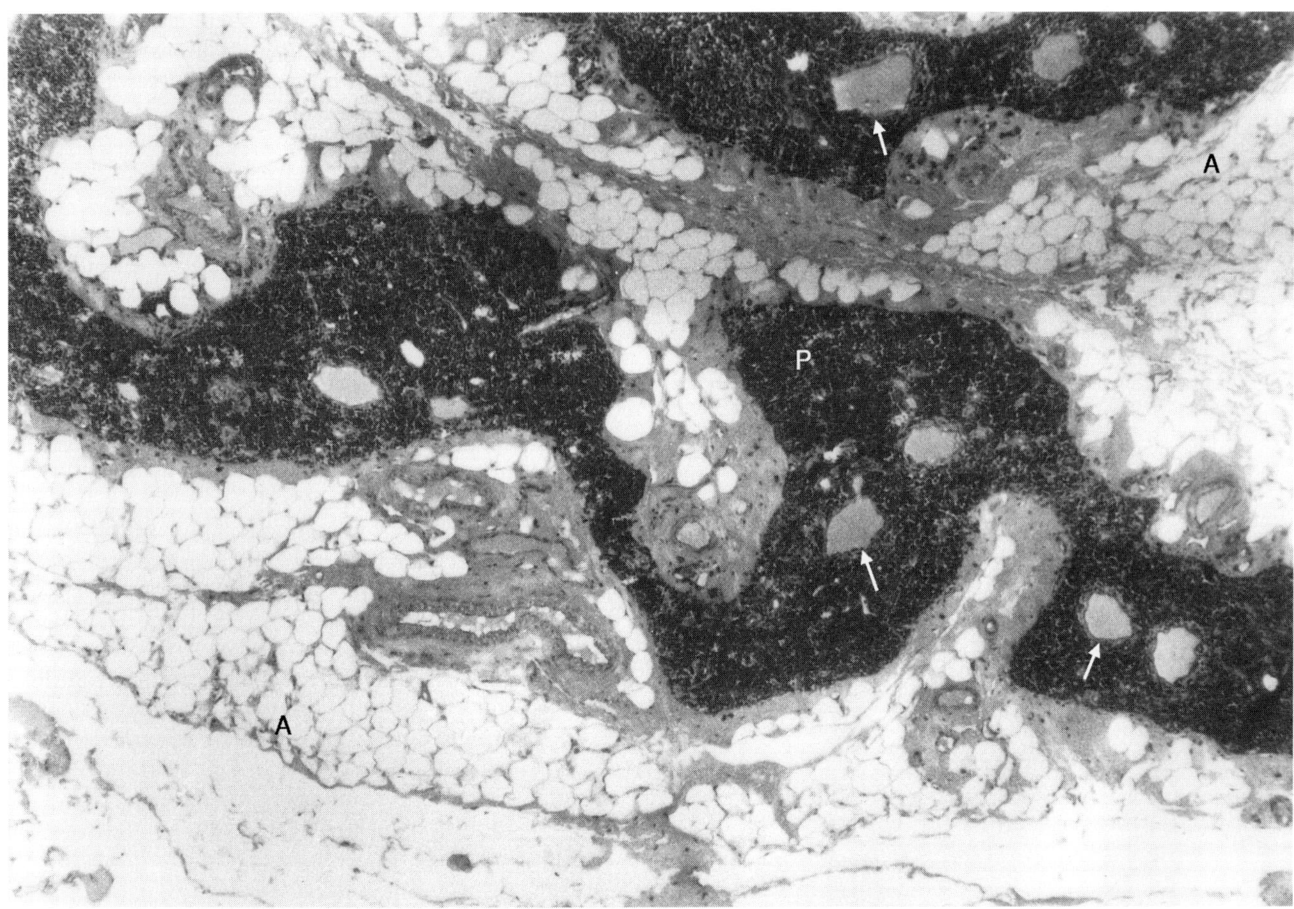

Figure 8.7. *A partially involuted thymus (adult dog). The parenchyma (P) has been replaced by adipose tissue (A). A cortex and medulla cannot be distinguished in the remaining parenchyma and cysts are prominent (arrows). Hematoxylin and eosin (×45).*

tions. Although this untemplated mechanism of diversity generation is somewhat different from that operating in the avian bursa, the effect is the same. There seem to be processes of positive and negative selection ensuring the suitability of the lymphocytes that are permitted to leave the patch. As with the avian bursa, the epithelium covering the patch is very efficient in transporting luminal macromolecules into the nodules. The rabbit appendix also shows similarities to the avian bursa, and the diversity-generating mechanisms constitute a combination of gene conversion and somatic mutation.

It should be noted that the earliest immigrants to both the single large aggregate of lymphatic nodules in the ileum of sheep and the avian bursa are already committed to the B-cell lineage, so strictly, neither organ is a primary lymphatic organ, i.e., B cells do not develop de novo from uncommitted precursors by progressively rearranging their immunoglobulin genes. These organs represent sites of postrearrangement diversification.

Secondary Lymphatic Organs

Primary lymphatic organs produce lymphocytes committed to either the B-cell or T-cell lineage. The processes of development and differentiation that occur in these organs are independent of foreign antigen. Thus, the lymphocytes leaving a primary lymphatic organ are said to be **naive** or **virgin cells**. The encounter with foreign antigen is most likely to occur in secondary lymphatic organs, which are strategically situated in the body at sites of entry of antigen and are well equipped with specialized microenvironments populated by the antigen-presenting cells necessary to induce an immune response. The secondary or peripheral lymphatic organs include lymph nodes, spleen, tonsils, mucosa-associated lymphatic tissue, and hemal nodes.

GENERAL STRUCTURE AND FUNCTION

Primary lymphatic nodules consist of a stromal network of immature follicular dendritic cells and associated reticular fibers. Small, tightly packed lymphocytes and some medium lymphocytes are evenly distributed throughout the stromal network and represent predominantly naive recirculating B cells.

Secondary lymphatic nodules appear in response to the recognition of antigen and have a germinal center in which lymphoblastic activity is marked (Fig. 8.8). Their formation begins in a primary nodule with an ac-

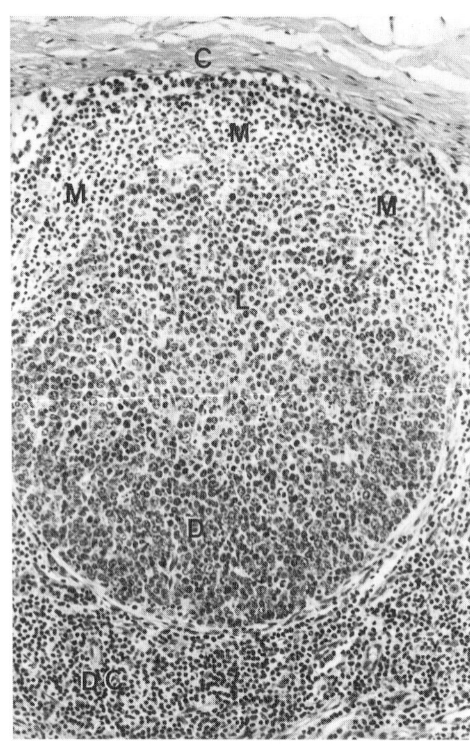

Figure 8.8. *Lymph node (goat). Secondary lymphatic nodule with germinal center. Dark area (D); light area (L); mantle (M); capsule (C); deep cortex (DC). Hematoxylin and eosin (×150).*

cumulation of large, basophilic lymphoblasts and tingible body macrophages. Differentiated follicular dendritic cells form the stroma of the secondary nodules. An established **germinal center** consists of a light zone and a dark zone. The germinal center is usually oriented so that the light zone is closest and the dark zone is farthest from the subcapsular sinus in lymph nodes or the surface epithelium in mucosal nodules or the marginal zone in the spleen. The **dark zone** is composed of large B-cell blasts engaged in intense mitotic activity and is delineated basally by several layers of flattened reticular cells that become less distinct laterally. The **light zone** is populated by smaller, less basophilic lymphocytes with few mitoses. Along the periphery of the light zone is a thin layer of small lymphocytes that often form a thicker cap over the apex of the germinal center. This layer is called the **mantle**. When cellular activity declines late in an immune response, the germinal center recedes.

The **diffuse extranodular lymphatic tissue** adjacent to the nodules contains dense accumulations of small T cells, mingled with some lymphoblasts (often seen in mitosis) and macrophages. A special type of cell, the interdigitating cell of bone marrow origin, is characteristic of these T-cell areas, as are specialized postcapillary venules that are sites of lymphocyte recirculation. The stroma of diffuse lymphatic tissue consists of a three-dimensional network of reticular cells.

Foreign antigens are transported from their site of entry into the body to the secondary lymphatic tissues via blood or lymph either free or associated with cells such as Langerhans cells. The antigens arrive in the extranodular lymphatic tissues, which are sites of both lymphocyte recirculation and the specialized antigen-presenting cells, the interdigitating cells. The conjunction of antigen, antigen-specific lymphocytes, and antigen-presenting cells results in the recognition of antigen and the initiation of a specific immune response. The outcome of a particular immune response depends on many factors, including the nature and amount of antigen, the type and number of antigen-presenting cells, and the presence or absence of the products of a nonspecific immune response, but the major influence is the origin of the antigen-specific lymphocyte. The recognition of antigen by B cells results in a humoral immune response, whereas recognition by T cells leads to a cell-mediated immune response.

B cells can respond to some antigens directly, but for other antigens, B cells require the assistance of antigen-specific T cells. Antigen recognition activates the B cells, inducing cell proliferation. The activated B lymphoblasts either undergo terminal differentiation toward plasma cells or migrate into primary nodules or the dark zone of germinal centers. The plasma cells resulting from extranodular differentiation secrete IgM, characteristic of a primary humoral immune response. Antigen or antigen–antibody complexes are transported into primary follicles and are held on the surface of follicular dendritic cells. The B lymphoblasts showing high affinity for this antigen proliferate intensely, displacing the resting nodular B cells, which form the mantle of the secondary nodule. After the initial expansion and establishment of a secondary nodule, the germinal center reaction continues with proliferation but no increase in cell number in the dark zone of the germinal center. Lymphoblast proliferation in the dark zone is accompanied by random mutation of the variable region of the antigen-receptor genes. The mutated lymphoblasts cease to proliferate and move into the basal light zone of the germinal center, which is characterized by an extensive follicular dendritic cell network and very few T cells. The survival of the mutated B cells is dependent on their binding to the low levels of antigen–antibody immune complexes exposed on the surface of follicular dendritic cells. Low-affinity mutants that do not bind to antigen and autoreactive mutants die by apoptosis and are eliminated by tingible body macrophages. High-affinity mutants bind antigen, process it, and present it to T cells that are localized mainly within the apical light zone. The T cells are induced to express accessory molecules and secrete cytokines, which are important for the further survival, proliferation, and isotype switching of B cells. These T-cell-derived signals also determine whether the high-affinity, isotype-switched B cells differentiate into memory B cells or plasma cells. The differentiation to plasma cells occurs in the medullary cords of lymph nodes, the mucosal lamina propria, and the bone marrow. Upon reexposure to antigen and the induction of a secondary humoral immune response, recirculating memory B cells can be activated in extranodular tissues, giving rise to plasma cells and cells capable of founding a germinal center reaction.

In a primary cell-mediated immune response, interdigitating cells in the extranodular lymphatic tissues present foreign antigen to naive recirculating T helper cells. Antigen is presented to T helper cells bound to MHC class II molecules on the surface of the antigen-presenting cell. Other cell types, including B cells and macrophages, may also present antigen to T cells, particularly in a secondary immune response. Antigen recognition results in cytokine secretion and rapid proliferation by the T cells. The proliferating cells acquire various effector functions or become long-lived memory cells and are eventually released into the circulation and efferent lymphatic vessels.

MUCOSA-ASSOCIATED LYMPHATIC TISSUE

Solitary lymphatic nodules, as well as aggregates of nodules, are common in the subepithelial connective tissue of most mucous membranes. Nodules are especially numerous in the digestive and respiratory systems and are also present in the urogenital tract and around the eye. Organlike **aggregated lymphatic nodules** are prominent in the intestine and the pharyngeal region. Those in the pharynx and the caudal oral cavity are referred to as tonsils. The **tonsils** are located adjacent to the lumen of the host organ and are covered by stratified squamous (oropharynx) or pseudostratified columnar (nasopharynx) epithelium. The tonsillar surface may be relatively smooth (e.g., palatine tonsil of dogs and cats), or it may have deep surface invaginations, referred to as tonsillar fossulae (e.g., lingual tonsil in horses, palatine tonsil in horses and small ruminants). These invaginations allow a high concentration of lymphatic tissue in a given area.

The epithelium is usually infiltrated to a variable degree with lymphocytes, neutrophils, and macrophages. This infiltration is particularly pronounced in the tonsils of the oropharynx. Leukocytes that reach the lumen are referred to as salivary corpuscles. When they are not washed out of the fossulae by secretions from the surrounding salivary glands, these cells, along with microorganisms, may obstruct the fossulae and cause inflammation.

Beneath the epithelium, diffuse lymphatic tissue with plasma cells surrounds lymphatic nodules, which frequently possess germinal centers and a cap of small lymphocytes (mantle) adjacent to the epithelium. The tonsil is separated from the surrounding tissue by a distinct connective tissue capsule, which makes the "enucleation" of the tonsil possible (e.g., pharyngeal tonsil of the dog). Tonsillar blood vessels have essentially the same distribution and character as those of lymph nodes (see following section). Afferent lymph vessels are lacking. A plexus of lymph capillaries is present in the deep layers of the tonsil and drains into the larger efferent lymph vessels in the tonsillar capsule.

The tonsils are often the site of an early encounter with infectious agents and other antigens, and the local production of antibodies is important in a rapid initial response and the subsequent elaboration of a generalized immune response.

GALT is the acronym for gut-associated lymphatic tissue, which includes solitary and aggregated lymphatic nodules, subepithelial lymphocytes, plasma cells and macrophages, and intraepithelial lymphocytes. The aggregates of lymphatic nodules occurring in the small intestine, seen grossly as elevations in the mucosa, are called **Peyer's patches**. These patches are most conspicuous in the ileum, appearing in ruminants, pigs, and carnivores as a single large patch that involutes in young age and may have a function different from that of the smaller patches (cf., earlier). The numerous discrete small intestinal Peyer's patches and scattered aggregated or solitary nodules of the colon and rectum persist into adulthood.

Peyer's patches may be compartmentalized into *(a)* submucosal lymphatic nodules with a high rate of lymphopoiesis, *(b)* a zone of small lymphocytes that caps the submucosal lymphatic nodule (the corona or mantle), *(c)* an internodular region rich in T cells and postcapillary venules through which lymphocytes recirculate, *(d)* the elevated region overlying lymphatic nodules (the dome), and *(e)* the nodule-associated epithelium (Fig. 8.9). At the level of the dome, villi and crypts are absent. The nodule-associated epithelium lacks goblet cells but includes a special cell that has numerous microfolds at its luminal surface, the M cell (Fig. 8.10). M cells typically enfold groups of lymphocytes and occasionally macrophages and dendritic cells. M cells are able to capture and transcytose particulate antigen, thereby enabling the initiation of an immune response. Precursors of plasma cells leave the submucosal nodules and migrate through the propria into the lymph vessels and mesenteric lymph nodes to reach the general circulation. Many of these cells migrate to other organs lined by a mucous membrane, such as bronchi(-oles), mammary glands, and the female reproductive tract. Thus, the term **MALT**, i.e., mucosa-associated lymphatic tissue, is used. At their final destination, many of these plasma cells produce immunoglobulin A (IgA), which is then combined with a secretory component in the epithelium that mediates transcellular transport and exocytosis of IgA-secretory-component complex into the lumen.

LYMPH NODE

Lymph nodes, situated along the extensive drainage system of lymph vessels, filter the lymph before returning it to the bloodstream. Lymph nodes are the only

Figure 8.9. *Schematic drawing of part of a Peyer's patch (small intestine). Submucosal lymphatic nodules (N) are capped by a mantle (M) and lie beneath the dome (D). The nodule-associated epithelium overlying the dome contains many M cells interspersed among absorptive cells but lacks goblet cells. Postcapillary venules (P) and T lymphocytes are present in the internodular region (I), which, along with the lamina propria of the villi, is drained by lymphatic vessels (L).*

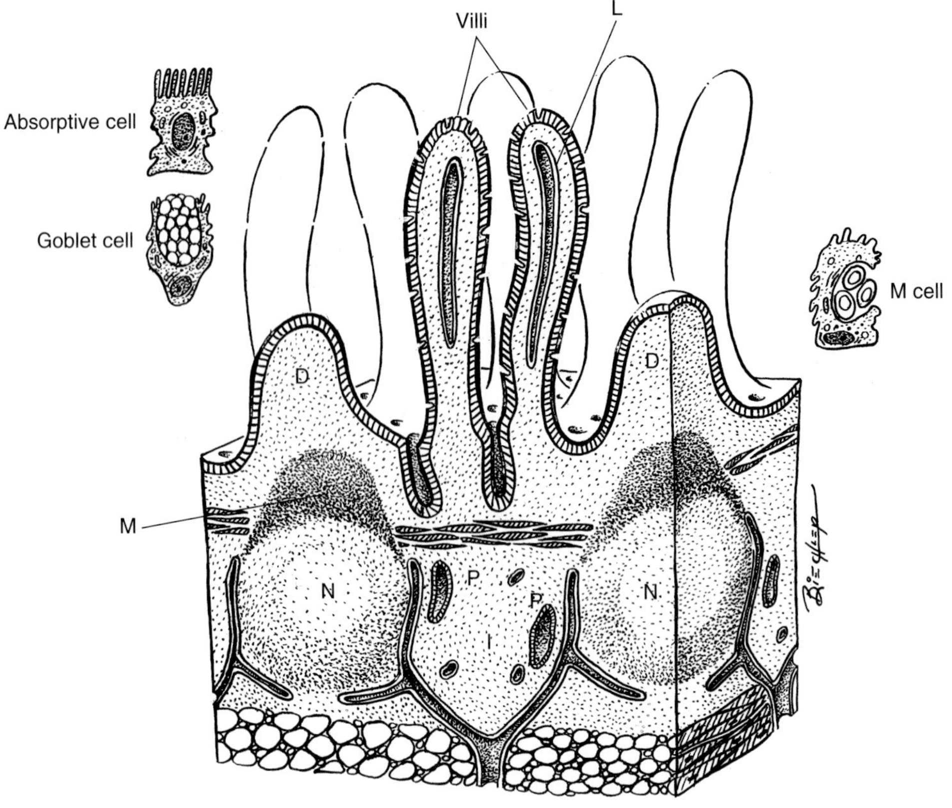

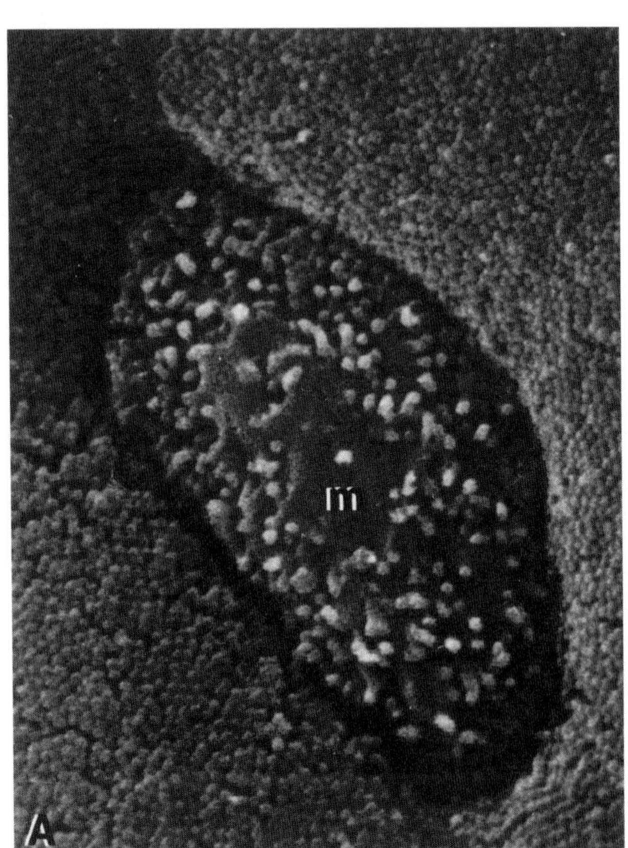

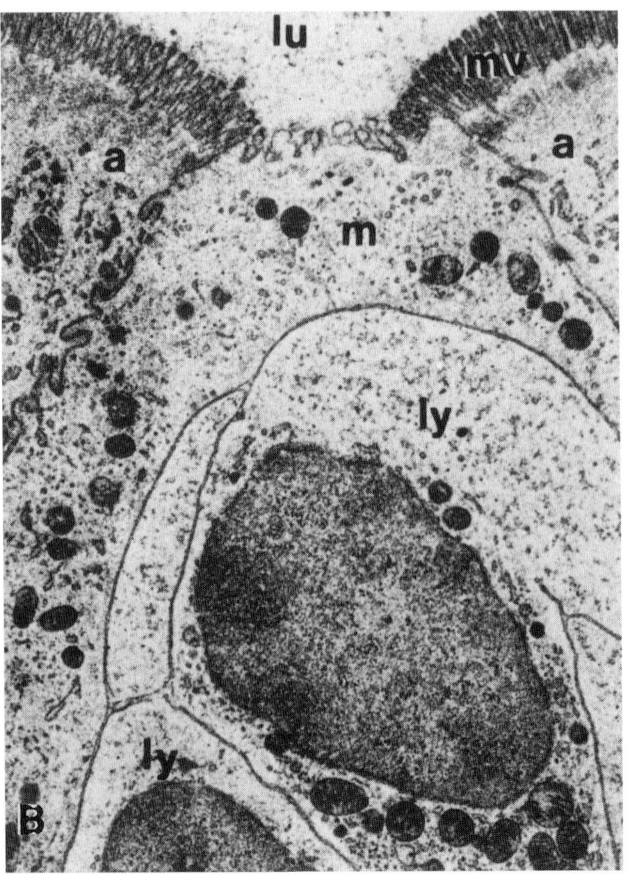

Figure 8.10. *Jejunal Peyer's patch (3-week-old calf).* ***A.****, Short microfolds are present on an M cell (m) at the dome surface; adjacent absorptive cells have densely packed microvilli (×10,000).* ***B.****, An M cell (m) with microfolds is wedged between two microvilli-bearing (mv) absorptive cells (a) and envelops lymphocytes (ly) (×7,500). lu = lumen.*

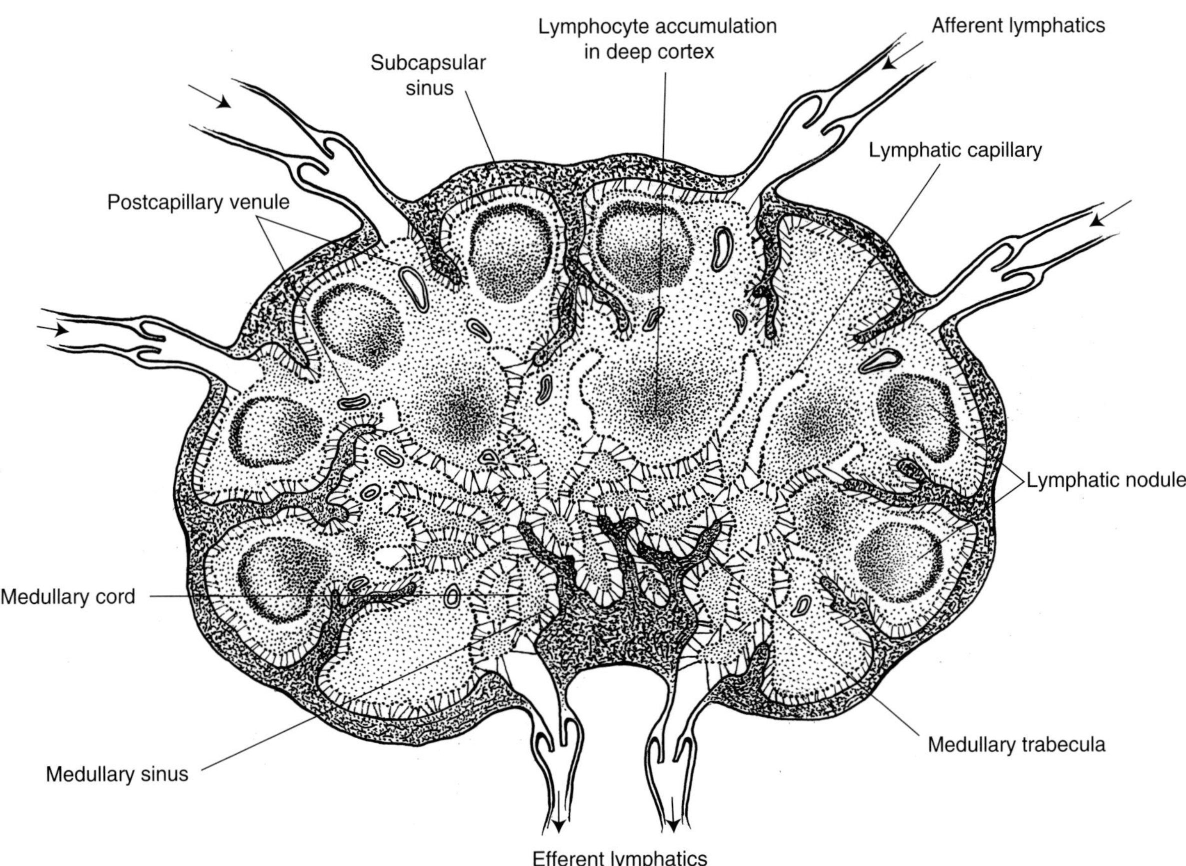

Figure 8.11. *Schematic drawing of a lymph node. The direction of lymph flow is shown with arrows.*

lymphatic organ with both afferent and efferent lymph vessels and sinuses. These organs usually have a slight indentation, the hilus, where blood and lymph vessels enter or leave the lymph node. The parenchyma is organized into a cortex of lymphatic nodules and diffuse lymphatic tissue, and a medulla of diffuse lymphatic tissue arranged in cords (Fig. 8.11). Lymph nodes provide the environment in which lymphocytes are able to respond to lymphborne antigens.

Structure

Lymph nodes are surrounded by a **capsule** composed primarily of dense irregular connective tissue with a few scattered elastic fibers. In ruminants, smooth muscle cells are also present. **Trabeculae** extend from the capsule into the parenchyma as irregular septa (Fig. 8.12). They provide support for the entire node, carry blood vessels and nerves, and are surrounded by cortical and medullary sinuses. The **stroma** of the lymph node is composed of reticular cells and fibers. **Lymphocytes**, **macrophages**, and **plasma cells** are supported by this reticular meshwork.

LYMPH VESSELS AND SINUSES. **Afferent lymph vessels** enter the lymph node at its periphery, penetrating the capsule at several different sites, and open into the subcapsular sinus. At the hilus, the subcapsular sinus is continuous with the efferent lymph vessels. Valves are present in both the afferent and the efferent lymph vessels, thereby ensuring a one-way flow of lymph (Fig. 8.11). From the **subcapsular sinus** arise sinuses that accompany the **trabeculae** and continue into the **medullary sinuses**. These sinuses form a network of branching and anastomosing channels that converge toward the hilus to open into the efferent lymph vessels. Most lymph circulates through the subcapsular, trabecular, and medullary sinuses, but some percolates through the cortex and medullary cords to reach the medullary sinuses. All lymph leaves the node through the efferent lymph vessels (Fig. 8.11).

The sinuses are lined by flattened endothelio-like reticular cells that form a continuous lining toward the capsule and trabeculae but often a discontinuous lining toward the parenchyma of the node. The lumina of the sinuses are traversed by a dense network of interconnected reticular cells similar to the lining cells and attached to the sinus walls through numerous slender processes (Fig. 8.13). Many macrophages are attached to this network.

Lymphocytes, macrophages, and dendritic cells lie free within the stromal mesh and in the sinus lumen. The reticular cells probably function as a baffle to slow lymph flow within the sinuses to facilitate antigen–cell

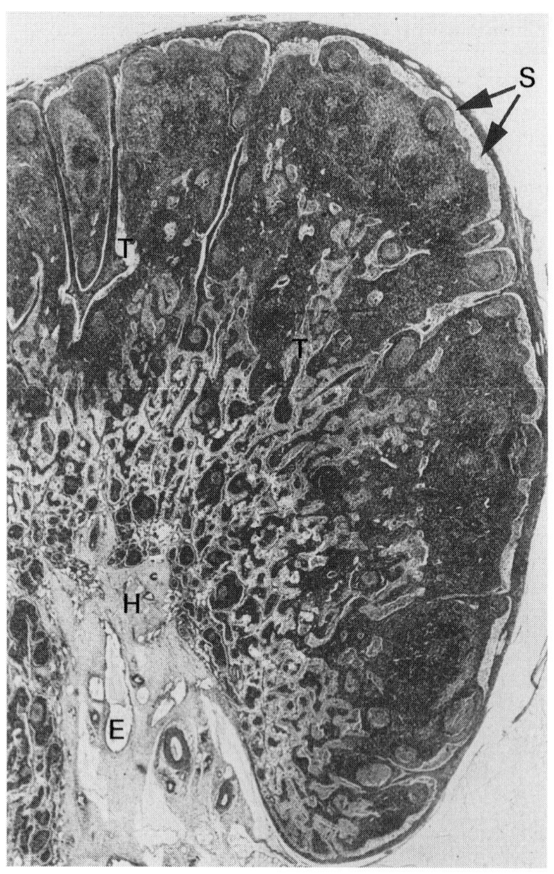

Figure 8.12. *Lymph node (cow). The dark cortex with lymphatic nodules lies adjacent to the lighter-appearing medulla. Subcapsular (S) and trabecular (T) sinuses drain toward the hilus (H) containing efferent lymph vessels (E). Hematoxylin and eosin (×10). (Courtesy of A. Hansen.)*

interactions, as well as the phagocytic activities of macrophages. Lymph percolates into the parenchyma through gaps in the sinus walls, thereby giving the parenchymal cells access to lymphborne antigens, cells, and particulate matter.

CORTEX. Most of the **outer cortex** consists of primary and secondary lymphatic nodules separated by diffuse lymphatic tissue (Fig. 8.12). The **deep cortex** is composed of diffuse lymphatic tissue and is drained by lymph capillaries (Fig. 8.11). Because most lymphocytes in the deep cortex originate from the thymus, this area is referred to as a T-cell area. The term **paracortex** has been applied variously to the deep cortex or to the diffuse lymphatic tissue of both the deep and outer cortex.

MEDULLA. The medulla is much less organized than the cortex. The lymphatic tissue extends from the cortical T cell areas as **medullary cords**, which branch and anastomose throughout the medulla (Fig. 8.11). These medullary cords are separated by a network of sinuses and connective-tissue trabeculae and are composed of lymphocytes, plasma cells, and macrophages held in a stromal mesh (Fig. 8.14).

BLOOD VESSELS AND NERVES. The major arteries enter the lymph node at the hilus, whereas smaller vessels penetrate the capsule at various sites. Upon entering the hilus, the arteries give off some branches that supply the medullary cords directly; other branches enter the trabeculae to supply the connective tissue and capsule. Those vessels supplying the medullary cords give off capillaries along their course, and the main vessels enter the cortex where branches feed capillary networks between and within the nodules. The internodular branches form capillary arcades below the subcapsular sinus and then continue inward to form postcapillary venules in the deep cortex that are lined in most species by a cuboidal endothelium (Fig. 8.15). The postcapillary venules join veins in the medullary trabeculae, which in turn empty into large veins that leave at the hilus.

Nerve fibers supply the capsule and trabeculae, and vasomotor nerves form perivascular networks throughout the lymph node.

SPECIES DIFFERENCES. Porcine lymph nodes are different from those of most other mammals (Fig. 8.16). The cortical tissue is centrally located, and most nodules occupy a deep position along trabecular sinuses. Areas similar to the deep cortex in conventional lymph nodes, with many postcapillary venules, are seen near the groups of nodules, but the periphery of the

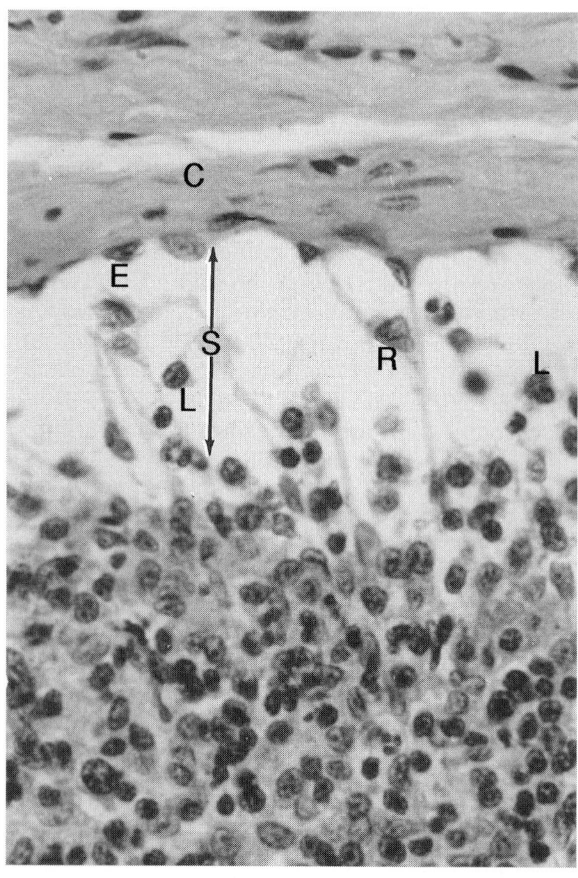

Figure 8.13. *Lymph node (dog). Beneath the connective-tissue capsule (C) is the subcapsular sinus (S) lined by flattened endothelial-like reticular cells (E). Reticular cells (R) and lymphocytes (L) are present in the sinus. Crossman's trichrome (×600).*

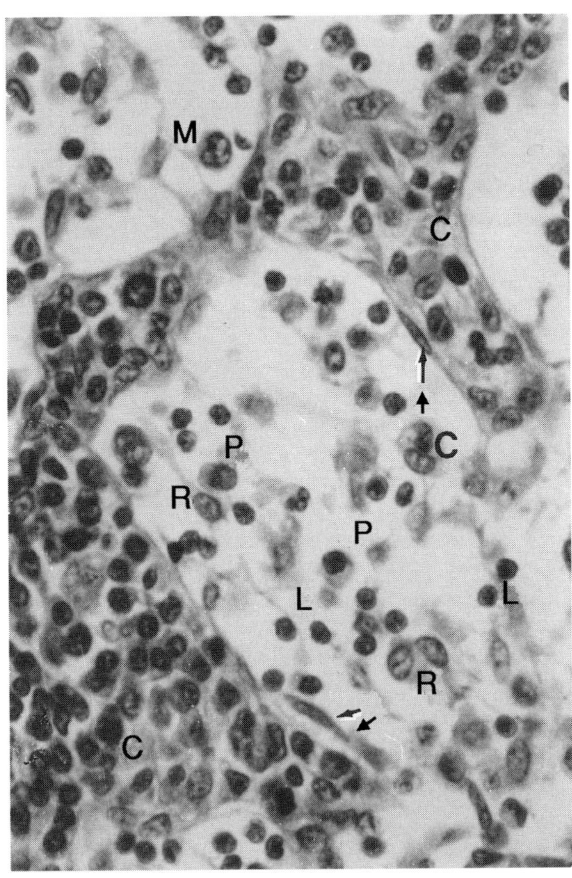

Figure 8.14. *Lymph node, medulla (dog). Flattened endothelial-like reticular cells (arrows) line the sinus containing lymphocytes (L), macrophages (M), plasma cells (P), and reticular cells (R). Lymphatic cords (C) are composed of lymphocytes, macrophages, and plasma cells. Crossman's trichrome (×600).*

node is occupied primarily by loose lymphoreticular tissue containing macrophages and only a few plasma cells. The sinuses are narrow, and medullary cords are absent. Moreover, the afferent lymph vessels enter the capsule at one or more sites and penetrate via the trabeculae deep into the area occupied by the lymphatic nodules, where they join the trabecular sinuses. The lymph then filters into the peripheral sinuses, which converge and form several efferent vessels at the periphery of the node. Functionally, the flow of the lymph is identical to that in lymph nodes of other animals because the incoming lymph first reaches the area of the node that is rich in lymphatic nodules. The efferent lymph, however, is poor in lymphocytes compared with that of other species and recirculating lymphocytes are believed to leave the porcine lymph node via the blood.

The blood vessels enter with the afferent lymph vessels and exit with the efferent vessels. As a result, a definitive hilus may not always be seen; instead, microscopic hilus-like indentations are apparent wherever afferent lymph vessels enter. Many small lymph nodes may fuse, thereby forming a large cluster of nodes, which often contributes to the difficulty in locating a hilus in porcine lymph nodes.

Immunologic function

The architecture of the lymph node represents a coarse mesh through which lymph collected from a large drainage area percolates to come in contact with lymphocytes, reticular cells, and macrophages. Any particulate

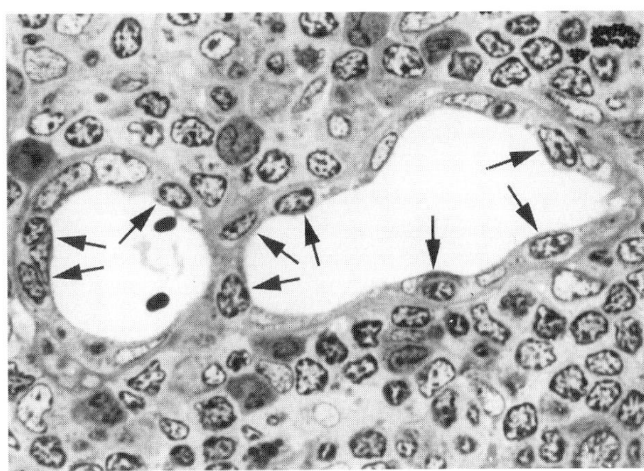

Figure 8.15. *Lymph node (goat). High endothelium in postcapillary venules with many migrating lymphocytes (arrows). Vascular perfusion. Epon. Toluidine blue (×1000).*

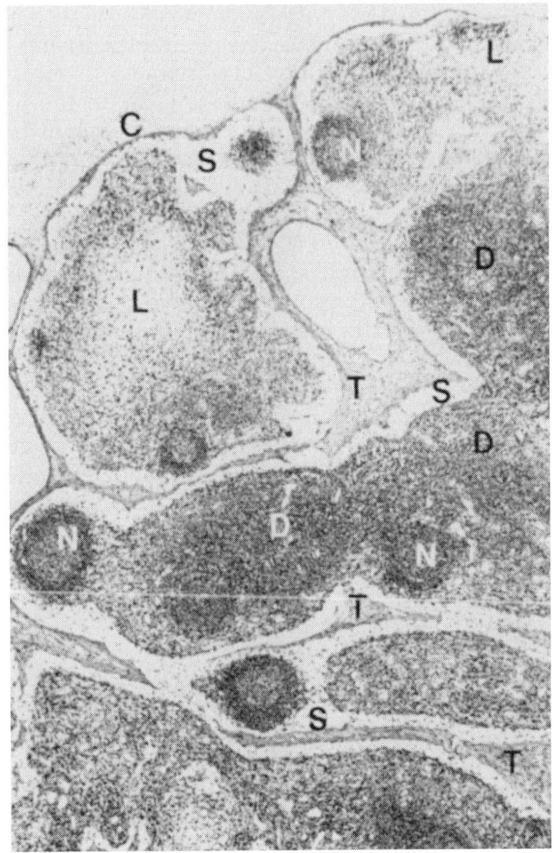

Figure 8.16. *Lymph node (pig). Capsule (C); trabeculae (T); nodules (N) along trabecular sinuses (S); "deep" cortex (D); loose peripheral tissue (L). Vascular perfusion. Hematoxylin and eosin (×100).*

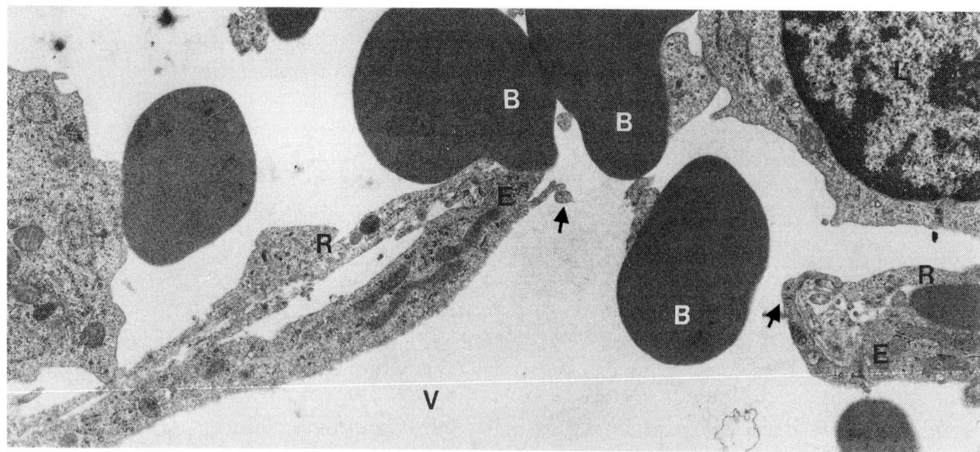

Figure 8.17. *Spleen (sheep). Electronmicrograph of a venule with erythrocytes (B) passing through an opening in the wall. Lumen (V); endothelium (E); reticular cells (R); lymphocyte (L). Arrowheads indicate the edges of the endothelial opening (×8000).*

matter in the lymph is filtered out and engulfed by the macrophages of the medullary sinus, whereas antigenic material in the lymph is made available to cortical macrophages, dendritic cells, and lymphocytes for processing. Antigen also arrives in the lymph node associated with cells. Dendritic cells, such as Langerhans cells in the skin, capture antigen in the periphery and migrate through the afferent lymphatics as veiled cells. Upon arrival in the lymph node, these antigen-laden dendritic cells move to the deep cortex to become interdigitating cells. Interdigitating cells, which are important for the presentation of antigen to T cells, persist and die in the lymph node, as very few are present in efferent lymph or blood. The arrival of antigen-laden dendritic cells in the T-cell areas of the lymph node results in the closing of valves of the efferent lymph vessels, causing the accumulation of recirculating lymphocytes and facilitating the selection of antigen-specific T cells and B cells. The initial cell proliferation and differentiation associated with antigen recognition by both T cells and B cells occur in the diffuse lymphatic tissue of the lymph node cortex. Plasmablasts move to the medullary cords to become mature plasma cells and some activated B cells colonize the primary nodules or dark zone of secondary nodules to initiate a germinal center reaction (see above). The expanded clones of T helper cells move into the circulation and lymphatic tissues as effector cells or to assist other cells such as T cytotoxic cells or B cells in mounting an immune response.

SPLEEN

The spleen serves as a filter for the blood, removing bloodborne particles and substances and aged blood cells. It also serves to store erythrocytes and platelets, as well as iron for reuse in hemoglobin synthesis, and engages in erythropoiesis in the fetus. The spleen is the major secondary lymphatic tissue involved in the clearance and mounting of immune responses against bloodborne antigens. The spleen can be divided into two compartments: a **red pulp** involved in the storage of red blood cells and antigen trapping, and a **white pulp** rich in lymphocytes and active in immune responses.

Structure

CAPSULE AND SUPPORTIVE TISSUE. The spleen is surrounded by a thick connective-tissue capsule invested by the peritoneum. The capsule has two ill-defined layers of connective tissue and smooth muscle. The total thickness and relative amount of smooth muscle vary with the species. Trabeculae composed of collagen and elastic fibers and smooth muscle cells extend from the capsule and the hilus. The trabeculae contain arteries, veins, lymph vessels, and nerves. The capsule, trabeculae, and reticular fibers support the splenic parenchyma composed of red and white pulp.

RED PULP. Most of the splenic parenchyma is red pulp, owing to the vast amount of blood held within the reticular network. The red pulp is composed of venous sinuses or venules, splenic cords, pulp arterioles, and sheathed and terminal capillaries. Two main types of red pulp are present in mammalian spleens, depending on the type of postcapillary vessels: sinusal and nonsinusal. Among the domestic animals, only dogs have typical venous sinuses, similar to those in human and rat spleens.

The **splenic sinuses** are wide vascular channels lined with elongated, longitudinally oriented endothelial cells that contain contractile microfilaments aligned in bands parallel and adjacent to the lateral cell margins. Gaps or slits are created upon contraction of these filaments, thus allowing erythrocytes to migrate from the splenic cords into the sinus lumen. The lining cells rest on a fenestrated basal lamina and are supported by reticular fibers, some of which form hooplike structures encircling the sinus at right angles to the long axis. In most domestic mammals, venules rather than venous sinuses are present. Their wide lumina are lined with a thin endothelium and discontinuous basal lamina supported by reticular cells and fibers. Openings between endothelial cells in this wall are common (Fig. 8.17).

The narrow **splenic cords** situated between the sinuses form a vast three-dimensional network composed of reticular fibers with enmeshed reticular cells, erythrocytes, macrophages, lymphocytes, plasma cells, and other leukocytes. The membranous processes of the reticular cells tend to form channel-like structures that may function to conduct blood toward the endothelial slits in the sinus walls. In nonsinusal spleens, the splenic cords are wider than in sinusal spleens. The red pulp of ruminant and porcine spleens contains numerous smooth muscle cells, whereas that of horses and dogs has myofibroblasts, which are cells that resemble fibroblasts but have some features of smooth muscle, e.g., actin filaments and dense bodies.

WHITE PULP. White pulp is lymphatic tissue that is distributed throughout the spleen and consists of diffuse lymphatic tissue, called the **periarterial lymphatic sheaths** (PALS), and lymphatic nodules (Fig. 8.18). Throughout the white pulp, reticular cells and associated reticular fibers form a three-dimensional stroma containing lymphocytes, macrophages, and dendritic cells similar to those seen in lymph nodes. The **nodules** may or may not have germinal centers, depending on their functional state. In the PALS, T cells are concentrated adjacent to the tunica media of the artery of the white pulp, whereas the peripheral region of the sheaths contains a more diverse mixture of T cells and B cells, macrophages, and dendritic cells.

MARGINAL ZONE. The marginal zone lies between the white pulp and the red pulp. The periphery of the white pulp is bounded by a circumferential reticulum, the reticular cells of which branch into the marginal zone. The marginal zone blends into the cords of the red pulp (Figs. 8.19 and 8.20).The reticular network of the marginal zone receives capillaries from the white pulp and some terminal capillaries of the red pulp. The capillaries empty into a marginal sinus (Fig. 8.21), which is a series of anastomosing channels, not equally apparent in all species. From here, the blood is drained slowly toward the venous sinuses or venules of the red pulp. Many macrophages and B cells are in the marginal zone. All elements of the blood, as well as antigens and particles, are brought into contact with the local macrophages and lymphocytes, facilitating phagocytosis and the initiation of an immune response.

BLOOD VESSELS. The circulation of blood through the spleen has important functional implications, particularly with respect to antigenic stimulation and the extraction of hemoglobin and iron from red blood cells (Fig. 8.22). Branches of the splenic artery enter the capsule and extend into the large trabeculae as **trabecular arteries**. As the artery leaves the trabecula, it is called the **artery of the white pulp**, and the externa becomes heavily infiltrated with lymphocytes (PALS). As the artery of the white pulp becomes finer, the PALS and marginal zone attenuate and eventually the circumferential reticulum disappears, allowing strands of white pulp to stretch across the attenuated marginal zone to the red pulp, forming bridging channels. Branches of the white pulp artery continue to feed capillary beds in the nodule and terminate in the marginal zone or enter the red pulp forming a **penicillus** (brushlike tuft). Some branches enter the red pulp as **pulp arterioles** and continue into distinctive structures called **sheathed capillaries** or **ellipsoids** (Figs. 8.21 and 8.22). Here, the vessel lumen narrows, and the endothelium is tall, with permeable junctions and a discontinuous basal lamina. The vessel is surrounded by a sheath of macrophages sequestered in a meshwork of reticular cells and fibers, called a pericapillary macrophage sheath.

The junction of the terminal capillaries with the venous system is controversial, and currently, three theories exist regarding the type of connection. The **first theory** is that the terminal capillaries expand, form an ampulla, and open directly into the splenic sinuses or venules. This is called the "closed" theory because the connection forms a continuous tubular structure.

The **second theory**, or "open" theory, suggests that the capillaries open into the spaces between the reticular cells of the red pulp and the blood then enters the venous sinuses through the slits in their walls.

The **last theory** proposes the existence of both an "open" and a "closed" circulation, depending on the physiologic state. When the spleen is distended, the spaces between the endothelial cells lining the sinuses or venules are pulled apart, and the blood leaks through the open meshwork from the terminal capillaries to the sinuses or venules. In a contracted spleen, the cells in

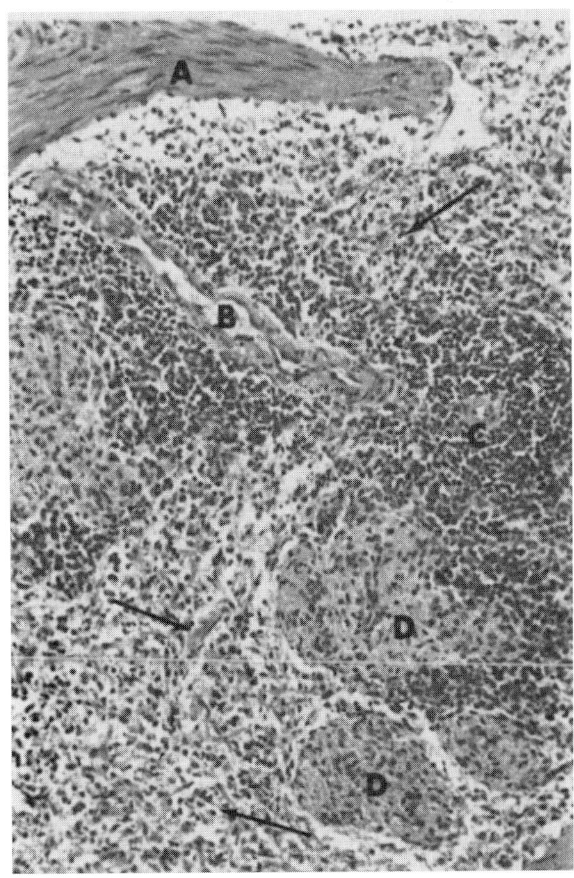

Figure 8.18. *Spleen (pig). Trabecula (A). An artery of the white pulp (B) is ensheathed with lymphocytes that constitute the periarterial lymphatic sheath; it continues into a nodule to become a nodular artery (C). Sheathed capillaries are surrounded by a wide macrophage sheath (D). Hematoxylin and eosin (×80).*

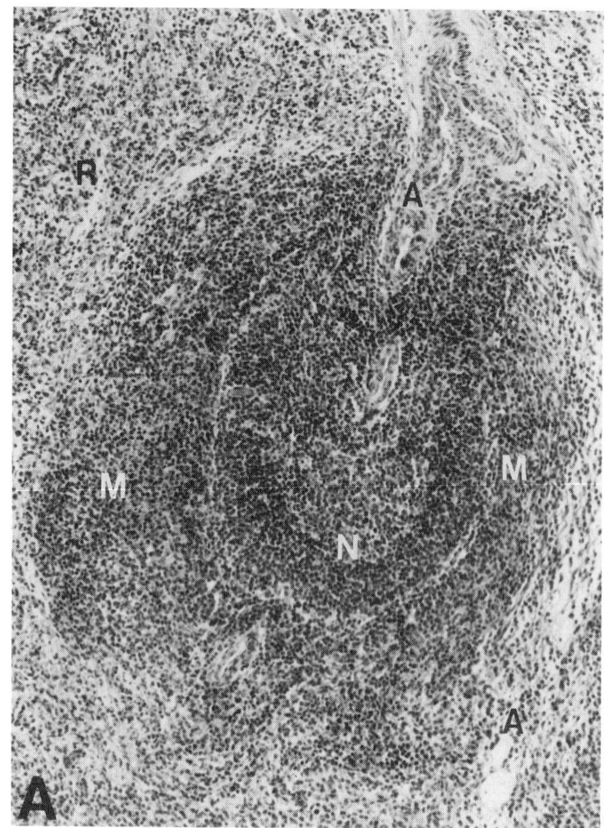

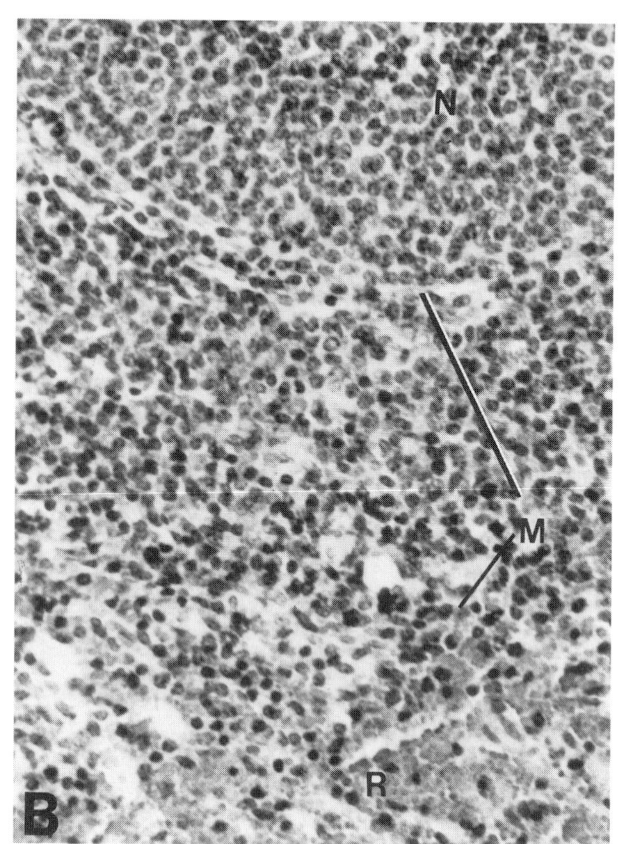

Figure 8.19. *Spleen (sheep).* ***A.,*** *Lymphatic nodule (N) with artery (A), surrounded by marginal zone (M) and red pulp (R). Hematoxylin and eosin (×90).* ***B.,*** *Marginal zone (M) between mantle of nodule (N) and red pulp with many red blood cells (R). Hematoxylin and eosin (×270).*

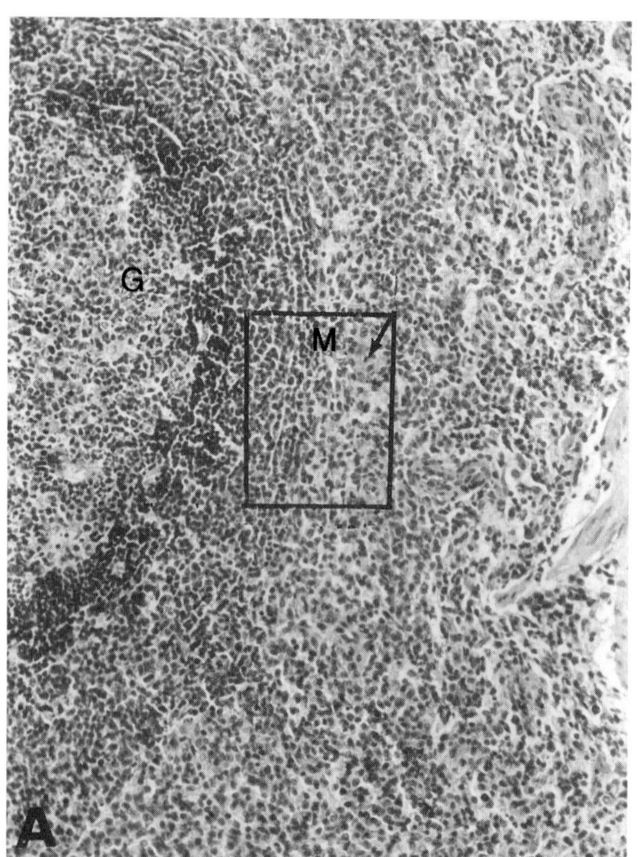

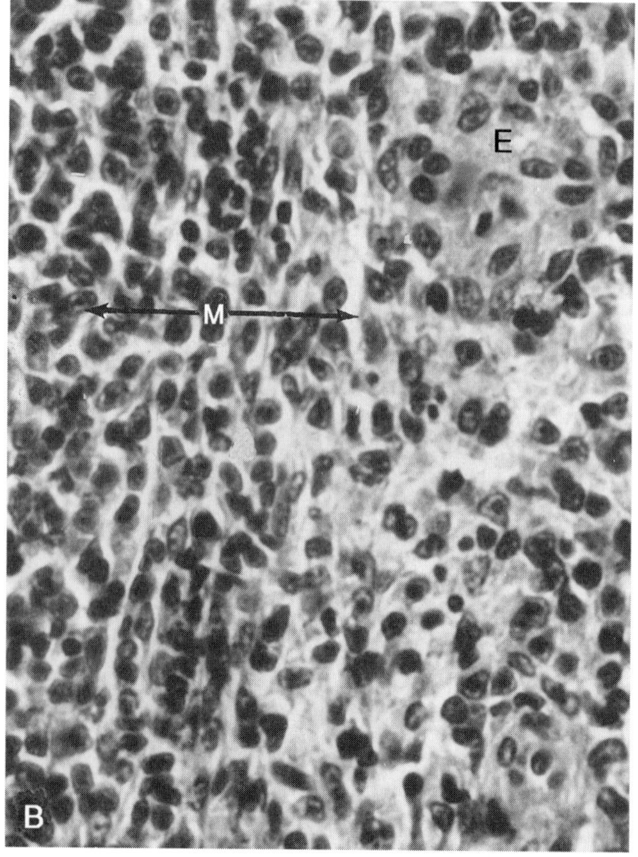

Figure 8.20. *Spleen (dog).* ***A.,*** *Lymphatic nodule with germinal center (G), marginal zone (M), and an ellipsoid at arrow. Hematoxylin and eosin (×80).* ***B.,*** *Enlargement of rectangle in* ***A;*** *marginal zone (M) and an ellipsoid (E). Hematoxylin and eosin (×870).*

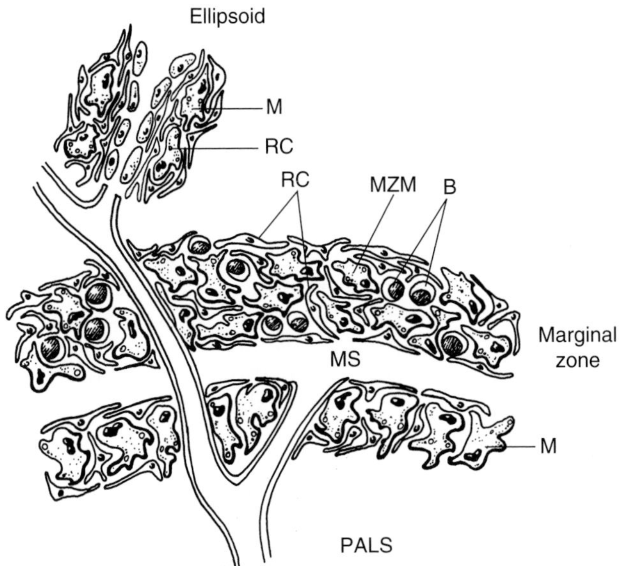

Figure 8.21. *Schematic drawing of the marginal zone and an ellipsoid. Blood vessels leave the periarterial lymphatic sheath (PALS) to pass through a rim of macrophages (M) and empty into the marginal sinus (MS), which represents the inner limit of the marginal zone. The marginal zone is composed of reticular cells (RC), B cells (B), and marginal zone macrophages (MZM). Some blood vessels pass through the marginal zone and terminate in the red pulp as sheathed capillaries or ellipsoids. These structures are surrounded by a meshwork of reticular cells and macrophages.*

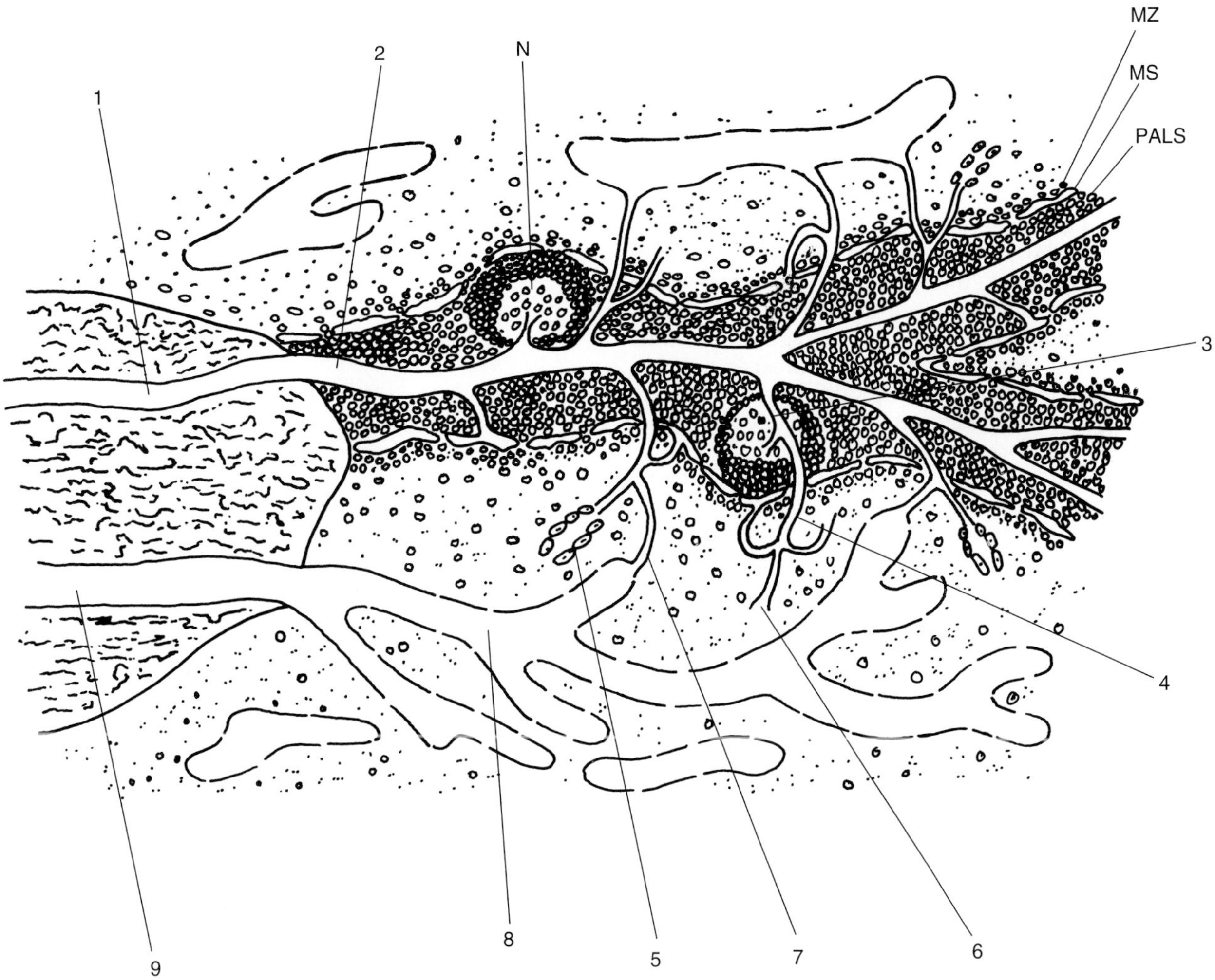

Figure 8.22. *Schematic drawing of the splenic parenchyma with emphasis on the vasculature. Trabecular artery (1); artery of the white pulp with lymphatic sheath (2); nodular artery (3); pulp arteriole (4); sheathed capillary (ellipsoid) (5); terminal capillaries emptying into reticular mesh (open circulation) (6); terminal capillaries emptying into venous sinus or venule (closed circulation) (7); venous sinus or venule (8); trabecular vein (9). Arrows indicate openings in the wall of sinuses or venules. MS = marginal sinus; MZ = marginal zone; N = nodule; PALS = periarterial lymphatic sheath.*

the venous sinuses or venules are pushed together to form a continuous uninterrupted connection with the terminal capillaries. Thus, the circulatory flow is closed. The last theory is widely accepted for sinusal spleens, but nonsinusal spleens seem to have an open circulatory flow. Whatever the exact nature of the capillary–venous junction, the blood in the small vessels eventually drains into the trabecular veins and leaves by the splenic vein.

LYMPH VESSELS AND NERVES. The spleen has no afferent lymph vessels. Efferent capsular and trabecular lymph vessels originate in the white pulp and are an exit route for some lymphocytes from the white pulp. The efferent lymph vessels drain into the splenic lymph nodes.

SPECIES DIFFERENCES. The spleens of horses, dogs, and pigs have abundant lymphatic nodules and periarterial lymphatic sheaths, but in the cat and ruminant spleens, lymphatic tissue is less abundant and occurs mainly as lymphatic nodules; the periarterial lymphatic sheaths are short.

The size and number of the sheathed capillaries also vary considerably among the domestic animals. In pigs and cats, the pericapillary macrophage sheaths are large and abundant and often particularly numerous near the white pulp. The pericapillary macrophage sheaths are smaller in horses and dogs and small and narrow in ruminants.

Immunologic function

The ability of the spleen to filter the blood is enhanced by the vast reticular fiber network filled with reticular cells and macrophages. Almost any section of red pulp contains numerous macrophages filled with engulfed red blood cell fragments and an iron pigment called hemosiderin. The marginal zone is the most important filter encountered by the blood. Bloodborne foreign particulate matter is first phagocytized by macrophages in the marginal zone. Foreign particulate matter, as well as erythrocytes and platelets, may also be phagocytized within the pericapillary macrophage sheath.

Bloodborne antigens are trapped within the marginal zone and transported by marginal zone macrophages to the outer PALS, an environment rich in recirculating lymphocytes and dendritic cells. The spleen lacks postcapillary venules and both B cells and T cells enter the white pulp through terminal capillaries that open into the marginal zone. The recirculating lymphocytes migrate rapidly into the outer edge of the PALS. B cells then move along the outer edge of the PALS to enter the primary nodules or the mantle of the secondary nodules, whereas T cells move toward the center of the PALS. Both lymphocyte populations return to the blood within the red pulp by migrating through bridging channels.

Antigen-containing macrophages and interdigitating cells of the PALS activate T cells, which is a prerequisite for the activation of antigen-specific naive B cells. Proliferating lymphoblasts appear first along the outer edge of the PALS, and then a germinal center reaction is initiated in lymphatic nodules. T-cell proliferation and differentiation continue in the inner PALS, whereas antigen-specific memory B cells appear in large numbers in the marginal zone. These nonproliferating, long-lived B cells do not recirculate. Many of the large resident population of B cells in the marginal zone are able to respond to antigens without the assistance of T cells, mounting rapid primary humoral immune responses.

Blood storage and hemopoiesis

Many erythrocytes are stored in the red pulp of the spleen of horses and, to a lesser extent, in the spleen of dogs. Many platelets are also stored in the splenic cords.

The major hemopoietic activity of the spleen in adult animals is lymphopoiesis. Erythropoiesis is a major function of the fetal spleen and persists in newborn horses and ruminants for several weeks postpartum.

HEMAL NODE

Hemal nodes are only described in ruminants. They are generally small, brown to dark red organs, but their size, number, and histologic characteristics vary within wide limits. They develop during fetal life from lymph node primordia that lose all their lymph vessels. Therefore, hemal nodes receive all their cells and antigens from the blood.

In young animals, the accumulation of lymphocytes is distinct, resembling the deep cortex of a lymph node, but few nodules are present (Fig. 8.23). In healthy adults, the

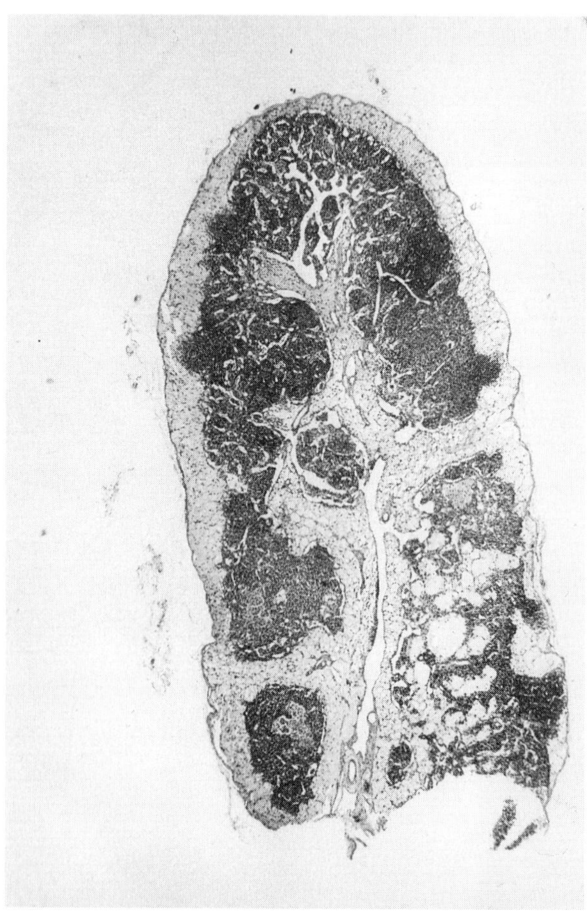

Figure 8.23. *Hemal node (young goat). Wide sinuses (S) under capsule (C) and around central veins (V). Many small venules (arrows) in lymphatic tissue. Vascular perfusion. Hematoxylin and eosin (×35).*

whole node is generally filled with red blood cells. As a result of antigenic stimulation, many nodules may form, and only a few red blood cells are present. There is no typical medulla. The sinuses are wide, with few macrophages and few lymphocytes. The diffuse lymphatic tissue contains relatively few lymphocytes but has many macrophages that digest erythrocytes and granulocytes.

The vascular supply is similar to that of lymph nodes, but all venules have a thin endothelium. Many lymphocytes and erythrocytes pass through this endothelium. The functional significance of the hemal node is not clear, although it is probable that they respond to bloodborne antigen.

REFERENCES

Bélisle C, Sainte-Marie G. Topography of the deep cortex of the lymph nodes of various mammalian species. Anat Rec 1981;201:553.

Blue J, Weiss L. Electron microscopy of the red pulp of dogs spleen including vascular arrangement, periarterial macrophage sheaths (ellipsoids), and the contractile, innervated reticular meshwork. Am J Anat 1981;161:198.

Griebel P, Hein W. Expanding the role of Peyer's patches in B-cell ontogeny. Immunol Today 1996;17:30.

Halleraker M, Landsverk T, Press C. Development and cell phenotypes of primary follicles in sheep fetal lymph nodes. Cell Tissue Res 1994;275:51.

Kraal G. Cells in the marginal zone of the spleen. Int Rev Cytol 1992;132:31.

Landsverk T, Halleraker M, Aleksandersen M, et al. The intestinal habitat for organized lymphoid tissues in ruminants; comparative aspects of structure, function and development. Vet Immunol Immunopathol 1991;28:1.

Liu Y-J, Banchereau J. The paths and molecular controls of peripheral B-cell development. Immunologist 1996;4:55.

Maybaum T, Reynolds J. B cells selected for apoptosis in the sheep ileal Peyer's patch have enhanced mutational diversity in the Ig V lambda light chain. J Immunol 1996;157:1474.

Morris B. The ontogeny and comportment of lymphoid cells in fetal and neonatal sheep. Immunol Rev 1986;91:219.

Nicander L, Nafstad P, Landsverk T, Engebretsen R. A study of modified lymphatics in the deep cortex of ruminant lymph nodes. J Anat 1991;178:203.

Nicander L, Halleraker M, Landsverk T. Ontogeny of reticular cells in the ileal Peyer's patch of sheep and goats. Am J Anat 1991;191:237.

Press CM, Halleraker M, Landsverk T. Ontogeny of leukocyte populations in the ileal Peyer's patch of sheep. Dev Comp Immunol 1992;16:229.

Pulendran B, van Driel R, Nossal G. Immunological tolerance in germinal centres. Immunol Today 1997;18:27.

Rajewsky K. Clonal selection and learning in the antibody system. Nature 1996;381:751.

Reynaud C, Weill J. Postrearrangement diversification processes in gut-associated lymphoid tissues. Curr Top Microbiol Immunol 1996;212:7.

Roitt I, Brostoff J, Male D. Immunology. 4th ed. London: Mosby, 1996.

Tizard IR. Veterinary immunology. An introduction. 5th ed. Philadelphia: WB Saunders, 1996.

Van Rooijen N, Claassen E, Kraal G, et al. Cytological basis of immune functions of the spleen. Immunocytochemical characterization of lymphoid and non-lymphoid cells involved in the 'in situ' immune response. Prog Histochem Cytochem 1989;19:1.

Westermann J, Pabst R. How organ-specific is the migration of 'naive' and 'memory' T cells? Immunol Today 1996;17:278.

9

Respiratory System

DONALD R. ADAMS
H. DIETER DELLMANN

The primary function of the respiratory system is to provide the exchange of respiratory gases (oxygen and carbon dioxide) between the organism and the environment. The conducting airways provide a series of air passages for moving air to and from the gas exchange area in the lungs. The conducting airways also serve a protective function by conditioning incoming (inspired) air. This conditioning includes heating the air to body temperature, saturating it to 100% relative humidity, and filtering out noxious gases and particulates. The conducting airways also conserve body heat and water by extracting them from the air during expiration. The mucociliary blanket, which covers the mucosal surface of conducting airways, serves to trap inhaled particles and conveys them and cellular debris out of the system. Other structures, such as the nasolacrimal duct, vomeronasal organ, paranasal recesses and sinuses, auditory tube, and equine guttural pouch, are associated with the conducting airways.

The distal, smallest conducting airways connect to the gas exchange area, which includes the respiratory bronchioles, alveolar ducts, and alveolar sacs. Gas exchange occurs in alveoli, where only a thin blood–air barrier is present between pulmonary capillary blood and respired air. An extensive pulmonary capillary bed receives the entire output of the right ventricle of the heart.

NASAL CAVITY, VOMERONASAL ORGAN, AND PARANASAL SINUSES

Nasal Cavity

CUTANEOUS REGION

The skin of the nasal apex is continuous through a tissue gradient with the mucous membrane of the nasal cavity proper. Rostrally, the **cutaneous region** (nasal vestibule) is lined by a relatively thick keratinized stratified squamous epithelium. At **midvestibule**, the epithelium is thinner and nonkeratinized (Fig. 9.1). Superficial cells have microridges on their free surface. The caudal portion of the cutaneous region and the rostral third of the nasal cavity proper are a **transitional zone** lined by an epithelium that varies from stratified cuboidal to nonciliated pseudostratified columnar. Surface epithelial cells in the transitional zone contain multilobated nuclei, possess microvilli on their free surface, and are frequently spherical (Fig. 9.2).

The propria-submucosa of the cutaneous region interdigitates via papillae with the epithelium. The papillae contain small vessels and numerous free cells, including mast cells, plasma cells, lymphocytes, macrophages, and granulocytes. Lymphocytes are also frequently observed

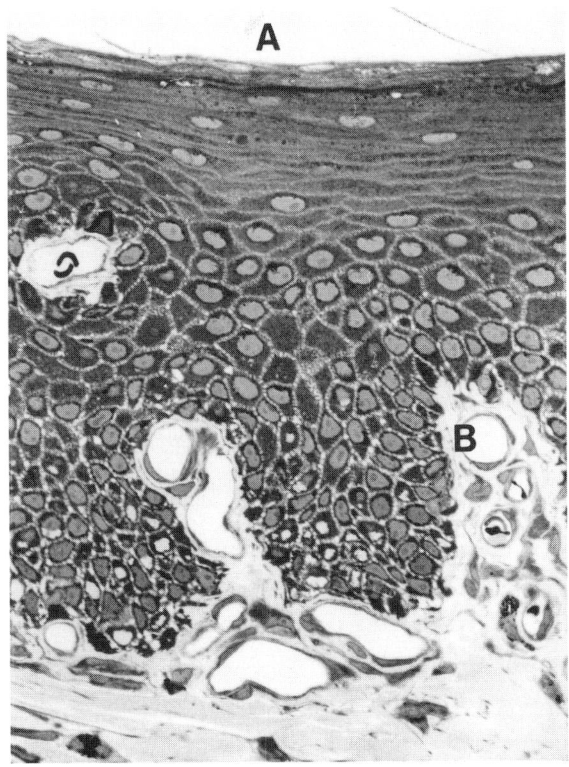

Figure 9.1. *Stratified squamous epithelium in the cutaneous region of the canine nasal cavity. Airway lumen (A); dermal papilla (B). 1 μm. Azure II (×385). (With permission from Adams DR, Hotchkiss DK. The canine nasal mucosa. Zentralbl Veterinarmed C Anat Histol Embryol 1983;12:111.)*

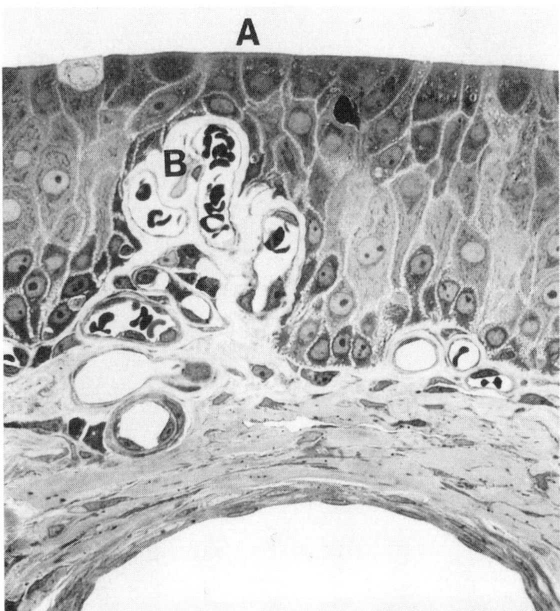

Figure 9.2. *Stratified cuboidal epithelium in the transitional zone of the canine nasal cavity. Airway lumen (A); connective-tissue papillae (B). 1 μm. Azure II (×385). (With permission from Adams DR, Hotchkiss DK. The canine nasal mucosa. Zentralbl Veterinarmed C Anat Histol Embryol 1983;12:113.)*

in the basal portion of the epithelium. Bundles of collagen fibers, larger blood vessels, and serous glands are located deep in the propria-submucosa.

In horses, a nasal diverticulum lined with skin opens into the cutaneous region of the nasal vestibule; this region is lined by an integument containing vibrissae, sebaceous glands, and sweat glands. The papillary layer of the vestibular dermis in dogs has particularly numerous papillae and capillary loops.

RESPIRATORY REGION

Epithelium lining the caudal two-thirds of the nasal cavity proper, with the exception of the olfactory region, is classified as **respiratory epithelium**, i.e., ciliated pseudostratified columnar; that lining the middle nasal meatus is thinner and contains fewer ciliated and goblet cells. The ciliated pseudostratified epithelium of the nasal cavity contains several cell types, including ciliated, secretory, brush, and basal cells (Figs. 9.3, 9.4, and 9.5).

Individual **ciliated cells** are columnar and have 200 to 300 motile cilia and numerous microvilli projecting into the nasal lumen. The supranuclear portion of the cell contains basal bodies, a Golgi complex, and numerous mitochondria; small strands of rough endoplasmic reticulum (rER) are scattered throughout the cell. Defects in the fine structure of cilia may result in ineffective ciliary

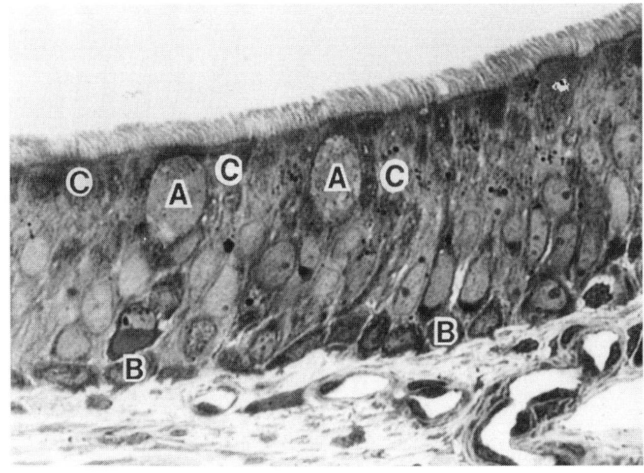

Figure 9.3. *Ciliated pseudostratified columnar epithelium with goblet cells lining the respiratory region of the nasal cavity. Goblet cells (A); basal cells (B); ciliated cells (C). 1 μm. Azure II (×590).*

beat or immotility. Immotile cilia syndrome is a condition associated with congenital ciliary abnormality, resulting in respiratory tract infections.

Secretory cells of the respiratory epithelium extend from the basal lamina to the epithelial surface. Their luminal surface bears microvilli. The morphologic and histochemical appearance of these cells is both species and regionally variable. Their description as mucous or serous is based on their glycoprotein content. Granules of mucous epithelial cells are relatively electron-lucent and contain sialated or sulfated acid glycoproteins. The

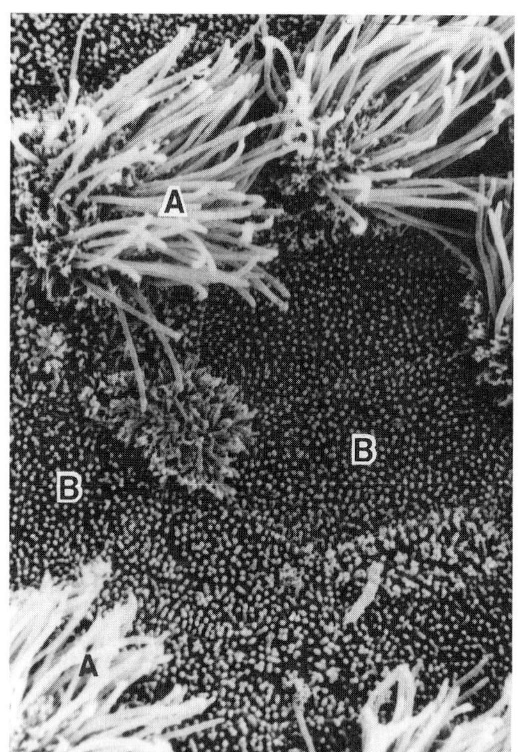

Figure 9.4. *Scanning electron micrograph of respiratory epithelium (ciliated pseudostratified columnar epithelium). Ciliated cells with cilia and microvilli (A); nonciliated cells with apical microvilli (B) (×3500).*

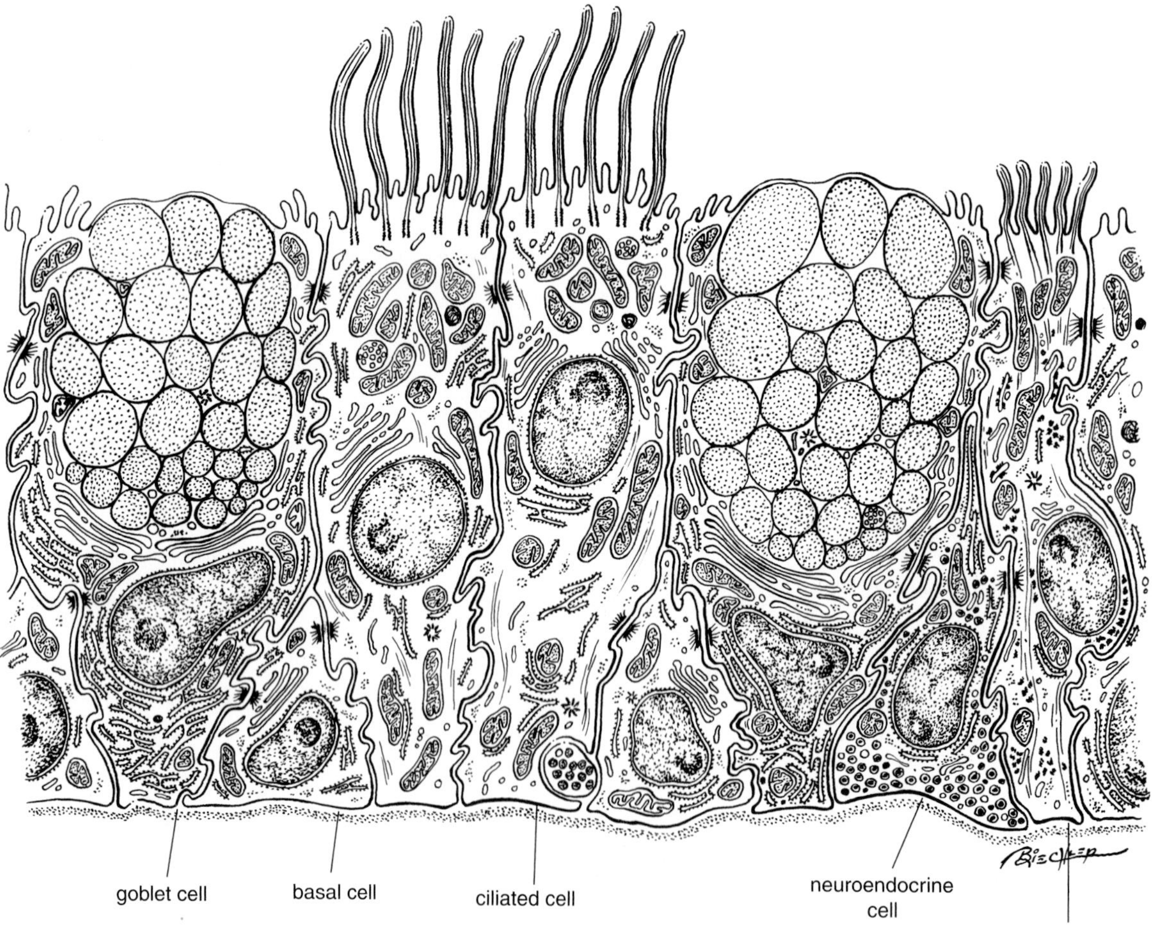

Figure 9.5. *Drawing of the fine structural characteristics of respiratory epithelial cells.*

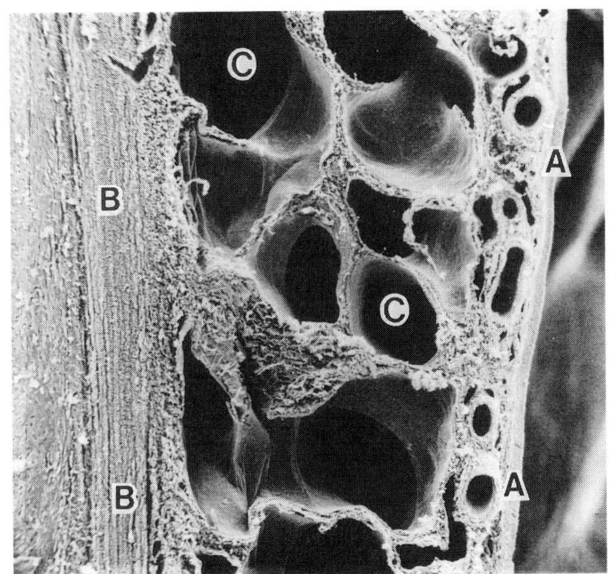

Figure 9.6. *Scanning electron micrograph of a section of the respiratory mucosa of the bovine nasal cavity. Epithelium (A); perichondrium (B); lumina of blood vessels (C) in the cavernous stratum (×40).*

supranuclear portion of mucous epithelial cells varies in appearance with the secretory phase from tall and slender with few granules to wide and globular with numerous mucous granules. Globular cells, known as **goblet cells**, have nuclei pressed to the base of the cell by the supranuclear mass of large mucous granules. Organelles usually present in the perinuclear region of the goblet cell include a Golgi complex, rER, and mitochondria. Goblet cells of most species secrete primarily a sulfated glycoprotein as a major component of mucus.

Granules of serous epithelial cells have electron-dense cores, contain neutral glycoproteins, and are smaller than those of mucous cells.

Brush cells have long, thick microvilli and a cytoplasm containing mitochondria and many filaments. These cells may be sensory receptors associated with endings of the trigeminal nerve. Another nonciliated cell type in the nasal mucosa has surface microvilli and contains much smooth endoplasmic reticulum (sER) and little secretory material; this unnamed cell type is believed to function in the metabolism of xenobiotic compounds (see below).

Basal cells are small polyhedral cells located along the basal lamina. The cytoplasm of basal cells contains numerous bundles of tonofilaments and free ribosomes. By division and differentiation, these cells may replace other epithelial cell types lost through attrition.

The respiratory mucosa of the nasal cavity is more vascular than the mucosae of the cutaneous, transitional, or olfactory regions. The highly vascular propria submucosa is called the **cavernous stratum** (Fig. 9.6), in which arteries and large thin-walled veins are oriented rostrocaudally. The veins interconnect profusely and are called **capacitance vessels** because they determine the degree of mucosal congestion and, inversely, nasal patency. Constriction of nasal blood vessels is effected by α-adrenergic stimulation via the sympathetic nervous system. Periods of vascular engorgement varying from 30 minutes to 4 hours followed by periods of decongestion normally occur in the cavernous stratum of mammals; during this nasal cycle, the vascular activity in one side of the nose alternates with that in the other side.

Serous or mixed nasal glands are present between the numerous veins of this stratum (Fig. 9.7). Acini of nasal glands also secrete secretory immunoglobulin A (IgA), lysozyme, and odorant-binding protein.

Nerves in the nasal mucosa include sensory fibers of the terminal, olfactory, vomeronasal, and maxillary division of the trigeminal nerve and efferent fibers of the autonomic nervous system. Intraepithelial nerve endings are frequently observed adjacent to juxtaluminal junctional complexes of adjacent cells.

Lymphatic nodules are commonly present in the caudal part of the nasal cavity, adjacent to the opening between nasal cavity and nasopharyngeal meatus.

Metabolically active exogenous compounds (xenobiotics) that reach nasal tissues via air or blood pathways may remain firmly bound to tissue elements unless degraded. Cytochrome P-450-dependent monooxygenase enzymes in surface epithelium and in acinar cells of the lateral nasal gland actively metabolize endogenous compounds (e.g., progesterone and testosterone) and exogenous compounds. These enzymes convert lipid-solu-

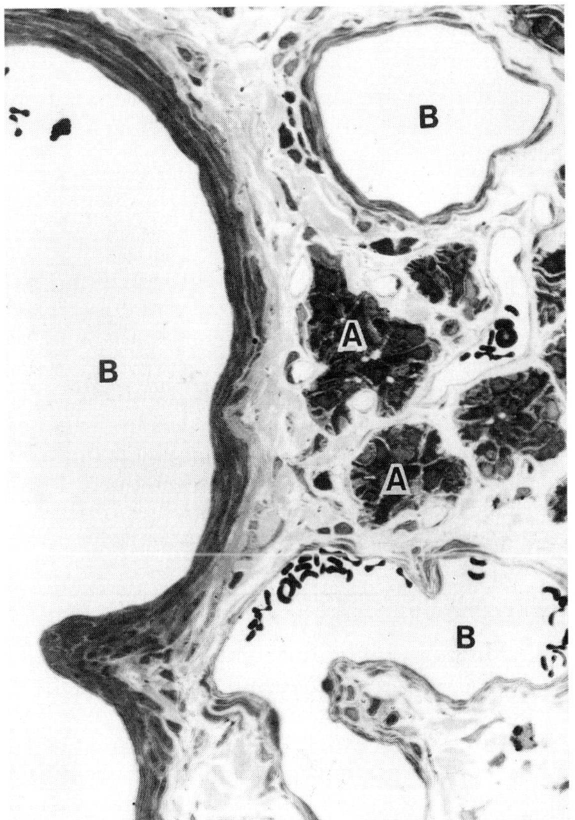

Figure 9.7. *Nasal gland acini (A) occupy the connective tissue between the veins of the cavernous stratum (B) of the respiratory mucosa. 1 μm. Azure II (×425)*

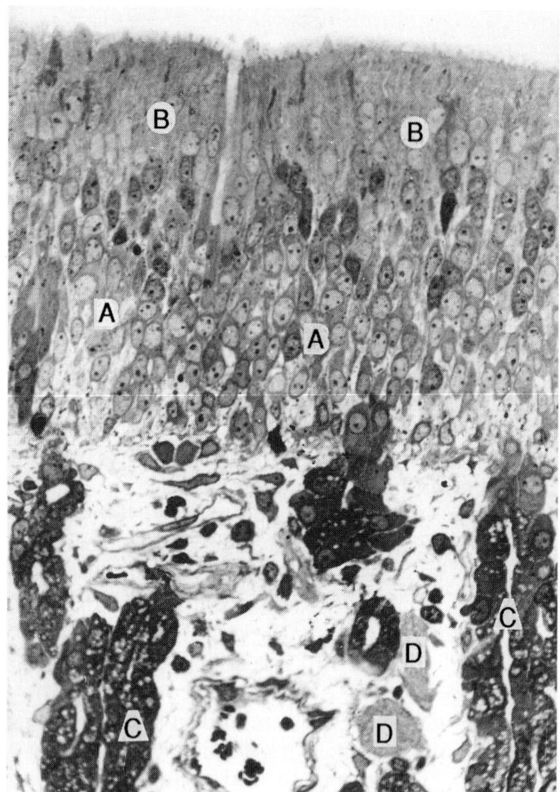

Figure 9.8. *Mucosa of the canine olfactory region. Nuclei of neurosensory cells (A); nuclei of sustentacular cells (B); olfactory glands (C); olfactory nerves (D). 1 μm. Azure II (×410).*

ble exogenous compounds to water-soluble metabolites, some of which are highly toxic (e.g., formaldehyde and acetaldehyde).

OLFACTORY REGION

The olfactory region comprises the dorsocaudal portion of the nasal cavity, including some of the surfaces of the ethmoid conchae, dorsal nasal meatus, and nasal septum. Olfactory mucosa may be discerned from adjacent respiratory mucosa because it has a thicker epithelium, numerous tubular glands, and many bundles of nonmyelinated nerve fibers in the lamina propria.

The olfactory mucosa is lined by a ciliated pseudostratified columnar epithelium consisting of three primary cell types: neurosensory, sustentacular, and basal (Fig. 9.8).

Neurosensory olfactory cells are bipolar neurons with perikarya in a wide basal zone of the epithelium, dendrites extending to the lumen, and axons reaching the olfactory bulb of the brain. A club-shaped apex, the **dendritic bulb**, protrudes from each dendrite into the lumen (Fig. 9.9), from which 10 to 30 cilia emanate. Each cilium is 50 to 80 μm long and consists of a wide, short basal portion and a long, thin, tapering distal portion. The number of microtubules decreases from the typical nine peripheral doublets (fused pairs of microtubules) plus two single central microtubules in the basal portion to singlets of one to four microtubules distally. The perikaryon has typical neuronal structural characteristics. Individual axons converge as they pass into the lamina propria, thereby forming bundles of nonmyelinated nerve fibers. Neurosensory cells are continuously replaced during the life of the animal by cells derived from basal cells.

Sustentacular cells are columnar cells with a narrow base and a wide apical portion. Their lightly staining nuclei form the most superficial nuclear layer in the epithelium. Microvilli, often branched, cover the luminal surface of sustentacular cells. Juxtaluminal junctional complexes occur between sustentacular cells and the adjacent dendrites of neurosensory cells. Pigment granules are present in the infranuclear cytoplasm. Sustentacular cells are also replaced by basal cells.

Basal cells of the olfactory mucosa are similar in structure to those of the nonolfactory epithelium.

Mixed **olfactory glands**, the cells of which contain pigment granules, are located in the propria submucosa. The intraepithelial portion of their ducts is lined by squamous cells.

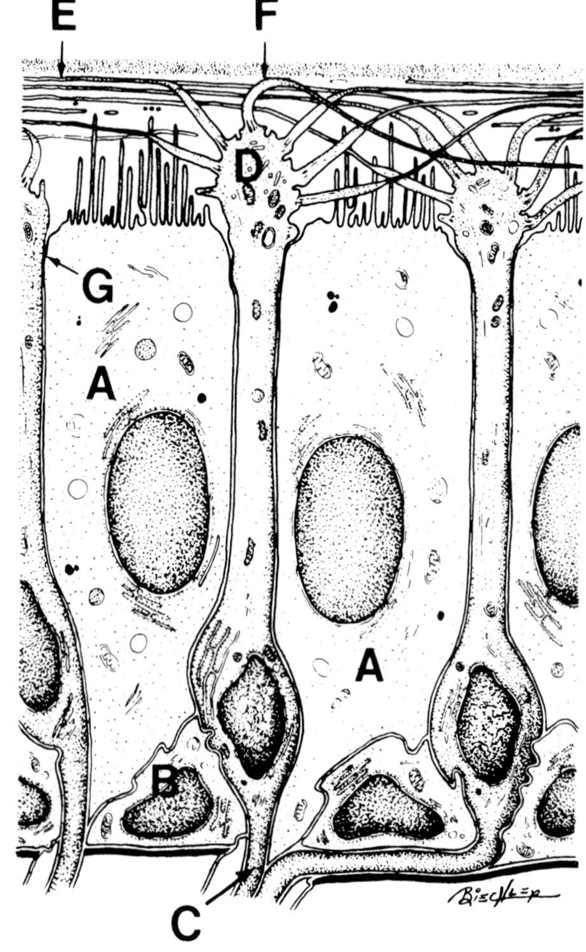

Figure 9.9. *Schematic drawing of the olfactory epithelium. Sustentacular cell (A); basal cell (B); axon of the receptor cell (C); dendritic bulb (D); thin distal portion of cilium (E); thick proximal portion of cilium (F); junctional complex between receptor and sustentacular cells (G).*

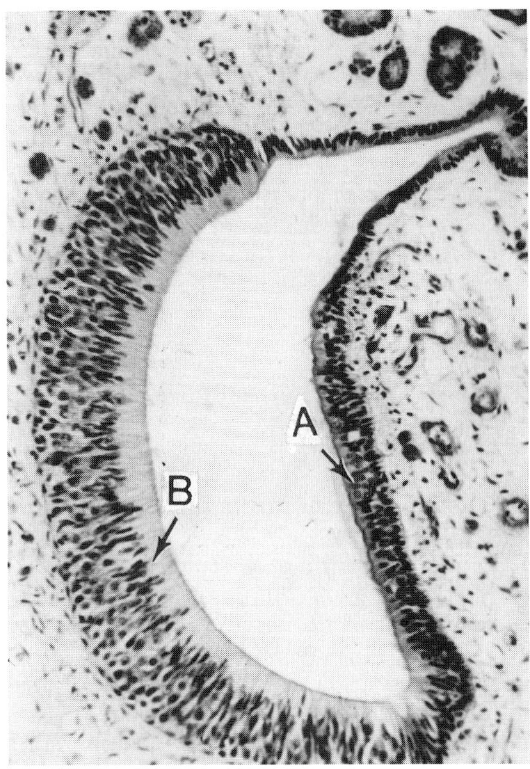

Figure 9.10. *Canine vomeronasal duct. The lateral epithelium (A) includes ciliated and nonciliated cells, whereas the medial epithelium (B) contains neurosensory and sustentacular epithelial cells (×158). (Courtesy of A.W. Stinson.)*

Vomeronasal Organ

Located in the mucosa of the ventral portion of the nasal septum, the tubular, blind-ending bilateral vomeronasal organ consists of an internal epithelial duct (vomeronasal duct), a middle propria submucosa, and an external cartilaginous support. Rostrally, the organs open into incisive ducts, except in horses, in which they are blind-ending ventrally.

The vomeronasal duct is crescent-shaped in transverse section with a lateral convex and a medial concave mucosal wall. The epithelium passes through a transition from a stratified cuboidal lining rostrally near the incisive duct to a ciliated pseudostratified columnar epithelium over much of the caudal portion of the vomeronasal duct. The medial pseudostratified columnar epithelium has neurosensory, sustentacular, and basal cells (Fig. 9.10). The dendritic portions of vomeronasal neurosensory cells lack dendritic bulbs and, with the exception of those in dogs, have microvilli instead of cilia on their apical surfaces. Neurosensory cells are periodically replaced in the adult mammal. The lateral pseudostratified columnar epithelium has ciliated and nonciliated columnar, goblet, and basal cells.

Vomeronasal glands, located in the highly vascular propria submucosa, secrete into the vomeronasal duct most commonly through the commissures between lateral and medial mucosal walls. Secretory granules of the acinar cells contain neutral glycoproteins. The hyaline **vomeronasal cartilage** is J-shaped, enclosing all but the dorsolateral portion of the organ.

The vomeronasal organ functions in the chemoreception of liquidborne compounds of low volatility. Sensing of these compounds is believed to function in sexual behavior of both the female and the male, in maternal behavior, and in the interaction of the fetus with its amniotic environment. In several mammals, vomeronasal detection of the odor of a female results in an elevation of plasma testosterone in the male. The vomeronasal organ is associated with the lip-curl type of facial grimace (Flehmen) action used by some male mammals to sample substances in the urine of the female; odorant particles may reach the incisive duct with inhaled air, through contact with the tongue, or during passage through the mouth with food or water. These substances, dissolved in fluid in the incisive duct, are sucked into the vomeronasal duct by constriction of blood vessels within the propria submucosa of the vomeronasal organ. Upon dilatation of these vessels, the dissolved substances are expelled from the vomeronasal lumen.

Paranasal Sinuses

The mucosae of the paranasal sinuses are thinner than those of the respiratory region of the nasal cavity with which they are continuous. Glands and blood vessels in the propria submucosa are scant. The epithelium is ciliated pseudostratified columnar, containing a few goblet cells. The ciliary beat carries mucus toward openings connecting the sinuses with the nasal cavity.

The **lateral nasal gland** (Fig. 9.11) is a relatively large compound gland that secretes neutral glycoproteins via a long duct into the nasal vestibule. The lateral nasal gland is present in the maxillary recess of carnivores, in the maxillary sinus of pigs, and at the nasomaxillary aperture in horses and small ruminants; in addition, separate maxillary recess glands are present in carnivores.

NASOPHARYNX

The nasopharynx is that portion of the pharynx that is located dorsal to the soft palate, extending from the nasal cavity to the laryngopharynx. The lining of the nasopharynx consists mostly of respiratory epithelium but is stratified squamous epithelium over the caudodorsal portion of the soft palate that makes contact either with the dorsal wall of the nasopharynx during deglutition or with the epiglottis. The propria submucosa is loose connective tissue containing mixed glands. Lymphatic nodules are prominent in the dorsal portion of the nasopharynx, where they aggregate as the pharyngeal tonsil.

LARYNX

The larynx opens rostrally into the laryngopharynx and is continuous caudally with the trachea (Fig. 9.12). It is lined by mucosa and supported by cartilage.

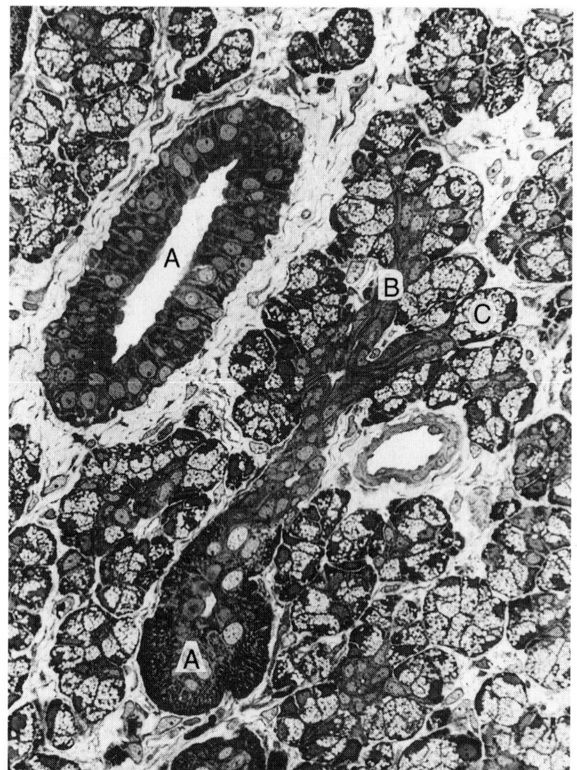

Figure 9.11. *Two striated ducts (A), an intercalated duct (B), and acinar cells (C) in the canine lateral nasal gland. 1 μm. Azure II (×425).*

The epithelium lining the epiglottis, laryngeal vestibule, and vocal folds is nonkeratinized stratified squamous; the laryngeal epithelium caudal to the vocal fold gradually changes into respiratory epithelium (Fig. 9.3). Respiratory epithelium also lines the equine laryngeal ventricle. The epithelium on the laryngeal surface of the epiglottis, aryepiglottic folds, and arytenoids may contain taste buds in all species except horses. Sensory receptors of the cranial laryngeal nerve in the epithelium respond to the presence of fluids, such as water, milk, gastric fluid, and saliva; stimulation of these receptors results in reflex apnea.

The propria-submucosa beneath the stratified squamous epithelium is a dense, irregular connective tissue; the propria-submucosa beneath the respiratory epithelium is a loose connective tissue. It is rich in elastic fibers, leukocytes, plasma cells, and mast cells. Diffuse lymphatic tissue or solitary lymphatic nodules are frequently observed. In pigs and small ruminants, a paraepiglottic tonsil is present on either side of the base of the epiglottis; this tonsil occurs occasionally in cats. Mixed glands (Fig. 9.13) occur in the propria-submucosa but are absent in the vestibular and vocal folds. Numerous elastic fibers are present in the vocal ligament and, to a lesser extent, in the vestibular ligament.

The laryngeal cartilages are connected to each other, to the trachea, and to the hyoid apparatus by ligaments. Extrinsic skeletal muscles move the larynx during swallowing; intrinsic skeletal muscles move individual laryngeal cartilages during respiration and phonation. Most of the laryngeal cartilages are of the hyaline type. The epiglottis, the cuneiform and corniculate cartilages or processes, and the vocal process of the arytenoid cartilage contain elastic cartilage. The epiglottis of carnivores often consists of a peripheral cartilaginous wall enclosing adipose tissue, strands of elastic fibers, and small areas of elastic cartilage. A loose connective tissue forms the tunica adventitia surrounding the laryngeal cartilages and muscles.

TRACHEA AND EXTRAPULMONARY BRONCHI

The trachea provides the air passageway between the larynx and the bronchi. It is a semiflexible and semicollapsible tube that extends from the larynx into the thoracic cavity.

The lining epithelium of the tracheobronchial tree is respiratory epithelium (Fig. 9.14), containing ciliated cells, brush cells, secretory cells, Clara cells, and neuroendocrine cells. Ciliated cells, brush cells, and secretory cells of the trachea are similar to those of the upper respiratory system (see "Respiratory region" earlier in this chapter). **Goblet cells** are the predominant secretory cell type in domestic mammals. **Clara cells** (also called bronchiolar exocrine cells) are relatively scarce or even absent in the larger airways; they are described on page 156. **Neuroendocrine cells** are APUD cells, i.e., they are characterized by **a**mine **p**recursor **u**ptake and **d**ecarboxylation; they are typically pyramid-shaped with their bases on the basal lamina; they are identified with histochemical methods and, at the fine-structural level, contain dense-cored, argyrophilic granules, abundant ER, Golgi complex, ribosomes, and many filaments. These cells are most abundant in young animals and are sometimes associated with nerve endings.

A variety of **migratory cells** are also observed in the ep-

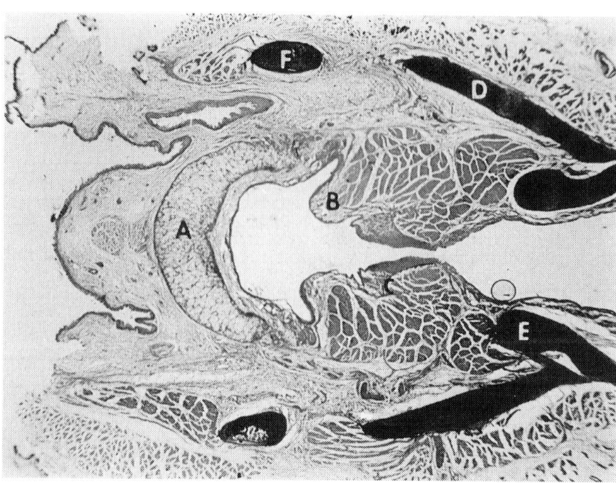

Figure 9.12. *Horizontal section through a feline larynx. Epiglottis cartilage (A); ventricular ligament (B); vocal ligament (C); thyroid cartilage (D); cricoid cartilage (E); stylohyoid bone (F). Hematoxylin and eosin (×8.3). (From Dellmann HD. Veterinary histology: an outline text–atlas. Philadelphia: Lea & Febiger, 1971.)*

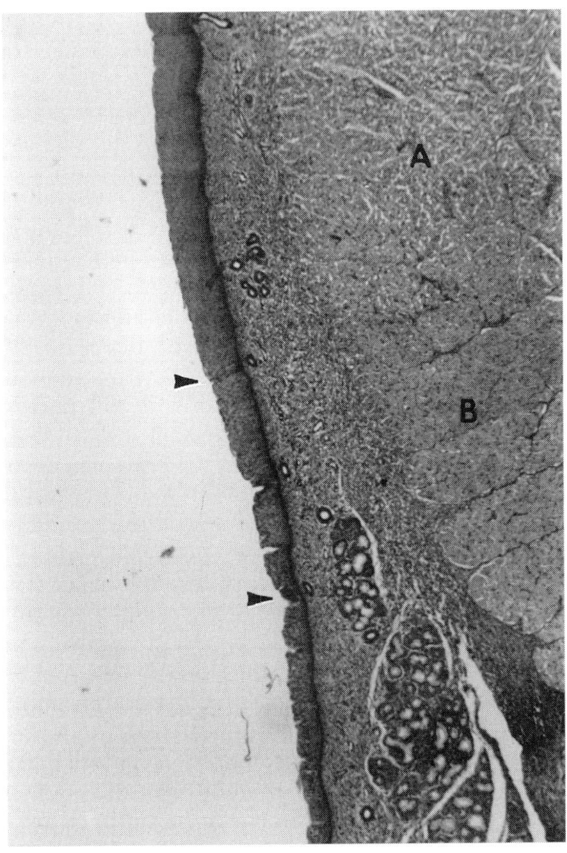

Figure 9.13. *Horizontal section through the caudal portion of a feline vocal fold. Vocal ligament (A); vocal muscle (B). Note the thick stratified squamous epithelium on the vocal fold and its gradual decrease in height toward the trachea. After a short transitional zone (between arrows), the epithelium becomes respiratory in nature. Hematoxylin and eosin (×39).*

ithelium. These include lymphocytes, globule leukocytes, and mast cells. **Globule leukocytes** are cells of unknown function that contain relatively large acidophilic, metachromatic granules.

The propria submucosa consists of loose connective tissue and a subepithelial layer of longitudinally oriented elastic fibers; cells include fibrocytes, lymphocytes, plasma cells, globule leukocytes, and mast cells. The propria submucosa contains tubuloacinar seromucous glands that open into the lumen via ducts, which are lined with ciliated cells, mucus-secreting cells, and various intermediate cells. The tubular portions of the tracheal glands are lined by mucus-secreting cells, and their acinar portions are lined primarily by serous secretory cells. The mucus-secreting cells generally secrete sulfated acid glycoproteins. Serous cells are the major secretory cells of the glands in most species; their secretory product is a neutral glycoprotein that is sometimes sulfated. Tracheal glands provide most of the secretory material that lines the ciliary surface in the trachea. These glands are abundant in the proximal portions of the trachea of virtually all domestic mammalian species.

The most distinctive feature of the trachea is hyaline cartilage (Fig. 9.14), which in most species occurs as roughly C- or U-shaped separate pieces. In some individuals, however, they are fused in places so they form a continuum. The dorsal free ends of the cartilages are bridged by the trachealis muscle, a band of smooth muscle. In most species, the muscle attaches to the perichondrium on the internal side of the cartilage. In carnivores, this attachment is on the external surface of the cartilage. Nerves and large blood vessels are generally associated with the smooth muscle band. The external perichondrium is surrounded by the loose connective tissue of the adventitia.

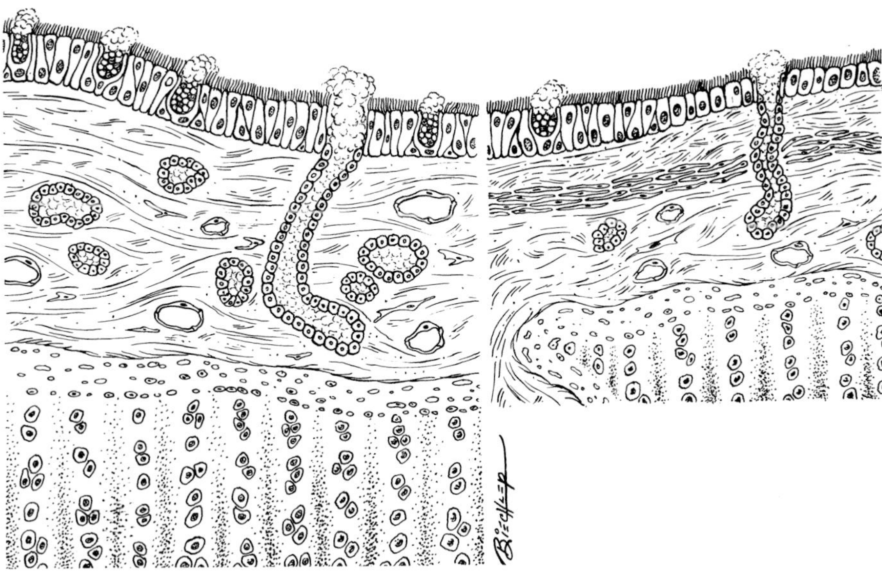

Figure 9.14. *Schematic drawing of cross sections through parts of the wall of the trachea and a bronchus. Note the differences in the height of the epithelium, the thickness of the propria-submucosa, the glandular density, and the presence of smooth muscle.*

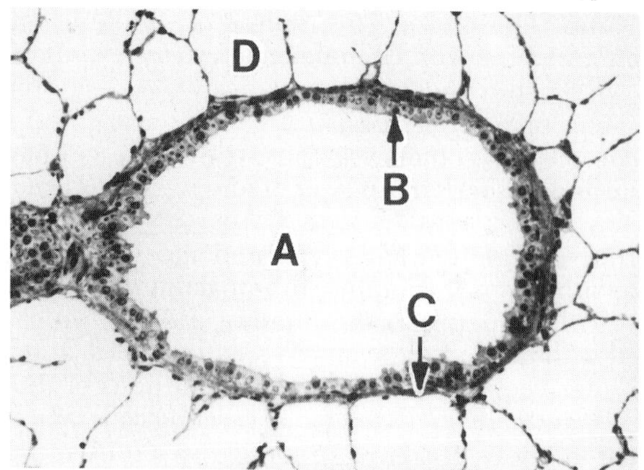

Figure 9.15. *Cross section of a bronchiole. The airway lumen (A) is lined by simple cuboidal epithelium (B) followed by a thin layer of smooth muscle (C). Alveoli (D) surround the bronchiole. Toluidine blue (×135).*

Within the thoracic cavity, the trachea terminates by bifurcating into two primary bronchi. Distal to the bifurcation, the primary bronchi provide branches that enter the lungs. The structural characteristics of primary bronchi are the same as those of the trachea, except that cartilage is here in the form of irregular plates.

LUNG

Most of the thoracic cavity is occupied by right and left lungs. The lung of mammals may be divided into intrapulmonary conducting airways, gas exchange area (parenchyma), and pleura. The intrapulmonary conducting airways (bronchi and bronchioles) compose approximately 6% of the lung. The gas exchange area, consisting of respiratory bronchioles and alveolar ducts (also referred to as transition zone), alveolar sacs, and alveoli, comprises approximately 85% of the lung. The lung is encapsulated by a layer of connective tissue and mesothelial cells termed the **visceral pleura**. Along with the pleura, the intrapulmonary nervous and vascular tissue (pulmonary arteries, pulmonary veins, and bronchial arteries) comprise the remaining 9 to 10% of the lung.

Intrapulmonary Conducting Airways

BRONCHI

The bronchial tree is formed by a primary bronchus and the various orders of airways that it supplies. The largest segments of the intrapulmonary conducting airways are called **lobar bronchi**, each of which enters a lobe of the lung at its hilum. Each of the lobar bronchi divides into two smaller branches, each of which divides again, and this process continues until the gas exchange area is reached. Each of the first two or three generations of branching from a lobar bronchus supplies portions of the lung lobe called **bronchopulmonary segments**. Each succeeding generation of branching is made of a greater number of airways and has a larger total cross-sectional area than the generation before it.

The histologic appearance of a bronchus is generally similar to that of the trachea, except that the various layers are thinner (Fig. 9.14). Bronchi are lined by a respiratory epithelium composed primarily of ciliated cells, secretory cells, and basal cells. Proximodistally, the composition of the epithelium changes; mucous cells and basal cells decrease and Clara cells increase in number. At the same time, the epithelial height and the thickness of the propria submucosa progressively decrease.

The propria-submucosa is loose connective tissue containing mixed submucosal glands in all species except goats; bronchial glands are less abundant in distal bronchi. The hyaline cartilage of the proximal bronchi is in the form of irregular plates, and the smooth muscle is interspersed either between or on the luminal side of the plates. The muscle cells are generally arranged in a circular fashion perpendicularly to the long axis of the airway. The amount of cartilage decreases proximodistally, whereas smooth muscle becomes relatively more abundant. The adventitial connective tissue is primarily loose, with many collagen fibers and variable numbers of elastic fibers. Many of the fibers are oriented longitudinally, whereas others are oriented perpendicularly to the long axis of the airway. Adventitial and submucosal nerve plexus and intraepithelial nerve endings are present.

BRONCHIOLES

Bronchioles arise from bronchi, branch into several generations, and terminate as terminal bronchioles. Several generations of terminal bronchioles are present in horses, cows, and sheep, whereas generally only one or two generations are present in carnivores.

Bronchioles have roughly circular cross-sectional profiles and are lined with simple columnar or cuboidal epithelium (Fig. 9.15) composed of ciliated cells and **bronchiolar exocrine cells** (Clara cells). These cells have characteristics of both secretory cells and cells capable of metabolizing xenobiotic compounds. The secretory granules contain either neutral glycoprotein or low-molecular-weight protein. Smooth endoplasmic reticulum is abundant in cells from horses and sheep and is minimally present in those from carnivores, cows, and pigs. Glycogen is the predominant feature of bronchiolar exocrine cells in carnivores and cows and is rarely observed in most other species. In carnivores, the epithelium of terminal bronchioles consists primarily of bronchiolar exocrine cells.

The propria-submucosa is sparse loose connective tissue; glands and cartilage are absent. The smooth muscle is arranged in separate circular and oblique fascicles. Numerous nerve fibers occur in the area immediately below the epithelium and interspersed between muscle fascicles.

The adventitia is loose connective tissue, including elastic fibers oriented circularly or obliquely.

Gas Exchange Area

The gas exchange area, also referred to as parenchyma, can be organized into either functional or structural units. The functional unit of the gas exchange area is called the acinus, or terminal respiratory unit (see Fig. 9.16). The acinus includes all air spaces distal to a single terminal bronchiole, including branching respiratory bronchioles, alveolar ducts, alveolar sacs, and alveoli.

The lobule is a structural unit rather than a functional unit. It comprises a cluster of acini that is separated from adjacent clusters by connective-tissue septa. These connective-tissue septa are termed **interlobular septa** and are composed of collagen and elastic fibers and blood vessels. Both bronchial arteries and pulmonary veins are located in interlobular septa. The lungs of cows, sheep, and pigs are highly lobulated and have complete septa. The lungs of horses have incomplete septa and are considered poorly lobulated. Carnivores do not have interlobular septa.

RESPIRATORY BRONCHIOLES

Bronchioles in which the walls possess outpocketings of gas exchange tissue, i.e., alveoli, are termed **respiratory bronchioles**. They are also called the transition zone, which is the focus of most lung disorders. The histologic appearance of respiratory bronchioles is similar to that of terminal bronchioles, with the exception that the epithelium is interrupted by alveoli (Figs. 9.16 and 9.17). The smooth muscle is arranged in fascicles that underlie the simple columnar or cuboidal epithelium. The alveoli open between these muscle bundles.

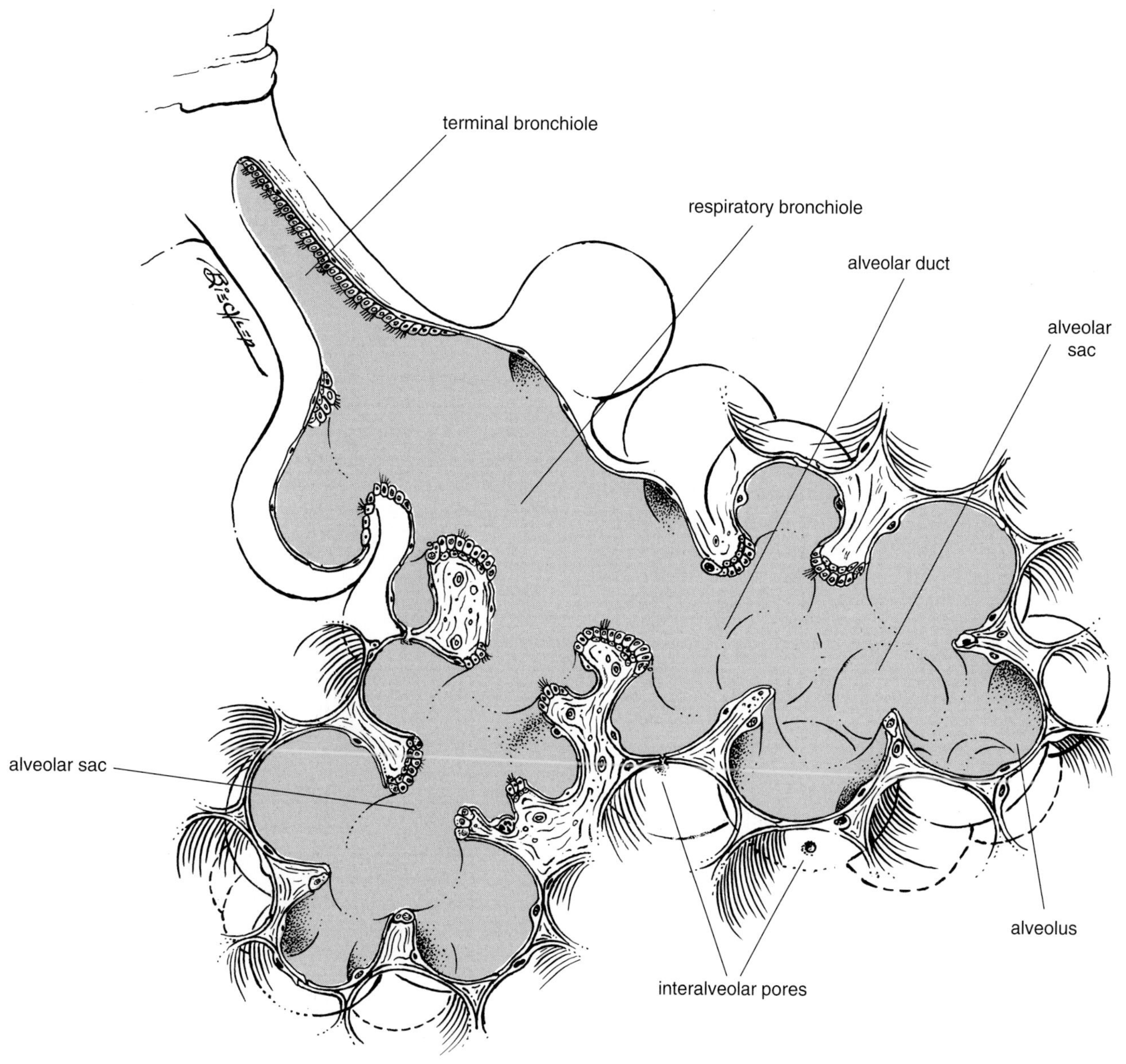

Figure 9.16. *Schematic illustration of the gas exchange area originating from a terminal bronchiole.*

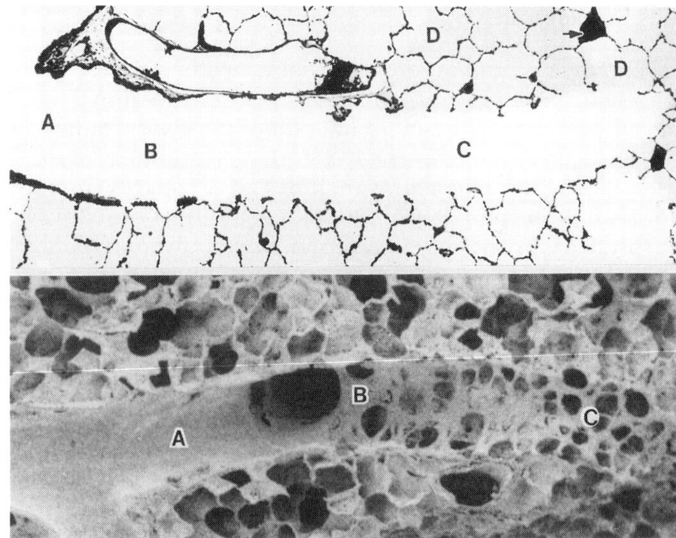

Figure 9.17. *Light microscopic and scanning electron microscopic appearance of a terminal bronchiole and gas exchange area in the feline lung. Terminal bronchiole (A), respiratory bronchiole into which open a few alveoli (B), alveolar duct, completely surrounded by alveoli (C), alveoli (D). Methylene blue; Azure II (top: ×55; bottom: ×70).*

In respiratory bronchioles of carnivores, extensive alveolarization occurs (Fig. 9.17); generally, there are fewer alveoli per generation of branching proximally than distally; the epithelium consists almost entirely of bronchiolar exocrine cells. In horses, cows, sheep, and pigs, respiratory bronchioles are short or absent (Fig. 9.18).

ALVEOLAR DUCTS AND ALVEOLAR SACS

Respiratory bronchioles branch into tubular structures termed **alveolar ducts** (see Figs. 9.16, 9.17, and 9.18). They are comparable to hallways lined by doorless rooms on all sides. Each of these doorless rooms is an alveolus. Between one and five generations of alveolar ducts are supplied by a single respiratory bronchiole. The walls of an alveolar duct are composed of the open sides of alveolar air spaces and the terminations of the interalveolar septa that separate these alveoli. Spiraling bands of smooth muscle and elastic fibers, perpendicular to the long axis of the alveolar ducts, lie underneath the epithelium at the terminations of the interalveolar septa.

The alveolar ducts terminate in clusters of alveoli called **alveolar sacs** (see Fig. 9.16). A shared space into which several alveolar sacs open is called an **atrium**.

ALVEOLI

The basic unit for gas exchange in the pulmonary parenchyma is the alveolus (Figs. 9.16, 9.19, and 9.20). Alveoli are epithelium-lined spheroid air spaces that open into an alveolar sac, alveolar duct, or respiratory bronchiole; they are separated by interalveolar septa.

The alveolar epithelial lining comprises two epithelial cell types, forming the air side of the blood–air barrier, type I and type II alveolar epithelial cells. The **type I** or **squamous alveolar epithelial cell** (respiratory epithelial cell) is a flat cell with a central nucleus, based on a continuous basal lamina (see Fig. 9.19). It has the shape of a fried egg. The flat sheet of cytoplasm that comprises

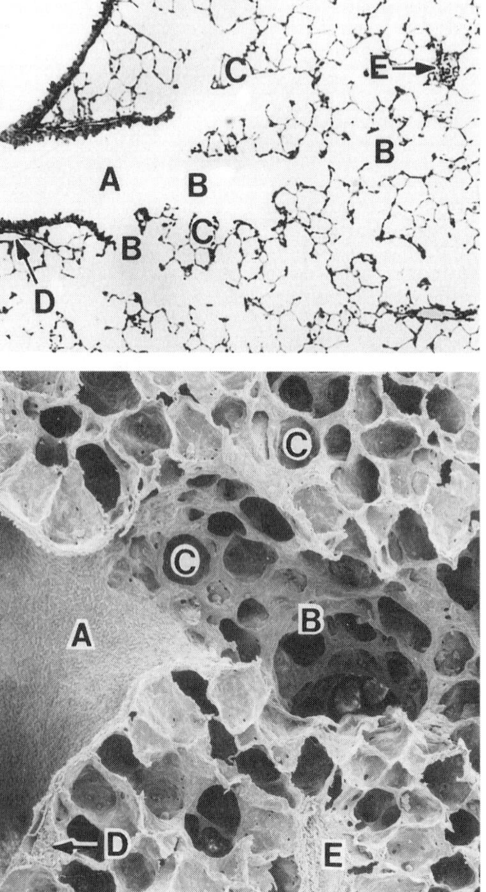

Figure 9.18. *Light microscopic and scanning electron microscopic appearance of the terminal air spaces of the mouse (top) and the rat (bottom). Terminal bronchiole (A); alveolar duct that is completely surrounded by alveoli (B); alveoli (C); pulmonary arteriole (D); pulmonary venule (E). Toluidine blue (top: ×85; bottom: ×110).*

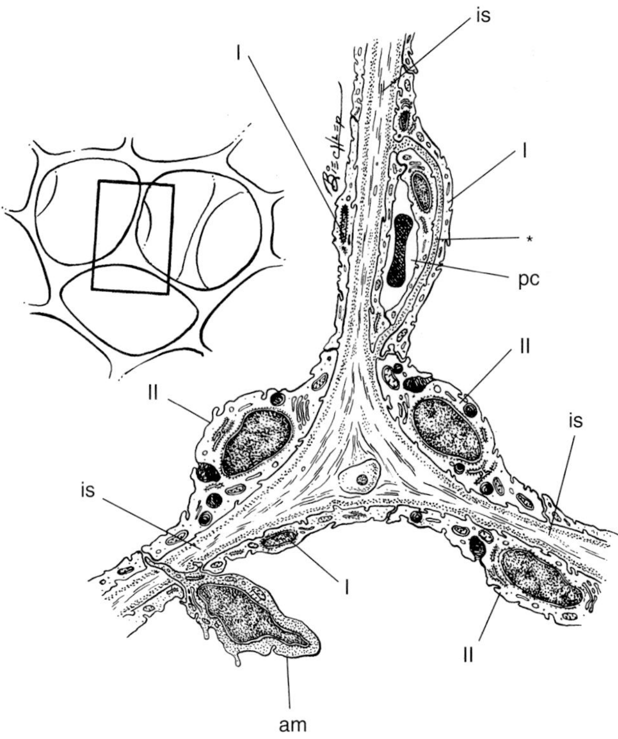

Figure 9.19. *Schematic illustration of parts of three adjacent alveoli, as outlined in the rectangle (inset): type I alveolar epithelial cell (I); type II alveolar epithelial cell (II); interalveolar septum (is); pulmonary capillary (pc); alveolar macrophage (am). Note the merger of the basal laminae of the pulmonary capillary and adjacent alveolus. (*)*

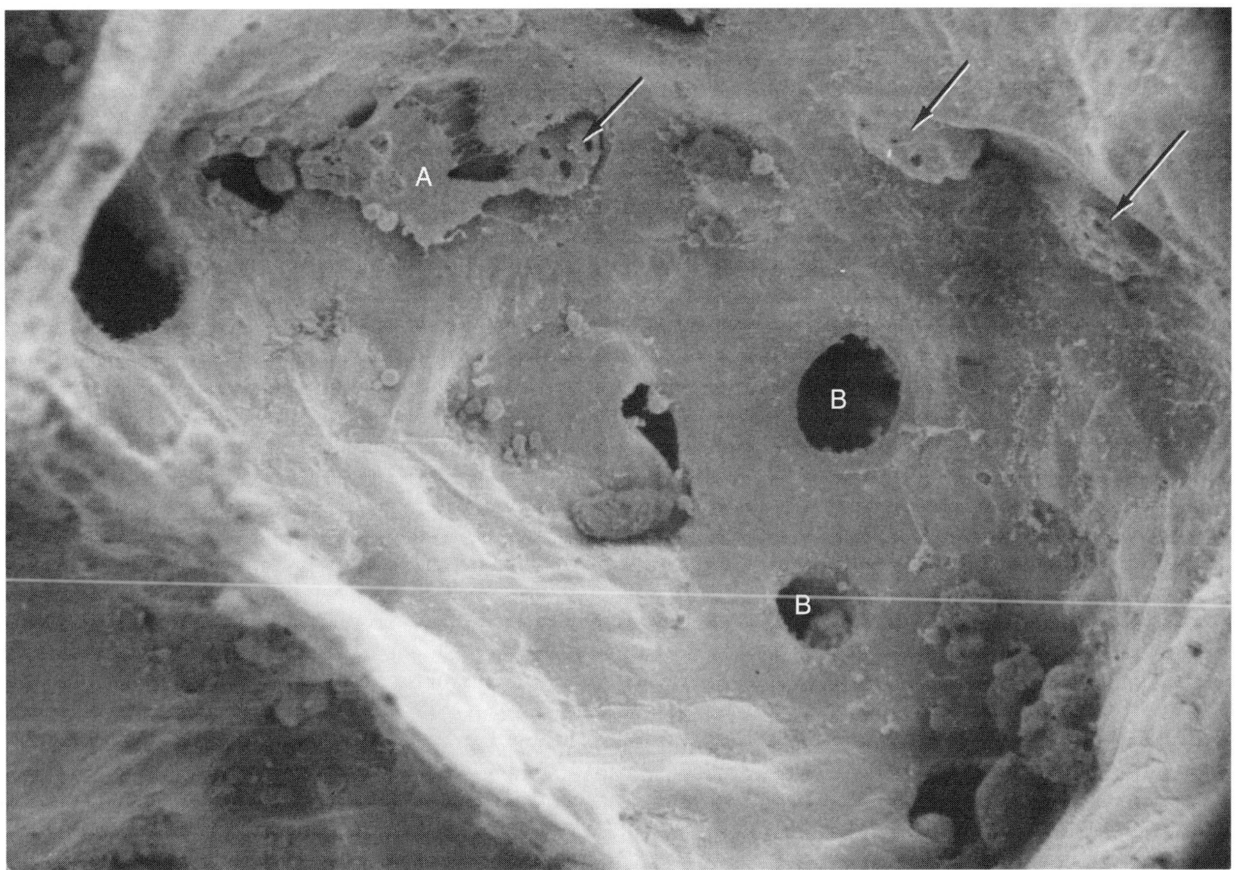

Figure 9.20. *Scanning electron micrograph of portion of an alveolus in the equine lung. Type II (granular) alveolar epithelial cells bulge into the lumen (arrows). On the left is a pulmonary alveolar macrophage (A). Note the pores in the interalveolar septum (B) (×1232). (Courtesy of W.S. Tyler.)*

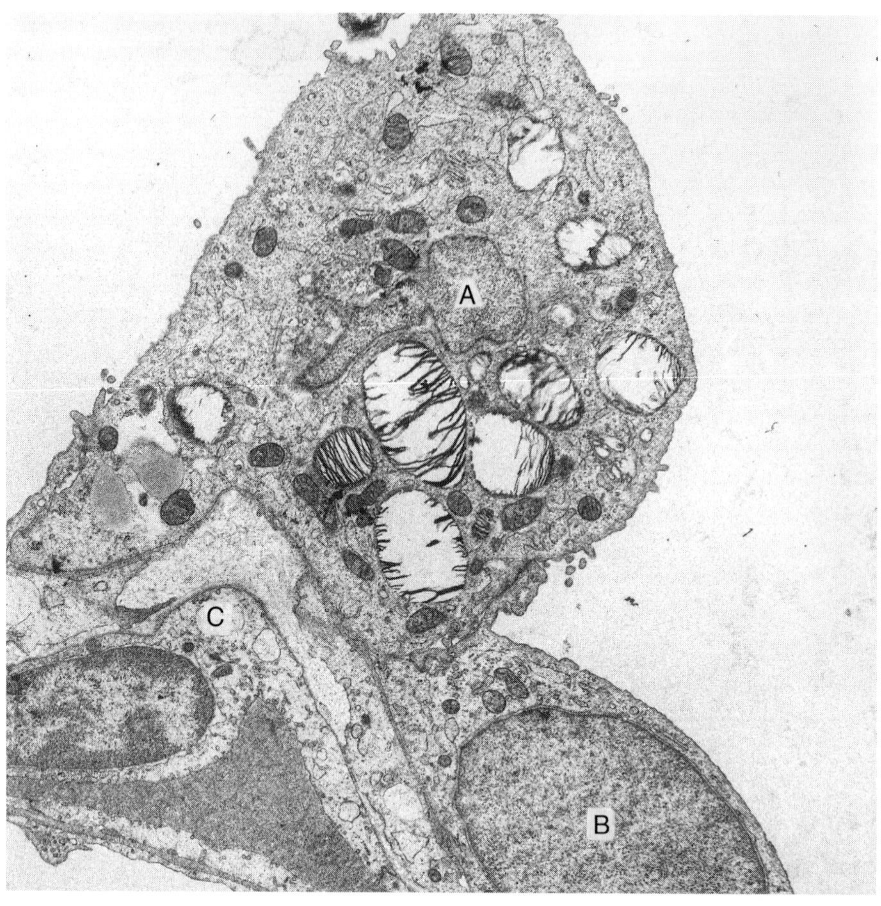

Figure 9.21. *Electron micrograph of a type II (granular) alveolar epithelial cell (A) containing numerous characteristic lamellar bodies and a type I (squamous) alveolar epithelial cell (B). Capillary endothelial cell (C) (×8200). (From Tyler WS, Gillespie JR, Nowell JA. Modern functional morphology of the equine lung. Equine Vet J 1971;3:84.)*

most of the cell has few mitochondria, minimal amounts of rER, and a moderate number of endocytotic vesicles. This cell type covers approximately 97% of the interalveolar septal surface in all the species studied thus far. The average surface area of a type I cell ranges from 5000 to 7000 μm^2.

The **type II** or **granular (great) alveolar epithelial cell** (Fig. 9.21) is a cuboidal cell with a central nucleus. This cell type covers the remainder of the interalveolar septal surface area (approximately 3%). Its alveolar cell surface bears microvilli and ranges from 100 to 280 μm^2 per cell. This cell contains mitochondria, rER, microvesicles, and a Golgi complex. Its characteristic feature are many osmiophilic vesicles called lamellar bodies. These lamellar bodies are believed to be primarily phospholipid and are the source of phospholipids that compose the **pulmonary surfactant** that lines the air spaces. The type II alveolar cell is the progenitor cell for both type I and type II cells.

Pulmonary **alveolar macrophages** are likewise present on the air side of the interalveolar septa (Fig. 9.22). As active phagocytic cells, they are part of the mononuclear phagocyte system distributed throughout the body.

Interalveolar septa are thin sheets of connective tissue containing a capillary plexus (see Fig. 9.19). The interalveolar **interstitial connective tissue** contains collagen and elastic fibers and fibrocytes; pericytes, monocytes (resident macrophages), lymphocytes, and plasma cells may be present.

The capillary bed of the interalveolar septa is an intermeshed network of short, branching vessels. Individual capillary beds traverse the walls of from three to seven alveoli in passing from a pulmonary arteriole to a pulmonary venule. Most endothelial cells have attenuated cytoplasm in the region adjacent to type I alveolar epithelial cells. In these attenuated areas, the basal laminae of alveolar epithelial cells and endothelial cells fuse. Capillary endothelial cells (see Fig. 9.19) are characterized by few organelles and relatively numerous endocytotic vesicles. The intercellular junctions tend to be loose or leaky; the tight junctions have few anastomosing ridges. The surface area of the gas exchange capillary bed is between 66 and 75% of the surface area of the air side of the interalveolar septa.

The alveoli contain a small amount of fluid, consisting of a biphasic layer of plasma filtrates overlaid by a thin layer of phospholipids. This phospholipid layer or **pulmonary surfactant** reduces the intra-alveolar surface tension, preventing alveolar collapse. The **blood–air barrier** prevents the massive release of fluid filtrate from capillaries into the air space while permitting diffusion of oxygen and carbon dioxide between blood capillaries and alveoli (see Fig. 9.19). The average thickness of this barrier is 1.5 μm in most species. At its thinnest, the blood–air barrier consists of the surface-lining layer of pulmonary surfactant and fluid, the alveolar type I cell, fused basal laminae of the alveolar epithelial cell and the underlying capillary endothelial cell, the capillary endothelial cell, and the plasmalemma of a red blood cell (see Fig. 9.19). The thickness of the thinnest areas ranges from 0.2 to 0.7 μm. At its thickest, this barrier consists of the above-mentioned layers and interstitial connective tissue and cells between the basal laminae of epithelial and endothelial cells. Openings in the interalveolar septa interconnect adjacent alveoli. These openings, called **alveolar pores** (Fig. 9.20), are lined by epithelial cells and permit air and alveolar macrophages to pass from one alveolus to another.

Pleura

The visceral, or pulmonary, pleura is a serous membrane that completely covers both lungs, except at the hilum and pulmonary ligament. This covering layer consists of squamous to cuboidal mesothelial cells overlaying varying amounts of elastic fibers and dense irregular connective tissue. Pleural mesothelial cells contain large amounts of rER and mitochondria; their free surfaces are covered by microvilli. At its thickest, the connective-tissue elements of the pleura consist of two or more layers of elastic laminae, many dense irregular bundles of collagen fibers, pulmonary capillaries, and two additional sets of vessels. These two sets of vessels include capillaries and small arterioles from the bronchial circulatory system and lymph vessels. The pulmonary capillaries supply the superficial portion of the gas exchange area. The connective tissue of the pulmonary pleura is continuous with that of the interalveolar septa. The thickness of the pulmonary pleura varies from species to species and within different regions of the same species. The pleura is thinnest in the dog and cat. In these species, the subpleural connective tissue is minimal, and the only blood supply derives from the pulmonary artery. The pleura is thick in large domestic mammals.

Blood Vessels and Lymphatics

Blood is supplied to the lungs through two different circulatory systems: **pulmonary** and **bronchial**. **Pulmonary arteries** carry the entire output of unoxygenated blood from the right ventricle. Pulmonary arteries and their branches are under low pressure; thus, their walls have fewer elastic and collagen fibers and fewer smooth muscle cells than vessels of comparable size in the systemic circulatory system. Pulmonary arteries and the tracheobronchial tree have a common adventitia.

The **bronchial arteries** are under high pressure as a part of the systemic arterial circulatory system. The blood vessels in this system have the same wall structure as those of other systemic arteries of the same size. In all species, the bronchial artery supplies

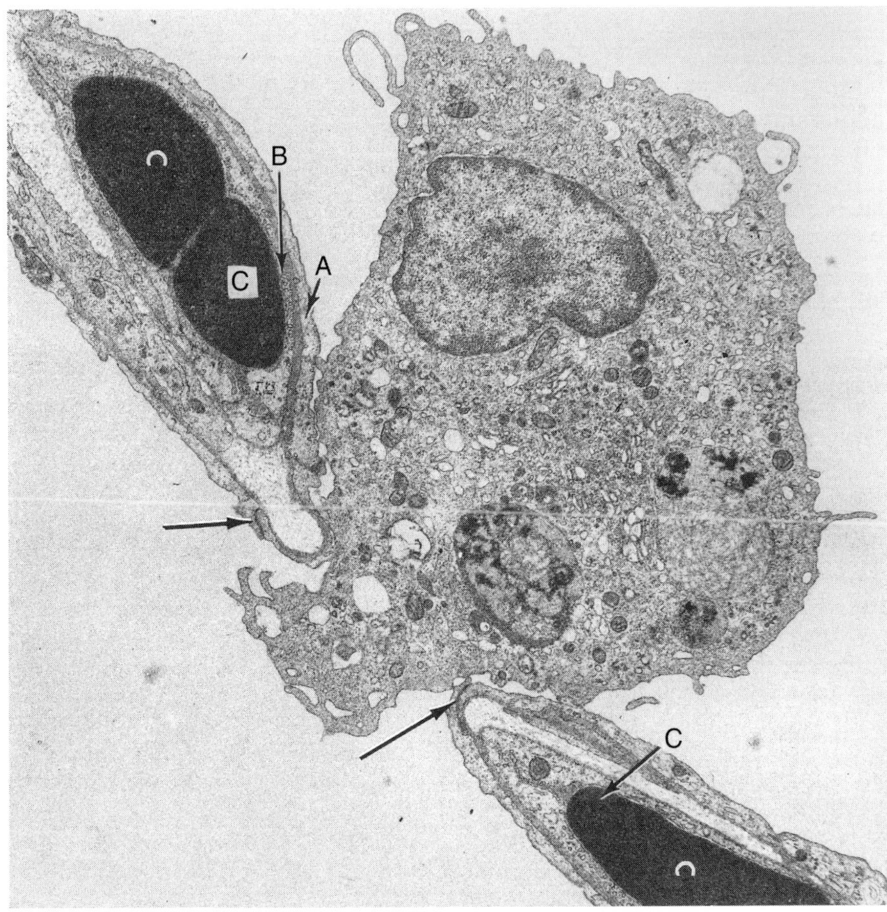

Figure 9.22. *Electron micrograph of an alveolar macrophage projecting through an alveolar pore. The macrophage has numerous filopodia, phagosomes, and phagolysosomes. The thin layer of cytoplasm of the type I (squamous) alveolar epithelial cells (A) is separated by a basal lamina from the capillary endothelium (B). Erythrocytes (C) are in the capillary lumen. The dark lines (arrows) are tight junctions betweeen adjacent squamous alveolar epithelial cells (×8100). (From Tyler WS, Gillespie JR, Nowell JA. Modern functional morphology of the equine lung. Equine Vet J 1971; 3:84.)*

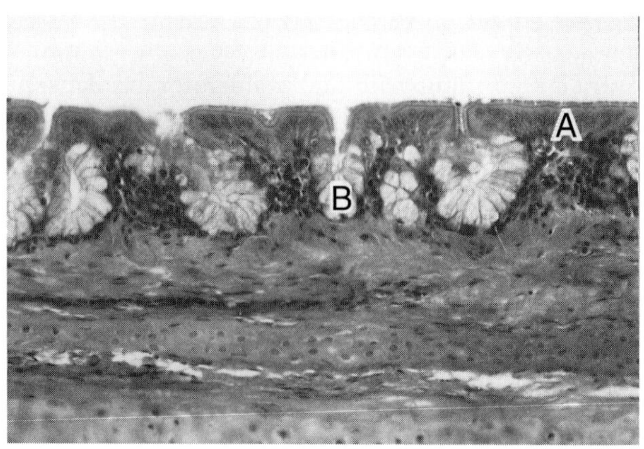

Figure 9.23. *Epithelium from the trachea of a chicken. Most epithelial cells (A) that line the surface of the conducting airways of birds are ciliated. Groups of goblet cells are from intraepithelial glands (B) that open onto the luminal surface. Hematoxylin and eosin (×270).*

blood to the large bronchi, the major pulmonary vessels, and the pulmonary lymph nodes. Anastomoses between bronchial and pulmonary arterial circulatory systems have been identified in the walls of medium-sized bronchi and bronchioles of horses, cows, and sheep.

All blood from the lungs is carried back to the heart by **pulmonary veins**, a low-pressure system. The pulmonary veins have thin walls with little smooth muscle in dogs, cats, horses, and goats. Pulmonary veins with large muscle bundles are present in cows and pigs. In most species, the pulmonary veins are located at the periphery of lobules and course to the hilum in interalveolar interstitium or interlobular septa. In cows, horses, pigs, and sheep, the pulmonary veins accompany the bronchial tree on the side opposite that of pulmonary arteries.

The **pulmonary lymphatics** begin as lymph capillaries, located throughout the interstitium, except for the interstitium of interalveolar septa. Collecting lymph vessels are found throughout the connective tissue of the lung, with the exception of that surrounding alveoli, alveolar sacs and ducts, and respiratory bronchioles.

Innervation

The innervation is from two sources: the parasympathetic system (via the vagus nerve) and the sympathetic system (via the middle cervical and cervicothoracic ganglia). General visceral afferent sensory fibers from pulmonary tissue are also contained in the vagus nerve. Fibers from vagus nerves intermingle to form a plexus along the walls of the airway tree and the pulmonary vasculature, with ganglia present in the adventitia of large airways. Individual nerve fibers are distributed irregularly over the wall of arteries, veins, and airways. Free nerve endings are present near glands, within smooth muscle bundles, and in the interalveolar septa.

AVIAN RESPIRATORY SYSTEM

In contrast to the mammalian respiratory system, the respiratory system of birds contains a simpler larynx, a syrinx, only four orders or generations of conducting airways, a compact spongy lung, and air sacs. The highly efficient avian respiratory system comprises lung tissue positioned between conducting airways and air sacs. During inspiration, air is drawn into the nasal cavity and through the lung tissue to the air sacs; during expiration, the reverse occurs. Birds breathe more slowly and deeply than mammals, and unlike that of mammals, the lung volume of birds remains relatively constant while the volume of their air sacs changes during ventilation.

The nasal cavity is lined by epithelia similar to those of mammals, with stratified squamous epithelium rostrally, olfactory epithelium dorsocaudally, and respiratory epithelium lining most of the remaining areas. In the respiratory epithelium, groups of goblet cells form intraepithelial glands (Fig. 9.23). Large air spaces, the paired infraorbital sinuses, are often clinically involved in respiratory infections; these sinuses, which drain into the nasal cavity, are lined by respiratory epithelium.

The larynx, devoid of vocal folds, produces little sound. The trachea is similar in structure to that in mammals, except that the tracheal cartilages form complete rings encircling the airway; the cartilage rings overlap and interlock with adjacent rings. The trachealis muscle is absent, and intraepithelial glands are numerous. As a result of differences in cartilage structure and smooth muscle content, the trachea of birds, unlike that of mammals, does not undergo phasic changes in diameter during breathing.

Vocalization occurs in the avian **syrinx**, a diverticulum near the tracheobronchial junction with considerable species-dependent structural variation. The intrasyringeal (tympanic) membranes, which vibrate during production of sound, are lined by stratified squamous epithelium.

The lungs comprise primary, secondary, and tertiary bronchi, atria, and air capillaries. Extrapulmonary primary bronchi continue as intrapulmonary **primary bronchi** or **mesobronchi**, each of which terminates by opening into an abdominal air sac. Epithelium of the primary bronchi is similar to that of the trachea. The bronchial cartilages are incomplete medially in the proximal portion of the bronchi and are patchlike more distally. **Secondary bronchi** arise from each intrapulmonary primary bronchus, and many open into other air sacs. **Tertiary bronchi** or **parabronchi**, approximately 100 to 150 μm in diameter, interconnect the secondary bronchi. The epithelium varies from respiratory epithelium in the secondary bronchi to simple cuboidal or squamous epithelium in the tertiary bronchi. A network of spiraling bundles of smooth muscle occurs in the lamina propria of the secondary and tertiary bronchi. Numerous small air spaces, or **atria**, open into tertiary bronchi; the projecting tips of these interatrial septa contain smooth muscle and are lined by squamous cells (Fig. 9.24).

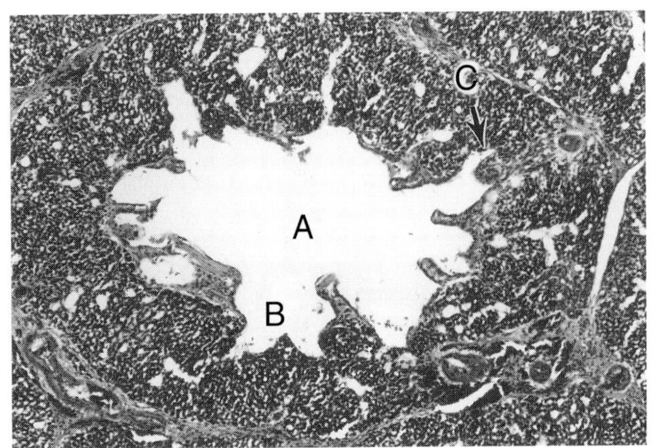

Figure 9.24. *Tertiary bronchus of a chicken lung. Atria (B) open into the lumen (A) of the tertiary bronchus. Air capillaries (C) open into the atria. Hematoxylin and eosin (×110).*

Gas exchange in the avian lung occurs between blood and **air capillaries**. These capillaries, 5 to 15 μm in diameter, open into the atria. Simple squamous epithelium lines the greater portion of the atria and air capillaries. The epithelial portion of the gas exchange area consists of both type I and type II cells similar to those of mammals; a biphasic fluid lining layer, similar to surfactant of mammals, is also observed in birds.

The terminal **air sacs** are lined by a simple squamous to cuboidal epithelium; epithelial surfaces adjacent to ostia of bronchi are ciliated.

REFERENCES

Adams DR, Hotchkiss DK. The canine nasal mucosa. Zentralbl Veterinärmed C Anat Histol Embryol 1983;12:109.

Adams DR, Wiekamp MD. The canine vomeronasal organ. J Anat 1984;138:771.

Berendsen PB, Ritter AB, DeFouw DO. An ultrastructural morphometric comparison of the peripheral with the hilar air-blood barrier of dog lung. Anat Rec 1984;209:535.

Breeze RG, Wheeldon EB. The cells of the pulmonary air ways. Am Rev Respir Dis 1977;161:705.

Crapo JD, Young SL, Frane EK, et al. Morphometric characteristics of cells in the alveolar region of mammalian lungs. Am Rev Respir Dis 1983;128:S42.

Frasca JM, Auerbach O, Parks VR, et al. Electron microscopic observations of the bronchial epithelium of dogs. I. Control dogs. Exp Mol Pathol 1968;9:363.

Gladysheva O, Martynova G. The morphofunctional organization of the bovine olfactory epithelium. Gegenbaurs Morphol Jahrb 1982; 128:78.

Jacobs VL, Sis RF, Chenoweth PJ, et al. Structure of the bovine vomeronasal complex and its relationships to the palate: tongue manipulation. Acta Anat 1981;110:48.

Jeffery PK. Morphologic features of airway surface epithelial cells and glands. Am Rev Respir Dis 1983;128:S14.

Kay JM. Comparative morphologic features of the pulmonary vasculature in mammals. Am Rev Respir Dis 1983;128:S53.

Leak LV, Jamuar MP. Ultrastructure of pulmonary lymphatic vessels. Am Rev Respir Dis 1983;128:S59.

Mariassy AT, Plopper CG. Tracheobronchial epithelium of the sheep. I. Quantitative light microscopic study of epithelial cell abundance and distribution. Anat Rec 1983;205:263.

Mariassy AT, Plopper CG. Tracheobronchial epithelium of the sheep. II .Ultrastructural and morphometric analysis of the epithelial secretory types. Anat Rec 1984;209:523.

Mariassy AT, Plopper CG, Dungworth DL. Characteristics of bovine lung as observed by scanning electron microscopy. Anat Rec 1975;183:13.

McLaughlin RF. Bronchial artery distribution in various mammals and in humans. Am Rev Respir Dis 1983;128:S57.

Phalen RF, Oldham MJ. Tracheobronchial airway structure as revealed by casting techniques. Am Rev Respir Dis 1983;128:51.

Plopper CG. Comparative morphologic features of bronchiolar epithelial cells: the Clara cell. Am Rev Respir Dis 1983;128:S37.

Plopper CG, Mariassy AT, Lollini LO. Structure as revealed by airway dissection: a comparison of mammalian lungs. Am Rev Respir Dis 1983;128:S4.

Plopper CG, Mariassy AT, Wilson DW, et al. Comparison of nonciliated tracheal epithelial cells in six mammalian species: ultrastructure and population densities. Exp Lung Res 1983;5:281.

Reid L, Jones R. Bronchial mucosal cells. Fed Proc 1979;38:191.

Robertson B, Van Golds LMG, Batenberg JJ, eds. Pulmonary surfactant. Amsterdam: Elsevier Science Publishers, 1984.

Tandler B, Sherman JM, Boat TF. Surface architecture of the mucosal epithelium of the cat trachea. I. Cartilaginous portion. Am J Anat 1983;168:119.

Tandler B, Sherman JM, Boat TF, et al. Surface architecture of the mucosal epithelium of the cat trachea. II. Structure and dynamics of the membranous portion. Am J Anat 1983;168:133.

Tyler WS. Comparative subgross anatomy of lungs: pleuras, interlobular septa and distal airways. Am Rev Respir Dis 1983;128:S32.

Wysocki CJ. Neurobehavioral evidence for the involvement of the vomeronasal system in mammalian reproduction. Neurosci Biobehav Rev 1979;3:301.

10

Digestive System

BRIAN L. FRAPPIER

The digestive system consists of a series of tubular organs and associated glands, the main function of which is to break down the ingested food into smaller units that can be absorbed into the circulation and used for the maintenance of the organism.

Morphologic adaptations for specialized functions are characteristic of the digestive systems of the domestic species. Considerable variations in the teeth, stomachs, and large intestines result mainly from the variety of food consumed. For example, the teeth of carnivores are adapted for tearing flesh, whereas those of herbivores are specialized for grinding roughage. The forestomach of ruminants and the cecum and colon of horses reflect structural variations that facilitate the microbial digestion of rough, fibrous food.

Although the large accessory digestive glands — salivary glands, liver, and pancreas — are located outside the tubular portion of the digestive system, they originate as epithelial evaginations from the digestive tube. Their ducts penetrate the walls of the tubular organs and discharge their secretory products into the lumina.

GENERAL STRUCTURE OF TUBULAR ORGANS

A general structural pattern exists for all tubular organs of the digestive, respiratory, urinary, and reproductive systems (Fig. 10.1). Familiarity with this general pattern is helpful in understanding the specific characteristics of each organ. The wall of a typical tubular organ is composed of four coats or tunics.

Tunica Mucosa

The tunic next to the lumen is the tunica mucosa. The tunica mucosa is also referred to as a mucous membrane or simply, the mucosa. A mucosa lines all organs that communicate to the outside of the body and is protected by a layer of mucus, a viscous material containing cast off epithelial cells and leukocytes, in addition to mucin, a product of specialized glands. Structures associated with or in the oral cavity, such as the lips, cheeks, and tongue, are considered to possess a mucosa, even though they are not typical tubular organs. The mucosa is composed of three layers or laminae: an epithelium, a lamina propria, and a lamina muscularis.

The **epithelium** is constantly present and may consist of any of the types of surface epithelia, depending on the function of the specific organ. The epithelium rests on a basement membrane.

The **lamina propria** is a layer of connective tissue immediately beneath the epithelium. In most organs, this is a loose connective tissue containing fine collagen, elastic, and reticular fibers as well as all of the cells typical of loose connective tissue (see Chapter 3). The lamina propria can also be classified as diffuse lymphatic tis-

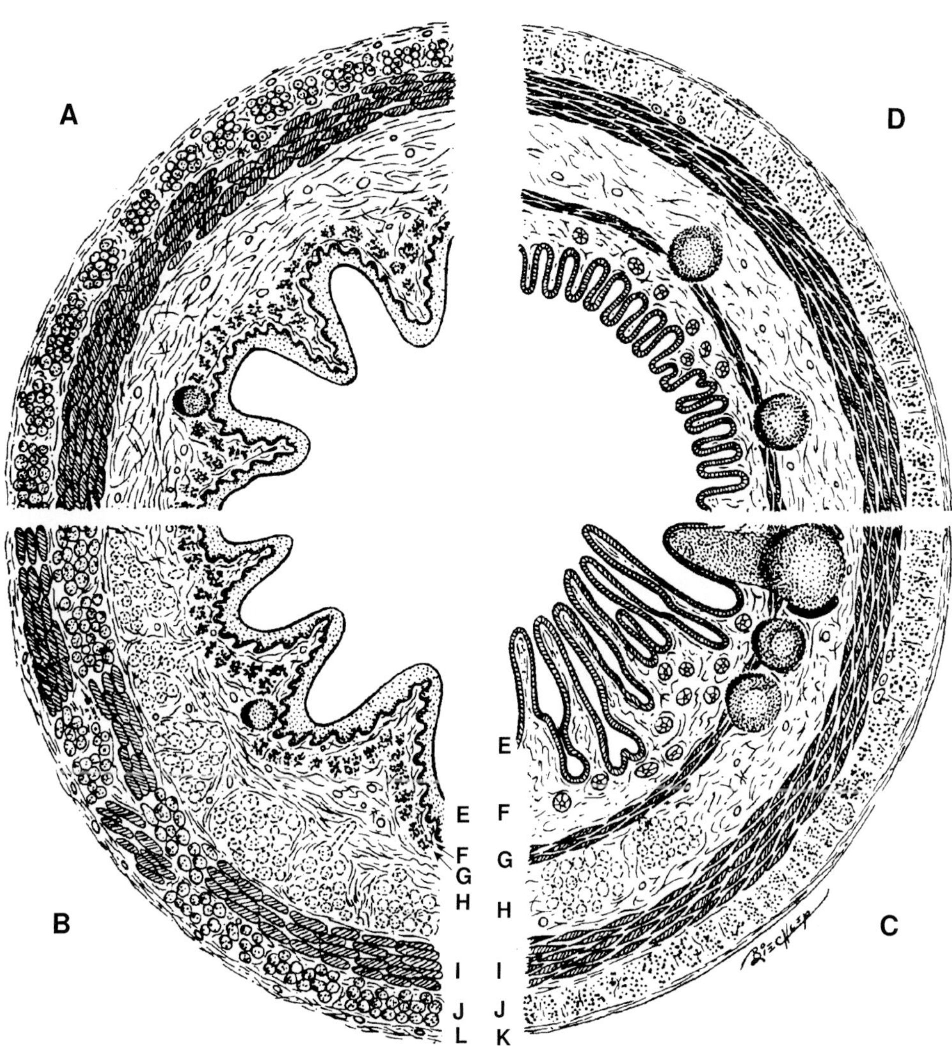

Figure 10.1. *Schematic drawing of cross sections through various portions of the digestive tract. Esophagus without submucosal glands (A). Esophagus with submucosal glands (B). Small intestine with and without submucosal glands and with aggregated lymphatic nodules (C). Large intestine (D). Tunica mucosa: epithelium (E), lamina propria (F), lamina muscularis (G). Tela submucosa (H). Tunica muscularis: circular layer (I), longitudinal layer (J). Tunica serosa (K). Tunica adventitia (L).*

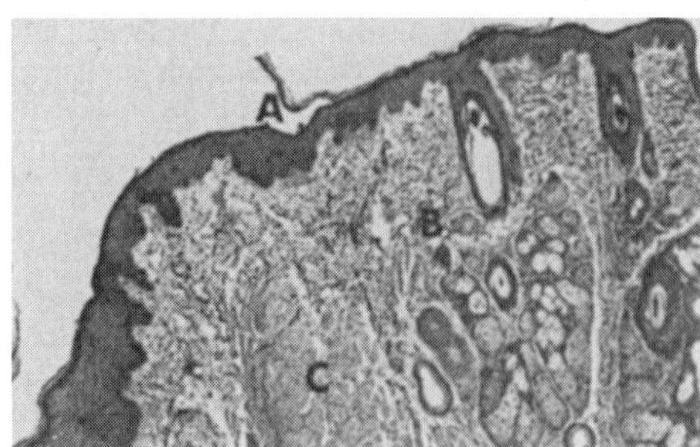

Figure 10.2. *Lip (cat). Junction of keratinized stratified squamous epithelium of skin and mucosa (A); junction of dermis and lamina propria of lip (B); orbicularis oris muscle (skeletal) of lip (C). Hematoxylin and eosin (×45).*

sue, because immunocompetent T and B lymphocytes are present. The lymphocytes initiate the immune response to injurious agents that have penetrated the epithelium. Blood vessels essential for the nourishment of the epithelium, along with lymph capillaries and nerves, are also present in the lamina propria. In some organs, the lamina propria contains glands that are referred to as **mucosal glands** because they are confined to the mucosa.

The **lamina muscularis** is inconstantly present. It consists of one to three layers of smooth muscle. The lamina muscularis allows independent movement of the mucosa, possibly to facilitate the movement of luminal contents or to assist in the expression of secretions from mucosal glands.

Tela Submucosa

The **tela submucosa**, or simply **submucosa**, is a layer of connective tissue that may contain glands (**submucosal glands**). In most organs, the connective tissue of the submucosa is more dense than that of the lamina propria. Also present are blood vessels, lymph vessels, and the **submucosal (Meissner's) plexus**, a ganglionic nerve plexus of the autonomic nervous system. In organs without a lamina muscularis, the lamina propria and submucosa blend without a clear line of demarcation, forming a **propria-submucosa**.

Tunica Muscularis

The **tunica muscularis** is the coat of smooth muscle or skeletal muscle responsible for moving the ingesta through the tract and for mixing the ingesta with glandular secretions. Usually, two layers of muscle are present in the tunica muscularis of the tubular organs of the digestive system. The muscle fibers of the inner layer are oriented circularly or in a tightly coiled pattern, whereas those of the outer layer are arranged longitudinally or in a loosely coiled pattern. Between these two layers is a ganglionic nerve plexus of the autonomic nervous system, the **myenteric (Auerbach's) plexus**.

Tunica Serosa/Adventitia

The outermost tunic may be either a tunica serosa or tunica adventitia. The **tunica serosa** (serosa or serous membrane) is composed of a layer of connective tissue with a covering of mesothelium. Organs that border the pleural, pericardial, and peritoneal cavities are covered by a serosa. In each of these locations, the serosa is given a special name: pleura, epicardium, and peritoneum, respectively. All organs not bordering these cavities, such as the cervical part of the esophagus, do not have a mesothelium. They do possess a layer of connective tissue, called a **tunica adventitia (adventitia)**, which blends with the surrounding fascia (Fig. 10.1).

ORAL CAVITY

Lips

The junction between the integument and the digestive system occurs on the lips. They are covered on the outside by skin and on the inside by a mucosa. Near the junction (the **mucocutaneous junction**), the skin is devoid of hair follicles and the epidermis is thicker, with a more elaborate interdigitation with the underlying connective tissue (Fig. 10.2). The mucosa of the lips is covered by stratified squamous epithelium that is keratinized in ruminants and horses but nonkeratinized in carnivores and pigs. The lamina propria and submucosa blend without a clear junction. Aggregates of **labial glands**, usually serous or seromucous, are distributed in the propria-submucosa. The tunica muscularis consists of skeletal muscle fibers of the orbicularis oris muscle.

Cheeks

The cheeks, like the lips, are composed of an external covering of skin, a middle muscular layer (the buccinator muscle), and an internal mucosa lined by stratified squamous epithelium that may or may not be keratinized, depending on the particular area or species. In ruminants, the mucosa is studded with macroscopic conical **buccal papillae** that facilitate the prehension and mastication of food (Fig. 10.3). The **buccal glands** are minor salivary glands located in the propria submucosa and among the skeletal muscle bundles of the cheek, with some secretory units extending into the dermis. The glands are compound tubuloacinar glands and may be serous, mucous, or seromucous, depending on the location and the species.

Hard Palate

The bones of the hard palate are covered by a mucosa, which exhibits a series of transverse ridges called **rugae**. The mucosa is covered by a keratinized stratified squamous epithelium, which is particularly thick in ruminants (Fig. 10.4). The lamina propria has a well-developed papillary layer that blends with the submucosa without an intervening lamina muscularis, forming a propria submucosa. The propria-submucosa is composed of a dense network of collagen and reticular

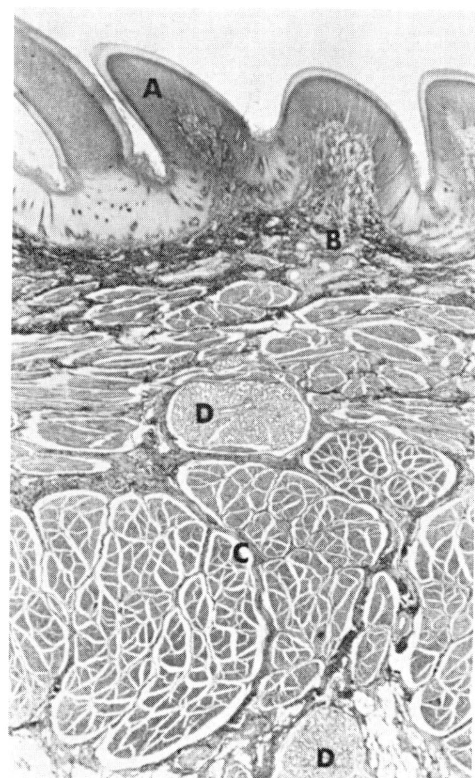

Figure 10.3. *Cheek, bucca (large ruminant). Conical buccal papillae covered with keratinized stratified squamous epithelium (A); lamina propria (B); skeletal muscle (C); buccal glands (D). Hematoxylin and eosin (×12).*

fibers and blends with the adjacent periosteum. A dense network of capillaries and veins, especially well developed in horses, permeates the propria-submucosa. Branched tubuloacinar mucous and seromucous glands (**palatine glands**) are located in the caudal part of the hard palate in all domestic mammals except pigs. The rostral portion of the mucosa of the hard palate is especially thick in ruminants and forms the dental pad (**pulvinus dentalis**). The dental pad consists of a heavily keratinized stratified squamous epithelium overlying a thick layer of dense irregular connective tissue (Fig. 10.5). The lower (inferior) incisor teeth press against the pad, forming a tight grip on forage during grazing.

Soft Palate

The soft palate consists of a core of skeletal muscle fibers with a mucosa covering both surfaces. The ventral surface, the oropharyngeal surface, is covered by a stratified squamous epithelium. The nasopharyngeal surface is covered by a stratified squamous epithelium caudally and a ciliated, pseudostratified columnar epithelium rostrally. Between these two types, a narrow transition zone consisting of transitional epithelium is present. The propria-submucosa contains branched tubuloacinar mucous and seromucous **palatine glands**. Lymphatic tissue occurs in the mucosa of both the oropharyngeal and the nasopharyngeal surfaces; in pigs and horses, a macroscopically visible **tonsil** is present on the oropharyngeal surface. Longitudinally oriented skeletal muscle fibers (the palatinus muscle) and connective tissue are located between the two mucous membranes.

Tongue

The tongue is a muscular organ covered by a mucosa. It is important in the prehension, mastication, and deglutition of food.

The epithelium covering the tongue is stratified squamous. It is thickest, and keratinized, on the dorsum and thinnest on the ventral surface, where it is typically nonkeratinized. The dorsum bears numerous macroscopic **lingual papillae**. These papillae differ somewhat in shape, are named according to their morphologic characteristics, and serve either a mechanical or a gustatory function. The

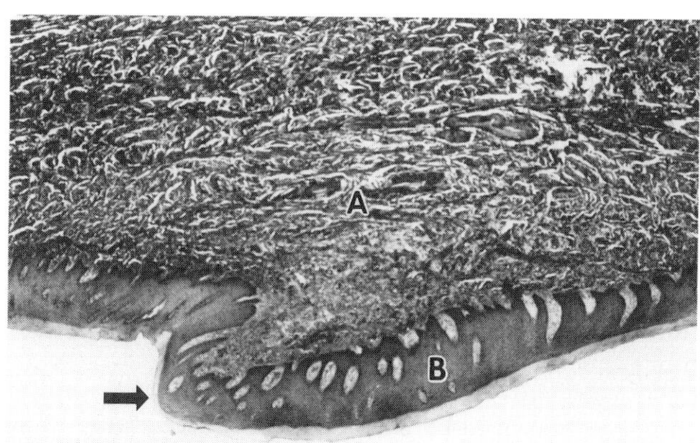

Figure 10.4. *Hard-palate mucosa (large ruminant). Propria-submucosa (A); keratinized stratified squamous epithelium (B); caudal surface of ruga (arrow). Hematoxylin and eosin (×22).*

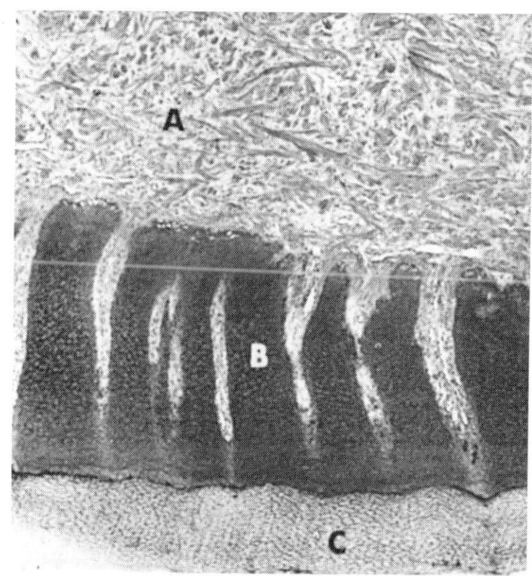

Figure 10.5. *Dental pad (sheep). Propria-submucosa (A) with papillae interdigitating with stratified squamous epithelium (B); stratum corneum (C). Trichrome (×48).*

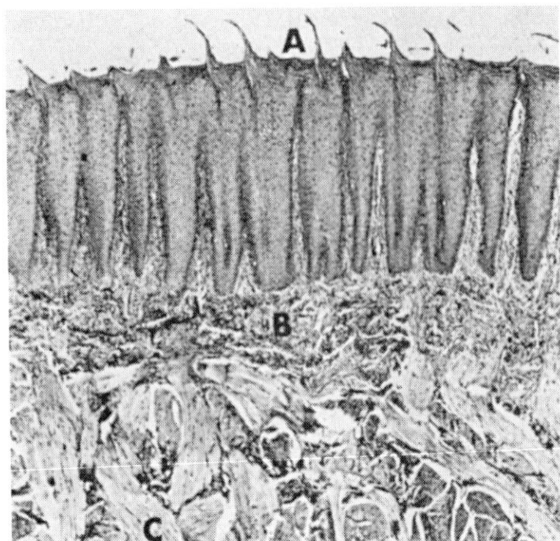

Figure 10.6. *Tongue (horse). Filiform papillae are keratinized threads extending from the surface of the stratified squamous epithelium on the dorsum of the tongue (A); lamina propria (B); skeletal muscle (C). Hematoxylin and eosin (×26).*

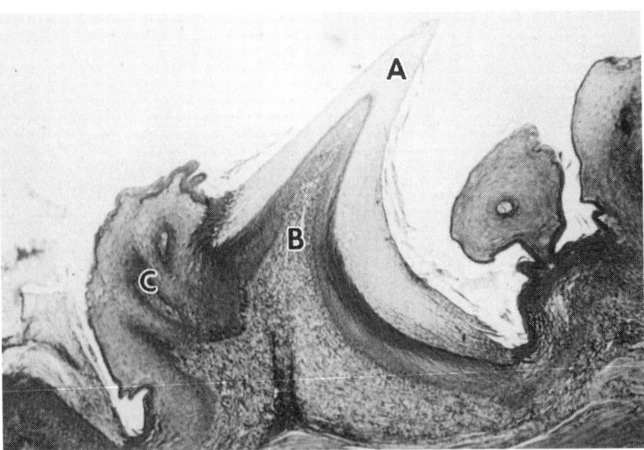

Figure 10.7. *Tongue (cat). Filiform papilla with a caudally directed keratinized spine arising from the caudal prominence (A); lamina propria (B); supporting rostral papilla (C). Hematoxylin and eosin (×35).*

filiform, conical, and lenticular papillae are purely mechanical; they facilitate the movement of ingesta within the oral cavity. The fungiform, vallate, and foliate papillae are gustatory, i.e., they contain the taste buds, which are responsible for mediation of the sense of taste.

The **filiform papillae** are the most numerous type. They are slender, threadlike structures that project above the surface of the tongue and are covered by a keratinized stratified squamous epithelium with a thick stratum corneum. They are supported by a highly vascularized connective tissue core. Equine filiform papillae consist of very fine keratinized threads projecting above the surface (Fig. 10.6). The connective tissue core ends at the base of the thread. In ruminants, a keratinized cone projects above the surface, and the connective tissue core has several secondary papillae. Cats have large papillae with two prominences of unequal size (Fig. 10.7). The caudal prominence is especially large and gives rise to a caudally directed keratinized spine, supported by a more rounded rostral papilla with a thinner stratum corneum. The filiform papillae of dogs may have two or more apices; the caudal apex is largest and has a stratum corneum thicker than that of the other(s) (Fig. 10.8).

Conical papillae occur on the root of the tongue in dogs, cats, and pigs, and on the **torus linguae** of ruminants (see "Special lingual structures" section below). They are larger than the filiform papillae and usually are not highly keratinized. They contain both primary and secondary connective tissue papillae. In pigs, these papillae are more correctly referred to as **tonsillar papillae**, because they contain a core of lymphatic tissue and, therefore, collectively constitute the **lingual tonsil**.

Lenticular papillae are flattened, lens-shaped projections that are found on the torus linguae of ruminants. They are covered by keratinized stratified squamous epithelium and have a core of dense irregular connective tissue.

The **fungiform papillae** are scattered among the filiform papillae and have a dome-shaped upper surface in horses and pigs (Fig. 10.9). The shape is suggestive of a

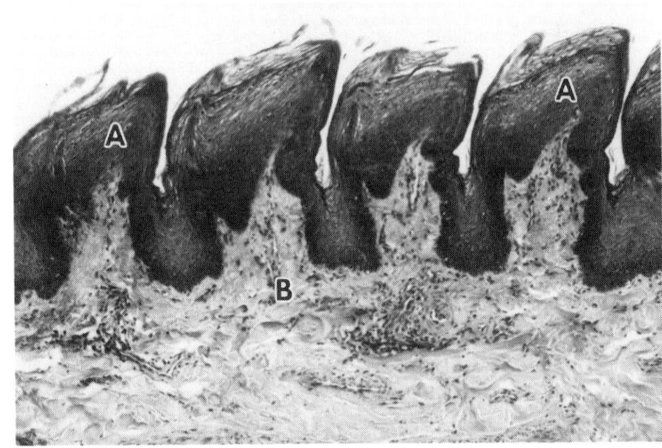

Figure 10.8. *Tongue (dog). Filiform papillae with caudally directed apices (A); lamina propria (B). Hematoxylin and eosin (×75).*

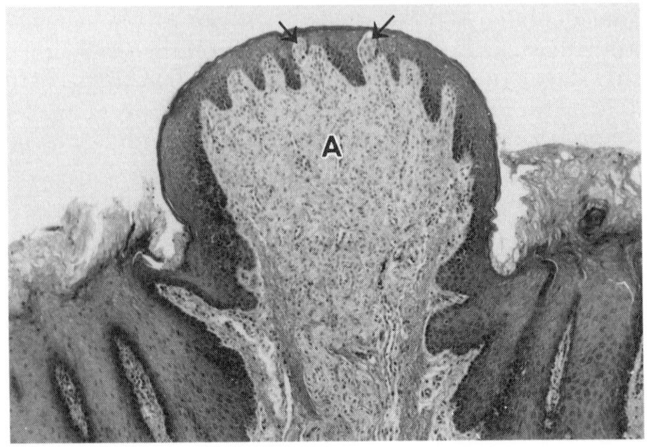

Figure 10.9. *Tongue (pig). Fungiform papilla (A) with taste buds (arrows). Hematoxylin and eosin (×75).*

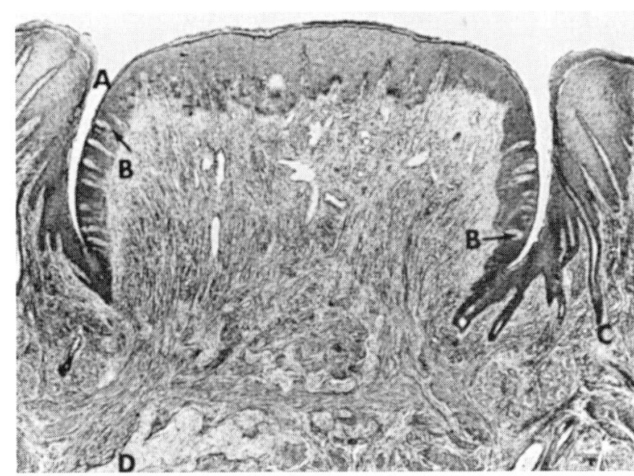

Figure 10.10. *Tongue (large ruminant). Vertical section of a vallate papilla with a surrounding sulcus (A); taste buds in the epithelium (B); a gustatory gland duct opening into the sulcus (C); gustatory gland (D). Hematoxylin and eosin (×30). (From Stinson AW, Brown EM. Veterinary histology slide sets. East Lansing, MI: Michigan State University, Instructional Media Center, 1970.)*

mushroom, and thus the name fungiform. The papillae are covered by a nonkeratinized stratified squamous epithelium containing one or more taste buds on the upper surface. The taste buds are sparse in these papillae in the tongues of horses and cattle, more numerous in those of sheep and pigs, and abundant in those of carnivores and goats. The connective tissue core is rich in blood vessels and nerves.

The **vallate papillae**, located on the dorsum and just rostral to the root of the tongue, are large, flattened structures completely surrounded by an epithelium-lined sulcus (Fig. 10.10). They extend only slightly, if at all, above the lingual surface and are covered by a stratified squamous epithelium. The epithelium on the papillary side of the sulcus contains many taste buds, and deep to the sulcus lie groups of serous gustatory glands, the ducts of which open into the sulcus at various levels (Fig. 10.10). Mucous glands may also be found beneath the papillae, but their secretory products are emptied directly onto the lingual surface. The connective tissue core is rich in blood vessels and nerves.

The **foliate papillae** are parallel folds of the lingual mucosa located on the margin of the tongue just rostral to the palatoglossal arch. Taste buds are located in the epithelium on the sides of the folds. The folds are separated by gustatory sulci (Figs. 10.11 and 10.12). Deep to the sulci lie serous gustatory glands, the ducts of which empty into the sulci. Foliate papillae are absent in ruminants and are rudimentary and without taste buds in cats.

The **taste buds** are ellipsoid clusters of specialized epithelial cells embedded in the stratified squamous epithelium of the fungiform, vallate, and foliate papillae of the tongue (Fig. 10.12). They also occur widely dispersed in the soft palate, epiglottis, or other areas of the oral cavity and pharynx. The taste bud consists of a cluster of spindle-shaped epithelial cells that extend from the basement membrane to a small opening, the **taste pore**, at the epithelial surface (Fig. 10.12). In most mammalian species, three cell types have been identified. They are referred to as type I cells, type II cells, and type III cells. Type I and type II cells have apical microvilli that project into the taste pore; type III cells have a club-shaped apex that also projects into the taste pore. The type III cell is characterized by clusters of cytoplasmic vesicles, resembling synaptic vesicles, adjacent to intraepithelial nonmyelinated afferent nerve fibers. Therefore, the type III cell is considered to be the **chemoreceptor (taste) cell**,

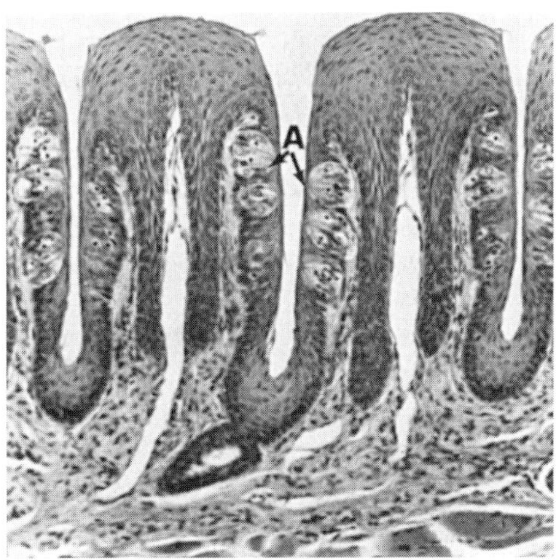

Figure 10.11. *Tongue (rabbit). Foliate papillae with prominent taste buds (A). Hematoxylin and eosin (×110).*

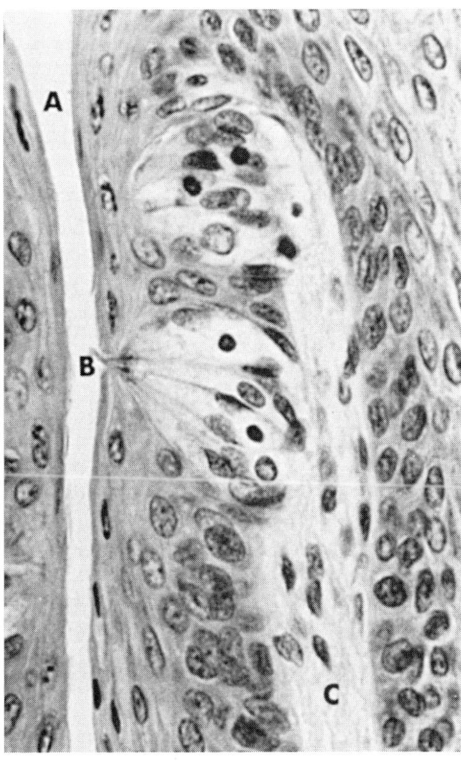

Figure 10.12. *Taste buds (rabbit). Gustatory sulcus (A); taste pore (B); nonmyelinated nerve fibers (C). Hematoxylin and eosin (×615).*

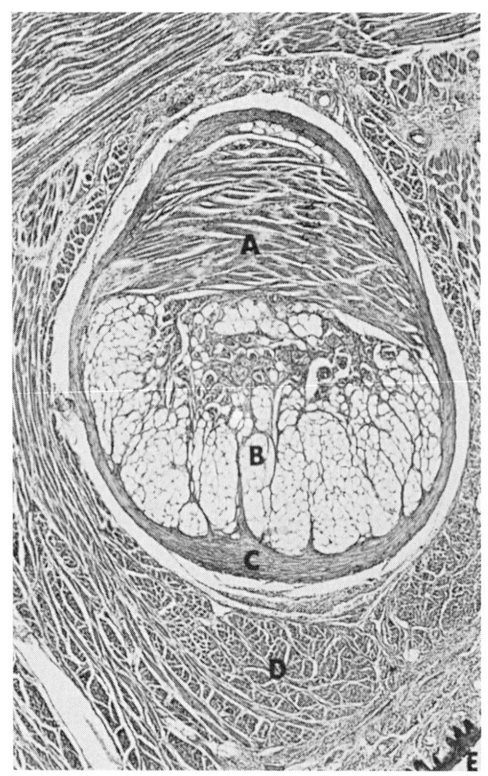

Figure 10.13. *Lyssa (dog). Skeletal muscle (A); white adipose tissue (B); dense irregular connective tissue capsule (C); intrinsic lingual muscles (D); ventral surface of tongue (E). Hematoxylin and eosin (×28).*

whereas the type I and type II cells are believed to serve a **sustentacular (supportive)** role. The average life span of the cells is approximately 10 days. New cells are recruited from mitotically dividing cells in the perigemmal region (Latin "*gemma*," meaning "a bud").

The proper (intrinsic) lingual muscles consist of longitudinally, transversely, and perpendicularly arranged bundles of skeletal muscle (Fig. 10.6). Because of the diverse arrangement of these muscle fibers, the tongue has extensive mobility to facilitate movement of food into and within the oral cavity.

The ventral surface of the tongue is covered by nonkeratinized stratified squamous epithelium. The mucosa contains an abundance of capillaries, arteriovenous anastomoses, and branches of the lingual artery and vein. They participate in thermoregulation.

Scattered among the muscle fibers and in the propria-submucosa of the tongue are clusters of seromucous minor salivary glands, which are collectively referred to as the **lingual glands**.

SPECIAL LINGUAL STRUCTURES

The **lyssa** of the tongue of carnivores is a cordlike structure enclosed in a dense irregular connective tissue capsule and extends longitudinally, in the midline, near the ventral surface of the apex of the tongue. The lyssa of dogs is filled with white adipose tissue, skeletal muscle, blood vessels, and nerves, but that of cats contains mainly white adipose tissue (Fig. 10.13). The tongue of pigs contains a similar structure. A mid-dorsal fibroelastic cord with hyaline cartilage, skeletal muscle, and white adipose tissue is present in the tongue of horses. It is termed the **dorsal lingual cartilage**.

The ruminant tongue has a large prominence covering the caudal portion of the dorsum, the **torus linguae**, characterized by a thickened mucosa. Connective tissue papillae extend almost to the surface of the epithelium, which is thicker than that on the other regions of the tongue. Flattened lenticular papillae are scattered over the surface of this area.

Teeth

Teeth are highly mineralized structures in the oral cavity that serve the domestic mammals in procuring, cutting, and crushing food and as weapons of offense and defense. The tooth consists of a highly mineralized outer part surrounding the **pulp cavity**, which contains the **dental pulp**, a core of connective tissue, blood vessels, lymph vessels, and nerves (Fig. 10.14).

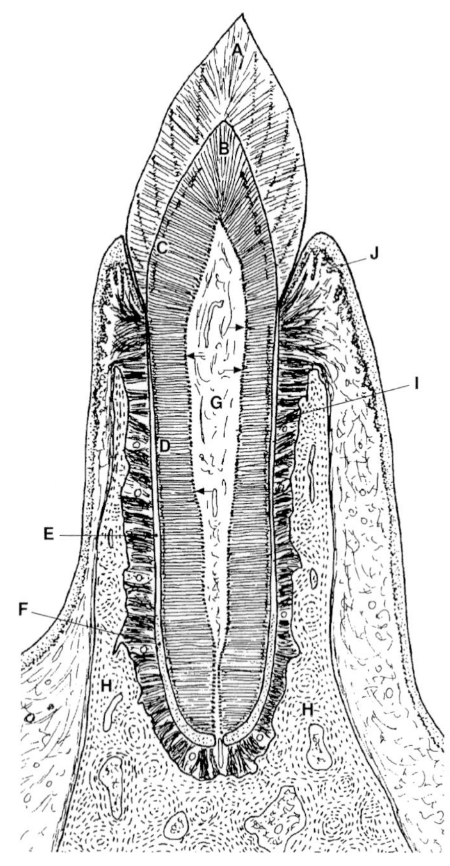

Figure 10.14. *Schematic drawing of a longitudinal section through a brachydont tooth in situ. Enamel (A); dentin (B) with interglobular dentin (C) and the stratum granulosum of the root (D); acellular (E) and cellular (F) cementum; dental pulp (filling the pulp cavity) with peripherally located odontoblasts (arrows); alveolar bone (H); periodontal ligament (I); gingiva (J). (From Dellmann H-D. Veterinary histology: an outline text–atlas. Philadelphia: Lea & Febiger, 1971.)*

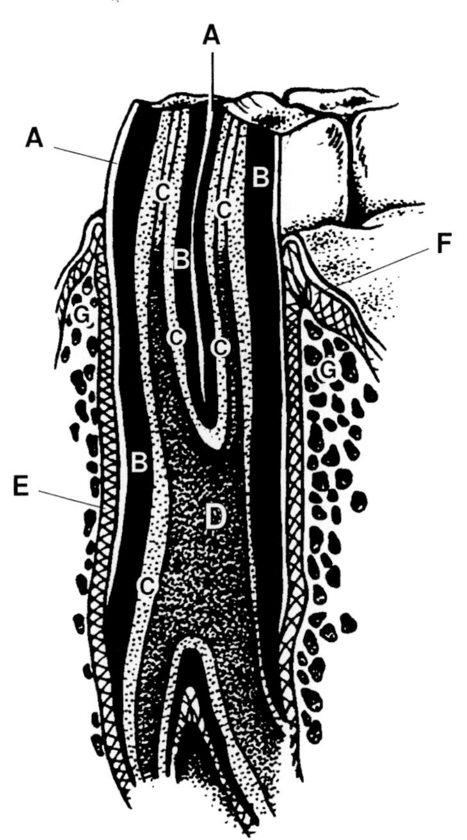

Figure 10.15. *Schematic drawing of a longitudinal section through a hypsodont tooth in situ. Cementum (A); enamel (B); dentin (C); dental pulp (filling the pulp cavity) (D); periodontal ligament (E); gingiva (F); alveolar bone (G).*

BRACHYDONT AND HYPSODONT TEETH

Two types of teeth occur in the domestic mammals: **brachydont** and **hypsodont**. These teeth differ in their rates of growth and in the arrangement of the layers of mineralized tissue.

Brachydont teeth are short and cease to grow after eruption is completed (Fig. 10.14). They have a **crown** (the portion above the gingiva), a **neck** (the constricted region just below the gingival line), and one or more **roots** embedded in a bony socket called the **alveolus**. The crown is covered by a cap of enamel that extends down to the neck. The root is covered by a layer of cementum that may slightly overlap the enamel on the neck. Beneath both the enamel and the cementum is a thick layer of dentin. Brachydont teeth include all those of carnivores and man, the incisor teeth of ruminants, and the teeth of pigs, except for the canine teeth.

Hypsodont teeth are much longer than brachydont teeth and continue their growth throughout a portion, if not all, of the adult life of the animal (Fig. 10.15). They do not have a crown and neck but, instead, have an elongated **body**; in some species, the roots and neck form only after a delayed period. The tusks of the boar continue to grow throughout life and never develop roots. **Cementum** covers the outside of the tooth both above and below the gingiva. Beneath the cementum is a layer of enamel extending throughout the length of the body and almost to the apex of the root. The enamel, in turn, lies on a thick layer of dentin. Hypsodont teeth differ from brachydont teeth in that the hypsodont cementum and enamel invaginate into the dentin. **Infundibula** form where these invaginations occur from the occlusal surface down into the tooth, whereas those infolding along the sides form the **enamel plicae**, characteristic of the cheek teeth (premolars and molars). The occlusal surface of each cheek tooth is corrugated as a result of the irregular wearing of the mineralized tissues. Because enamel is the hardest of the mineralized tissues, it is most resistant to wear and projects above the surface as sharp **enamel crests**. Dentin and cementum are less resistant than enamel and wear away more readily. The enamel crests make the occlusal surface effective for grinding food. Hypsodont teeth include all those of horses, the cheek teeth of ruminants, and the canine teeth of pigs.

STRUCTURE

The mineralized tissues of the teeth are enamel, dentin, and cementum. Each of these has a separate origin and differs morphologically and in degree of mineralization.

Enamel covers the crown of brachydont teeth but lies beneath a layer of cementum in hypsodont teeth. It is the hardest substance in the body, composed of 99% mineral (**hydroxyapatite**) and 1% organic matrix by weight. Histologically, enamel is composed of long, slender rods, **enamel prisms**, held together by **inter-rod enamel**. Parallel bundles of rods pursue a wavy or oblique course from the inner to the outer surface of the enamel layer (Fig. 10.16). Curved lines appear where these bundles change directions. Enamel is produced by ameloblasts that differentiate from the inner

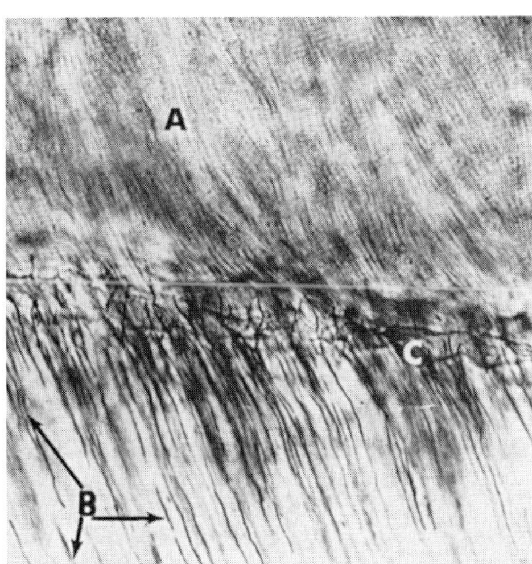

Figure 10.16. *Ground tooth (human being). Junction of enamel (A) and dentin (B) with the odontoblastic processes penetrating the dentinal tubules; interglobular dentin (C). Unstained (×235).*

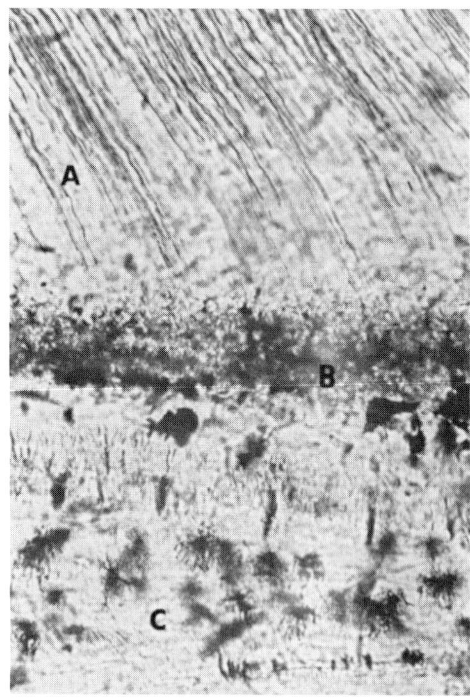

Figure 10.17. *Ground tooth (human being). Dentinocemental junction. Dentin (A) containing dentinal tubules (the dark lines); stratum granulosum of the root (B); cementum (C) with lacunae. Unstained (×185).*

enamel epithelium of the enamel organ (see "Development" section below).

Dentin is a highly mineralized tissue that constitutes the major part of the tooth. It underlies the enamel of the crown and the cementum of the root in brachydont teeth and the enamel of the body in hypsodont teeth and forms the wall of the **pulp cavity**. It consists of a matrix of organic material, mainly randomly oriented collagen fibrils and glycoprotein, upon which are deposited minerals, mainly hydroxyapatite, with some carbonate, magnesium, and fluoride. The composition is approximately 70% mineral and 30% organic matter. The dentin is perforated by roughly parallel anastomotic channels, the **dentinal tubules**, that extend from the inner to the outer surface of the dentin. The dentinal tubules contain long cytoplasmic processes of the odontoblasts, the **odontoblast processes**. The **peritubular dentin** immediately surrounds the odontoblast processes and is more highly mineralized than is the **intertubular dentin**, which constitutes the remainder of the dentin. The odontoblasts form a layer of columnar cells beneath the dentin and produce the organic matrix of dentin. This unmineralized organic material, termed **predentin**, lies between the apex of the cell body of the odontoblasts and the mineralized dentin. **Interglobular dentin** is composed of small, unmineralized or incompletely mineralized areas within the dentin at its periphery, immediately adjacent to the enamel or cementum. These areas are more numerous in the root of the tooth and form the stratum granulosum of the dental root at the dentinocementum junction (Fig. 10.17). The odontoblasts continue to produce dentin throughout the life of the tooth, although at a slower rate after the tooth erupts.

Cementum resembles bone in all its structural features. It is composed of lamellae oriented parallel to the surface of the tooth, with **cementocytes** occupying the lacunae (Fig. 10.18). Cytoplasmic processes of the cementocytes extend into anastomosing canaliculi similar to those of bone. The cementum covering the upper part of the root may be devoid of cells, thus forming **acellular cementum**. Bundles of collagen fibers, called **cementoalveolar (Sharpey's) fibers**, extend from the alveolar bone into the cementum of the tooth (Fig. 10.18). Collectively, these fibers form the **periodontal ligament**, which anchors the tooth in the alveolus.

Dental pulp occupies the pulp cavity of the tooth. It is composed of connective tissue cells and fibers, amorphous ground substance, numerous blood and lymph vessels, and nerves. It resembles embryonic connective tissue in texture, with delicate collagen fibers coursing through the amorphous ground substance. The most peripheral part is the layer of odontoblasts, from which the odontoblast processes extend into the dentinal tubules. Basal processes from the odontoblasts extend into the amorphous ground substance or unite with similar processes from neighboring cells. Because dentin is continuously deposited on the inside of the tooth, the size of the pulp cavity is gradually reduced as the animal ages.

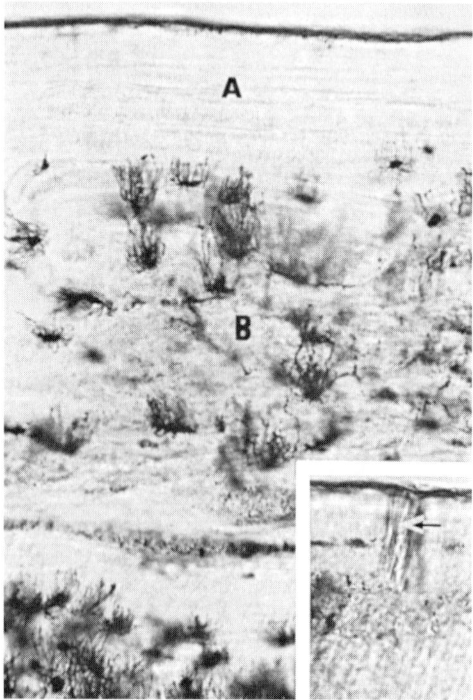

Figure 10.18. *Ground tooth (human being). Lamellae of acellular cementum (A) oriented parallel to the surface of the root. Cellular cementum with cementocytes (B) (×185). Inset: cementoalveolar (Sharpey's) fibers (arrow) embedded in the cementum. Unstained (×185).*

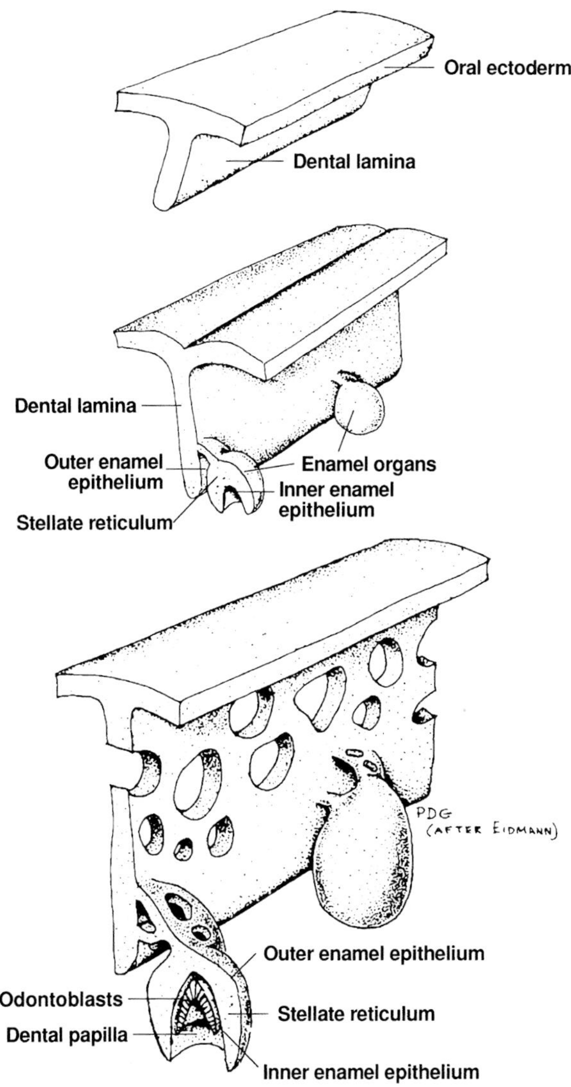

Figure 10.19. *Stages in the development of the tooth. The dental lamina degenerates (holes) as the teeth mature.*

DEVELOPMENT

In the embryo, an invagination of the oral ectoderm into the underlying mesenchyme forms the **dental lamina** (Fig. 10.19), a continuous, arch-shaped sheet of epithelial cells extending along the future site of the gingiva in both the upper and lower jaws. Isolated thickenings arise on the labial side of the dental lamina, where each deciduous and permanent tooth develops. These thickenings are the primordia of the enamel organ, which eventually gives rise to the enamel.

As the **enamel organ** develops, it takes on the appearance of an inverted cup, attached to the dental lamina by a thin stem (Figs. 10.19 and 10.20). The epithelial cells lining the inside of the cup form the **inner enamel epithelium**, and those covering the outside form the **outer enamel epithelium**. The epithelial cells between these two layers become stellate and take on the appearance of connective tissue, thus forming the **stellate reticulum** of the enamel organ. The mesenchyme (derived from mesoderm) enclosed by the cup of the enamel organ condenses to form the **dental papilla**, the future dental pulp. The internal contour of the cup is a replica of the shape of the tooth crown to be produced (Fig. 10.21).

As the enamel organ enlarges, the cells of the inner enamel epithelium take on a distinct columnar shape and differentiate into **ameloblasts**, which later produce the enamel. The mesenchymal cells of the dental papilla immediately adjacent to the ameloblasts differentiate into **odontoblasts**, which produce dentin. Dentin is deposited as sheaths of mineralized material around the odontoblast processes that are anchored to the basement membrane of the inner enamel epithelium. As more dentin is produced, the cell body of the odontoblast recedes toward the developing pulp cavity. Shortly after the first dentin is deposited, the ameloblasts begin to produce the enamel matrix (Figs. 10.21 and 10.22). The deposition of the dentin and enamel begins at the apex of the crown and continues down the sides of the crown to the neck of the tooth.

The formation of the root begins shortly before the eruption of the tooth. The root is formed by a downward growth of a sheet of cells originating from the enamel organ at the junction of the inner and outer enamel epithelia. This downward-growing sheet of cells, the **epithelial sheath of Hertwig**, surrounds the connective tissue of the dental pulp and induces the formation of odontoblasts. The dentin of the root is produced by these odontoblasts.

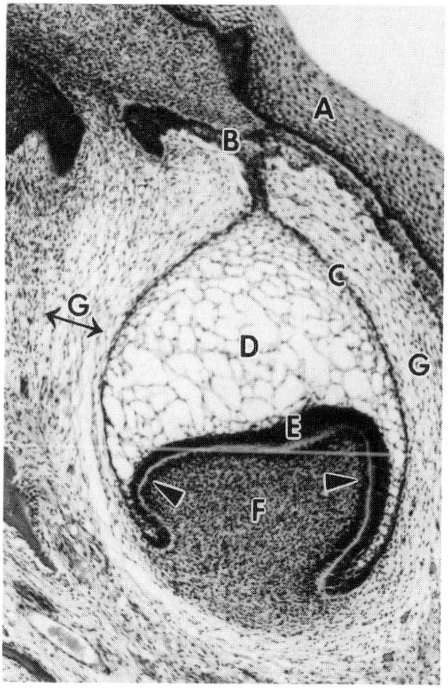

Figure 10.20. *Developing tooth (dog). Oral ectoderm (A); dental lamina (B); outer enamel epithelium of enamel organ (C); stellate reticulum of enamel organ (D); inner enamel epithelium of enamel organ (E); dental papilla (F) with peripheral odontoblasts (arrowheads); developing dental sac (G). Hematoxylin and eosin (×85).*

The entire enamel organ and developing tooth are enclosed by the **dental sac**, a thickened connective tissue layer that completely surrounds the developing tooth (Fig. 10.20). In brachydont teeth, the crown erupts through the dental sac, which then collapses against the dentin of the root. The cells of the collapsed dental sac then differentiate into **cementoblasts**, which deposit a covering of cementum over the roots. In hypsodont teeth, the dental sac collapses before the tooth erupts, and therefore, cementum covers the entire tooth.

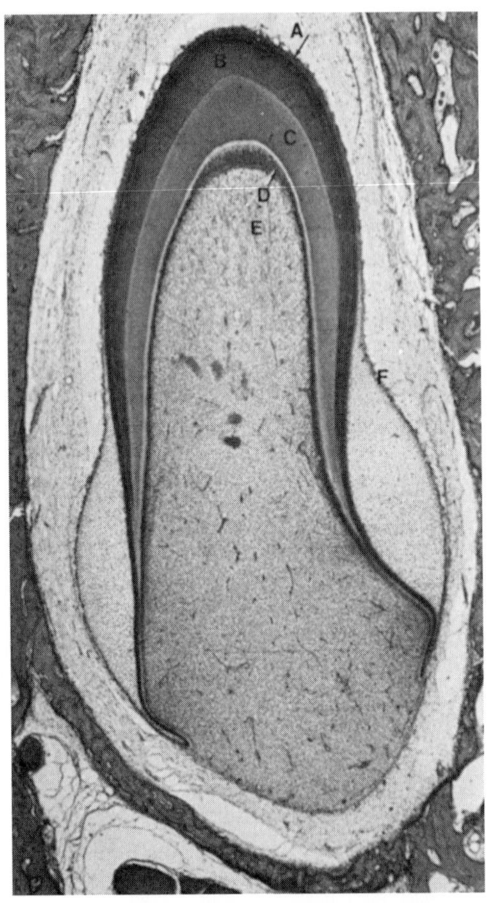

Figure 10.21. *Developing permanent tooth (dog). Ameloblasts (A); enamel (B); dentin (C); odontoblasts (D); dental pulp (E); outer enamel epithelium (F) (×25). (Courtesy of A. Hansen.)*

SALIVARY GLANDS

General Characteristics

The salivary glands comprise a series of secretory units (glandular epithelium) that originate from the oral ectoderm and grow into the underlying mesoderm as large aggregates of compound glands (see Chapter 2). The **major salivary glands** include the parotid, mandibular, and sublingual glands. The **minor salivary glands** are named according to their location, e.g., labial, lingual, buccal, palatine, molar (cats), and zygomatic (carnivores).

Saliva is a mixture of both serous and mucous secretory products of salivary glands. It is important in the moistening of the ingested food and the lubrication of the surface of the upper digestive organs, thus enhancing the flow of ingesta into the stomach. Saliva dissolves water-soluble components of food, thereby facilitating access to the taste buds. Consequently, the sense of taste is somewhat dependent on the saliva. Saliva in domestic mammals is considered to play only a minor role in the digestion of food before it reaches the stomach. Ruminants, however, produce a large volume of saliva, which is an important source of fluids in the rumen.

Parotid Salivary Gland

The parotid salivary gland in domestic mammals is predominantly serous, although occasional isolated mucous secretory units may occur in dogs and cats. Structurally, it is a compound acinar gland composed of numerous lobules separated by thin connective tissue septa. The lobule consists of acini formed by pyramid-

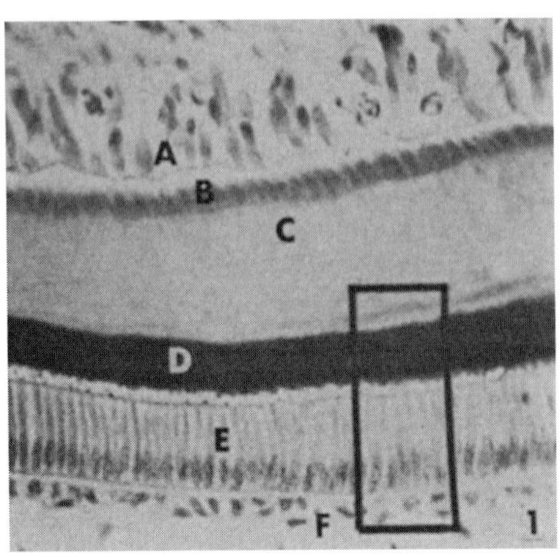

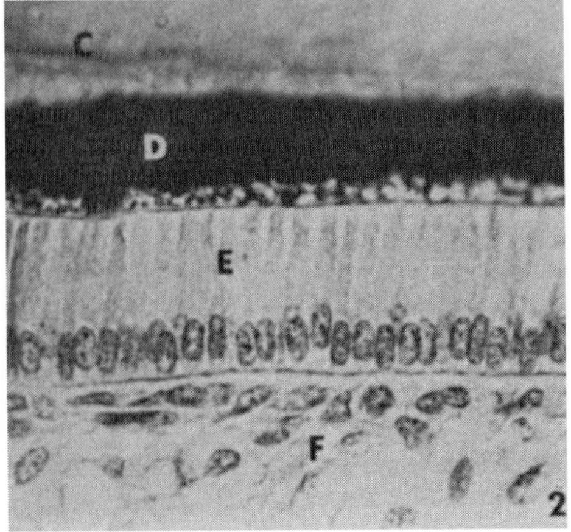

Figure 10.22. *Developing tooth (dog). **1.**, Odontoblasts (A); predentin (B); dentin (C); enamel (D); ameloblasts (E); stellate reticulum (F) (×200). **2.**, Area marked in **1**. Trichrome (×300).*

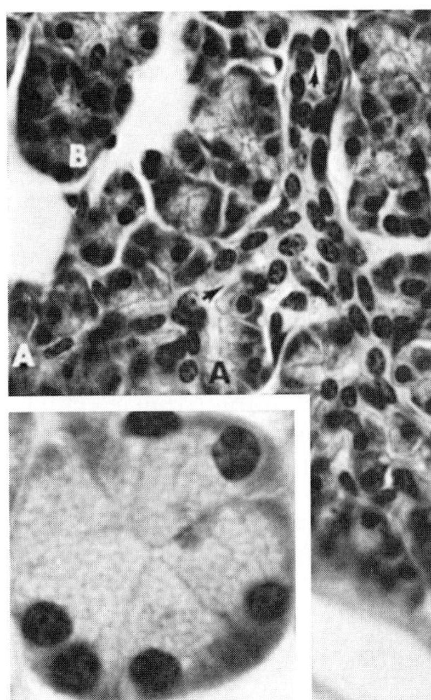

Figure 10.23. *Parotid salivary gland (horse). Serous acini (A) opening into intercalated ducts (arrows); serous acinus (B). Hematoxylin and eosin ((440). Inset: serous acinus. Hematoxylin and eosin (×1382).*

shaped cells with basal nuclei surrounded by basophilic cytoplasm (Fig. 10.23). The apex of each cell is filled with secretory granules, referred to as **zymogen granules**, containing precursors of digestive enzymes. Myoepithelial cells are located between the secretory cells and the basement membrane.

The narrow lumen of the acinus opens into a short **intercalated duct** lined by low cuboidal epithelium (see Fig. 2.16). The intercalated duct joins a large **striated or salivary duct** lined by simple columnar epithelium that is characterized by striations in the basal portion of the cells (Figs. 2.16 and 10.24). This appearance results from perpendicularly oriented mitochondria within numerous cytoplasmic compartments formed by deep infoldings of the basal cell membrane. This arrangement creates a large basal membrane surface area containing energy-requiring ion pumps located near energy-producing mitochondria, thus facilitating active transport of substances between the cells and the underlying tissue. The striated ducts are easily recognized as the largest structures within the lobule and participate in the secretory process. The striated ducts extend to the edge of the lobule, where they join **interlobular ducts** located in the connective tissue septa between lobules (see Fig. 2.16).

Interlobular ducts are lined by simple columnar epithelium, which changes to stratified columnar epithelium as the ducts become larger and fuse with similar ducts draining other lobules. The interlobular ducts converge to form the parotid duct. The epithelium changes from stratified columnar to stratified squamous where the parotid duct opens into the vestibule of the oral cavity.

Mandibular Salivary Gland

The mandibular salivary gland is a seromucous (mixed) compound tubuloacinar gland. The morphologic structure of the secretory unit is somewhat variable from one species to another but generally consists of a tubular unit with an enlarged terminal acinus. Mucus-secreting cells border the lumen of the tubule and acinus, and serous demilunes occur at the periphery (Fig. 10.25). The serous secretory product reaches the lumen through

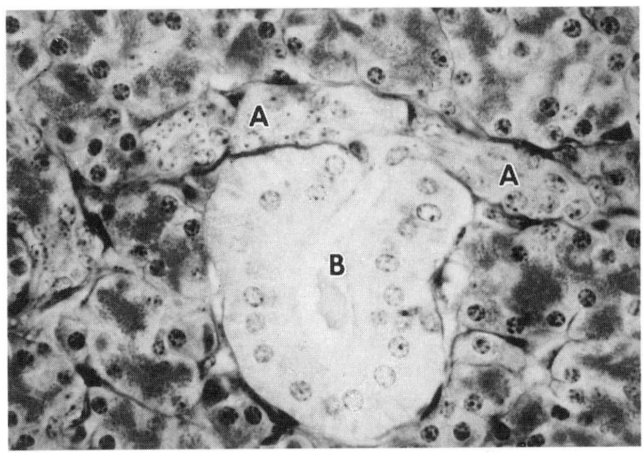

Figure 10.24. *Parotid salivary gland (horse). Intercalated ducts (A) joining striated duct (B). Hematoxylin and eosin (×425).*

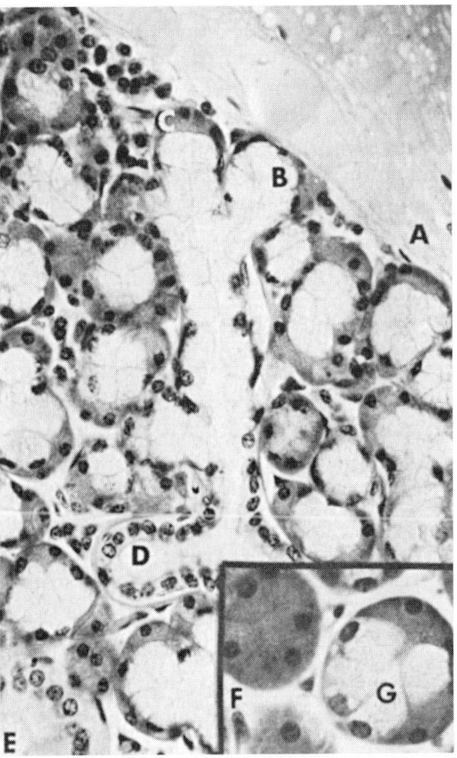

Figure 10.25. *Mandibular salivary gland (horse). Capsule (A); mucous acinus (B) and serous demilunes (C); intercalated duct (D); striated duct (E). Hematoxylin and eosin (×384). Inset: serous acinus (F); mixed acinus (G). Hematoxylin and eosin (×530).*

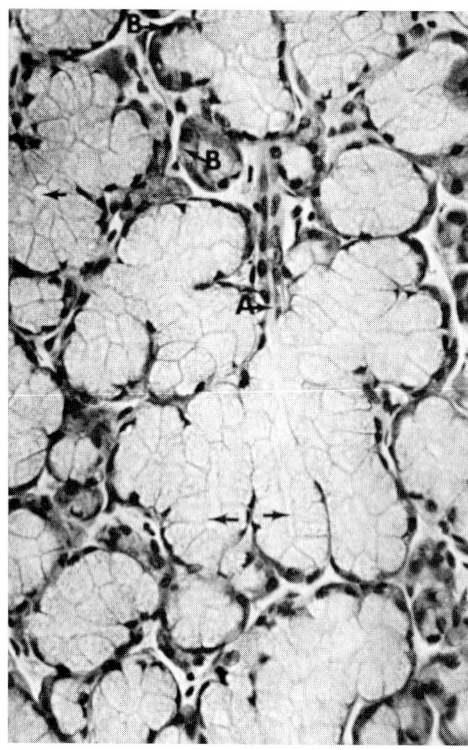

Figure 10.26. *Sublingual salivary gland (dog). Mucous acini with lumina (arrows) emptying into intercalated duct (A); serous demilunes (B). Hematoxylin and eosin (×280).*

intercellular canaliculi between the mucous cells. Variations in this basic pattern may include separate serous and mucous acini or mucous tubular units with enlarged, serous, acinar end pieces. In dogs and cats, the mucous elements predominate. **Myoepithelial cells** are present around the secretory units (see Fig. 2.17). The duct system is like that of the parotid salivary gland. In the epithelium of the main duct, goblet cells may occur.

Sublingual Salivary Gland

Like the mandibular salivary gland, the sublingual salivary gland is also a seromucous (mixed) compound tubuloacinar gland (Fig. 10.26). The number of mucous acini and serous demilunes and the seromucous nature of their secretory product varies among species. Sublingual glands of cattle, sheep, and pigs are almost entirely mucous, with relatively few serous demilunes. In addition to the typical mucous acini and demilunes, the glands of dogs and cats contain clusters of serous acini with periodic acid-Schiff (PAS)-positive granules in their basal portion (Fig. 10.27). The mucous cells form tubular secretory units that connect the serous acini with intercalated ducts. Striated and intercalated ducts are present, but not prominent, in cats and dogs. In horses, ruminants, and pigs, however, they are well developed. The interlobular ducts have, at their origin, a low simple columnar epithelium that increases in height and becomes two-layered in larger ducts. The main duct is lined with stratified cuboidal epithelium, and goblet cells occur in cattle and pigs.

Minor Salivary Glands

Clusters of serous, seromucous, or mucous minor salivary glands, occurring throughout the oral cavity, are generally named according to their location. The **lingual glands** are located in the propria submucosa and between the intrinsic muscle bundles of the tongue. The **gustatory glands**, associated with the vallate and foliate papillae (Fig. 10.10), are entirely serous and their ducts open into the sulcus at the base of the papillae. The **labial**, **buccal**, **palatine**, and **pharyngeal glands** also contribute mucous and serous secretory products to the saliva. Histologically, the secretory units resemble those of the major salivary glands and occur in a variety of forms, i.e., acinar, tubuloacinar, or tubular. Mucous tubules and acini frequently have serous demilunes associated with them; however, striated ducts are not characteristic of the minor salivary glands. The duct system is lined with simple cuboidal epithelium within the lobules and two-layered cuboidal epithelium in the larger interlobular ducts. The stratification of the duct epithelium increases as it reaches the oral cavity, where it changes to a stratified squamous type.

Among the domestic species, the **zygomatic salivary gland** is present only in carnivores. The parenchyma is composed of long, branched tubuloacinar secretory units that are predominantly mucus-secreting (Fig. 10.28). Intercalated and striated ducts are almost nonexistent. The interlobular and main ducts are similar to those of the other glands.

The **molar salivary gland** of cats is histologically similar to the zygomatic salivary gland. It is a compound tubuloacinar gland that is predominantly mucus-secret-

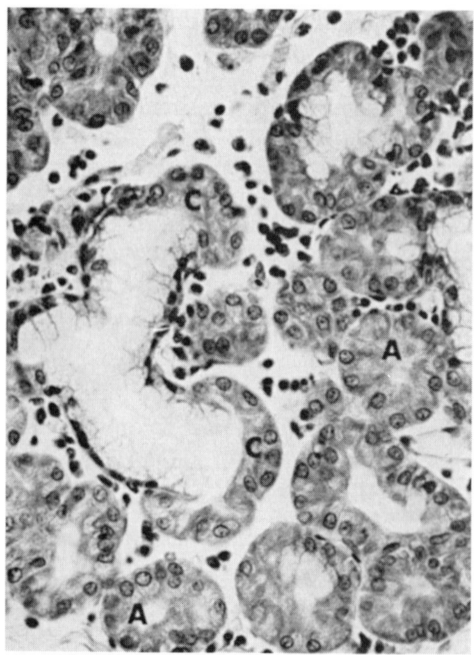

Figure 10.27. *Sublingual salivary gland (dog). Serous acini (A); serous demilunes (C) on tubular mucous secretory unit. Hematoxylin and eosin (×275).*

ing. Intercalated and striated ducts are not present, and the interlobular ducts have a two-layered cuboidal epithelium. Several main ducts empty into the vestibule of the oral cavity opposite the molar teeth.

PHARYNX

The pharynx connects the oral cavity to the esophagus and contains openings to the oral cavity (**oropharynx**), nasal cavity and auditory tubes (**nasopharynx**), and larynx (**laryngopharynx**). A mucosa, a tunica muscularis of skeletal muscle, and an adventitia make up the wall. The mucosa is lined by a stratified squamous epithelium, except for a portion of the nasopharynx, which is lined by a ciliated, pseudostratified columnar epithelium. A lamina muscularis is absent. The propria-submucosa contains collagen and elastic fibers intermingled with lymphatic tissue and mucous glands. The tunica muscularis consists entirely of skeletal muscle. The adventitia is dense irregular connective tissue that attaches the pharynx to the surrounding tissue.

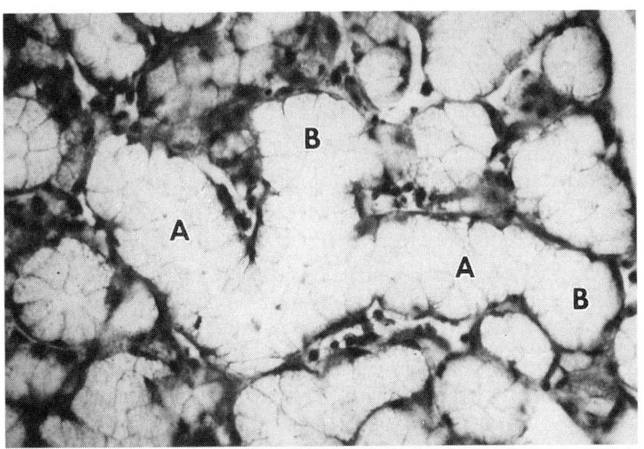

Figure 10.28. *Zygomatic salivary gland (dog). Mucous tubules (A); mucous acini (B). Hematoxylin and eosin (×300).*

ESOPHAGUS

The esophagus (Table 10.1) joins the laryngopharynx with the stomach and contains all the layers of a typical tubular organ of the digestive system (Fig. 10.1). An internal annular fold, the **pharyngoesophageal limen**, marks the junction of the laryngopharynx and esophagus in carnivores.

The mucosa is composed of three layers: a stratified squamous epithelium, a lamina propria, and a lamina muscularis. The degree of keratinization of the stratified squamous epithelium varies with the species. It is usually nonkeratinized in carnivores, slightly keratinized in pigs, more so in horses, and keratinized to a high degree in ruminants. The lamina propria consists largely of a dense feltwork of fine collagen fibers with an

Table 10.1.
Characteristics of the Esophagus

	Horses	*Pigs*	*Cattle*	*Goats*	*Sheep*	*Dogs*	*Cats*
Stratified squamous epithelium[a]	Keratinized	Keratinized	Keratinized	Keratinized	Keratinized	Nonkeratinized	Nonkeratinized
Lamina propria papillae	+	+	+	‡	+	—	—
Lamina muscularis	[b]	Absent in cranial part. Highly developed in caudal part.	[b]	[b]	[b]	Absent in cranial part. Interrupted in middle part.	[b]
Submucosal glands	[c]	More abundant in cranial than in caudal half.	[c]	[c]	[c]	Present throughout and extends into stomach.	[c]
Tunica muscularis[d]	Cranial two-thirds striated. Caudal one-third smooth.	Cranial part striated. Middle part mixed. Caudal part smooth.	Striated throughout and extends into the reticular sulcus.			Striated throughout.	Cranial part striated. Caudal one-third to one-fifth is smooth.
Tunica adventitia	Loose connective tissue cells and fibers with blood and lymph vessels and nerves surround the esophagus. A tunica serosa may be present in the thoracic cavity (mediastinal pleura) or near the stomach (visceral peritoneum).						

[a] Related to character of food: coarse food, highly keratinized; soft food, slightly keratinized to nonkeratinized.
[b] Longitudinal only: isolated bundles of smooth muscle near pharynx, increases in thickness near stomach.
[c] Present only at the pharyngoesophageal junction.
[d] Inner circular muscle layer becomes thicker at the cardiac ostium of the stomach (forming the cardiac sphincter muscle), especially in horses.

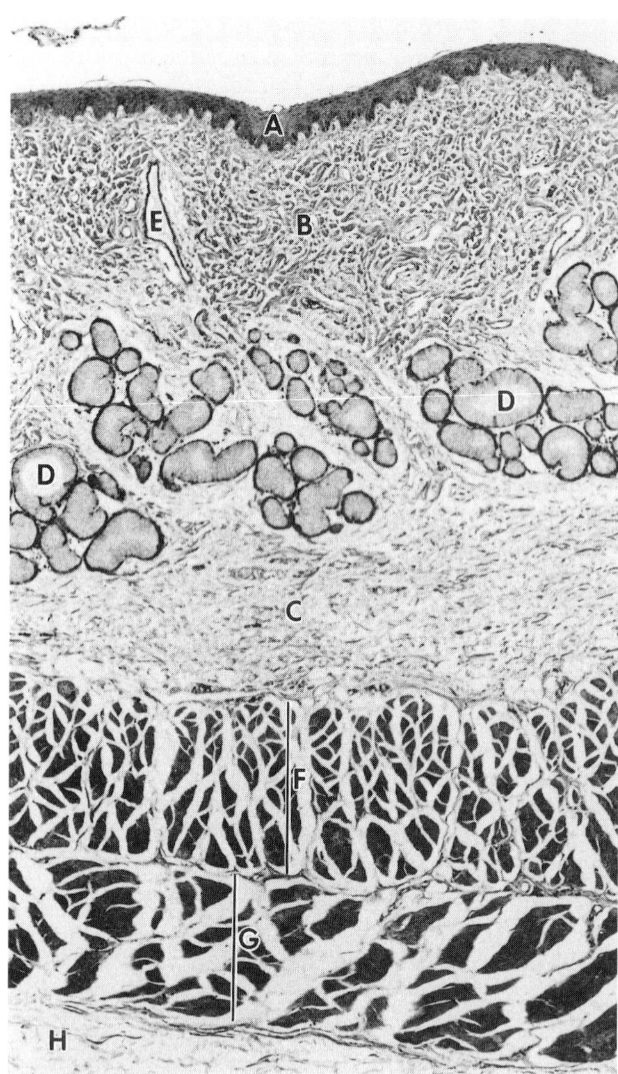

Figure 10.29. *Esophagus, midcervical region (dog). Nonkeratinized stratified squamous epithelium of the tunica mucosa (A); lamina propria of the tunica mucosa (B); submucosa (C); submucosal glands (D); submucosal gland duct (E); inner circular layer of the tunica muscularis (F); outer longitudinal layer of the tunica muscularis (G); adventitia (H). Note that a lamina muscularis is absent in this region of the canine esophagus. Hematoxylin and eosin (×88).*

abundance of evenly distributed elastic fibers; the esophagus is atypical in that the connective tissue of the lamina propria is more dense than the connective tissue of the submucosa (Fig. 10.29). The lamina muscularis contains only longitudinally oriented smooth muscle bundles. It is absent in the cranial end of the esophagus of pigs and dogs, but cats, horses, and ruminants have isolated smooth muscle bundles near the pharynx that increase in number and become confluent toward the stomach. In pigs, the lamina muscularis is especially well developed in the caudal end, where it is as thick as the outer layer of the tunica muscularis.

The submucosa is loose connective tissue containing large, longitudinally oriented arteries, veins, large lymph vessels, and nerves. Seromucous glands containing mucous acini with serous demilunes are present in this layer in pigs and dogs (Fig. 10.29). In pigs, the glands are abundant in the cranial half but do not extend into the caudal half, whereas in dogs, they are present throughout, extending into the cardiac gland region of the stomach. Density of the glands may be as much as four times greater near the stomach (caudally) than at the beginning of the organ (cranially). Glands are present only at the pharyngoesophageal junction in horses, cats, and ruminants. Mixed acini with serous demilunes occur in cattle. The loose nature of the submucosa allows the mucosa of the relaxed esophagus to form longitudinal folds.

The tunica muscularis of the esophagus consists of two layers of muscle. In ruminants and dogs, the tunica muscularis consists entirely of skeletal muscle (Fig. 10.29). In horses, skeletal muscle comprises the cranial two-thirds of the tunica muscularis but gradually changes to smooth muscle in the caudal third. The tunica muscularis of pigs is similar to that of horses except that the middle third has mixed smooth and skeletal muscle. In cats, the skeletal muscle may extend four-fifths of the length of the esophagus before changing to smooth muscle. At the cranial end of the esophagus, there is some interdigitation and spiraling of the two muscle layers, but more caudally, these layers change orientation to inner circular and outer longitudinal. The inner circular muscle layer thickens at the cardiac ostium of the stomach in all domestic mammals, forming the **cardiac sphincter muscle**. This muscle is especially prominent in horses, where it is 10 to 15 mm thick. In ruminants, skeletal muscle extends from the esophagus into the wall of the **reticular sulcus (groove)**.

In the cervical part of the esophagus, the tunica muscularis is surrounded by the adventitia, a loose connective tissue containing blood vessels, lymph vessels, and nerves (Fig. 10.29). The thoracic part of the esophagus is largely invested by a serosa (the mediastinal pleura) in most species. In horses, the abdominal part of the esophagus is approximately 2.5 cm in length and is also covered by a serosa (visceral peritoneum). In carnivores, the abdominal part is shorter but is also covered by visceral peritoneum, whereas in other species, the esophagus–stomach junction is at or near the diaphragm, and a mesothelial covering is lacking.

Esophagus–Stomach Junction

The morphologic characteristics of this junction vary considerably among species. In the carnivores, the junction of the stratified squamous epithelium of the esophagus with the simple columnar epithelium of the cardiac gland region is abrupt (Fig. 10.30). In cats, the junction is 3 to 5 mm cranial to the cardiac part (cardia) of the stomach, whereas in dogs, it is 1 to 2 cm cranial to the cardiac part. In horses and pigs, the stratified squamous epithelium extends throughout the nonglandular portion of the mucosa of the stomach, whereas in ruminants, it lines the entire forestomach. The glands of the esophagus may extend a short distance into the submucosa of the stomach in species in which they are present throughout the length of the esophagus. In species in which the skeletal muscle of the esophagus extends to the stomach (carnivores and ruminants), a gradual change from skeletal to smooth muscle occurs.

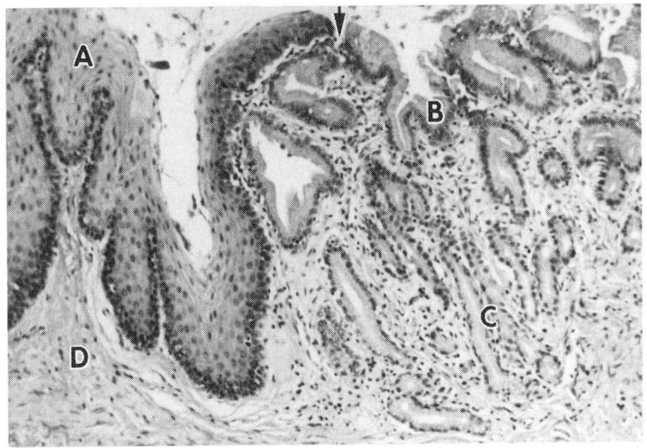

Figure 10.30. *Esophagus–stomach junction (dog). Epithelium of esophagus (A); epithelium of stomach (B); junction of nonkeratinized stratified squamous epithelium with simple columnar epithelium (arrowhead); cardiac glands (C); lamina propria (D). Hematoxylin and eosin (×180).*

STOMACH

The stomach is an enlarged part of the digestive tube specialized for initiating the enzymatic and hydrolytic breakdown of food into digestible nutrients. The tunica muscularis aids in mixing the ingesta with gastric secretions. The stomach is lined exclusively by a glandular mucosa in carnivores, whereas herbivorous animals have, in addition to a glandular region, a nonglandular region of the mucosa lined with stratified squamous epithelium.

The wall of the stomach has all the layers of a typical tubular organ (Fig. 10.31). The mucosa is composed of an epithelium, a lamina propria (of typical loose connective tissue), and a lamina muscularis. The submucosa contains collagen fibers, white adipose tissue, blood vessels, and the submucosal nerve plexus. The tunica muscularis has three layers: inner oblique, middle circular, and outer longitudinal. The myenteric plexus is located between the middle and outer muscle layers. The serosa is composed of mesothelium overlying a layer of loose connective tissue.

Nonglandular Region of the Tunica Mucosa

The nonglandular region of the mucosa is absent in carnivores and is small in pigs. In horses, the nonglandular region extends a considerable distance from the esophagus and ends at the **margo plicatus**. The nonglandular region reaches its greatest development in the ruminant stomach, where it lines the entire **forestomach**

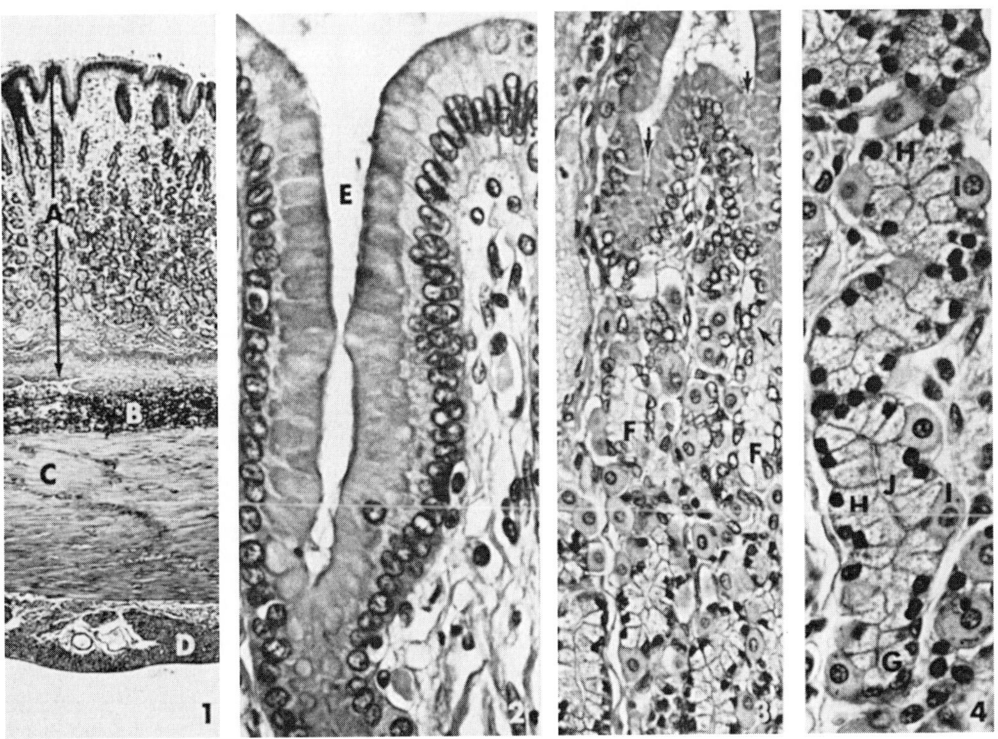

Figure 10.31. *Proper gastric (fundic) gland region of tunica mucosa, stomach (dog).* ***1.****, Section through proper gastric gland region. Trichrome (×48).* ***2.****, Gastric pit. Hematoxylin and eosin (×450).* ***3.****, Neck of proper gastric gland with mucous neck cells. Hematoxylin and eosin (×210).* ***4.****, Fundus of proper gastric gland with chief and parietal cells. Hematoxylin and eosin (×480). Tunica mucosa (A); tela submucosa (B); circular (C) and longitudinal (D) layers of tunica muscularis; gastric pit (E); gastric gland lumen opening into gastric pit (arrows); mucous neck cells (F); fundus of gastric gland (G); chief cells (H); parietal cells (I); gland lumen (J).*

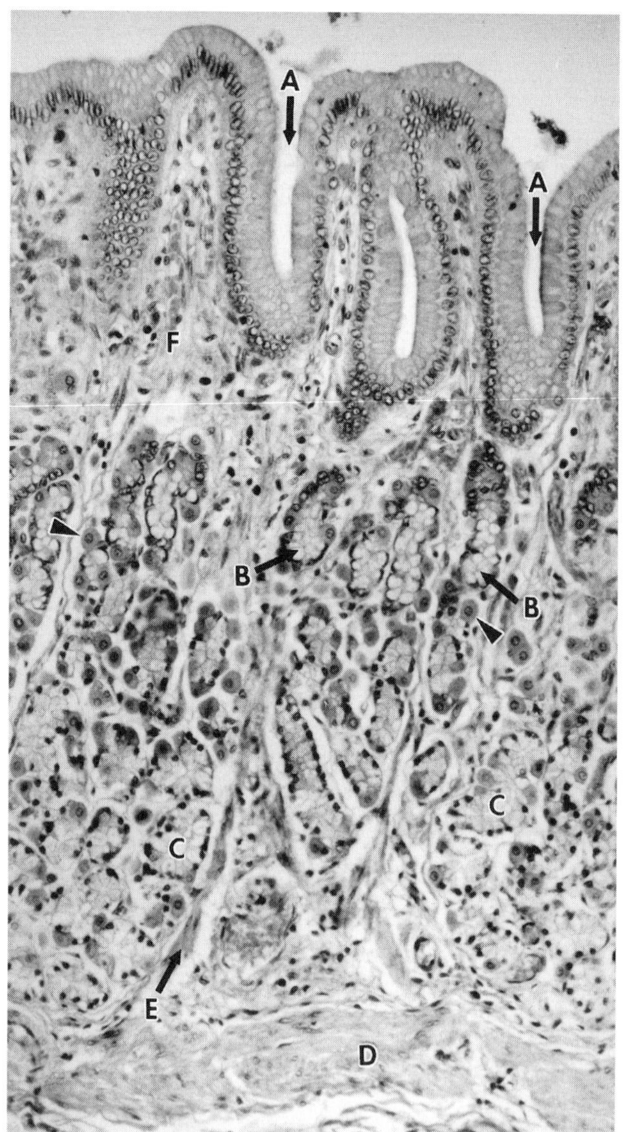

Figure 10.32. *Proper gastric gland region of tunica mucosa, stomach (dog). Gastric pits (A); mucous neck cells (B); chief cells (C); lamina muscularis (D); smooth muscle cells entering lamina propria (E); lamina propria (F); parietal cells (arrowheads). Hematoxylin and eosin (×180).*

(rumen, reticulum, and omasum) (Fig. 10.37). These parts are described in detail later in this chapter.

The lining epithelium of the nonglandular region of the mucosa is stratified squamous and may be keratinized, depending on species and diet. The lamina propria is composed of typical loose connective tissue. The lamina muscularis is distinct. The junction between the epithelial linings of the nonglandular and glandular regions of the mucosa is abrupt, with stratified squamous epithelium joining simple columnar epithelium.

Glandular Region of the Tunica Mucosa

The structure of the glandular region of the mucosa conforms to the general pattern described earlier. The mucosa has extensive folds (**gastric folds**), which flatten as the stomach fills. The surface is covered with small invaginations called **gastric pits**, which are continuous with the **gastric glands** and receive their secretory products (Figs. 10.31.2 and 10.32). The mucosal surface, including the gastric pits, is lined with tall simple columnar epithelial cells, the mucous secretory product of which is released continuously and serves as a protective coat that prevents digestion of the mucosa. The surface epithelial cells have a rapid turnover rate; within approximately 3 to 4 days, they are replaced by cells originating from mitosis in the gastric pit. The gastric glands are densely packed within the lamina propria (Figs. 10.31.3 and 10.32). The loose connective tissue in this area is often difficult to visualize because of the large amount of glandular epithelium. In carnivores, a layer of densely packed collagen fibers called the **stratum compactum** may be interposed between the bases of the gastric glands and the lamina muscularis (Fig. 10.33). The function of this layer may be to limit penetration of the stomach wall by sharp bones.

The lamina muscularis is relatively thick, usually comprising three layers (Fig. 10.33). Small bundles of smooth muscle cells extend into the mucosa, coursing between the gastric glands (Fig. 10.32).

The glandular region of the mucosa of the stomach is divided into three distinct smaller regions named according to the various glandular types present: **cardiac**, **proper gastric (fundic)**, and **pyloric**. The extent of the various glandular regions of the mucosa in the domestic mammals is illustrated in Figure 10.37.

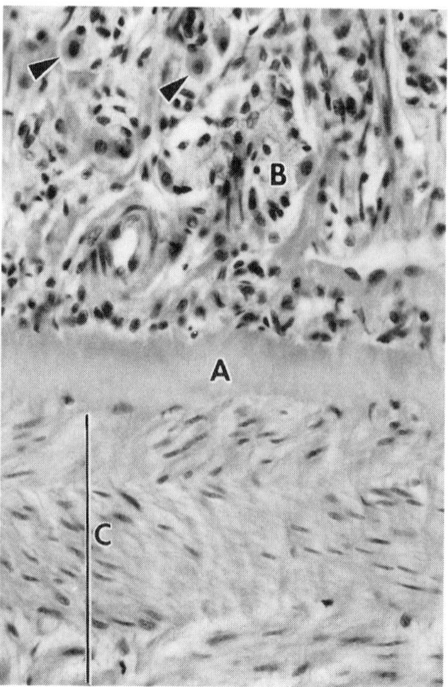

Figure 10.33. *Proper gastric gland region of tunica mucosa, stomach (cat). Stratum compactum of lamina propria (A); fundus of proper gastric gland (B); lamina muscularis (C); parietal cells (arrowheads). Hematoxylin and eosin (×355).*

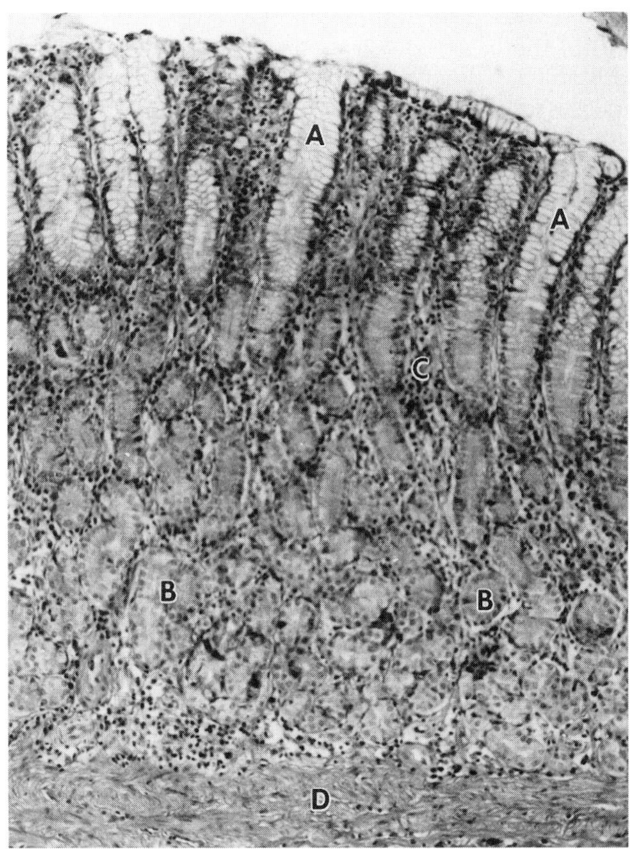

Figure 10.34. *Cardiac gland region of tunica mucosa, stomach (pig). Gastric pits (A); cardiac glands (B); lamina propria (C); lamina muscularis (D). Hematoxylin and eosin (×80).*

CARDIAC GLAND REGION

The cardiac gland region of the mucosa occupies a narrow strip at the junction of the glandular and nonglandular mucosae in all domestic mammals except pigs, in which it covers nearly half the stomach, including most of the **diverticulum ventriculi** (Fig. 10.37). The **cardiac glands** are relatively short, simple, branched, coiled tubular glands that release a mucous secretory product. The cells of the cardiac glands are cuboidal, and the nuclei are located in the basal portion of the cells. The cardiac glands empty into relatively shallow gastric pits (Fig. 10.34). Parietal cells (described below) may occur at the junction of the cardiac and proper gastric (fundic) gland regions.

PROPER GASTRIC (FUNDIC) GLAND REGION

The proper gastric (fundic) gland region of the mucosa is well developed in all domestic mammals (see Fig. 10.37). In carnivores, it occupies more than one-half of the stomach; in horses, it occupies more than one-third; and in pigs, it occupies approximately one-fourth. Two-thirds of the abomasum in ruminants is occupied by proper gastric glands. Also note in Figure 10.37 that this gland region actually occupies the fundus of the stomach only in dogs and cats, as in human beings; therefore, the term **proper gastric** is used to eliminate confusion as to location within the stomach.

Proper gastric glands are straight, branched tubular glands that extend to the lamina muscularis (Figs. 10.31.3 and 10.32). The gland consists of a short **neck**, a long **body**, and a slightly dilated blind end, the **fundus**. Four structurally and functionally distinct cell types comprise the secretory epithelium of the proper gastric gland: mucous neck cells, chief cells, parietal cells, and endocrine cells.

The **mucous neck cells** occupy the neck of the proper gastric gland (Figs. 10.31.3 and 10.32). They are typical mucous cells, with a flat nucleus located toward the cell base. They appear similar to the surface cells but have cytoplasm that is more basophilic. In addition, when treated with PAS, the mucous neck cells give an intensely positive reaction throughout, whereas the surface cells have PAS-positive material only in the upper two-thirds of the cell.

The **chief cells** are the most numerous of the gastric gland cells (Figs. 10.31.4 and 10.32). They are cuboidal or pyramidal, with a spherical nucleus near the base of the cell. The area between the nucleus and the free surface appears lacy owing to the clear spaces that remain after fixation. In the living state, zymogen granules occupy these vacuoles and are demonstrable with special fixation and staining. Thus, chief cells are also referred to as zymogen cells. The basal area of the chief cell has an extensive rough endoplasmic reticulum (rER), resulting in a basophilic staining reaction. Chief cells secrete **pepsinogen**, which is transformed into pepsin by hydrochloric acid.

The **parietal cells** are larger and less numerous than the chief cells. They have a tendency to occur singly and are peripheral to the chief cells (Figs. 10.31.4 and 10.32). Usually, only a narrow apex of the cell borders the gland lumen. Frequently, the base of the cell bulges outward from the external surface of the gland. The parietal cell has a spherical nucleus. The cytoplasm stains deeply with eosin and has a granular appearance due to the presence of numerous mitochondria. At the apex, the cell membrane invaginates to form a branching intracellular canaliculus that extends toward the center of the cell. Numerous microvilli of varying length project into the canaliculus, thereby providing an extensive surface area associated with the active transport system necessary for the production of free hydrochloric acid. Because parietal cells contain an abundance of carbonic anhydrase, it is believed that carbonic acid is formed, from which hydrogen ions are transported across the cell membrane and combine with chloride ions. Thus, free hydrochloric acid is formed within the canaliculus.

Throughout the glandular regions of the gastric mucosa and continuing into the small and large intestines is a series of **endocrine cells (enteroendocrine cells)** responsible for the production of gastrointestinal hormones, such as gastrin, secretin, cholecystokinin, and gastric inhibitory polypeptide. The hormone is released either into the blood or lymph vascular systems, where it circulates throughout the body or diffuses locally to its

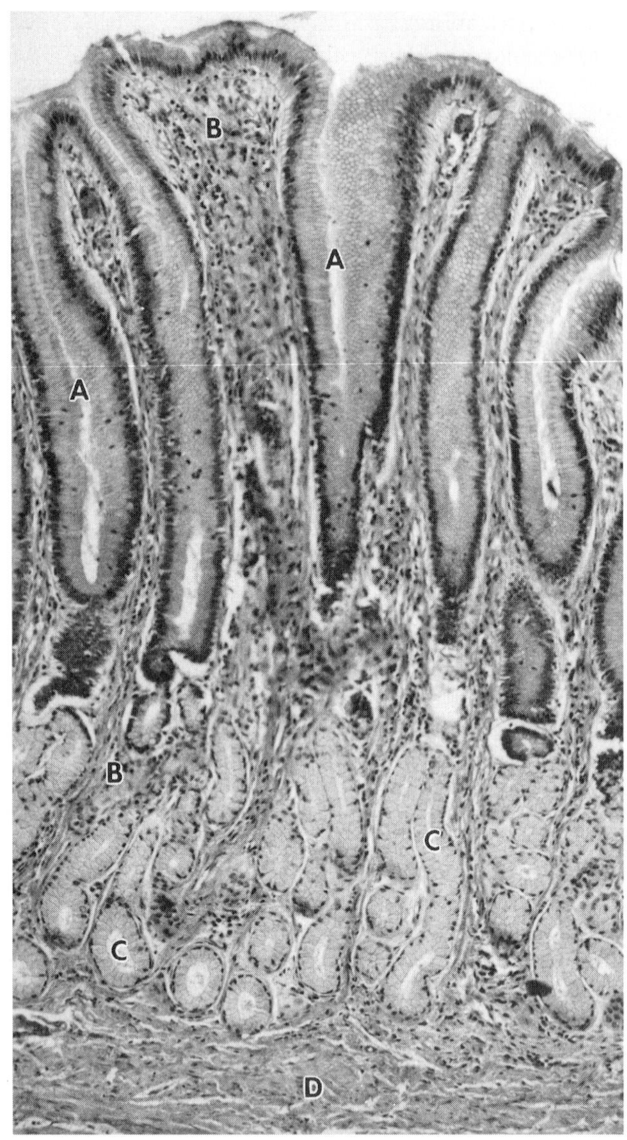

Figure 10.35. *Pyloric gland region of tunica mucosa, stomach (pig). Gastric pits (A); lamina propria (B); pyloric glands (C); lamina muscularis (D). Hematoxylin and eosin (×80).*

target cells, i.e., a paracrine mode of secretion. These cells are difficult to identify in routine hematoxylin and eosin sections and generally appear clear or poorly stained. Many of these cells demonstrate an affinity for silver stains and therefore have been referred to as **argentaffin cells** or **argyrophilic cells** (see Fig. 10.53). Some of these cells can also be demonstrated with potassium dichromate solutions and are therefore referred to as **enterochromaffin cells**. Most frequently, these cells are wedged between the basement membrane and the chief cells and do not reach the surface of the epithelium. Some of these cells, however, do extend to the lumen and are believed to monitor the luminal contents and respond with the release of hormones. At least 12 different endocrine cell types have been identified by electron microscopy in the gastrointestinal tract. They all possess numerous small membrane-bounded granules, mostly within the basal cytoplasm, and contain relatively little rER and small Golgi complexes. The endocrine cells of the gastrointestinal tract are part of a larger group of cells designated as amine precursor uptake and decarboxylation (APUD) cells (see Chapter 15).

PYLORIC GLAND REGION

The pyloric gland region of the mucosa occupies approximately one-half of the stomach in carnivores, but only one-third of the stomach in horses and one-third of the abomasum in ruminants. In pigs, the pyloric gland region is small, representing approximately one-fourth of the mucosa (see Fig. 10.37).

Pyloric glands are branched, coiled tubular glands that are relatively short compared to the other gastric glands (Fig. 10.35). The gastric pits are considerably deeper than those in the cardiac and proper gastric gland regions. The cells of the pyloric glands have the appearance of typical mucus-secreting cells with flat nuclei located at the base of the cell and a lightly stained apical cytoplasm.

At the pylorus–duodenum junction, **submucosal intestinal glands** extend into the submucosa of the pyloric gland region. The middle circular layer of the tunica muscularis thickens at the pylorus to form the **pyloric sphincter muscle**, which causes the submucosa and mucosa to bulge into the lumen. In ruminants and pigs, this protuberance, called the **torus pyloricus**, is especially prominent (Fig. 10.36).

Species Differences

In carnivores, the cardiac gland region is a relatively narrow area, with the proper gastric and pyloric gland regions occupying the remainder of the stomach. In dogs, the proper gastric gland region is divided into two zones. The light zone has a thinner mucosa with deep gastric pits and short tortuous glands that appear in groups and do not reach the lamina muscularis. The dark zone is adjacent to the pyloric gland region and has

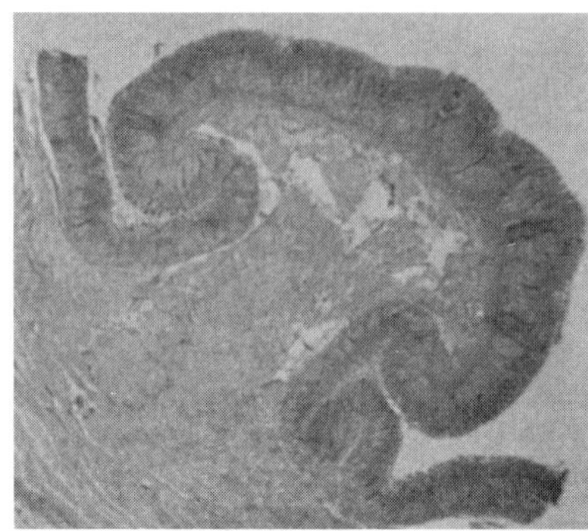

Figure 10.36. *Torus pyloricus, stomach (pig). Hematoxylin and eosin (×3.7). (From Dellmann H-D. Veterinary histology: an outline text–atlas. Philadelphia: Lea & Febiger, 1971.)*

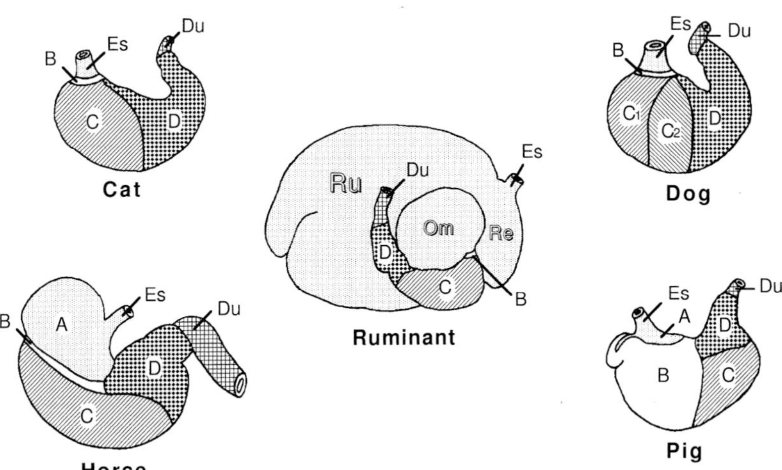

Figure 10.37. *Schematic drawing illustrating the regions of the gastric tunica mucosa. Nonglandular region of the mucosa lined by stratified squamous epithelium (A), including the rumen (Ru), reticulum (Re), and omasum (Om); cardiac gland region (B); fundic gland region (C), with light (C1) and dark (C2) zones in the dog; pyloric gland region (D); esophagus (Es); duodenum (Du).*

a thicker mucosa, shallow gastric pits, and proper gastric glands that more closely resemble those of the other species (Fig. 10.37).

The stomach of the pig has a very large cardiac gland region that contains numerous lymphatic nodules in the lamina propria. The parietal cells in the proper gastric gland region tend to occur in clusters.

The stomach of the horse has an extensive nonglandular region of the mucosa that terminates abruptly, forming the **margo plicatus**. The cardiac gland region is almost nonexistent, whereas the proper gastric and pyloric gland regions follow the normal pattern.

Ruminant Stomach

The stomach of ruminants is composed of four structurally distinct parts. The first three parts (the rumen, reticulum, and omasum) are collectively called the **forestomach** or **proventriculus** (Fig. 10.37). The forestomach is lined entirely by a nonglandular mucosa having a keratinized stratified squamous epithelium. The fourth part of the ruminant stomach, the **abomasum**, is lined by a glandular mucosa that is similar to the stomach of other species.

The forestomach is effective in breaking down the coarse, fibrous ingesta into absorbable nutrients by both mechanical and chemical action. The rumen acts as a fermentation vat where a large population of bacteria and protozoa act on the ingesta, thereby producing short-chain, volatile fatty acids, which are then absorbed through the mucosa into the blood. The reticulum and omasum exert a mechanical action on the ingesta that reduces the mass to fine particles. The wall of the omasum is especially well adapted for this function. In addition to fermentation and mechanical activities, considerable absorption occurs across the keratinized stratified squamous epithelium of all three portions of the forestomach. The enzymatic digestive processes in the abomasum further degrade the ingesta, along with accompanying microorganisms, to such substances as glucose and amino acids in a manner similar to that of the stomach of nonruminants.

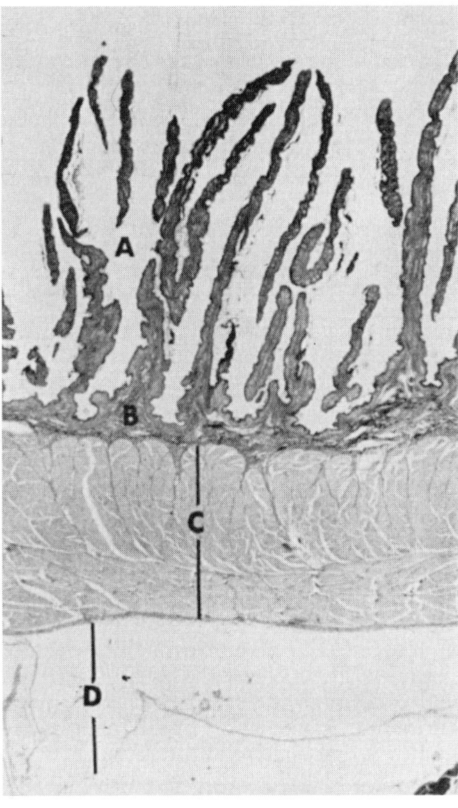

Figure 10.38. *Rumen (large ruminant). Papillae (A); propria-submucosa (B); tunica muscularis (C); tunica serosa (D). Hematoxylin and eosin (×7). (From Stinson AW, Brown EM. Veterinary histology slide sets. East Lansing, MI: Michigan State University, Instructional Media Center, 1970.)*

RUMEN

The mucosa of the rumen is characterized by small tongue-shaped **papillae** (Figs. 10.38 and 10.39), the size and shape of which vary considerably from one region of the rumen to another. They develop prenatally and remain small as long as the animal is on a milk diet. When roughage is included in the diet and fermenta-

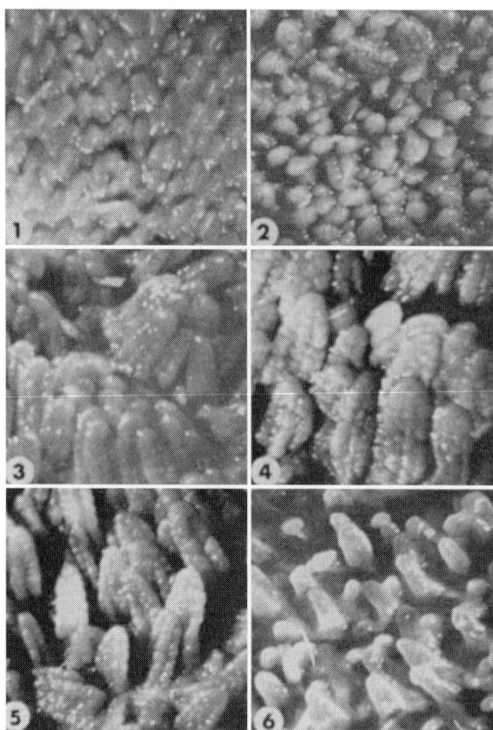

Figure 10.39. *Changes in ruminal papillae caused by age and diet (same steer) (×2). **1.**, Six months of age, milk since birth. Papillae are rudimentary. **2.**, Hay and grain for 3 weeks. Papillae are enlarged. **3.**, Hay and grain for 2 months. **4.**, Hay and grain for 3 months. Papillae have reached maximal length. **5.**, After return to milk diet for 3 days. Papillae are smaller. **6.**, After return to milk diet for 10 days. Papillae are strikingly reduced. (From Stinson AW, Brown EM. Veterinary histology slide sets. East Lansing, MI: Michigan State University, Instructional Media Center, 1970.)*

tion begins in the rumen, the papillae increase rapidly in size (Fig. 10.39).

The ruminal epithelium is keratinized stratified squamous and performs at least three important functions: protection, metabolism, and absorption (Figs. 10.40 and 10.41). The stratum corneum forms a protective shield against the rough, fibrous ingesta, whereas the deeper strata metabolize short-chain, volatile fatty acids, particularly butyric, acetic, and propionic acids, the chief products of fermentation. Sodium, potassium, ammonia, urea, and many other products are also absorbed from the ruminal contents.

The **stratum corneum** varies in thickness from one to two cells to as many as 10 to 20 cells. Stainable nuclei may or may not be present. The **stratum granulosum** is usually one to three cells thick. The cells are distinctly flattened, and keratohyalin granules are present in the cytoplasm. The cells of the stratum granulosum near the stratum corneum are frequently swollen and are characterized by a pyknotic nucleus surrounded by clear, electron-lucent cytoplasm. The peripheral cytoplasm of these cells contains keratohyalin granules, tonofilaments, and numerous membrane-bound, electron-dense granules (Fig. 10.41). The **stratum spinosum** consists of polyhedral cells that are slightly larger than the basal cells (Fig. 10.41). The thickness of this layer varies considerably from 1 to 10 cells. The cytologic features of these cells include numerous mitochondria and ribosomes distributed throughout the cytoplasm. Adjacent cells are connected through numerous desmosomes (Fig. 10.41). The cells of the **stratum basale** are columnar and extend numerous processes to the basement membrane, which greatly increases the basal cell membrane surface area. The cytologic features of the basal cells are similar to those of the stratum spinosum.

The intercellular spaces throughout the entire epithelium are distended to varying degrees. The spaces may be wide and contain flocculent material that is passing through the epithelium (Fig. 10.41), or in other areas, they may be collapsed with no flocculent material present, thus reflecting a period of little or no movement of material across the epithelium.

A lamina muscularis is absent; thus, the lamina propria blends with the submucosa, forming a propria-submucosa. Each papilla has a core (an extension of the propria-submucosa) containing a dense feltwork of collagen, elastic, and reticular fibers. A dense network of fenestrated capillaries lies just beneath the basement membrane of the epithelium. Near the tunica muscularis, the connective tissue of the propria-submucosa is more loosely arranged. A network of blood vessels and the submucosal plexus is located within this layer.

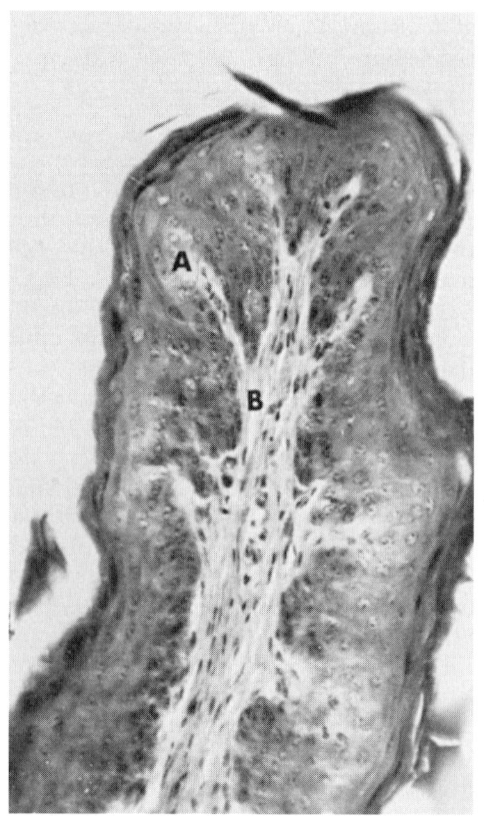

Figure 10.40. *Tip of ruminal papilla (large ruminant). Keratinized stratified squamous epithelium (A); lamina propria (B). Hematoxylin and eosin (×250). (From Stinson AW, Brown EM. Veterinary histology slide sets. East Lansing, MI: Michigan State University, Instructional Media Center, 1970.)*

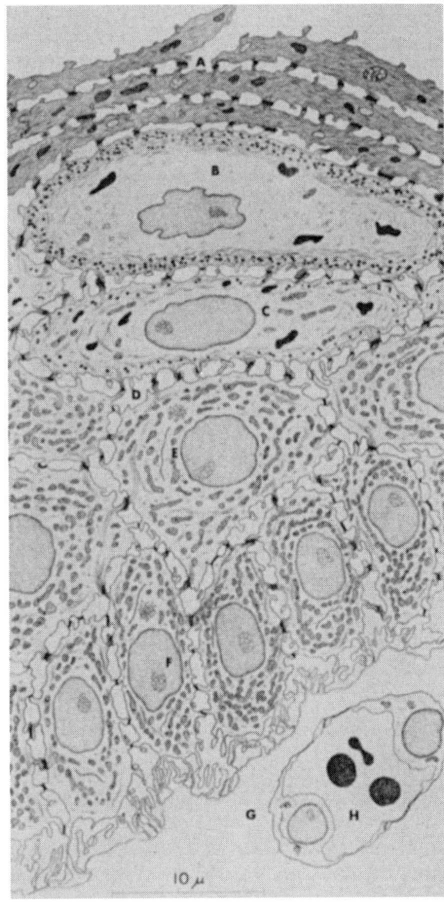

Figure 10.41. *Drawing from an electron micrograph of ruminal epithelium. Stratum corneum (A); swollen cells of the stratum granulosum (B); flat cells of the stratum granulosum (C); intercellular canaliculi (D); stratum spinosum with desmosomes (E); stratum basale (F); lamina propria (G); capillary in lamina propria (H). (From Stinson AW, Brown EM. Veterinary histology slide sets. East Lansing, MI: Michigan State University, Instructional Media Center, 1970.)*

The tunica muscularis is composed of inner circular and outer longitudinal layers of smooth muscle. The myenteric plexus is located between the layers.

The serosa of the rumen is a loose connective tissue covered by a mesothelium. Varying amounts of white adipose tissue, as well as blood vessels, lymph vessels, and nerves, are located in the loose connective tissue of the serosa.

RETICULUM AND RETICULAR SULCUS

The reticulum has a mucosa with permanent interconnecting folds, the **reticular crests**, giving it the appearance of a honeycomb (Fig. 10.42). These crests are of two different heights. The taller crests separate the mucosal surface into shallow compartments, the **reticular cells**, which are further divided into smaller areas by the shorter crests. The sides of the crests have vertical ridges, and the mucosa between the crests is covered by conical **reticular papillae** that project into the lumen.

The keratinized stratified squamous epithelium resembles that of the rumen. The propria-submucosa consists predominantly of a feltwork of collagen and elastic fibers. A lamina muscularis is located only in the upper part of the larger reticular crests; therefore, the lamina propria and the submucosa blend imperceptibly. The lamina muscularis is continuous with that of the esophagus (Fig. 10.43). The smooth muscle bundles pass from one crest into another where the crests intersect, thus forming a continuous network of smooth muscle throughout the reticular mucosa.

The tunica muscularis consists of two layers of smooth muscle cells that follow an oblique course and cross at right angles. The serosa is like that of the rumen.

The **reticular sulcus** (groove) begins at the cardiac ostium and passes ventrally on the medial wall of the reticulum to end at the reticulo-omasal ostium. The sulcus is bordered by two thick folds, the labia (lips).

The entire sulcus is lined by keratinized stratified squamous epithelium (Fig. 10.44). The propria submucosa consists predominantly of collagen and elastic fibers. The lamina muscularis, an extension of the esophageal lamina muscularis, is incomplete and is

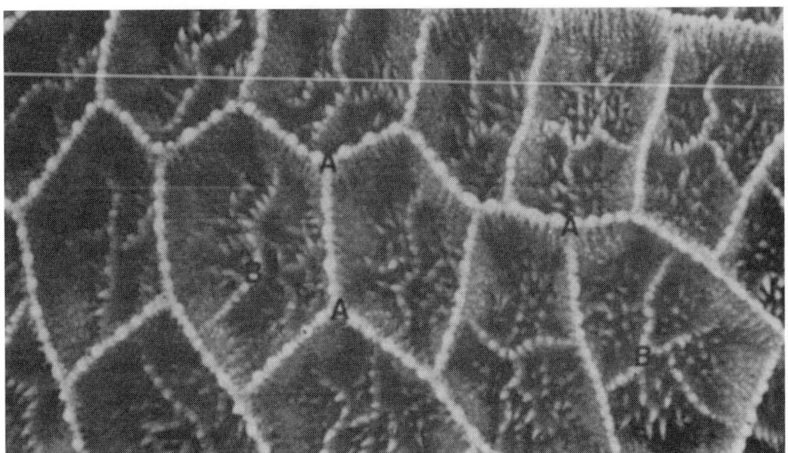

Figure 10.42. *Surface view of the reticulum mucosa. Primary crests (A) delineating the reticular cells; secondary crests (B). (Courtesy of A. Hansen.)*

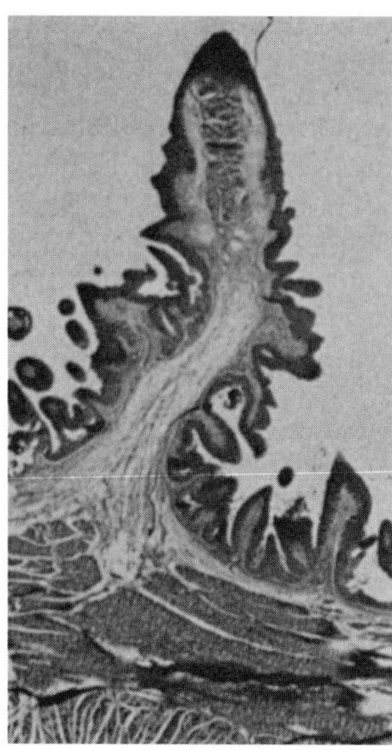

Figure 10.43. *Reticulum (large ruminant). Cross section through a primary crest with condensed lamina muscularis in the upper portion. Hematoxylin and eosin (×9.5). (From Dellmann H-D. Veterinary histology: an outline text–atlas. Philadelphia: Lea & Febiger, 1971.)*

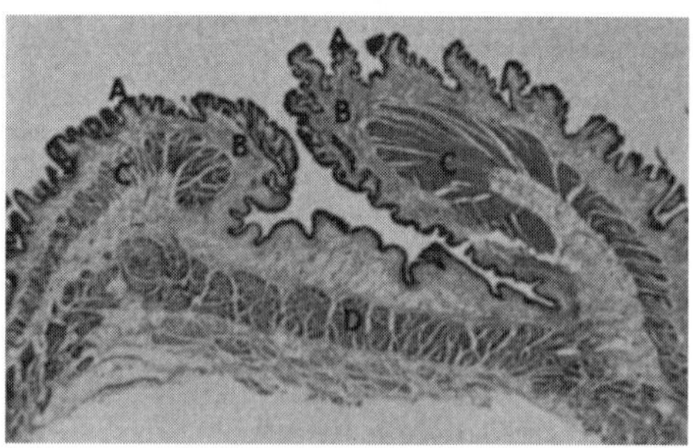

Figure 10.44. *Reticular sulcus (large ruminant). Keratinized stratified squamous epithelium covering the reticular papillae (A); lamina propria blending with the submucosa between scattered small bundles of the lamina muscularis (B); longitudinal musculature of the labia (C); transverse musculature of the floor (D). Hematoxylin and eosin (×12). (From Dellmann H-D. Veterinary histology: an outline text–atlas. Philadelphia: Lea & Febiger, 1971.)*

most conspicuous in the labia of the sulcus. It forms a complete layer near the omasum.

The tunica muscularis of the reticular sulcus is composed largely of smooth muscle fibers. Skeletal muscle fibers from the tunica muscularis of the esophagus are present near the cardiac ostium but fade out rapidly in the sulcus. Both longitudinally and transversely oriented smooth muscle fibers are found in the floor of the sulcus, whereas the labia contain mainly longitudinally oriented smooth muscle fibers. The longitudinal muscle fibers in the labia form a loop around the cardiac ostium corresponding to the cardiac loop of animals with simple stomachs. At the ventral end of the reticular sulcus, the muscle fibers pass into the sphincter of the reticulo-omasal ostium. In the young animal, the smooth muscle layers of the labia contract reflexly during suckling. As a result, the edges of the labia come together to create a channel that allows milk to bypass the reticulum and rumen. The milk passes through a very short omasal groove directly into the abomasum. The serosa of the reticulum is similar to that of the other parts of the forestomach.

OMASUM

The omasum is nearly filled with approximately 100 longitudinal folds, the **laminae**, that arise from the internal surface of the greater curvature and sides of the organ (Fig. 10.45). The largest laminae, approximately 12 in number, have a thick, concave, free edge that reaches to within a short distance of the lesser curvature. Second, third, fourth, and fifth orders of shorter laminae progressively decrease in length. The omasal contents are pressed into thin layers in the narrow spaces between the laminae (**interlaminar recesses**) and are reduced to a fine pulp by the numerous rounded, horny **omasal papillae** that stud the surface of the mucosa. The papillae are directed so that the movement of the laminae works the solid contents from the reticulo-omasal ostium into the interlaminar recesses and out at the omaso-abomasal ostium.

The lining is keratinized stratified squamous epithelium, and the aglandular lamina propria contains a dense subepithelial capillary network. A lamina muscularis forms a thick layer just beneath the lamina propria on both sides of the laminae. The submucosa is very thin.

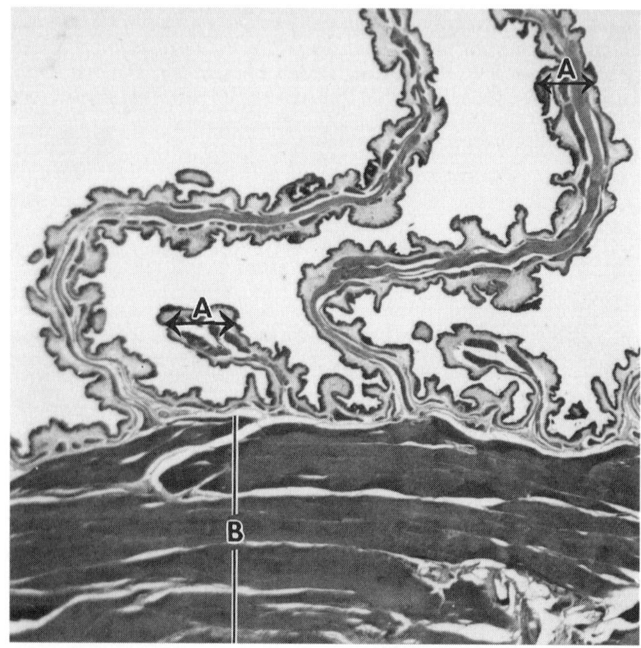

Figure 10.45. *Omasum (large ruminant). Portion of the wall including laminae of different sizes (A); tunica muscularis (B). Large laminae are penetrated by an extension of the tunica muscularis, whereas the smaller laminae have muscle originating from the lamina muscularis only. Hematoxylin and eosin (×6.5).*

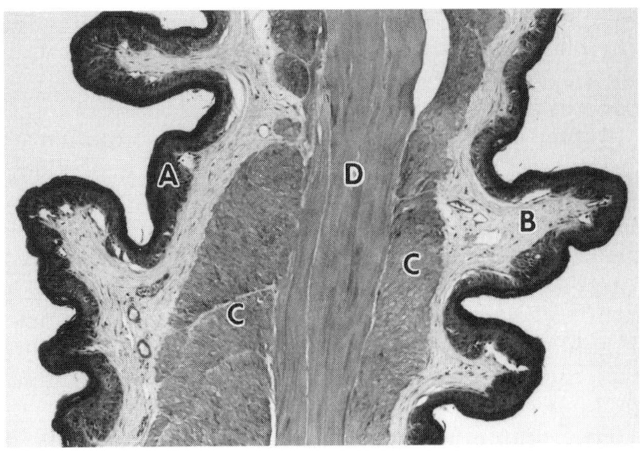

Figure 10.46. *Omasum (large ruminant). Portion of a large lamina containing three layers of muscle. Keratinized stratified squamous epithelium (A); lamina propria (B); lamina muscularis (C); extension of inner circular layer of tunica muscularis (D). Hematoxylin and eosin (×47).*

The tunica muscularis is composed of a thin, outer longitudinal layer and a thicker, inner circular layer of smooth muscle. The innermost fibers of the circular layer are continued into the large omasal laminae (first through third orders) as the intermediate muscle sheet (Fig. 10.46).

ABOMASUM

The omaso-abomasal ostium is marked by two mucosal folds, the **vela abomasica**, where the epithelium changes abruptly from keratinized stratified squamous to simple columnar. In cattle, this change is on the apex of the folds, whereas in small ruminants, the change occurs on the omasal side. The lamina propria becomes less dense on the abomasal side of the folds and frequently exhibits a lymphatic nodule beneath the epithelial junction. The mucosa of the abomasum has all the characteristic glandular regions of the stomach described previously (Fig. 10.37).

SMALL INTESTINE

The small intestine is divided into three parts: the **duodenum**, **jejunum**, and **ileum**. Intestinal digestion, or reduction of food to an absorbable form, begins when the contents from the stomach are acted on by the pancreatic secretions, bile, and intestinal secretions, and it continues throughout the length of the small intestine.

The digestive and absorptive functions of the small intestine are facilitated by several specialized structures. The digestive functions require voluminous amounts of digestive enzymes in addition to a copious supply of mucus to protect the lining cells from mechanical injury and irritating compounds. The enzymes are membrane-bound at the microvillous luminal surface of the columnar absorptive cells and are also provided by the pancreas. Mucus is produced by submucosal glands in the small intestine (Figs. 10.47 and 10.51) and by goblet cells, which are intermingled with the columnar absorptive cells throughout the entire intestine (Figs. 10.49 and 10.50).

The efficiency of the absorptive function is enhanced by three structural features that increase the surface area exposed to the intestinal contents. *(a)* The upper two-thirds of the small intestine has circularly disposed mucosal folds (**plicae circulares**) extending approximately two-thirds of the way around the lumen. In ruminants, these folds are permanent, but in all other domestic mammals, they disappear when the organ is distended (Fig. 10.47). *(b)* The surface of the mucosa is covered with fingerlike projections, the intestinal **villi** (Figs. 10.48 and 10.49). The villi vary in length, depending on the region of the small intestine and the

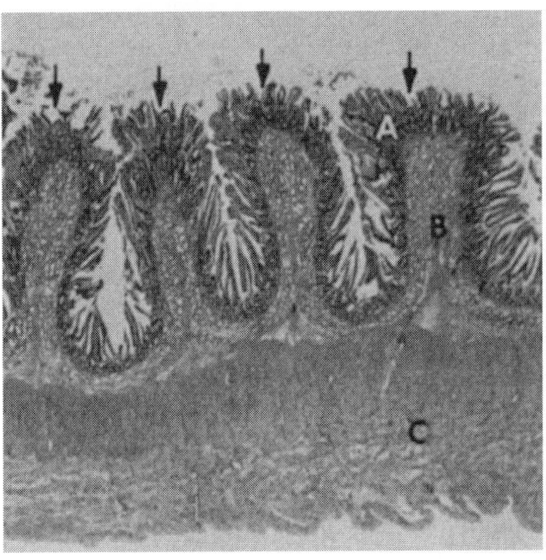

Figure 10.47. *Longitudinal section of duodenum, large ruminant. Circular folds (plicae circulares) (arrows). Mucosa (A); submucosal glands (B); tunica muscularis (C). Hematoxylin and eosin (×42).*

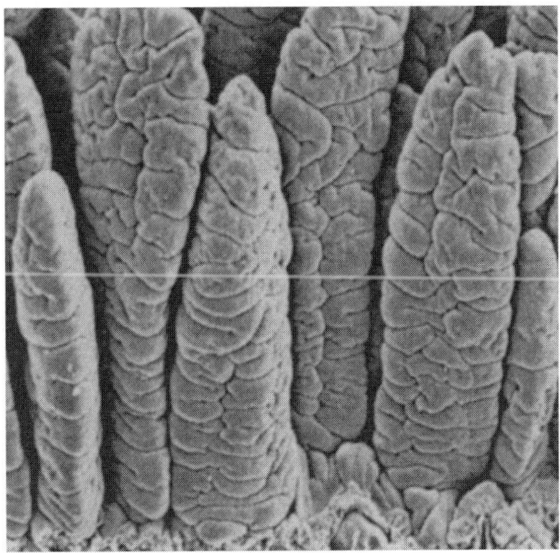

Figure 10.48. *Scanning electron micrograph of intestinal villi, ileum (calf). These villi are in a contracted state (×85). (Courtesy of J.F. Pohlenz.)*

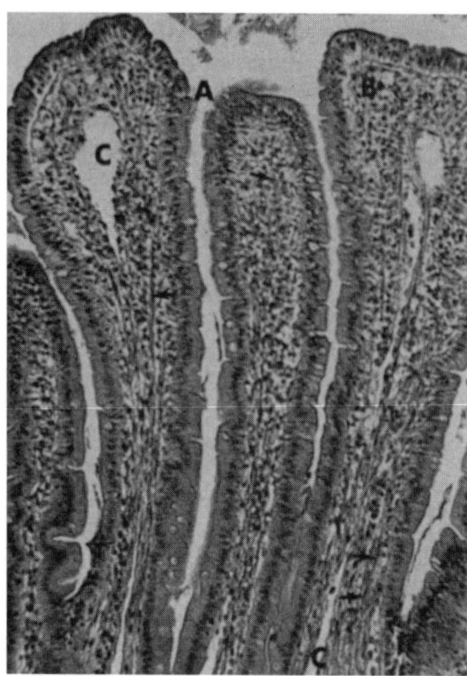

Figure 10.49. *Villi of the small intestine (dog). Simple columnar epithelium with goblet cells (A); lamina propria (B); lymphatic capillary (lacteal) (C); smooth muscle (arrows). Hematoxylin and eosin (×115). (From Titkemeyer CW, Calhoun ML. A comparative study of the structure of the small intestine of domestic animals. Am J Vet Res 1955;16:152.)*

species. They are long and slender in carnivores and short and wide in cattle. *(c)* Microvilli are present on the free surface of the simple columnar epithelial cells of the villi (Fig. 10.50).

Tunica Mucosa

The mucosa includes the lining epithelium, a lamina propria with glands, and a lamina muscularis. The villi are mucosal projections and are the most characteristic feature of the small intestine. The intestinal glands (crypts of Lieberkühn), which open between the bases of the villi, penetrate the mucosa as far as the lamina muscularis. These simple tubular glands are sometimes referred to simply as mucosal glands (Fig. 10.51).

The lumen of the small intestine is lined by a simple columnar epithelium containing numerous goblet cells interspersed among columnar absorptive cells (Fig. 10.50). Junctional complexes, located between the epithelial cells at the luminal surface, prevent the fluid of the intestinal contents from diffusing into the lamina propria without going through the cells. The columnar **absorptive cells** have ovoid nuclei situated near the cell base and have prominent microvilli forming a striated border. In electron micrographs, mitochondria are seen near the nucleus and in the basal region (Fig. 10.50). The apical cytoplasm contains a terminal web and extensive smooth endoplasmic reticulum (sER) necessary for the synthesis of triglycerides. A prominent supranuclear Golgi complex functions in digestive enzyme secretion as well as in the transformation of emulsified fats into chylomicrons, small droplets of fat transported by the blood. Free ribosomes and rER are located in the basal part of the cell.

Goblet cells are dispersed among the columnar absorptive cells (Fig. 10.50). As **mucinogen** is produced within the cell, the apical portion of the cell becomes distended, mucinogen droplets accumulate, and the nucleus and remaining cytoplasm are pushed into the narrow cell base that rests on the basement membrane (Fig. 10.50). (For more details, see Chapter 2.) The number of goblet cells is decreased at the tips of the villi; however, the density of the goblet cells is two to three times greater in the ileum than in the duodenum.

The simple tubular **intestinal glands (crypts of Lieberkühn)** are lined by a variety of cell types. The principal cell type of the intestinal glands is the undifferentiated columnar cell. These cells multiply, differentiate, and migrate onto the villus, giving rise to the columnar absorptive cells and the goblet cells. They are pushed toward the tip of the villus by succeeding cells, where they slough off into the lumen. Because of this continuous cell renewal, many mitotic figures occur among the cells lining the glands. The mitotic activity is constant and bears no relation to the amount of ingesta or enzyme activity. The epithelium is renewed approximately every 2 to 3 days.

Near the base of the intestinal glands, **acidophilic granular cells (of Paneth)** are present in ruminants and horses (Fig. 10.52). They are pyramid-shaped cells with prominent spherical, acidophilic granules located between the nucleus and the cell apex. They have all the characteristics of enzyme-producing cells, and substantial evidence shows that they produce peptidase and **lysozyme**, an antibacterial compound. These cells also contain zinc, which has been reported to be important in the activation of peptidase. **Enteroendocrine cells** are also present in the intestinal glands. They were described earlier in the "Proper gastric (fundic) gland region" section (Fig. 10.53).

The lamina propria forms the cores of the villi and surrounds the intestinal glands. It is composed of loose connective tissue with a prominent reticular fiber framework. Within this extensive fiber network are blood and lymph vessels, leukocytes, fibrocytes, smooth muscle cells, plasma cells, and mast cells. Globule leukocytes are found in the intestinal mucosa of most domestic species. They contain large eosinophilic globular material surrounding a small nucleus. Their function is unknown. Diffuse lymphatic tissue and solitary lymphatic nodules are present throughout the lamina propria of the small intestine. The number of lymphatic nodules increases toward the ileum. A **stratum compactum** similar to that found in the stomach may be found between the bases of the intestinal glands and the lamina muscularis of carnivores.

A single lymphatic capillary, the **lacteal**, is located in the center of the lamina propria of the villus (Fig. 10.49). This vessel has a blind terminal end at the tip of the villus and is the origin of the lymph vessels that form a plexus at the bases of the villi. This basal plexus gives rise to a larger plexus surrounding the intestinal glands and the lymphatic nodules. Longitudinally oriented smooth muscle cells that originate from the lamina muscularis extend to the tip of the villus (Fig. 10.49). Contraction of these muscle cells causes the villus to shorten and undoubtedly is responsible for lateral movements as well. Muscle contraction also aids in pumping the lymph out of the lacteal into the plexus below. A single arteriole from an arterial plexus in the submucosa penetrates the lamina muscularis and courses into the villus, where it forms an arteriovenular loop and a capillary network immediately beneath the surface epithelium. As a result of digestive activity, the vascular network becomes engorged with blood, thus causing the villus to lengthen. During muscular contraction, the blood is pumped out as the villus shortens. Thus, the villi act as pumping stations for moving blood and lymph into the general circulation.

The lamina muscularis is composed of inner circular and outer longitudinal layers of smooth muscle that tend to be thin and incomplete, except in dogs. The lamina muscularis may vary with the species, the individual animal, and the region.

Tela Submucosa

The submucosa is a layer of connective tissue that is more dense than that of the lamina propria. Tubu-

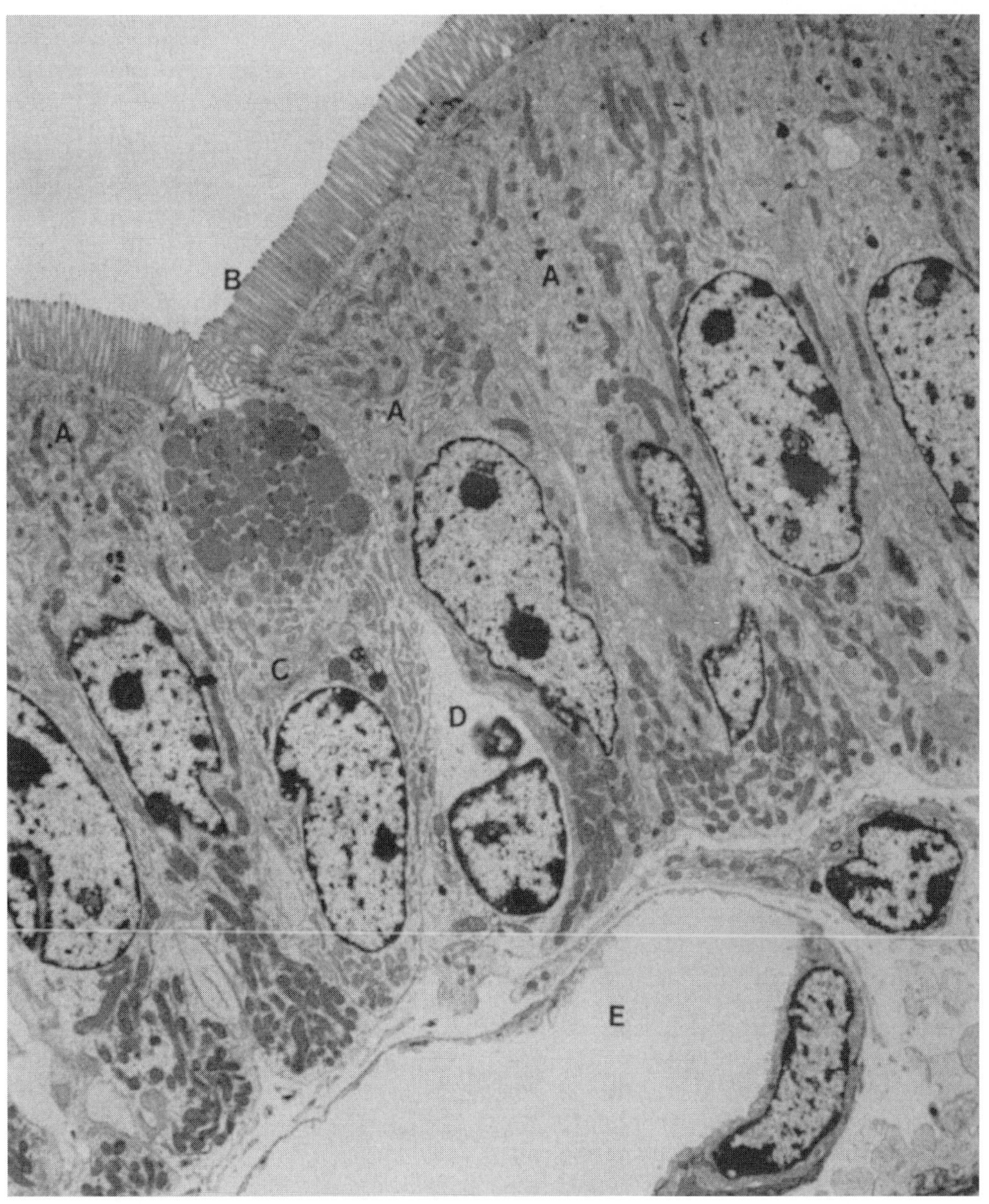

Figure 10.50. *Transmission electron micrograph of jejunum surface epithelium (calf). Simple columnar epithelial cells (A) with microvilli (B). One goblet cell (C) and a migrating lymphocyte (D) are also present. Immediately below the epithelium is a capillary (E) (×5000). (Courtesy of J.F. Pohlenz.)*

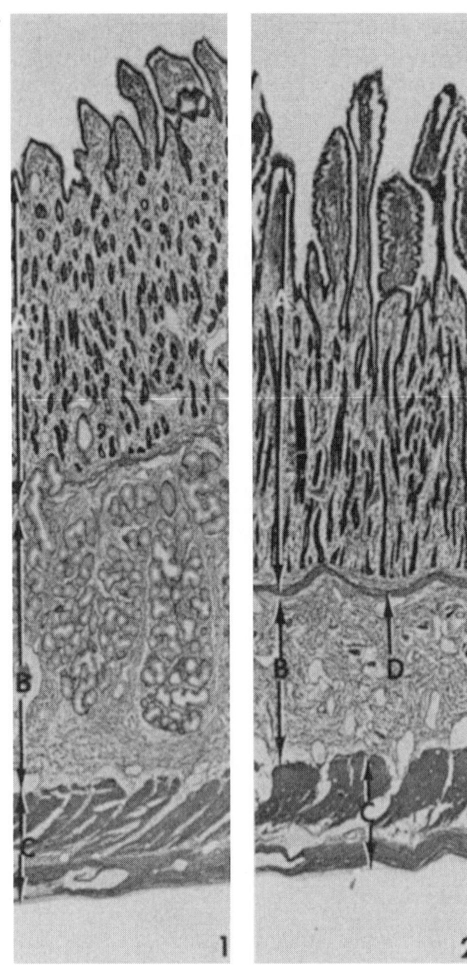

Figure 10.51. *Duodenum (dog). 1., Area near pylorus with submucosal glands. 2., More caudal area without glands. Tunica mucosa (A); tela submucosa (B); tunica muscularis (C); lamina muscularis (D). Hematoxylin and eosin (×28). (From Adam WS, Calhoun ML, Smith EM, et al. Microscopic anatomy of the dog: a photographic atlas. Springfield, IL: Charles C. Thomas, 1970.)*

loalveolar **submucosal glands (Brunner's glands)**, located within this connective tissue, open into the base of the intestinal mucosal glands. The submucosal glands are mucous in dogs and ruminants, serous in pigs and horses, and seromucous in cats (Fig. 10.61). The serous (proteinaceous) or mucous secretory product of these glands lubricates the surface epithelium and provides protection from the acidic gastric chyme. The glands are present in all domestic mammals, but their distribution varies with the species. For example, they are confined to the proximal portion of the duodenum in dogs, whereas in horses, they extend well into the jejunum.

Solitary (isolated) lymphatic nodules are present in the submucosa throughout the small intestine. Large **aggregated lymphatic nodules (Peyer's patches)** occur in all three segments of the small intestine, but they are usually considered to be more characteristic of the ileum (Figs. 10.54 and 10.55). These masses of lymphatic tissue can be located grossly, except in cats, because they create well-delineated elevations of the mucosal surface. Aggregated lymphatic nodules are largest in cattle and most numerous in horses. The intestinal glands may extend into the submucosa in areas of the small intestine where the lamina muscularis is disrupted by the aggregated lymphatic nodules. (See Chapter 8 for details on this gut-associated lymphatic tissue.)

The submucosa also contains the submucosal nerve plexus. Nerve fibers from this plexus extend into the villi.

Tunica Muscularis

In all species, the tunica muscularis of the small intestine consists of inner circular and outer longitudinal smooth muscle layers. The tunica muscularis is thickest in horses, in which the two layers are nearly equal in thickness. The connective tissue between the two muscle layers contains the myenteric plexus.

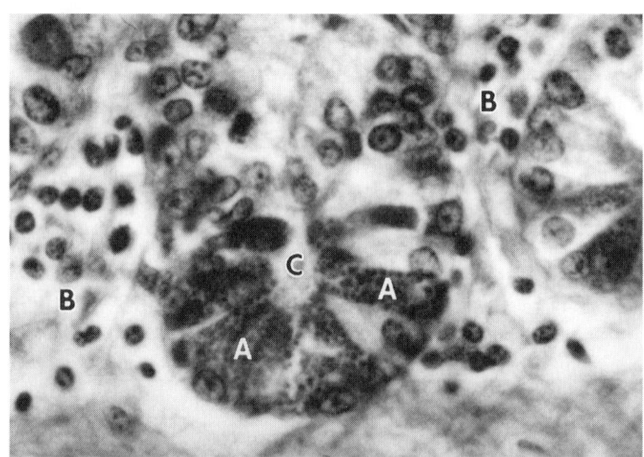

Figure 10.52. *Mucosal glands, small intestine (horse). Acidophilic granular cells (of Paneth) (A) in the base of an intestinal mucosal gland; lamina propria (B); lumen of intestinal mucosal gland (C). Hematoxylin and eosin (×560).*

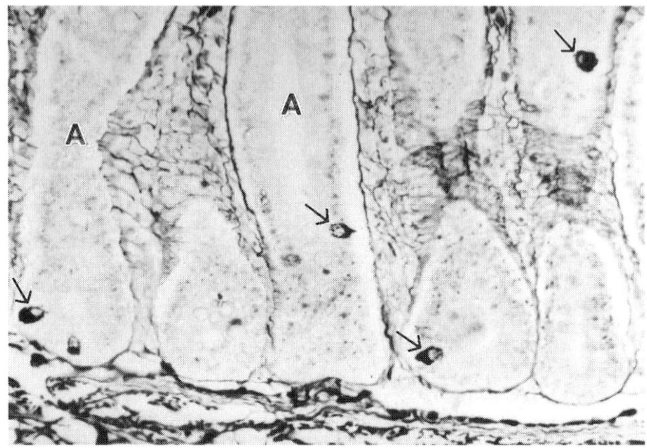

Figure 10.53. *Mucosal glands, small intestine (cat). Lumen of intestinal mucosal gland (A); enteroendocrine cells (arrows). Silver stain (×320).*

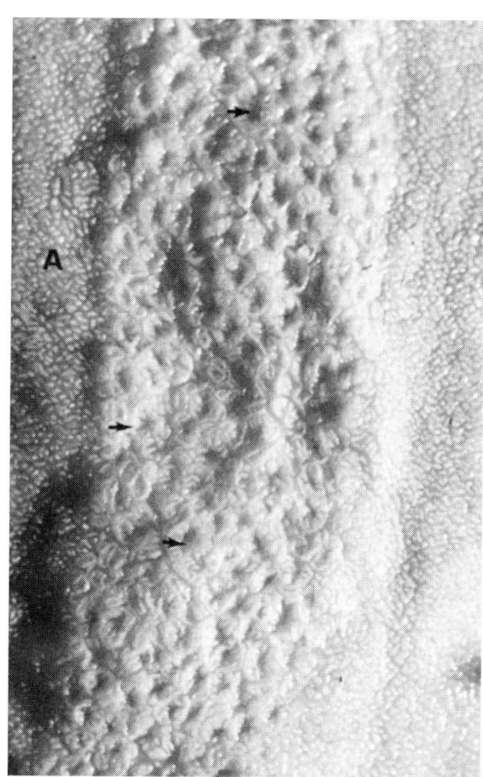

Figure 10.54. *Mucosa of small intestine with aggregated lymphatic nodules (pig). Villi (A); surface depressions over lymphatic nodules (arrows) (×6). (From Titkemeyer CW, Calhoun ML. A comparative study of the structure of the small intestine of domestic animals. Am J Vet Res 1955;16:152.)*

Tunica Serosa

A serosa covers the entire small intestine. It consists of a layer of loose connective tissue covered by mesothelium.

Blood Supply

Branches of the cranial mesenteric artery, coursing in the mesentery, penetrate the tunica muscularis along the line of mesenteric attachment. These arteries give off branches to supply the tunica muscularis and continue into the submucosa, where they form a submucosal arterial plexus. The plexus gives rise to short arterioles, which supply capillary beds around the lamina muscularis and intestinal (mucosal) glands, and long arterioles, which extend to the tips of the villi. In the villus, the single arteriole supplies a capillary network and continues to the tip of the villus, where it is continuous with a venule, forming an arteriovenular loop. Venules from the villi and the periglandular capillary bed combine to form a submucosal venous plexus. This plexus gives rise to veins that traverse the tunica muscularis parallel to the arterial supply and drain into the portal vein. The circulatory system in the small intestine of horses, carnivores, and pigs differs from the previously described pattern in that these animals lack arteriovenular loops in the villi but have arteriovenous (AV) anastomoses in the submucosa preceding the villous circulation. During digestion, circularly arranged smooth muscle cells in the AV anastomoses contract, shunting blood to the villi. When the digestive process is inactive, these AV anastomoses are open and a partial bypass of the villus circulation is created.

General Identifying Features

The various regions of the small intestine in the domestic mammals are not clearly defined microscopically, as they are in human beings. For example, the submucosal glands do not extend the full length of the duodenum in sheep, goats, and carnivores, whereas in horses, cattle, and pigs, these glands extend into the jejunum. Likewise, the aggregated lymphatic nodules (Peyer's patches), often considered an identifying feature of the ileum, may be seen anywhere along the small intestine of domestic mammals.

Because the length of the villi varies with physiologic activities and with species, it is not a reliable characteristic for the identification of the various segments.

LARGE INTESTINE

The large intestine is composed of the cecum, colon, rectum, and anal canal. It is a site for microbial action on the ingesta, absorption of water, vitamins, and electrolytes and secretion of mucus. Many gross and functional variations in the large intestine relate to the necessity of breaking down the large masses of

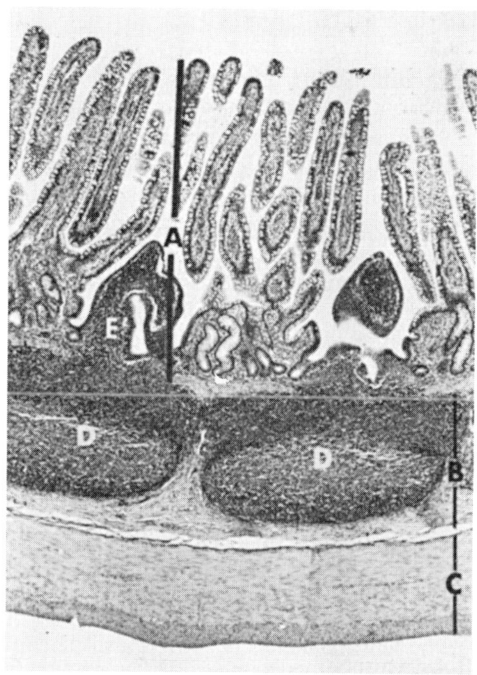

Figure 10.55. *Ileum (cat). Tunica mucosa (A); submucosa (B); tunica muscularis (C); aggregated lymphatic nodules (D); dome (E) (see Chapter 8). Hematoxylin and eosin (×48).*

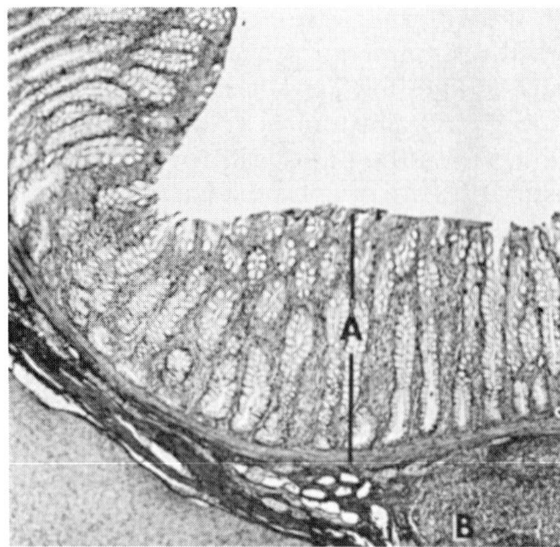

Figure 10.56. *Cecum (cat). Tunica mucosa (A) containing simple tubular glands; lymphatic nodule in submucosa (B). Trichrome (×45).*

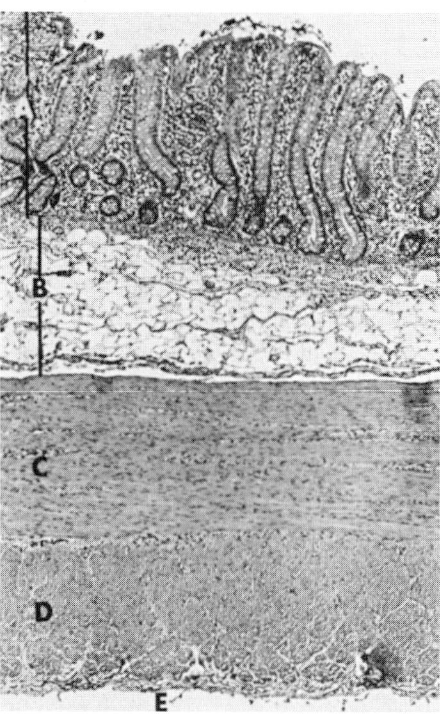

Figure 10.57. *Cecum (pig). Tunica mucosa (A); submucosa filled with white adipose tissue (B); inner circular (C) and outer longitudinal (D) layers of the tunica muscularis; serosa (E). Hematoxylin and eosin (×48).*

cellulose-containing material consumed by the herbivores. However, despite gross anatomic differences, the cecum, colon, and rectum are difficult to differentiate in histologic sections. Characteristics common to these three segments of the large intestine are the absence of villi, longer, less-coiled, simple tubular intestinal glands with many goblet cells (Fig. 10.56), the absence of Paneth cells, and an increased number of lymphatic nodules. Plicae circulares are absent in the large intestine, but longitudinal folds are present. Animals fattened for slaughter tend to accumulate white adipose tissue in the submucosa (Fig. 10.57).

Cecum

The **cecum** varies in size among the different species. In herbivores with simple stomachs, e.g., horses, the cecum is large and is an important bacterial fermentation reservoir, but in carnivores, it is small. In all domestic mammals, the cecum has a substantial number of lymphatic nodules scattered throughout its length (Fig. 10.56). Lymphatic nodules are located around the ileal ostium (the opening of the ileum into the cecum or colon) in pigs, ruminants, and dogs; however, in horses and cats, lymphatic nodules are concentrated near the apex of the cecum.

Colon

The mucosa of the **colon** is substantially thicker than that of the small intestine because of the increased length of the intestinal glands. Because villi are absent, the mucosal surface is smooth (Fig. 10.58). The number of goblet cells is increased. The submucosa is often distended by lymphatic tissue, which also disrupts the lamina muscularis. In such instances, intestinal glands may extend into the submucosa.

In pigs and horses, the outer longitudinal layer of the tunica muscularis of the cecum and colon forms large,

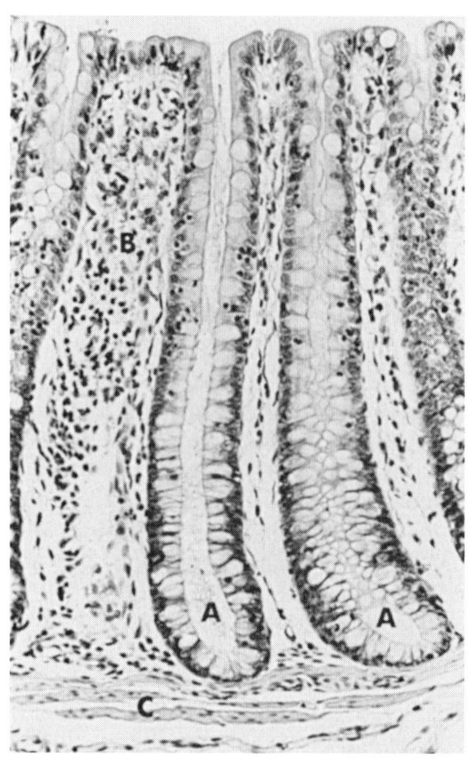

Figure 10.58. *Colon (pig). Tunica mucosa with intestinal glands and goblet cells (A); lamina propria (B); lamina muscularis (C). Hematoxylin and eosin (×200).*

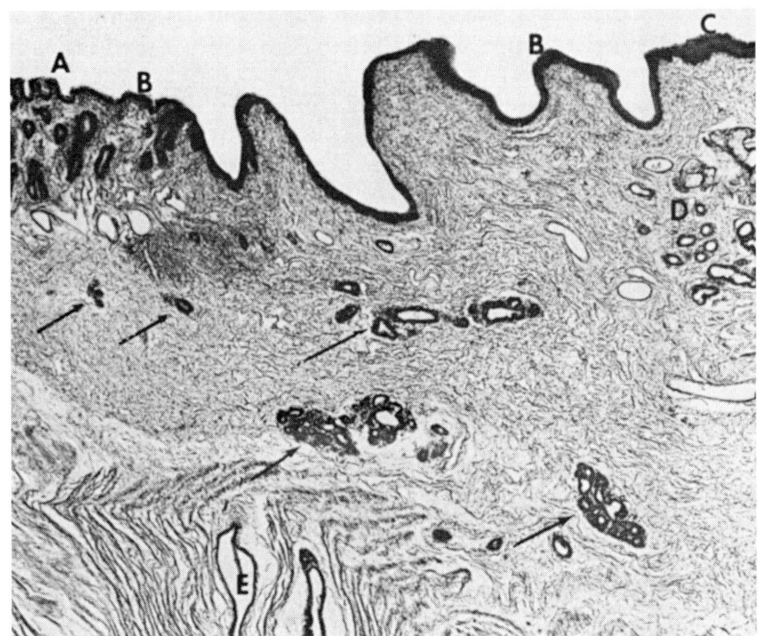

Figure 10.59. *Rectum and anal canal (dog). Rectum (A); anal canal (B); skin (C) with sweat and sebaceous glands (D); veins (E); anal glands (arrows). Hematoxylin and eosin (×66). (From Adam WS, Calhoun ML, Smith EM, Stinson AW. Microscopic anatomy of the dog: a photographic atlas. Springfield, IL: Charles C. Thomas, 1970.)*

flat muscle bands containing numerous elastic fibers, the **taenia ceci** and **taenia coli**. Those of the cecum and ventral colon of horses have more elastic fibers than smooth muscle cells.

Rectum

Like that of the cecum and colon, the mucosa of the **rectum** is smooth, and except for the increased number of goblet cells, the basic structures are similar as well. In horses and cattle, the rectal wall is thicker than the wall of the colon. In carnivores, the outer longitudinal layer of the tunica muscularis is thickened. Elastic fibers are most prominent in the rectum of horses and cattle and least prominent in the rectum of sheep and goats. The outer layer (circular) of the tunica muscularis contains more elastic fibers than does the inner layer (longitudinal). The cranial portion of the rectum is covered by a serosa, whereas the retroperitoneal portion is surrounded by an adventitia, which blends with the pelvic fascia.

Near its junction with the anal canal, the rectal mucosa in ruminants is thrown into longitudinal folds, the **rectal columns (columnae rectales)**. All domestic mammals have an extensive venous plexus in the lamina propria of this region of the rectum. In dogs, approximately 100 solitary lymphatic nodules are a prominent feature of the rectum. They are visible grossly because of pitlike depressions, **rectal pits**, in the mucosa overlying the lymphatic nodules.

Anal Canal

The **anal canal** is the terminal segment of the digestive tract, and at the **anorectal line**, the simple columnar epithelium of the rectum changes abruptly to nonkeratinized stratified squamous epithelium (Fig. 10.59). Also at the anorectal junction, the lamina muscularis of the rectum terminates. In ruminants, the short gland-free anal canal is continuous proximally with the rectal columns and ends distally at the **anocutaneous line**. In horses, the anal canal is also nonglandular and, at the anocutaneous line, joins the skin that covers the anal protuberance.

In pigs and carnivores, the anal canal is divided into three distinct zones: *(a)* columnar zone (zona columnaris ani); *(b)* intermediate zone (zona intermedia); and *(c)* cutaneous zone (zona cutanea). The **columnar zone** contains longitudinal folds, the **anal columns**, between which are grooves, and the **anal sinuses**. The **intermediate** zone is a narrow strip between the columnar zone and the cutaneous zone. The mucosa of both the columnar and intermediate zones is lined with nonkeratinized stratified squamous epithelium, and modified tubuloalveolar sweat glands, the **anal glands**, occupy the propria submucosa. The anal glands produce a lipid secretion in cats and dogs (Fig. 10.59) and a mucous secretion in pigs. The cutaneous zone is lined by keratinized stratified squamous epithelium. In carnivores, the ducts from the **anal sacs (paranal sinuses)** open at the junction of the intermediate and cutaneous zones. The anal sacs and ducts are bilateral evaginations of the anal mucosa. In dogs, the mucosa of the outermost part of the cutaneous zone, near the junction with the skin, contains large, modified sebaceous glands, the **circumanal glands**. The anal sacs and their associated glands and the circumanal glands are discussed with the integument in Chapter 16.

The outer longitudinal layer of the tunica muscularis of the rectum terminates at the anorectal junction. The inner circular layer continues into the anal canal and terminates as the internal anal sphincter muscle. The external anal sphincter muscle, which is circularly dis-

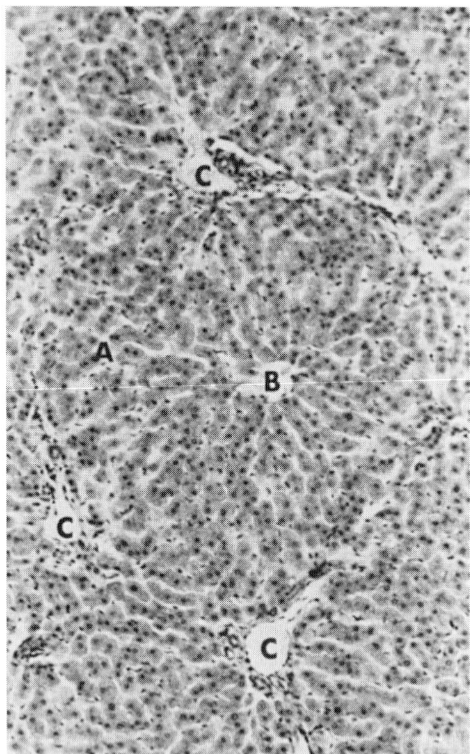

Figure 10.60. *Liver (calf). Lobule (A) with central vein (B) is not separated from adjacent lobules by connective tissue as is that of the pig in Figure 10.61. Interlobular portal venules (C) in portal canals (areas). Hematoxylin and eosin (×80).*

posed skeletal muscle, covers the internal anal sphincter muscle.

LIVER

The liver is the largest gland in the body and is characterized by a multiplicity of complex functions: excretion (waste products), secretion (bile), storage (lipids, vitamins A and B, glycogen), synthesis (fibrinogen, globulins, albumin, clotting factors), phagocytosis (foreign particulate matter), detoxification (lipid-soluble drugs), conjugation (toxic substances, steroid hormones), esterification (free fatty acids to triglycerides), metabolism (proteins, carbohydrates, lipids, hemoglobin, drugs), and hemopoiesis (in the embryo and potentially in the adult). An understanding of the structure of the liver is vital to the interpretation of these processes.

Capsule and Stroma

Each lobe of the liver is covered by a typical serosa (visceral peritoneum) overlying a thin connective tissue capsule. Connective tissue from the capsule extends into the liver lobes, as interlobular connective tissue, to surround individual liver lobules and support the vascular and bile duct systems. A fine network of reticular fibers surrounds the cells and sinusoids. Smooth muscle cells may be present in the capsule and interlobular connective tissue. Interlobular connective tissue is scant and difficult to see (Fig. 10.60), except in pigs, which have distinct interlobular connective tissue septa (Fig. 10.61). This difference accounts for the tougher nature of pork liver as a food, as opposed to beef liver.

Expanded areas of interlobular connective tissue supporting: *(a)* a **lymph vessel**; *(b)* branches of the **hepatic artery**; *(c)* branches of the **portal vein**; and *(d)* a **bile duct** appear throughout any section of liver. These groups of vessels and ducts, together with the supportive connective tissue, are called **portal canals** or **portal areas** (Fig. 10.62).

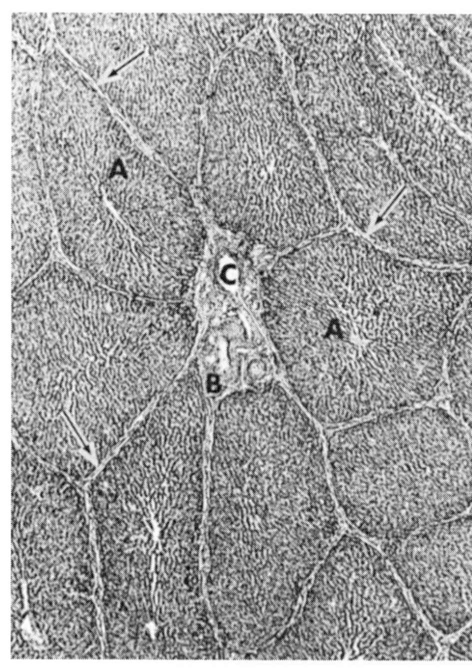

Figure 10.61. *Liver (pig). Liver lobules (A); portal canal (B); branch of the portal vein (C); interlobular connective tissue (arrows). Trichrome (×30). (From Stinson AW, Brown EM. Veterinary histology slide sets. East Lansing, MI: Michigan State University, Instructional Media Center, 1970.)*

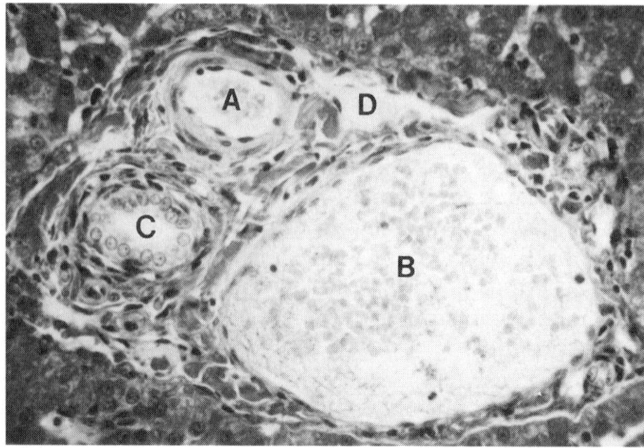

Figure 10.62. *Liver (pig). Portal canal (area). Branch of the hepatic artery (A); branch of the portal vein (B); bile duct (C); lymph capillary (D). Hematoxylin and eosin (×200).*

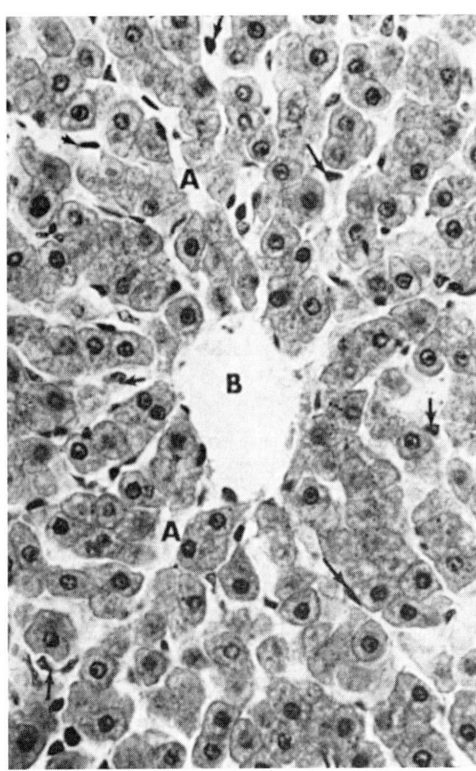

Figure 10.63. *Liver (calf). Hepatic sinusoids (A); central vein (B); stellate macrophages (Kupffer cells) (arrows). Hematoxylin and eosin (×384).*

The Classic Liver Lobule — The Anatomical Unit of the Liver

The clear delineation afforded by abundant interlobular connective tissue in the liver of pigs has led to the recognition of **hepatic lobules (classic liver lobules)**. This morphologic unit is organized around the central vein (Figs. 10.60 and 10.61). The lobule consists of a polyhedral prism of hepatic tissue measuring approximately 2 mm long and approximately 1 mm wide. Cross-sectional profiles of this lobule are roughly hexagon-shaped, with the sinusoids converging from the periphery to the central vein, into which they empty. Portal canals are present at approximately three of the six angles of the lobule. The parenchyma between the portal canals and the interlobular connective tissue on one hand, and the central vein on the other, consists of cells arranged in branching plates or laminae (Fig. 10.63). These laminae are one cell thick; the free surfaces of the cells face the sinusoids. An anastomosing network of bile canaliculi, formed by the apposed cell membranes of hepatocytes, is present throughout the laminae (Fig. 10.64).

The Portal Lobule and the Liver Acinus — Functional Units of the Liver

The **portal lobule** is a functional unit developed to emphasize the exocrine function (bile secretion) of the liver. The portal lobule is defined as a triangular area consisting of the parenchyma of three adjacent classic lobules that are drained by the bile ductule in the portal canal. Thus, the axis (center) of the portal lobule is the interlobular bile ductule in the portal canal and the angles are the central veins of the three adjacent lobules (Fig. 10.65).

The **liver acinus** is a functional unit that describes the vascular supply to the parenchyma. The liver acinus is a roughly diamond-shaped area made of parts of two classic lobules supplied by terminal branches of the interlobular portal venule and interlobular hepatic arteriole. The blood vessels course at right angles from a portal canal between two hepatic lobules to form the axis of the acinus, and the two central veins are at the two opposing points of the diamond (Fig. 10.65). Three ill-defined zones have been identified in the liver acinus. **Zone 1** is the nearest to the vascular axis of the acinus. In this zone, hepatocytes receive an excellent nutrient and oxygen supply and are metabolically most active. Cells in this zone may also be the first to be exposed to toxic substances entering the liver. **Zone 2** is one of intermediate activity, whereas **zone 3** borders the central vein and is the least favorably situated with respect to oxygen and nutrient supply and, therefore, is most susceptible to damage.

Parenchyma

The hepatic laminae consist of rows of **hepatocytes**. Hepatocytes have six or more surfaces that are of three different types: *(a)* microvillous surfaces that face the perisinusoidal space; *(b)* canalicular surfaces that border the bile canaliculi; and *(c)* contact surfaces between adjacent hepatocytes where apposed cell membranes may have gap junctions and desmosomes (Fig. 10.66). Hepa-

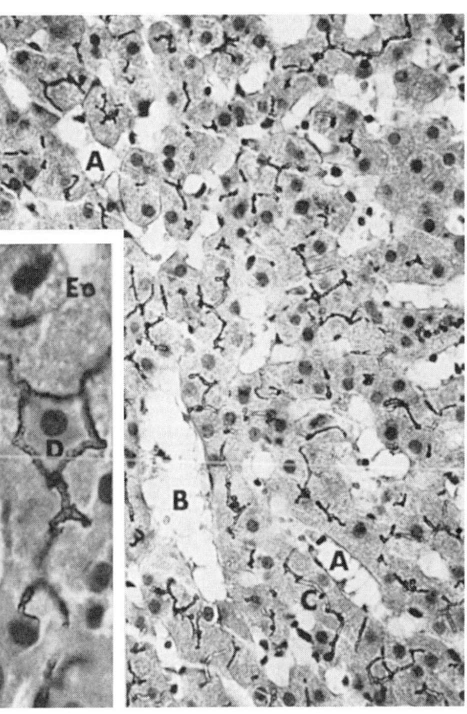

Figure 10.64. *Liver (pig). Sinusoids (A); central vein (B); liver laminae with bile canaliculi between the cells (C). Silver stain (×300). Inset: bile canaliculi surrounding a hepatocyte (D) and a cross section of a bile canaliculus (E). Silver stain (×768)*

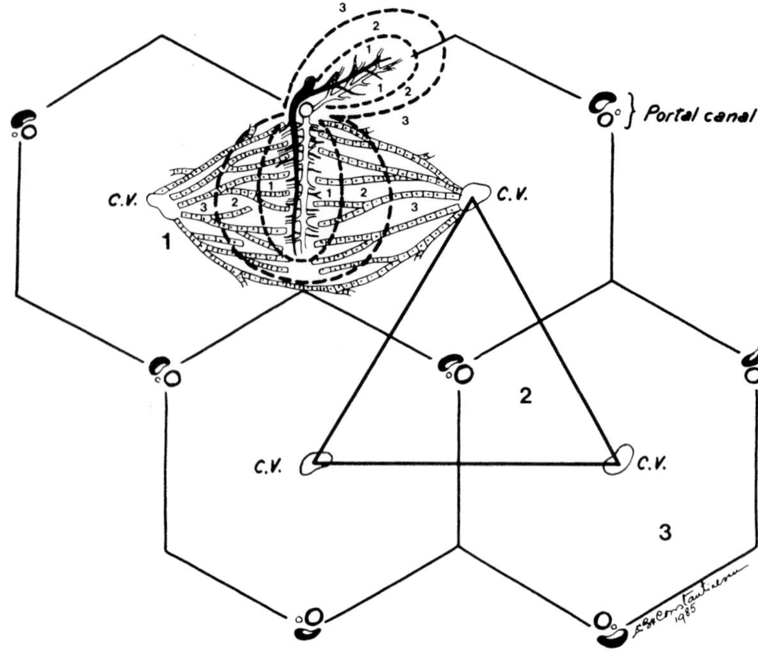

Figure 10.65. *Schematic drawing of the functional units of the liver in relation to the anatomic unit (classic lobule).* ***1.****, Liver acinus with three zones on each side of the vascular backbone.* ***2.****, Portal lobule with a portal area as the axis and one central vein at each point of the triangle.* ***3.****, Classic hepatic lobule (anatomic unit) with the central vein as its axis. (Modified and redrawn from Rappaport A, Borowy ZJ, Laugheed WM, Lotto WN. Subdivision of hexagonal liver lobules into a structural and functional unit; role in hepatic physiology and pathology. Anat Rec 1954;119:11.)*

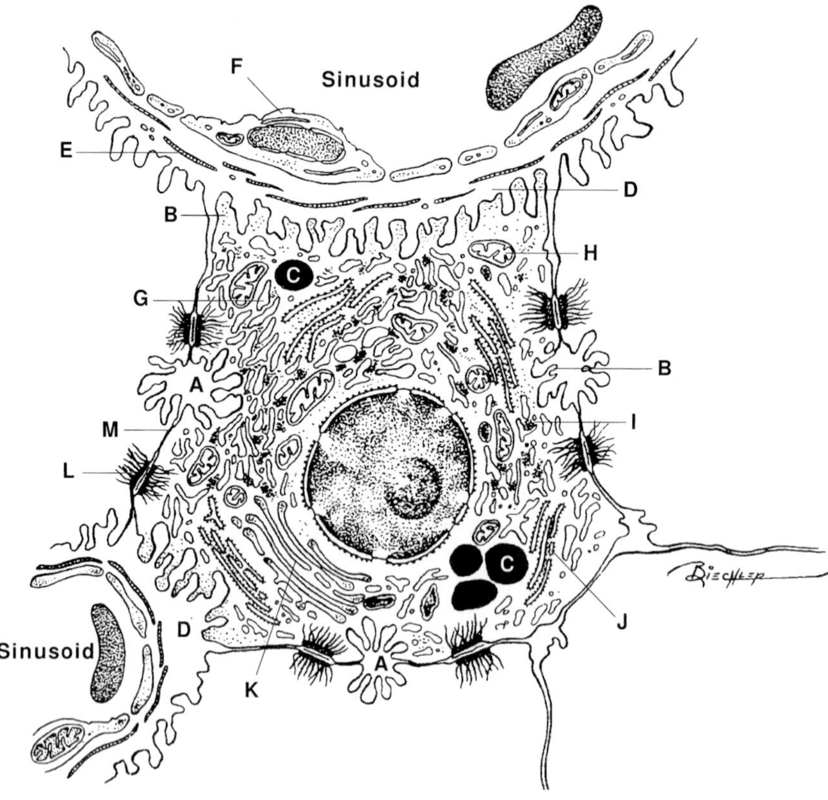

Figure 10.66. *Drawing of an electron micrograph of a hepatocyte and adjacent structures. Bile canaliculus (A); microvillus (B); lipid droplet (C); perisinusoidal space (of Disse) (D); reticular fiber (E); porous endothelial cell (F) lining the sinusoid; smooth endoplasmic reticulum (G); mitochondrion (H); glycogen (I); rough endoplasmic reticulum (J); Golgi complex (K); desmosome (macula adherens) (L); tight junction (zonula occludens) (M).*

tocytes are further characterized by a centrally located spherical nucleus with one or more prominent nucleoli and scattered clumps of heterochromatin. Occasionally, binucleated cells are seen. The appearance of the cytoplasm of hepatocytes varies within wide limits, depending on nutritional and functional changes. Mitochondria are abundant and the Golgi complex is usually near the bile canaliculus but may be juxtanuclear. There are numerous lysosomes, clusters of free ribosomes, and well-developed rER and sER, which are often contiguous with each other. At the ultrastructural level, glycogen is seen as dense granules in a rosette configuration (Fig. 10.66). In ordinary histologic preparations, glycogen-rich areas appear grainy or as irregularly shaped empty spaces, whereas sites occupied by lipids appear as round vacuoles. Bile pigments may be seen in normal hepatocytes.

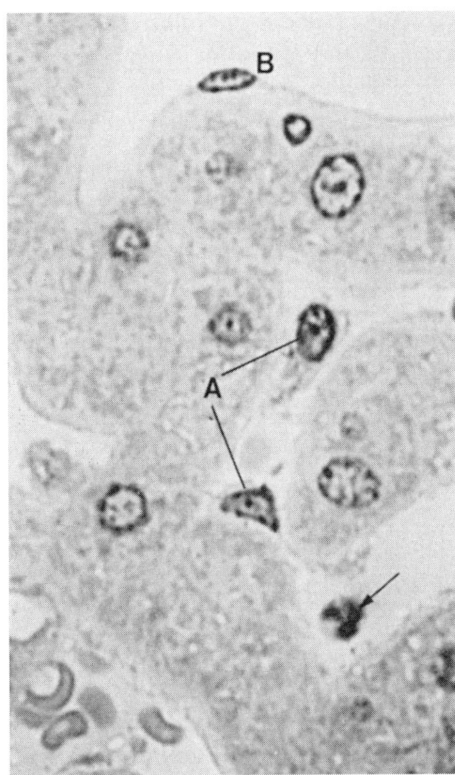

Figure 10.67. *Liver laminae and sinusoids (cat). Two stellate macrophages (Kupffer cells) (A) and one endothelial cell (B) comprise the sinusoidal lining cells. Notice the erythrocytes (lower left) and one neutrophil (arrow). Epon. Toluidine blue (×1600).*

Considerable evidence shows that all hepatocytes may not be functionally identical, but instead, certain enzyme patterns and metabolic systems may be related to the position of the cell within the lobule. Although metabolic activity of the hepatocytes is generally believed to be closely associated with blood supply, the extent to which hepatocytes are similar or dissimilar with respect to metabolic systems, susceptibility to insults, and nutritional needs remains to be resolved.

Bile Canaliculi and Bile Ducts

Hepatocytes absorb bilirubin (bile pigment) from the blood, conjugate it, and secrete it as one component of bile. Bile salts, protein, and cholesterol are the other components. Bile is secreted into minute canals (0.5 to 1.0 μm in diameter) between apposed hepatocytes, the bile canaliculi (Fig. 10.64). Bile canaliculi are simply areas in which the membranes of adjacent hepatocytes diverge, forming expanded intercellular spaces. The cell membranes bordering these spaces have short microvilli. Tight junctions adjacent to the bile canaliculi prevent bile from escaping into the narrow intercellular space adjacent to the canaliculus (Fig. 10.66).

Bile flows in the bile canaliculi to the periphery of the classic lobule, where it enters small **bile ductules** lined by low simple cuboidal epithelium. The bile ductules join **interlobular bile ducts** located in the portal canals. These ducts are lined by a simple cuboidal or simple columnar epithelium. Interlobular bile ducts converge to form progressively larger intrahepatic ducts, which finally leave the liver lobes through the **hepatic ducts**. The extrahepatic biliary passages are composed of the hepatic ducts, the cystic duct, the bile duct, and the gallbladder. Hepatic ducts drain the individual liver lobes. The **cystic duct** drains the gallbladder (absent in horses). The hepatic ducts and the cystic duct unite to form the **bile duct**, which empties into the duodenum. All of the extrahepatic biliary passages are lined by a tall simple columnar epithelium.

Blood Supply

The vascularity of the liver is directly related to its multitudinous functions. The liver has a dual blood supply. The portal vein brings blood from the intestines and associated organs, and the hepatic artery supplies the liver cells with oxygenated blood. These vessels enter the liver at a hilus on its visceral surface, the porta. Branches (rami) of these two vessels enter the lobes, where they ramify and follow the interlobular connective tissue. The small branches within the portal canal are termed the interlobular portal venule and the interlobular hepatic arteriole.

The interlobular portal venules give rise to small branches, sometimes referred to as distributing venules, which form the axis of the liver acinus. Short terminal venules arise from the distributing venules and end directly in the sinusoids. Most of the blood from the interlobular hepatic arterioles enters a capillary plexus within the portal canal and interlobular connective tissue; only a small portion of the blood reaches the sinusoids directly by way of terminal arterioles.

The **hepatic sinusoids** are blood capillaries, located between hepatic laminae, that course through the lobule carrying blood from terminal branches of the interlobular hepatic arteriole and interlobular portal venule to the central vein. They often communicate with each other via interruptions in the laminae. This ramifying arrangement ensures that hepatocytes have at least one surface adjacent to a sinusoid. Sinusoids are lined by two types of cells: endothelial cells and **stellate macrophages (Kupffer cells)** (Fig. 10.67).

The porous sinusoidal endothelium rests on a discontinuous basal lamina. The endothelial cells contain small pores that lack diaphragms. The pores are too small to allow the passage of blood cells, but blood plasma can flow through them freely. The endothelium is separated from the hepatocytes by a space, the **perisinusoidal space (of Disse)**. Hepatocyte microvilli extend into the perisinusoidal space, where they are bathed in plasma, allowing a direct exchange of substances between blood and hepatocytes. The sinusoids of the ruminant liver differ from those described above in that the endothelium is non-porous and the basal lamina is continuous.

Stellate macrophages are scattered among the sinusoidal endothelial cells, often sending long pseudopodia through the endothelial pores or between the cells. These highly phagocytic cells are derivatives of blood monocytes and, as such, are components of the monocyte–macrophage system.

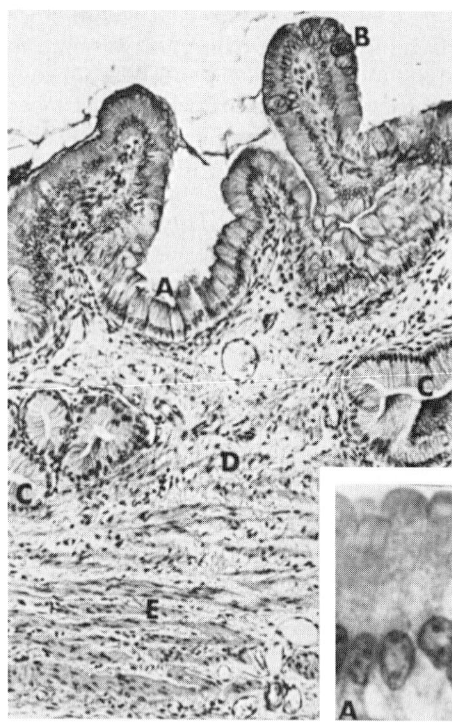

Figure 10.68. *Gallbladder (dog). Simple columnar epithelium (A); goblet cells (B); cross sections of mucosal crypts (C); propria submucosa (D); tunica muscularis (E). Hematoxylin and eosin (×120). Inset: simple columnar epithelial lining. Hematoxylin and eosin (×768).*

In addition to the hepatocyte microvilli, the perisinusoidal space contains reticular fibers as well as perisinusoidal adipocytes. These cells are believed to store vitamin A and synthesize type III collagen after injury to the liver.

Blood in the sinusoids leaves the lobule via the central vein. Central veins are lined by endothelium resting on a thin adventitia. The central veins connect with sublobular veins at the periphery of the lobules. Sublobular veins join to form progressively larger veins that eventually form the hepatic veins, which drain directly into the caudal vena cava.

Lymph and Lymph Vessels

Lymph in the liver is formed in the perisinusoidal space. It flows toward the periphery of the lobule and enters the intercellular spaces of the portal canal and interlobular connective tissue. Here, it diffuses into lymph capillaries within the portal canals. The lymph is carried from the portal canals by larger lymph vessels that ultimately leave the liver at the porta. These lymph vessels drain to the hepatic lymph nodes.

GALLBLADDER

The gallbladder is the storage site of bile produced by the liver. Although bile is stored in the gallbladder, it is also concentrated by the reabsorption of water and inorganic salts. In the contracted (empty) state, the gallbladder mucosa is thrown into numerous folds (plicae). As it fills and expands, these folds have a tendency to flatten, resulting in a smoother mucosal surface. A tall simple columnar epithelium lines the luminal surface and extends into mucosal crypts, which are small epithelial diverticula that sometimes give the impression of being glands (Fig. 10.68). Two types of columnar cells are located in the epithelium. The most numerous type is the "light" cell, which has a pale cytoplasm of uniform density. The cytoplasm of the apical region contains vesicles but is devoid of organelles. Electron-dense bodies with smooth outlines occur in the subapical and supranuclear cytoplasm. The less numerous "dark" cells are seen among the light cells. They have a narrow profile and contain a dark, dense cytoplasm with few organelles and a nucleus that is more heterochromatic than that of the light cells. The epithelial cell surface is covered with microvilli, and tight junctions (zonulae occludentes) between adjacent cells prevent the intercellular passage of fluids from the lumen of the organ. Goblet cells are characteristic of the epithelium of some species, such as cattle, and globule leukocytes may be found in the epithelium of cats. Endocrine cells, possibly of the APUD system, have been described in the epithelium of the gallbladder of cattle.

The propria-submucosa is composed of loose connective tissue. Lymphatic tissue, either diffuse or nodular, is often present. In some species, particularly ruminants, glands are present in the propria-submucosa. They may be serous or mucous, depending on the species, individual, or location in the mucosa (Fig. 10.69). The

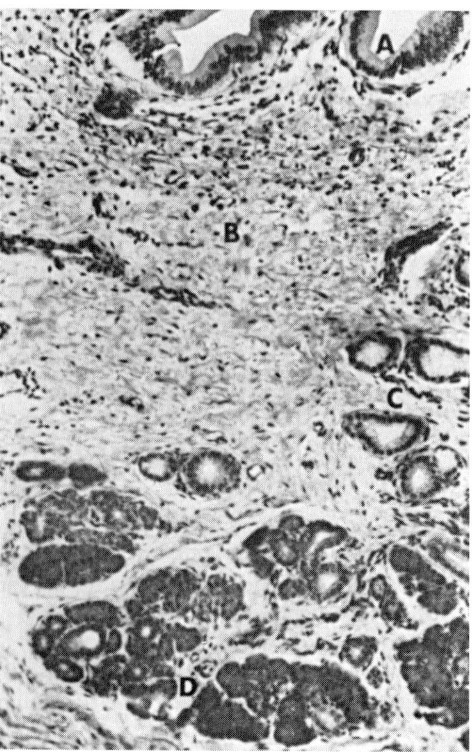

Figure 10.69. *Gallbladder (large ruminant). Simple columnar epithelium (A); propria-submucosa (B); mucous glands (C); serous glands (D). Hematoxylin and eosin (×120).*

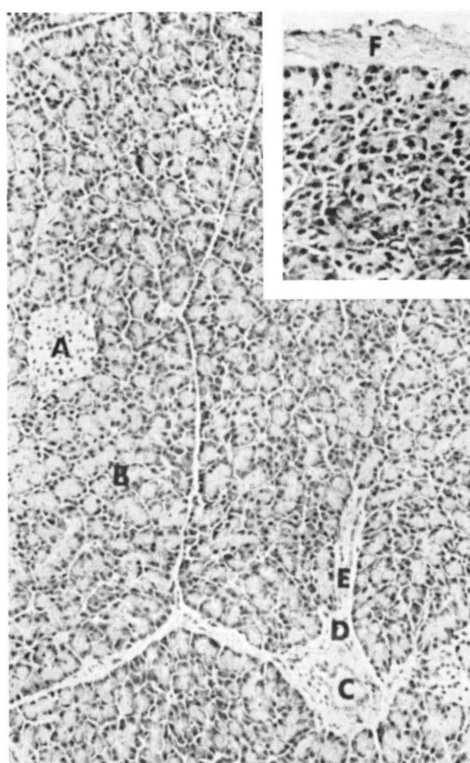

Figure 10.70. *Pancreas (pig). Pancreatic islet (A); pancreatic acini (B); interlobular duct (C) in interlobular connective tissue (D); intralobular duct (E). Hematoxylin and eosin (×120). Inset: capsule of sheep pancreas (F). Hematoxylin and eosin (×192).*

smooth muscle cells of the tunica muscularis generally course in a circular direction. The muscle is supplied by both sympathetic and parasympathetic nerves.

The walls of the hepatic, cystic, and bile ducts are composed of the same tunics as the gallbladder.

PANCREAS

The pancreas is an encapsulated, lobulated, compound tubuloacinar gland containing both exocrine and endocrine parts (Fig. 10.70). The function of the exocrine part is to produce a variety of enzymes, including amylase, lipase, and trypsin, which act on the products of gastric digestion as they reach the duodenum. The endocrine part, pancreatic islets (Fig. 10.71), produces mainly insulin and glucagon. The histologic structure of the islets is discussed in Chapter 15.

The stroma of the pancreas consists of a thin capsule that gives rise to delicate connective tissue septa separating the parenchyma into distinct lobules. The lobule is composed of secretory units and intralobular ducts. The secretory units are tubuloacinar, with the tubular portion more prominent in ruminants. The glandular epithelial cells are generally pyramid-shaped, with a spherical nucleus near the base of the cells (Figs. 10.72 and 10.73). The cytoplasm surrounding the nucleus is intensely basophilic and contains an extensive rER and numerous mitochondria. The apical region of the cells contains eosinophilic, membrane-bound zymogen granules, which are filled with the proenzymes synthesized in the rER. An extensive Golgi complex is located between the nucleus and the zymogen granules. The tubuloacinar secretory unit has a small lumen and is continuous with a short **intercalated duct**. This duct begins with flattened cells that extend into the lumen of the acinus; therefore, they are referred to as **centroacinar cells** (Fig. 10.73). These cells

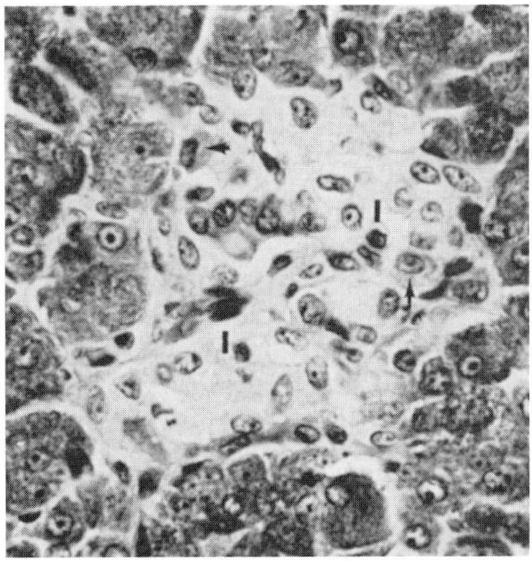

Figure 10.71. *Pancreatic islet surrounded by pancreatic acini (dog). A cells (arrows); B cells (I). Trichrome (×450).*

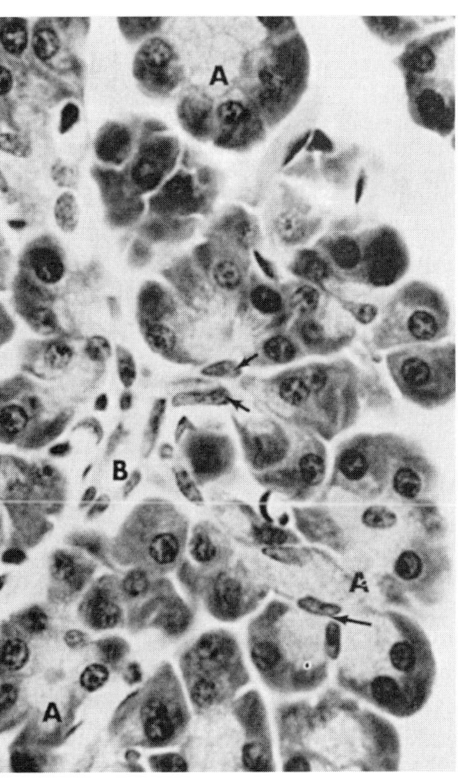

Figure 10.72. *Pancreas (dog). Pancreatic acini (A); intercalated duct (B); centroacinar cells (arrows). Hematoxylin and eosin (×768).*

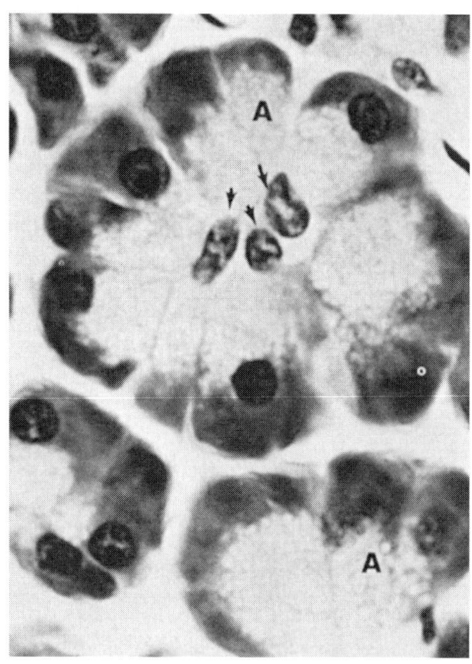

Figure 10.73. *Pancreatic acinus with three centroacinar cells at arrows. Zymogen granules (A). Hematoxylin and eosin (×1200).*

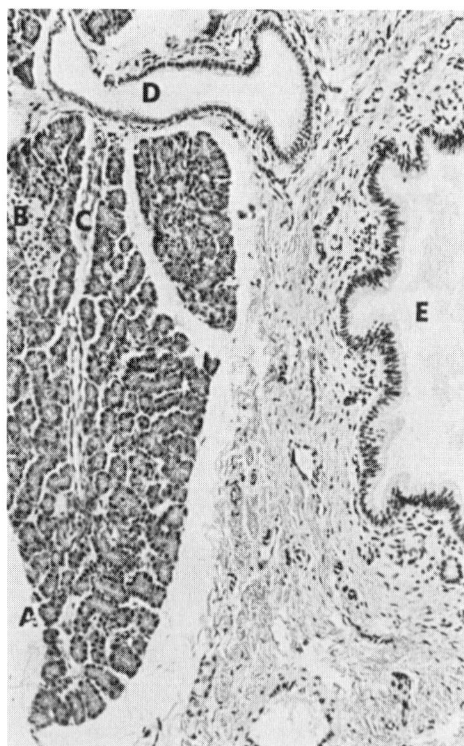

Figure 10.74. *Pancreas (goat). Pancreatic lobule (A); pancreatic islet (B); intralobular duct (C); interlobular duct (D); pancreatic duct (E). Hematoxylin and eosin (×145).*

secrete bicarbonate and water when stimulated by the polypeptide, **secretin**. Bicarbonate raises the pH of the intestinal contents, thereby facilitating the action of intestinal digestive enzymes. Intercalated ducts join **intralobular ducts**, which are lined by low simple cuboidal epithelium. The intralobular ducts of the pancreas are not "striated," as are the intralobular ducts of the parotid salivary gland. The intralobular ducts continue into **interlobular ducts** that are lined by simple columnar epithelium (Fig. 10.74). Interlobular ducts converge to eventually form the **pancreatic duct** and the **accessory pancreatic duct**, both of which empty into the duodenum. Goblet cells may be present in the larger ducts. Frequently, **lamellar (Pacini's) corpuscles** are present in the interlobular connective tissue of the pancreas of cats.

DIGESTIVE SYSTEM OF THE DOMESTIC FOWL

The oral cavity is lined throughout by a keratinized stratified squamous epithelium. The propria submucosa contains considerable diffuse lymphatic tissue and salivary glands. The tongue is covered by a keratinized stratified squamous epithelium and contains bundles of skeletal muscle, lingual salivary glands, and a bone, the **entoglossal bone**. Taste buds are found only on the base of the tongue and the floor of the oral cavity. All salivary glands are branched tubular mucous glands with openings into a common cavity from which an excretory duct leads to the oral cavity.

The esophagus is similar in structure both cranially and caudally to the crop. It is characterized by a thick keratinized stratified squamous epithelium. The lamina propria is a loose connective tissue containing large mucous glands. The lamina muscularis consists of longitudinally arranged smooth muscle fibers. The submucosa consists of a thin layer of loose connective tissue. The tunica muscularis is composed of a thick inner circular layer and a thin outer longitudinal layer of smooth muscle (Fig. 10.75).

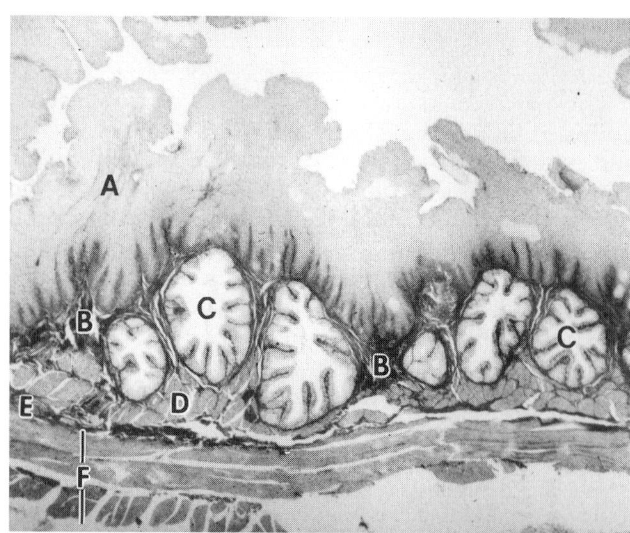

Figure 10.75. *Esophagus (chicken). Keratinized stratified squamous epithelium (A); lamina propria (B); mucous glands (C); lamina muscularis (D); submucosa (E); tunica muscularis (F). Hematoxylin and eosin (×45).*

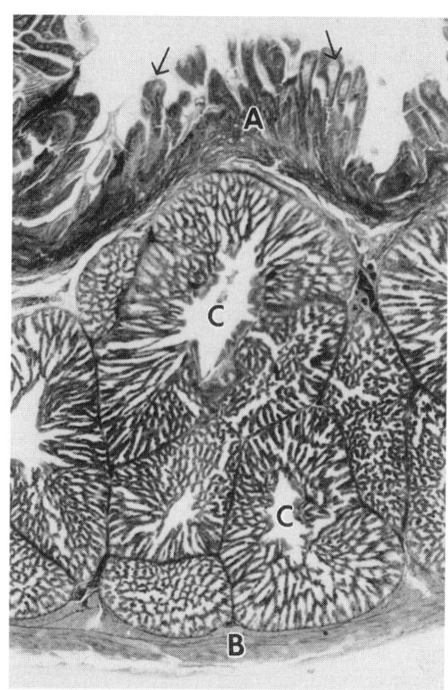

Figure 10.76. *Proventriculus (chicken). Papilla (A) with plicae (arrows); tunica muscularis (B); submucosal glands (C). Hematoxylin and eosin (×23).*

The **crop** is a saclike diverticulum of the esophagus. It is a storage organ where the ingested food is moistened by the mucous secretions of the esophageal and crop glands. Its histologic structure is similar to that of the esophagus. In the chicken, the glands are restricted to an area near its junction with the esophagus.

The bird does not have a glandular stomach similar to that of mammals, but instead has two separate organs between the esophagus and the duodenum. The **proventriculus**, or "glandular" stomach, and the **ventriculus**, or "muscular" stomach, perform many of the functions of the mammalian stomach.

The mucosa of the **proventriculus** is characterized by macroscopic papillae with numerous microscopic folds (plicae) of varying height that are arranged concentrically around the single duct opening at the apex of each papilla (Fig. 10.76). Simple columnar epithelium lines the lumen and continues into three generations of ducts of the submucosal glands (Fig. 10.76). The glands are lined by a simple cuboidal to low columnar epithelium in which the adjacent cells are in direct contact only on their basal half, thereby giving a serrated appearance to the luminal surface. Only one cell type is identifiable (**oxynticopeptic cells**), and this type presumably produces both pepsinogen and hydrochloric acid. The lamina propria is typical loose connective tissue. The lamina muscularis consists of scattered bundles of smooth muscle. The loose connective tissue of the submucosa is followed peripherally by a triple-layered tunica muscularis consisting entirely of smooth muscle (Fig. 10.76). The proventriculus is covered by a typical **serosa**.

The **ventriculus (gizzard)** is a highly muscular organ responsible for grinding and macerating the ingesta (Figs. 10.77 and 10.78). The lining of the ventriculus is referred to as the **cuticle**. It is a secretory product produced by mucosal glands; it is not a stratum corneum. A pattern of wavy lines running parallel to the surface, formed from consecutive layers of secretory product, and perpendicular colonnades or thickenings extending from the openings of the underlying glands, give a characteristic microscopic appearance to this layer. The surface epithelium is simple columnar and that of the branched tubular mucosal glands is simple cuboidal. The lumina of the glands are filled with secretory product, which stains bright red with keratohyalin stains. The lamina propria and submucosa are both composed of loose connective tissue. The lamina muscularis is very discontinuous. The tunica muscularis is a single thick layer of parallel smooth muscle cells that spreads from two aponeuroses at the center of the organ. It is crisscrossed by bands of dense connective tissue. The outermost tunic is a typical serosa.

The histologic structure of the **small intestine** is similar to that of the mammalian small intestine. The lamina propria and submucosa contain large amounts of dif-

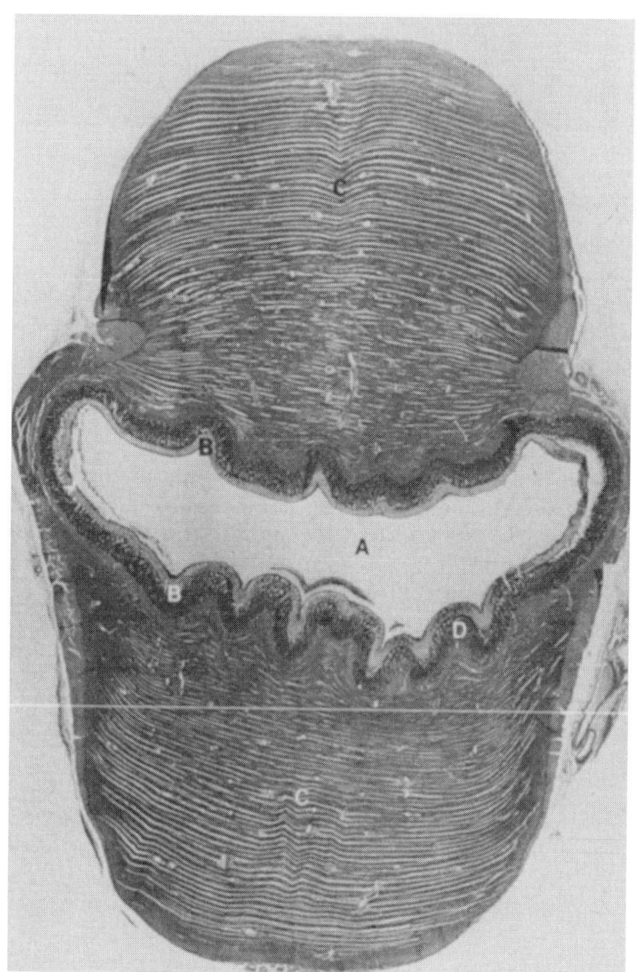

Figure 10.77. *Ventriculus, gizzard (chicken). Lumen (A); cuticle (B); smooth muscle of tunica muscularis (C); simple branched tubular ventricular glands (D). Hematoxylin and eosin (×10).*

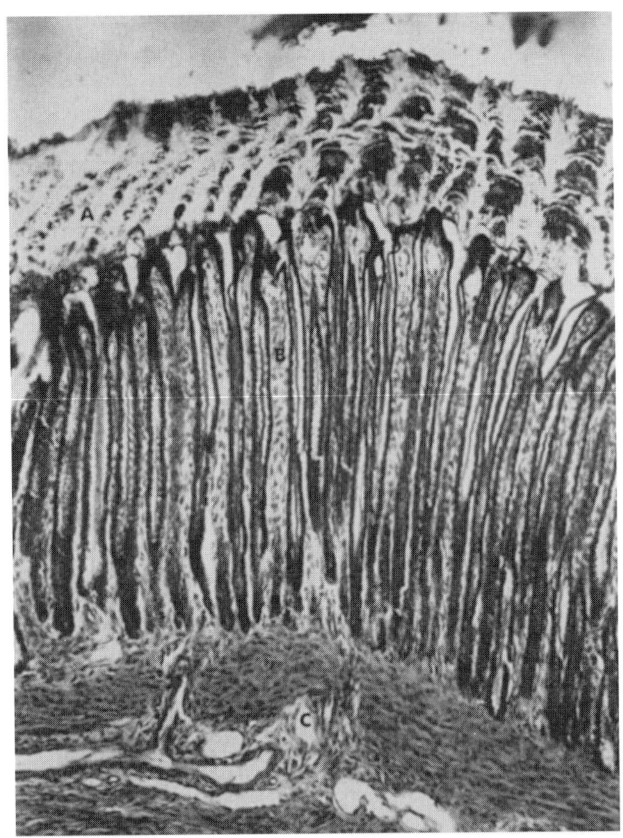

Figure 10.78. *Ventriculus, gizzard (chicken). Cuticle (A); lamina propria between the ventricular glands (B); submucosa (C). Trichrome (×88).*

fuse and nodular lymphatic tissue. Submucosal glands of the duodenum are generally absent. The tunica muscularis is composed of inner circular and outer longitudinal layers of smooth muscle. The outermost tunic is a typical serosa.

Two **ceca** open into the digestive tract at the junction of the ileum and rectum. Three regions of this organ present slightly different histologic features. The proximal portion contains prominent villi. In the adult bird, large masses of diffuse and nodular lymphatic tissue infiltrate the lamina propria and submucosa of this portion, forming grossly visible **cecal tonsils**. In the midportion, the villi are shorter and broader and mucosal folds are present. The distal ceca are devoid of villi. The surface epithelium of the mucosa is simple columnar with goblet cells.

The **rectum**, a part of the large intestine, extends from the ileum to the coprodeum of the cloaca. It resembles the small intestine in that villi are present. Scattered diffuse and nodular lymphatic tissues occur in the lamina propria and submucosa.

The **cloaca** is divided into three parts — the **coprodeum**, **urodeum**, and **proctodeum** — by transverse folds. All three parts have a similar structure. Villi are present and the epithelium of the mucosa is simple columnar. The **cloacal bursa** opens into the proctodeum.

Histologic features of the liver, gallbladder, and exocrine pancreas of the bird are not significantly different from those of the same organs in mammals.

REFERENCES

Adam WS, Calhoun ML, Smith EM, et al. Microscopic anatomy of the dog: a photographic atlas. Springfield, IL: Charles C. Thomas, 1970:102.

Boshell JL, Wilborn WH. Histology and ultrastructure of the pig parotid gland. Am J Anat 1978;152:447.

Budsberg SC, Spurgeon TL. Microscopic anatomy and enzyme histochemistry of the canine anal canal. Anat Histol Embryol 1983;12:295.

Chu RM, Glock RD, Ross RF. Gut-associated lymphoid tissue of young swine with emphasis on some epithelium of aggregated lymph nodules (Peyer's patches) of the small intestine. Am J Vet Res 1979; 40:1720.

Gemmell RT, Heath T. Fine structure of sinusoids and portal capillaries in the liver of adult sheep and the newborn lamb. Anat Rec 1972;172:57.

Gershon MD, Kirchgessner AL, Wade PR. Functional anatomy of the enteric nervous system. In: Johnson LR, ed. Physiology of the gastrointestinal tract, 3rd ed. New York: Raven Press, 1994;1:381

International Committee on Veterinary Gross Anatomical Nomenclature. Nomina anatomica veterinaria, 4th ed. Ithaca, NY: International Committee on Veterinary Gross Anatomical Nomenclature, 1994.

International Committee on Veterinary Histological Nomenclature. Nomina histologica, revised 2nd ed. Ithaca, NY: International Committee on Veterinary Histological Nomenclature, 1994.

Madara JL, Trier JS. The functional morphology of the mucosa of the small intestine. In: Johnson LR, ed. Physiology of the gastrointestinal tract, 3rd ed. New York: Raven Press, 1994;2:1577.

Rappaport AM, Borowy ZJ, Loughheed WM, et al. Subdivision of hexagonal liver lobules into a structural and functional unit. Role in hepatic physiology and pathology. Anat Rec 1954;119:11.

Titkemeyer CW, Calhoun ML. A comparative study of the structure of the small intestines of domestic animals. Am J Vet Res 1955;16:152.

Wünsche A. Anatomy of the liver lobule of pig. Anat Histol Embryol 1981;10:342.

11

Urinary System

CHARLES HENRIKSON

The urinary system is composed of two kidneys, two ureters, a urinary bladder, and a urethra. In general, the kidneys regulate the volume and composition of body fluids. They conserve fluid components necessary to maintain homeostasis while ridding the body of metabolic waste products, as well as excess water and electrolytes, in the form of urine. This process is accomplished by filtration of the blood, reabsorption, and secretion. The urinary bladder provides storage and intermittent release of urine, whereas the ureters and urethra provide conduits for urine.

KIDNEY

General Organization

EXTERNAL FEATURES

An understanding of the structure of the kidney, and especially the interrelationships of the renal tubules and renal vasculature, is essential to appreciate the diverse functions of the kidney. The kidneys of domesticated animals have a variety of shapes, including smooth and beanlike in cats, dogs, sheep, and goats; smooth, elongated, and flattened in pigs; smooth and heart-shaped in horses; and externally scalloped and oval in the ox. In all species, the renal artery and vein, lymphatics, nerves, and the ureter pass through a single indentation or hilus. Surrounding all kidneys is a connective tissue capsule, which is composed primarily of collagen fibers but also may contain varying amounts of smooth muscle. The retroperitoneal position of the kidney usually provides one surface with peritoneum (mesothelium and a thin layer of connective tissue), whereas the remaining surfaces are covered by adipose tissue, perirenal fat.

LOBATION

A longitudinal section through the kidney reveals the parenchyma divided into an outer, dark red **cortex** and an inner, lighter-colored **medulla** (Fig. 11.1). A varia-

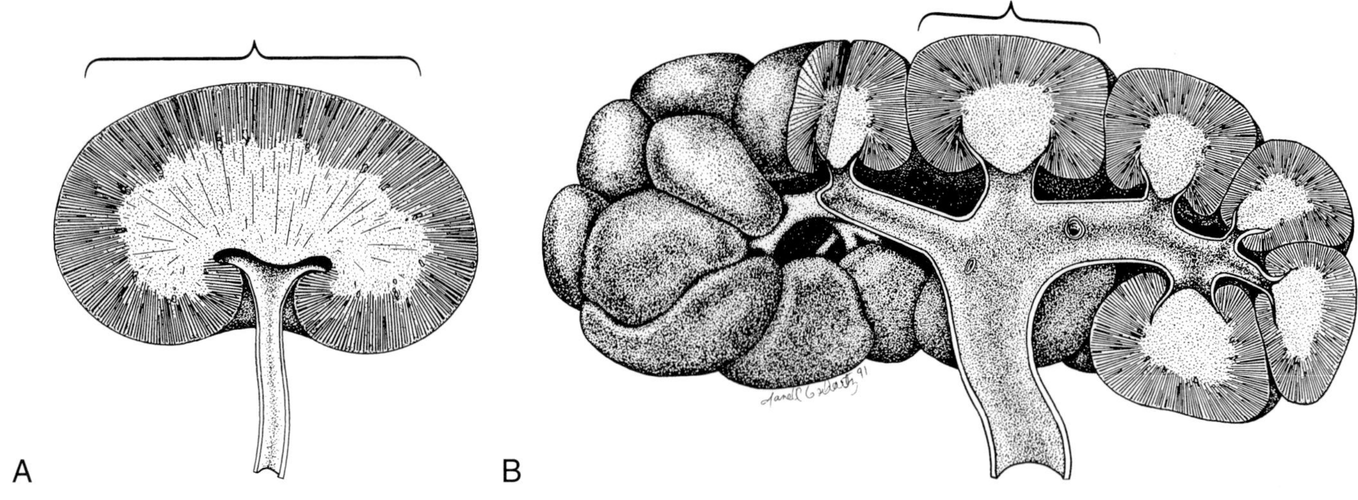

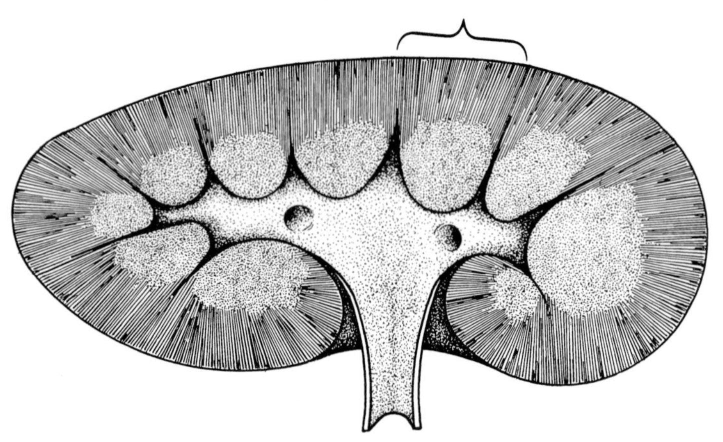

Figure 11.1. *Schematic drawing of the gross structure and lobation pattern in three different kidneys.* ***A.,*** *Unilobar kidney typical of carnivores.* ***B.,*** *Multilobar kidney typical of large ruminants. On the surface of the kidney, each lobe is distinctly outlined by deep invaginations. Note that this kidney lacks a renal pelvis.* ***C.,*** *Multilobar kidney of the pig. Note the smooth surface of kidney. (Redrawn from Dellmann H-D, Brown EM. Textbook of veterinary histology. Philadelphia: Lea & Febiger, 1987.)*

tion in the amount of fusion of the cortical and medullary components during embryonic development results in a diversity of structural arrangements in the adult kidneys of domesticated animals. The bovine kidney has the most distinct lobed arrangement, with external demarcation of the cortex and segmentation of the medulla into pyramids. The bases of the pyramids are adjacent to the cortex, and their apexes or papillae point toward the hilus. A renal lobe is composed of a renal pyramid plus its associated cap of cortex. Thus, the ox has an obvious, multilobed (multipyramidal) kidney. Pigs have a multilobed kidney with numerous, separate medullary pyramids; however, its single, continuous cortex has an outer smooth surface. Cats, dogs, horses, sheep, and goats have unilobar (unipyramidal) kidneys. The cortical and medullary components fuse into a single unit. Instead of a pointed pyramid, however, the linearly fused papillae form a renal crest.

CORTEX AND MEDULLA

With careful gross or low-magnification microscopic examination, the cortex and medulla can be further subdivided (Table 11.1, Figs. 11.2 and 11.3). The cortex has two basic divisions: the **cortical labyrinth** and the **medullary rays**. As the name suggests, the cortical labyrinth contains the tortuous tubular components, the **convoluted tubules**, as well as small granular structures, the **renal corpuscles**. The medullary rays are composed of straight tubules aligned perpendicular to the surface of the kidney. Although the medullary rays ap-

Table 11.1.
The Organization of Renal Parenchyma

Divisions of Renal Parenchyma	*Major Components in Each Division*
1. Cortex	
a. Cortical labyrinth	Renal corpuscles, proximal convoluted tubules, distal convoluted tubules (arched collecting ducts)
b. Medullary rays	Proximal straight tubules, distal straight tubules, collecting ducts
2. Medulla	
a. Outer medulla	
1. Outer stripe	Proximal straight tubules, distal straight tubules, collecting ducts
2. Inner stripe	Descending thin tubules, distal straight tubules, collecting ducts
b. Inner medulla	Descending and ascending thin tubules, collecting ducts

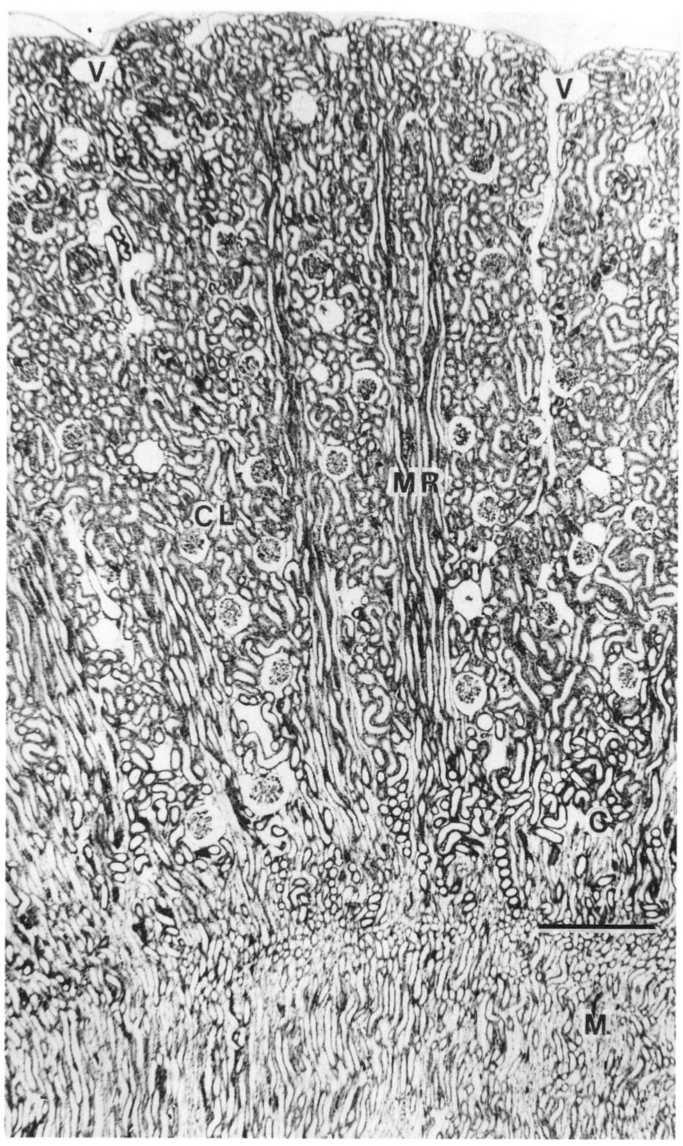

Figure 11.2. *Kidney (cat). Cortex (C) and small part of medulla (M). The cortex is composed of the cortical labyrinth (CL) and medullary rays (MR). The renal corpuscles and convoluted tubules are in the cortical labyrinth and the longitudinally sectioned, straight tubules are in the medullary rays. Note the capsular veins (V) at the surface of the kidney. In the lower right corner, a small bar indicates the approximate division between the cortex and medulla. Hematoxylin and eosin (×30).*

pear similar to the medulla, they are cortical structures. The medulla is composed of straight tubules and vessels and has a subtle striated appearance. The medulla can be divided into an **outer zone** nearest the cortex and an **inner zone** that includes the papilla or renal crest. The outer zone can be further subdivided into outer and inner stripes. These subdivisions of the medulla represent the location and orientation of the various segments of the renal tubules within the kidney (Fig. 11.4).

TYPES OF NEPHRONS

The **nephron** is often designated as the structural and functional unit of the kidney. Thousands of nephrons are present in each kidney. The number of nephrons per kidney varies with species, e.g., dogs have approximately 400,000 per kidney, whereas cats have approximately 200,000 per kidney. In carnivores and pigs, species in which the young are fairly immature when born, the formation of nephrons may continue for several weeks after birth. After renal maturity has been established, however, no new nephrons can be formed. Nephrons are classified either by the location of their renal corpuscles within the cortex as superficial, midcortical, or juxtamedullary or by the length of the loop of the nephron (Henle's loop) as **short-looped** or **long-looped**. Short-looped nephrons turn in the outer medulla, whereas long-looped nephrons turn in the inner medulla. The loops of the cortical nephrons in a few species, e.g., pigs, turn in the medullary ray of the cortex. In general, the two systems of classification overlap; the superficial and midcortical nephrons are short-looped, and the juxtamedullary nephrons are long-looped. Most species have both short- and long-looped nephrons. Some species, however, such as cats and dogs, have only long-looped nephrons, whereas other species, such as beavers, have only short-looped nephrons. This heterogeneity of types of nephrons indicates several functional differences among the various nephrons. In addition to the variation in types of nephrons, structural

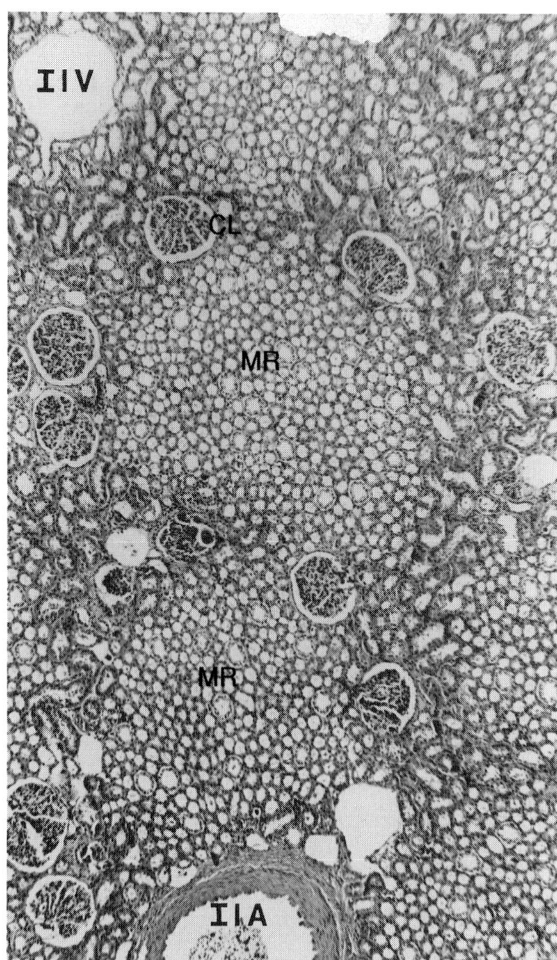

Figure 11.3. *Kidney (horse). Section cut parallel to the surface of the kidney, deep in the cortex. The medullary rays (MR), roughly circular profiles, contain straight tubules cut in cross section. The cortical labyrinth (CL) contains the renal corpuscles and convoluted tubules and surrounds the medullary rays. Note the interlobular artery (IlA) and vein (IlV) in the cortical labyrinth. Hematoxylin and eosin (×55).*

differences also occur along the length of a single nephron, thus dividing it into a variety of segments. The length of each segment differs with each type of nephron. Several nephrons empty into a single **collecting duct** and, as the collecting ducts descend through the medullary ray and the various layers of the medulla, they join to form larger and larger ducts. The largest collecting ducts are the papillary ducts. They terminate at the tip of the papilla, forming a perforated area called the **area cribrosa**.

NEPHRON VERSUS RENAL TUBULE

Classically, the collecting duct has not been considered part of the nephron because the duct has a separate origin during development. The collecting duct arises from the ureteric bud, whereas all of the components of the nephron develop from the metanephric blastema. During development, these two components fuse to become continuous tubules. The term **renal tubule** (uriniferous tubule) encompasses both the nephron and the collecting duct and may be a more appropriate term to describe the structural and functional unit of the kidney. Conversely, some investigators, recognizing the continuity of these tubular structures and the importance of the collecting duct in the formation of urine, include the collecting duct in the definition of the nephron and, thus, appropriately use the nephron as the structural and functional unit of the kidney. In this chapter, the classic separation of nephron and collecting duct system is maintained.

PARTS OF THE RENAL TUBULE

The segmentation of the renal tubule, as well as the sequence in which the filtrate flows from where it leaves the blood to where it drips as final urine from the renal parenchyma, includes the following (Fig. 11.4):

- I. Nephron
  - A. Renal corpuscle
    - 1. Glomerulus
      - a. Glomerular rete (capillary tuft)
      - b. Mesangium
    - 2. Glomerular capsule (Bowman's capsule)
  - B. Proximal convoluted tubule
  - C. Proximal straight tubule
  - D. Thin tubule
    - 1. Descending portion
    - 2. Ascending portion
  - E. Distal straight tubule (contains macula densa)
  - F. Distal convoluted tubule
- II. Collecting duct system
  - A. Arched collecting duct (connecting tubule)
  - B. Collecting duct (straight collecting tubule)
    - 1. Cortical collecting duct
    - 2. Outer medullary collecting duct
    - 3. Inner medullary collecting duct (includes papillary duct)

Renal Tubule

RENAL CORPUSCLE

General structure

The **renal corpuscle**, found in the cortical labyrinth (Figs. 11.5 and 11. 6), is the first part of the nephron. A filtrate of the blood is formed here. The renal corpuscle is spherical and varies in size, depending on species. Larger animals have larger renal corpuscles, e.g., 220 μm in diameter in horses, compared with 120 μm in diameter in cats. The renal corpuscle is composed of the glomerulus and the glomerular capsule. Strictly defined, the glomerulus includes only the capillary rete (capillary tuft) and the mesangium; however, the term **glomerulus** is used throughout the literature and in many different disciplines to refer to the entire renal corpuscle.

Glomerular rete

The **glomerular rete** or capillary tuft of the glomerulus is composed of several loops of branching and anastomosing capillaries that are fed by a single afferent arteriole and drained by a single efferent arteriole at the vascular pole of the renal corpuscle. These capillaries are lined by an extremely thin squamous epithelium of porous endothelial cells (Fig. 11.7). The endothelial pores (fenestrations) have a diameter of 50 to 150 nm.

Mesangium

The **mesangium** forms the core structure of the glomerulus and is located on the same side of the glomerular basement membrane (GBM) as the endothelial cells. The mesangium is made of mesangial cells embedded in a mesangial matrix. The mesangial cells are irregular in shape and have elongated cell processes (see Fig. 11.6). Bundles of microfilaments are found in the cytoplasm, especially within the processes. The occurrence and distribution of several contractile proteins correspond to the pattern of the microfilaments in the mesangial cells. The mesangial cells are connected to each other and to extraglomerular mesangial cells by gap junctions. They are believed to be derived from smooth muscle cells or pericytes. The mesangial matrix is characterized by a dense network of microfibrils surrounded by an amorphous material similar to the basal lamina. Of the proteins identified in the matrix, fibronectin is the most abundant and is associated with the microfibrils.

Glomerular basement membrane

The **glomerular basement membrane** (basal lamina) separates the endothelial and mesangial cells on its inner surface from the podocytes covering its outer surface (Figs. 11.6 and 11.7). The GBM is composed of three layers: the **lamina rara interna**, an electron-lucent

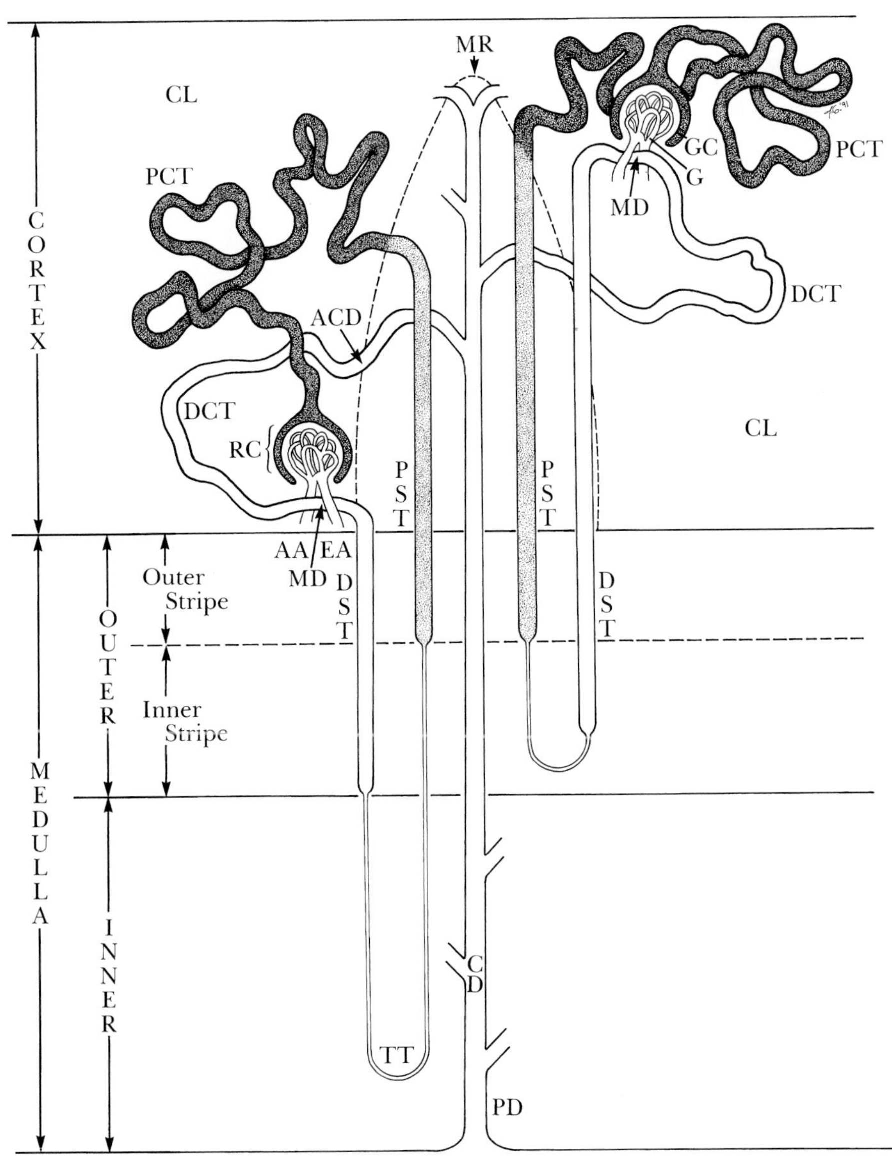

Figure 11.4. *Schematic drawing of the major divisions of the cortex and medulla as well as the major components of a long-looped (left) and a short-looped (right) nephron. The two divisions of the cortex are the cortical labyrinth (CL) and the medullary ray (MR, inside arched dashed lines). The afferent arteriole (AA) carries blood to the glomerulus (G) while the efferent arteriole (EA) carries blood away from it. A renal corpuscle (RC) is made up of a glomerulus and its surrounding glomerular capsule. A filtrate of the blood collects in the urinary space of the glomerular capsule (GC) and flows through the proximal convoluted tubule (PCT), proximal straight tubule (PST), thin tubule (TT), distal straight tubule (DST) containing the macula densa (MD), distal convoluted tubule (DCT), arched collecting duct (ACD), collecting duct (straight) (CD), and papillary duct (PD).*

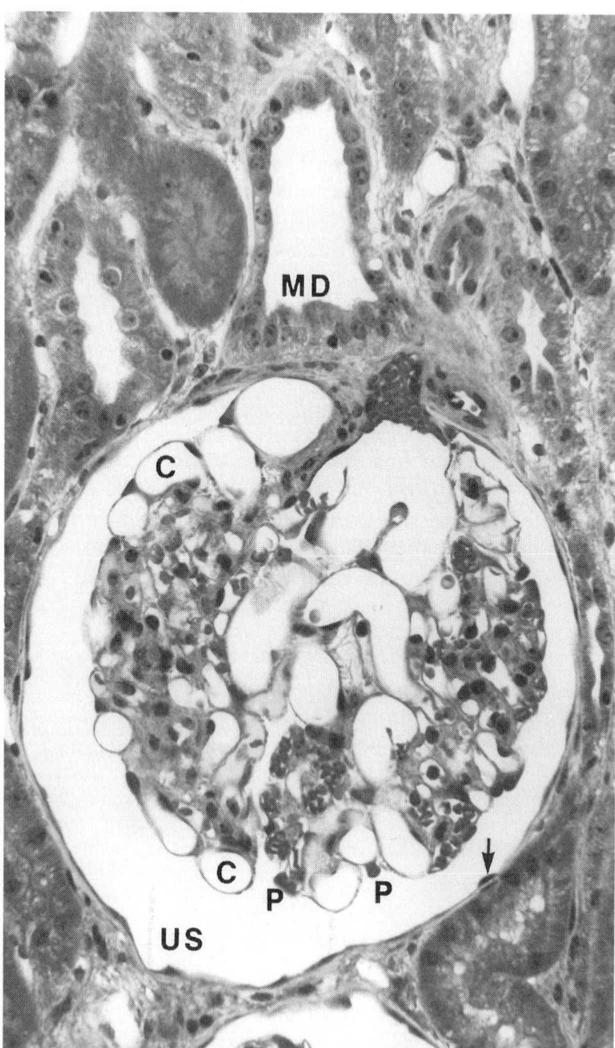

Figure 11.5. Renal corpuscle (horse). The glomerulus, composed of numerous capillary loops (C) and mesangial cells (not easily distinguished), is surrounded by the glomerular capsule made up of a visceral layer of podocytes (P) and a parietal layer of squamous cells (arrow). A filtrate of the blood first collects in the urinary space (US) of the glomerular capsule. Two components of the juxtaglomerular apparatus, the macula densa (MD) in the distal straight tubule and the extraglomerular mesangial cells, are found at the vascular pole of the renal corpuscle. JB-4 plastic. Hematoxylin and eosin and phloxine (×335).

layer beneath the endothelium; the **lamina densa**, an electron-dense layer in the middle; and the **lamina rara externa**, an electron-lucent layer beneath the podocytes. The GBM is 100 to 250 nm thick in dogs (320–340 nm thick in humans) and comprises many different substances, including type IV collagen, which is concentrated in the lamina densa, and proteoglycans, which contain glycosaminoglycans rich in heparan sulfate and are concentrated in the laminae rarae interna and externa. The GBM also contains glycoproteins, such as fibronectin, laminin, and entactin. The GBM stains positively with the periodic acid-Schiff (PAS) stain (see Fig. 11.12).

Glomerular capsule

The **glomerular capsule** (Bowman's capsule) surrounds the glomerulus and is composed of visceral and parietal layers (Figs. 11.8 through 11.10). The relationship of the glomerulus to the glomerular capsule has often been compared to a fist pushed into a partially inflated balloon. The fist represents the glomerulus, the part of the balloon directly covering the fist represents the **visceral layer**, and the rest of the balloon not touching the fist represents the **parietal layer**. The visceral layer of the glomerular capsule covers the outer surface of the GBM and is made of a continuous layer of octopuslike cells surrounding the capillaries. The cell body, where the nucleus is located, gives off several large, pri-

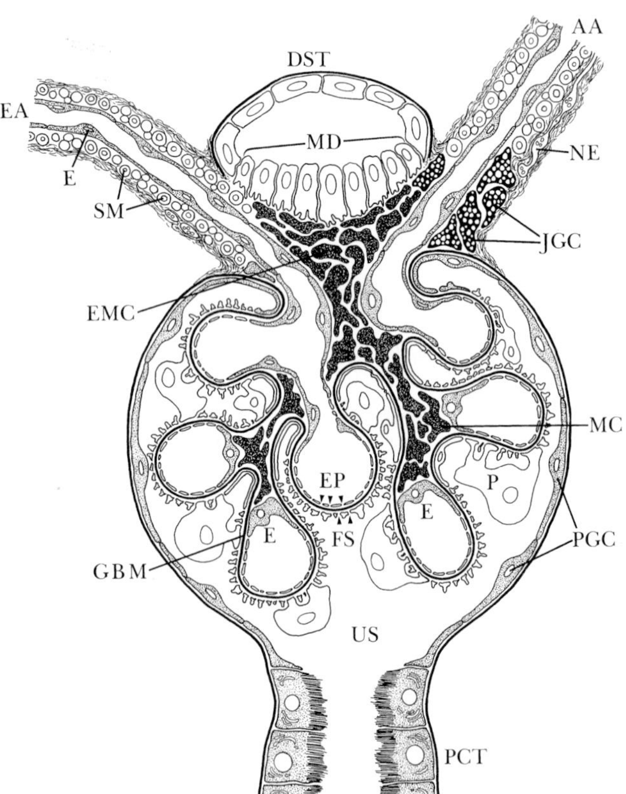

Figure 11.6. Schematic drawing of the renal corpuscle and juxtaglomerular apparatus. The afferent arteriole (AA) supplies the glomerulus while the efferent arteriole (EA) carries blood away from it. The endothelial cells (E) lining the arterioles are not porous, whereas those of the glomerulus have endothelial pores (EP). The mesangial cells (MC) of the glomerulus are found on the same side of the glomerular basement membrane (GBM) as the endothelial cells. The glomerular capsule surrounds the glomerulus and is composed of a visceral layer of podocytes (P) and a parietal layer (PGC) of flattened cells. The podocytes have foot processes that contact the GBM. The spaces between the foot processes are the filtration slits (FS). The urinary space (US) is continuous with the lumen of the proximal convoluted tubule (PCT). The juxtaglomerular apparatus includes the macula densa (MD) within the distal straight tubule (DST), the extraglomerular mesangial cells (EMC), and the JG cells (JGC). The JG cells are derived from the smooth muscle cells (SM) of the afferent arteriole. Nerve endings (NE) are found near the JG cells. (Redrawn from Koushanpour E, Kriz W. Renal physiology. Principles, structure and function. New York: Springer-Verlag, 1986.)

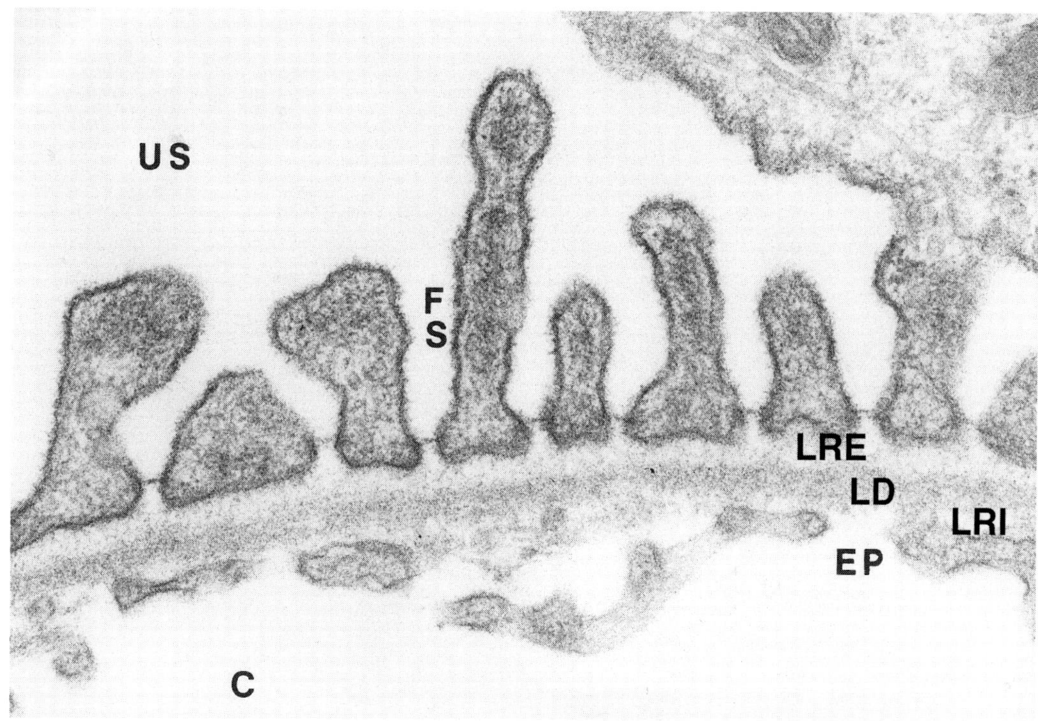

Figure 11.7. *Transmission electron micrograph of glomerular basement membrane (rat). The blood within the glomerular capillary (C) is selectively filtered as it passes through the endothelial pores (EP), the three layers of the glomerular basement membrane [lamina rara interna (LRI), lamina densa (LD) and lamina rara externa (LRE)] and the filtration slits (FS) between the podocytic foot processes to enter the urinary space (US). Note the filtration diaphragms, which bridge adjacent foot processes (×67,000). (Courtesy of J.W. Verlander.)*

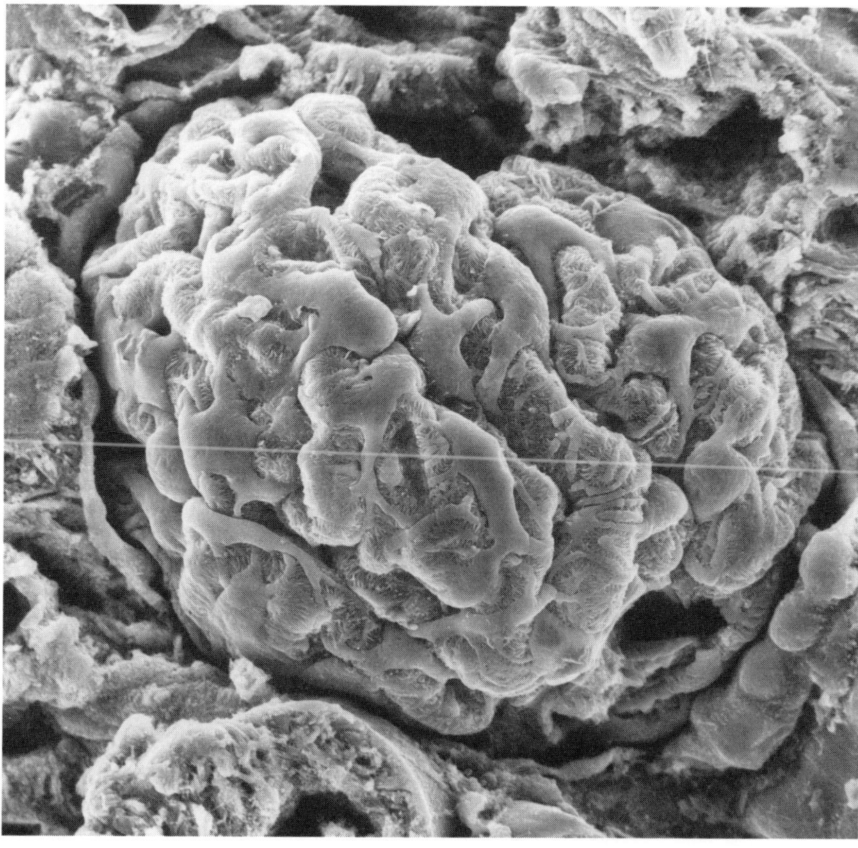

Figure 11.8. *Scanning electron micrograph of renal corpuscle (rat). This is a view of a renal corpuscle as seen from the urinary space. The parietal layer of the glomerular capsule has been removed, revealing the visceral layer of podocytes embracing the glomerular capillaries. The large, smooth-surfaced cell bodies of the podocytes project primary processes that branch to form secondary and tertiary processes. The terminal or smallest processes are the foot processes (×1300). (Courtesy of J.W. Verlander.)*

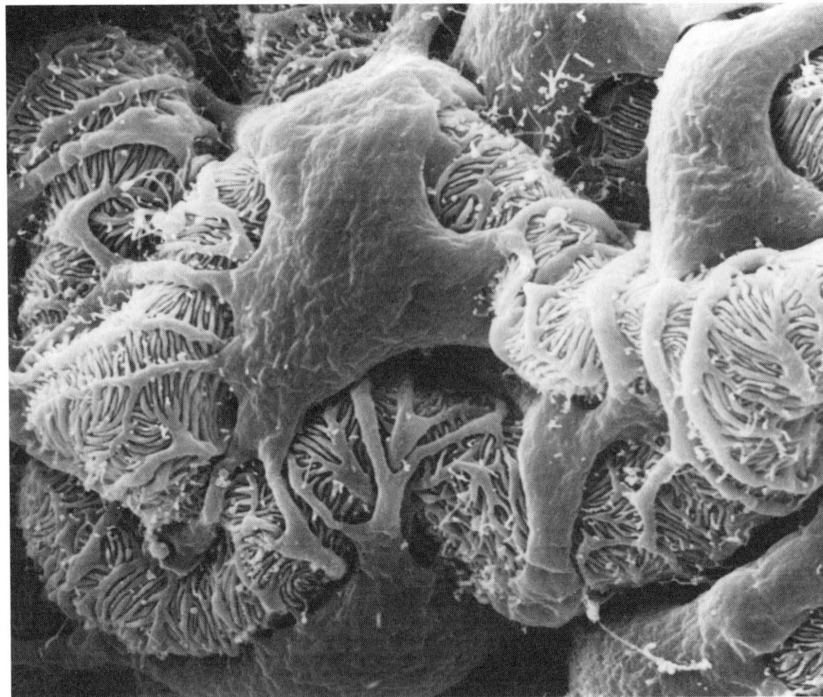

Figure 11.9. *Scanning electron micrograph of podocyte (rat). Detail of Figure 11.8. The cell body of one podocyte is in the center of the field. Numerous processes of varying size extend from the cell body and wrap around the glomerular capillaries. The foot processes are the smallest of the processes and are separated from each other by filtration slits (×4100). (Courtesy of J.W. Verlander.)*

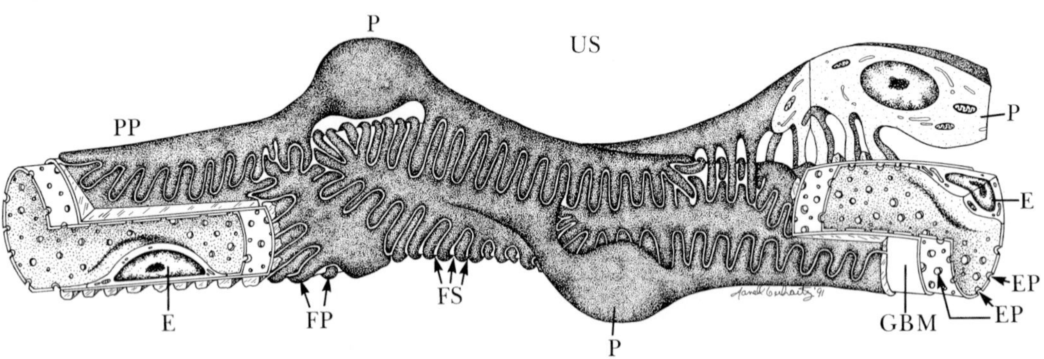

Figure 11.10. *Schematic drawing of the components of the filtration barrier of the kidney. The endothelium (E) lining the glomerular capillaries has numerous pores (EP). Surrounding the capillaries is the glomerular basement membrane (GBM) and covering its outer surface are the podocytes (P). The podocytes have processes of several different calibers. Only the primary processes (PP) and foot processes (FP) are shown here. Certain components of the plasma are allowed through the endothelial pores, the GBM, and the filtration slits (FS) to become the filtrate in the urinary space (US).*

mary processes from which smaller secondary processes emanate. The smallest of these processes are foot-shaped and referred to as **foot processes** or **pedicels**. Because of the foot processes, these visceral epithelial cells are often referred to as **podocytes**. The pedicels of one cell interdigitate with the pedicels of adjacent cells. The narrow spaces between the pedicels are called the filtration slits and form a complex switchback pattern. The filtration slits, measuring approximately 25 to 60 nm, are bridged by a thin electron-dense layer called the **slit diaphragm**.

The relationship of the components of the renal corpuscle can be best understood by considering its construction in the following way. The centrally located mesangium forms the axis of the renal corpuscle. Pushed into the sides of the mesangium are the endothelial-lined tubes of the capillary tuft. Around the tuft is wrapped the GBM, which mainly contacts the endothelial cells, but also, to a lesser degree, contacts the mesangial cells. Finally, the podocytes and their foot processes cover the exterior of the GBM. At the vascular pole of the renal corpuscle, the visceral layer of the glomerular capsule becomes continuous with the parietal layer (Fig. 11.6). The parietal layer is composed of a simple squamous epithelium overlaying a thick basal lamina (Fig. 11.11). The lumen created between the two epithelial layers is called the **urinary space** (Bowman's space). At the urinary pole of the renal corpuscle, opposite the vascular pole, the glomerular capsule opens into the proximal convoluted tubule (Fig. 11.12). Components of the plasma pass through the endothelial pores, the GBM, and the filtration slits to become the filtrate in the urinary space of the glomerular capsule.

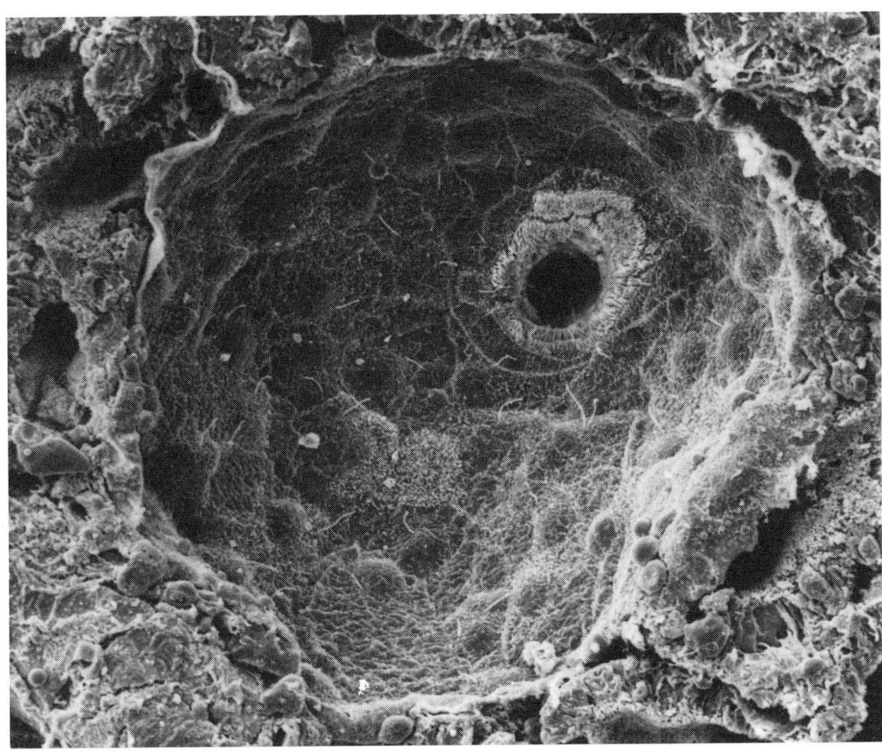

Figure 11.11. *Scanning electron micrograph of the parietal layer of the glomerular capsule (rat). All the components of the renal corpuscle have been removed except the parietal layer. Each squamous cell of the parietal layer is distinctly outlined and projects a single, centrally located cilium. Deep within the concavity formed by this epithelium is the opening into the proximal convoluted tubule. The microvilli covering the tubular epithelial cells are just visible (×1200). (Courtesy of J.W. Verlander.)*

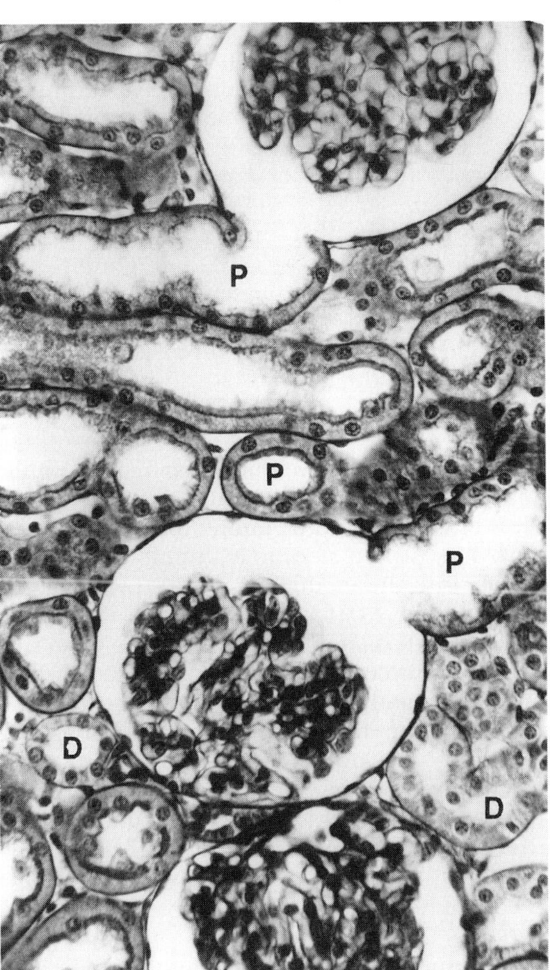

Figure 11.12. *Cortical labyrinth (perfused rat kidney). The three major components of the cortical labyrinth are the renal corpuscles, the proximal convoluted tubules (P), and the distal convoluted tubules (D). Two of the three renal corpuscles show continuity with proximal convoluted tubules. The PAS stain used on this section enhances the staining of the glomerular basement membrane, the basal laminae around the tubules, and the cell coat associated with the brush border of the proximal convoluted tubules. PAS (×335).*

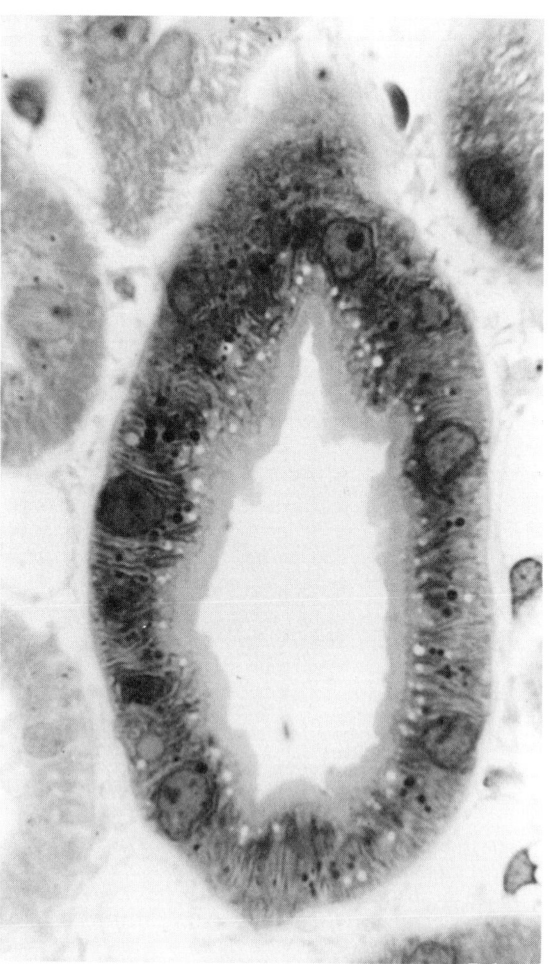

Figure 11.13. *Proximal convoluted tubule (dog). The brush border composed of microvilli covers the apical surface of the cells. White vacuoles near the lumen and dark, round granules deeper in the cytoplasm are endocytotic vacuoles and lysosomes, respectively. The elongated granules, oriented along the apex to base axis, are mitochondria. The nuclei are located more toward the base of the cell. Epon-Araldite. Azure II, methylene blue (×1320).*

PROXIMAL CONVOLUTED AND STRAIGHT TUBULES

The **proximal convoluted tubule** is located in the cortical labyrinth, whereas the **proximal straight tubule** is found in the medullary rays and extends into the outer stripe of the outer medulla. Because the proximal convoluted tubule is much longer than the distal convoluted tubule, the profiles of the proximal convoluted tubules dominate the cortical labyrinth (Fig. 11.12). The proximal convoluted tubule begins at the urinary pole of the renal corpuscle with an abrupt change in epithelium from the simple squamous epithelium of the parietal layer of the glomerular capsule to a simple cuboidal epithelium. The apical surface of this epithelium is covered by a continuous brush border of microvilli (Figs. 11.13 and 11.14). The microvilli are covered by an extensive, PAS-positive cell coat (Fig. 11.12). The lateral borders of the epithelial cells are characterized by an elaborate interdigitation of lateral cell processes. In addition, the basal surface of the cells has a remarkably folded membrane with processes from adjacent cells located between the folds. The arrangement of the epithelial cells can be likened to a group of highly corrugated tree stumps packed closely together with their roots growing beneath one another. Within the cytoplasm of the lateral processes and closely apposed to the cell membranes are numerous long mitochondria. The infolding of the membrane and the alignment of the mitochondria create the basal striations seen with the light microscope. This arrangement is typical of actively transporting cells. The surface modifications significantly increase the surface area of the cell to enhance its various transport processes, whereas the close association of the mitochondria provides a ready source of energy. Near the apical surface, the lateral sides of the cells are joined together by tight junctions, intermediate junctions, and desmosomes. Occasional gap junctions also link the cells. The tight junctions form continuous bands around the cells, but because of their simple structure, these junctions are considered leaky. An extensive endocytotic apparatus consists of numerous apical vesicles and large lysosomes. The peroxisome is a characteristic organelle of the proximal convoluted tubule. The rich complement of organelles tends to cause a more intense stain of the proximal convoluted tubule than of the distal convoluted tubule. The single nucleus is spherical and situated in the middle to basal part of the cell. (Two common fixation artifacts are associated with the proximal convoluted tubule. First, interruption of blood flow to the kidney, e.g., in immersion fixation, causes either collapse of the tubules or swelling of the epithelial cells with a resultant loss of tubular lumina. Patent lumina exist in the live animal and can only be preserved with careful perfusion fixation techniques. Second, if the kidney is not fixed rapidly, the labile brush border will disintegrate.)

The proximal convoluted tubule continues into the medullary ray to become the proximal straight tubule (Fig. 11.15). The proximal straight tubule, also referred to as the descending thick limb, forms the first part of the loop of the nephron (Henle's loop). The straight tubule retains many of features of the convoluted tubule, although in a less developed form. For example, its cells and microvilli are shorter, its basolateral membrane is less elaborate, and its endocytotic apparatus is diminished. The proximal straight tubule extends for some distance into the medulla and ends by becoming the thin tubule (Fig. 11.16). This transition most often occurs abruptly with the epithelium changing from simple cuboidal to simple squamous. The point at which this transition occurs is the division between the inner and outer stripes of the outer medulla. In dogs, the change occurs at the corticomedullary junction; therefore, the kidney of dogs lacks an outer stripe. Two unique species characteristics of the proximal straight and convoluted tubules are noteworthy. In cats, numerous lipid droplets are normally found in the cells of the proximal convoluted tubule (Fig. 11.17). Thus, the kidney of cats has a yellowish color. In dogs, the lipid droplets are found in the proximal straight tubule (see

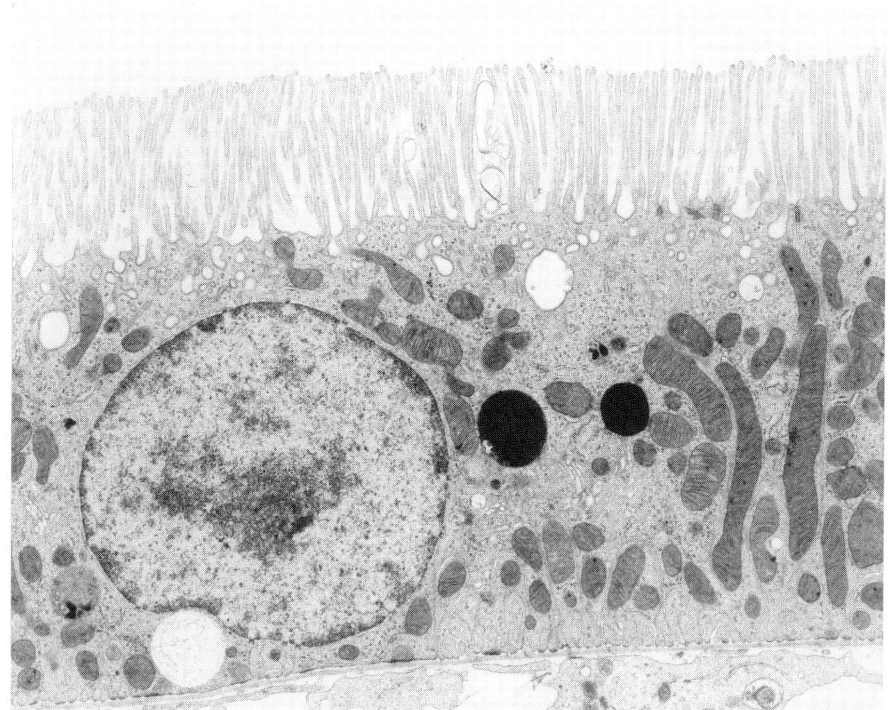

Figure 11.14. *Transmission electron micrograph of proximal convoluted tubule cell (rat). Numerous microvilli cover the apical surface. The endocytotic system of this cell consists of endocytotic vacuoles in the apical cytoplasm and two large, densely staining lysosomes in the middle of the cell. Mitochondria and basal infoldings of the cell membrane are prominent (×8800). (Courtesy of J.W. Verlander.)*

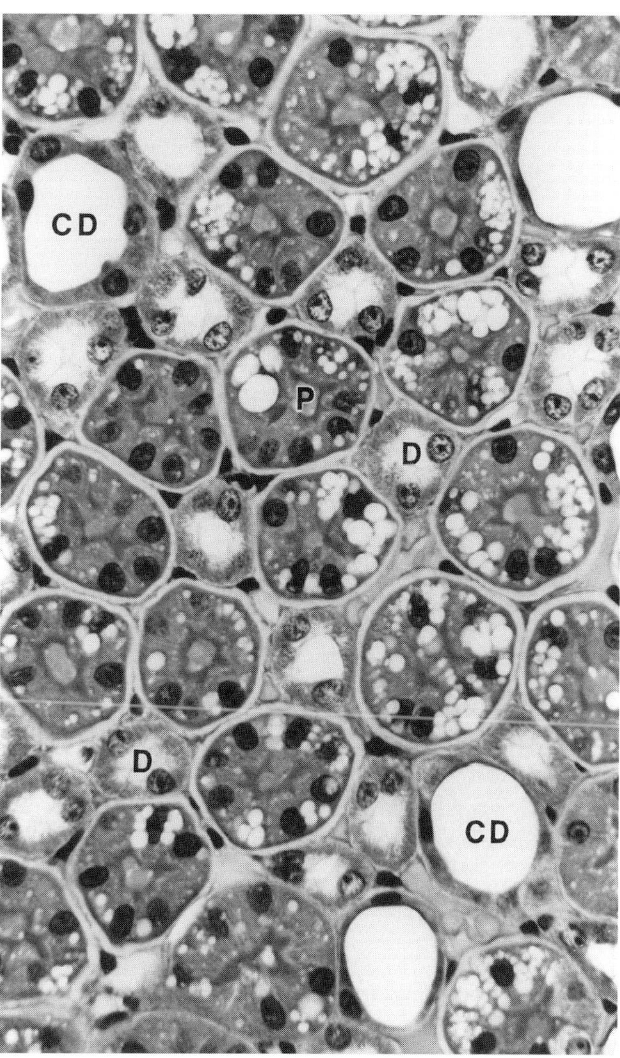

Figure 11.15. *Medullary ray (dog). The three major components of the medullary ray are the proximal straight tubules (P), distal straight tubules (D), and the collecting ducts (CD). Note the lipid droplets in the proximal straight tubules. This is normal in the dog. JB-4 plastic. Hematoxylin and eosin and phloxine (×530).*

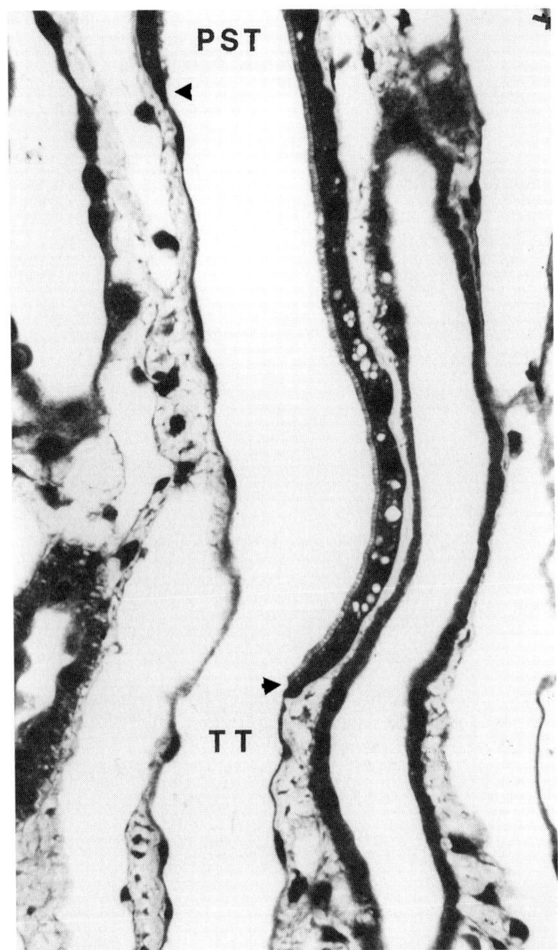

Figure 11.16. *Proximal straight tubule to thin tubule (dog). The simple cuboidal epithelium (note apical brush border) of the proximal straight tubule (PST) changes to a simple squamous epithelium in the thin tubule (TT). Note that the transition occurs at different points (arrows) around the circumference of the tubule. JB-4 plastic. Hematoxylin and eosin and phloxine (×510).*

Fig. 11.15) and can give the medullary rays on the cut surface of a gross kidney a much lighter appearance.

THIN TUBULE

The **thin tubule** begins at the border between the outer and inner stripes of the outer medulla, descends for a variable distance into the medulla (depending on the type of nephron), makes a hairpin turn (Fig.11.18), ascends in the medulla and ends at the border between the inner and outer medulla. The thin tubule forms the thin descending limb and the thin ascending limb of the **loop of the nephron** (Henle's loop). Investigators have described four different parts to the thin tubule. These parts vary somewhat with type of nephron and species studied. Distinction between various parts of the thin segment can be determined only at the electron-microscopic level and include differences in the height of the epithelium, the amount of amplification of the apical and basolateral cell membranes, the number of mitochondria, and the complexity of the tight junctions, all of which relate to functional differences along its length. In general, the thin tubule is lined by simple squamous epithelium. The change from simple squamous epithelium to simple cuboidal epithelium at the two ends of the thin segment may be abrupt or gradual, depending on the species. The nuclei, although somewhat flattened, protrude into the lumen to a greater degree than do the nuclei of the endothelial cells of adjacent capillaries. In addition, the nuclei are round as viewed from the lumen, whereas endothelial nuclei are elongated in the direction of the longitudinal axis of the vessel.

DISTAL STRAIGHT AND CONVOLUTED TUBULES

The **distal straight tubule** begins at the border of the inner and outer medulla (Fig. 11.19), ascends through both stripes of the outer medulla, ascends in the cortical medullary ray, passes by the vascular pole of its parent re-

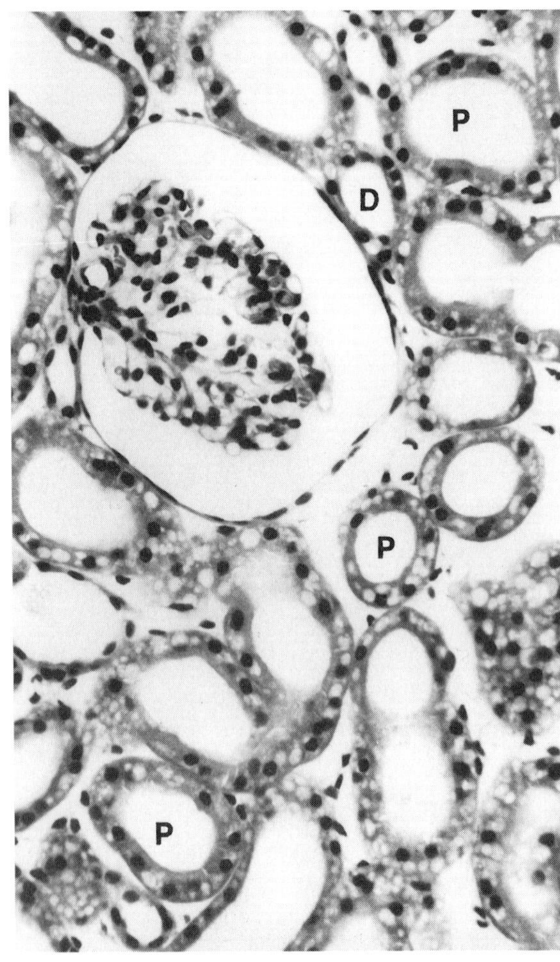

Figure 11.17. *Cortical labyrinth (cat). The proximal convoluted tubules contain numerous lipid droplets, which is normal in the cat. Note that the profiles of the proximal convoluted tubule (P) greatly outnumber those of the distal convoluted tubule (D) because of the proximal convoluted tubule's greater length. Hematoxylin and eosin (×335).*

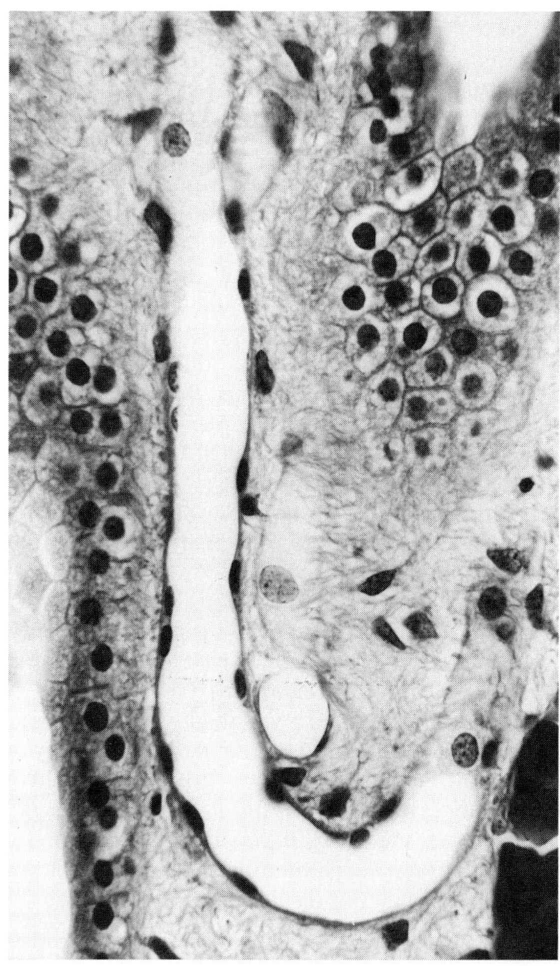

Figure 11.18. *Loop of the nephron (horse). The thin tubule makes a hairpin turn in the inner medulla. The nuclei of the simple squamous epithelial cell are flattened but rounded as viewed from the lumen. Glancing sections of two collecting ducts are also present near the thin tubule. Hematoxylin and eosin (×530).*

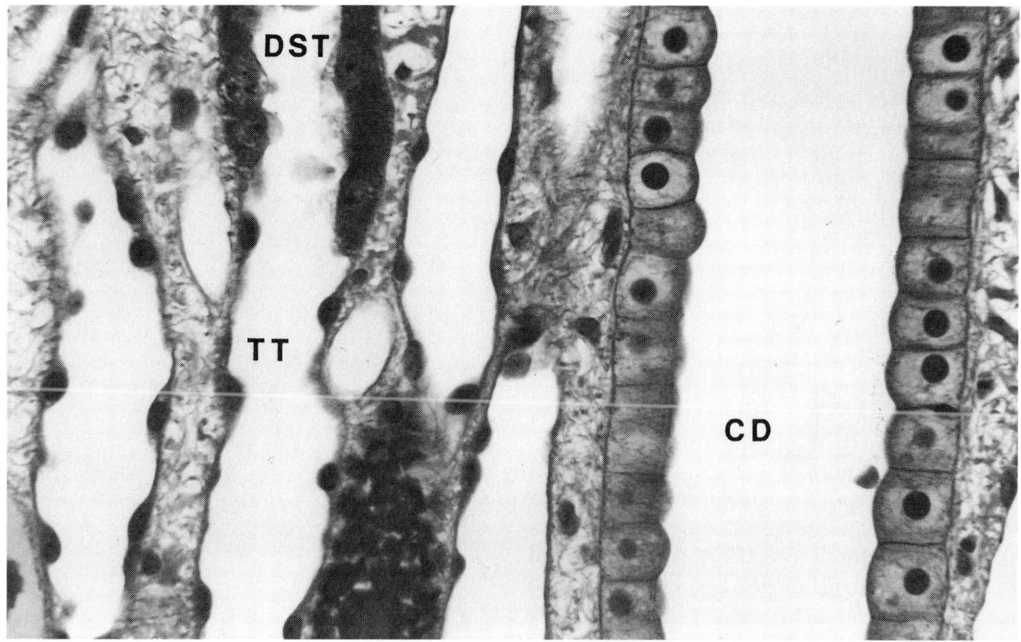

Figure 11.19. *Thin tubule to distal straight tubule (horse). This section was taken from the border of the inner and outer medulla. This is the location of the transition between the thin tubule (TT) with its simple squamous epithelium and the distal straight tubule (DST) with its simple cuboidal epithelium. Other thin tubules are present. The collecting duct (CD) is lined by simple cuboidal epithelium with distinct lateral cell borders. All of the cells of the collecting duct are principal cells. JB-4 plastic. Hematoxylin and eosin and phloxine (×530).*

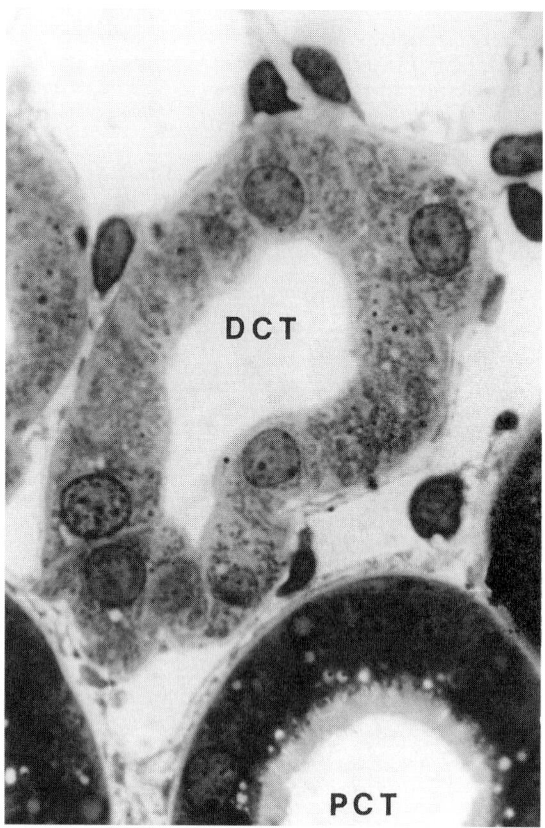

Figure 11.20. *Distal convoluted tubule (dog). The cells of the distal convoluted tubule (DCT) lack a brush border, contain numerous mitochondria, and have nuclei that tend to locate, more often, in the apical part of the cells. Note the proximal convoluted tubule (PCT) with its distinct brush border. Epon-Araldite. Azure II, methylene blue (×1320).*

nal corpuscle, and ends shortly beyond by becoming the **distal convoluted tubule**. The distal straight tubule forms the ascending thick limb and is the terminal part of the loop of the nephron (Henle's loop). As the distal straight tubule passes its glomerulus of origin, it forms a specialized patch of epithelial cells in its wall, called the **macula densa**.

The distal convoluted tubule is much shorter than the proximal convoluted tubule, and therefore, fewer profiles of the distal convoluted tubule are seen in the cortical labyrinth (Figs. 11.12 and 11.20). The distal straight and convoluted tubules are lined by simple cuboidal epithelium. The cells of these tubules lack a well developed brush border of microvilli; however, some short microvilli or microprojections can be seen with the electron microscope. The basolateral cell membranes are folded and are closely associated with elongated mitochondria. The nucleus is located in the apical part of the cell. The tight junctions are complex and therefore not leaky.

ARCHED COLLECTING DUCTS

The **arched collecting duct** (connecting tubule) is located in the cortical labyrinth and connects one to several distal convoluted tubules to a collecting duct in the medullary ray (see Fig. 11.4). Although distinct cell types have been identified in certain species, in general, these arched ducts have a structure that is transitional between the two tubules they connect and, therefore, are not easily distinguished.

COLLECTING DUCTS

Each **collecting duct** (straight collecting tubule) accepts tubular fluid from several nephrons. The collecting ducts extend throughout the medullary rays (Figs. 11.15 and 11.21), pass through the outer and inner medulla (see Fig. 11.19), and after fusing several times (Fig. 11.22), open as papillary ducts at the tip of the papilla (or at the edge of the renal crest). The collecting ducts are primarily lined with simple cuboidal epithelium. In carnivores, the epithelium remains low throughout its length, whereas in large animals, the epithelium in the medullary portions can be simple columnar or even transitional near the papillary openings. The collecting ducts are lined by two cell types: the **principal** (light) **cells** and the **intercalated** (dark) **cells** (Fig. 11.21). The principal cells are the most numerous and have a simple cuboidal shape. Their pale-staining cytoplasm lacks many organelles. The mitochondria are small, oval, and randomly oriented. The borders between the cells are easily distinguished because of the relatively straight, lateral cell membranes. Folding of the basolateral membranes is present but minimal. The in-

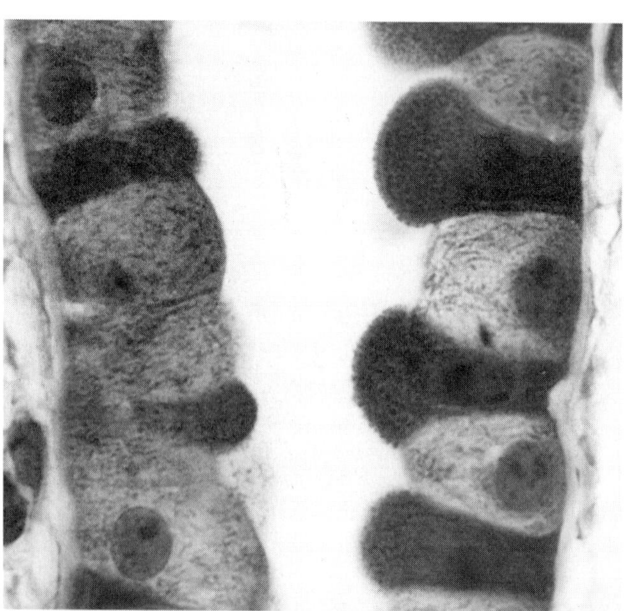

Figure 11.21. *Collecting duct in medullary ray (horse). This collecting duct is lined by two cell types. The principal cell stains lightly and contains relatively few irregularly shaped mitochondria. The intercalated cells are the dark staining cells and are in their protruded state. The apical part of the intercalated cell protrudes above and expands over the principal cell. The apical surface of the intercalated cell has numerous short projections. JB-4 plastic. Hematoxylin and eosin and phloxine (×1320).*

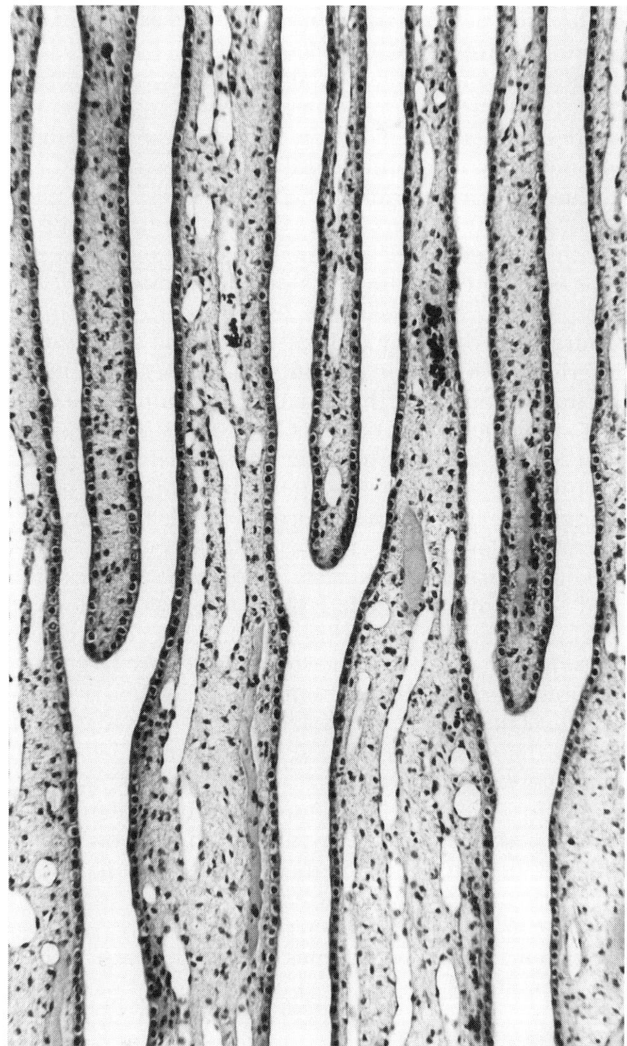

Figure 11.22. *Confluence of collecting ducts (horse). This section was taken from the inner medulla and contains only thin tubules and collecting ducts. Six smaller collecting ducts are coalescing to form three larger ones. A few blood vessels and a relatively extensive interstitium are also present. Hematoxylin and eosin (×170).*

tercalated cells are found throughout the collecting duct system; however, their numbers diminish distally. There are two types of intercalated cells that represent different functional states of the same cell. The first type is a dark-staining, tall cell that protrudes above the principal cell. Its apical surface is covered by numerous microplicae. The second form is a light-staining, retracted cell that is actually shorter than the surrounding principal cells. Its apical cytoplasm contains numerous vesicles. The transformation between the two types of cells is probably the result of a shuttling of membranes between the apical vesicles and the surface membrane. The cells of the collecting ducts are connected by complex tight junctions.

Vasculature of the Kidney

Each kidney is supplied by a single renal artery that arises directly from the abdominal aorta. Branching of the renal artery can occur near or within the hilus or within the renal sinus. These branches divide into **interlobar arteries**, which ascend in the substance of the kidney to the corticomedullary junction. Here, the interlobar arteries form variably arched vessels called **arcuate arteries** (Fig. 11.23). The arcuate arteries give off interlobular arteries, which radiate toward the surface of the

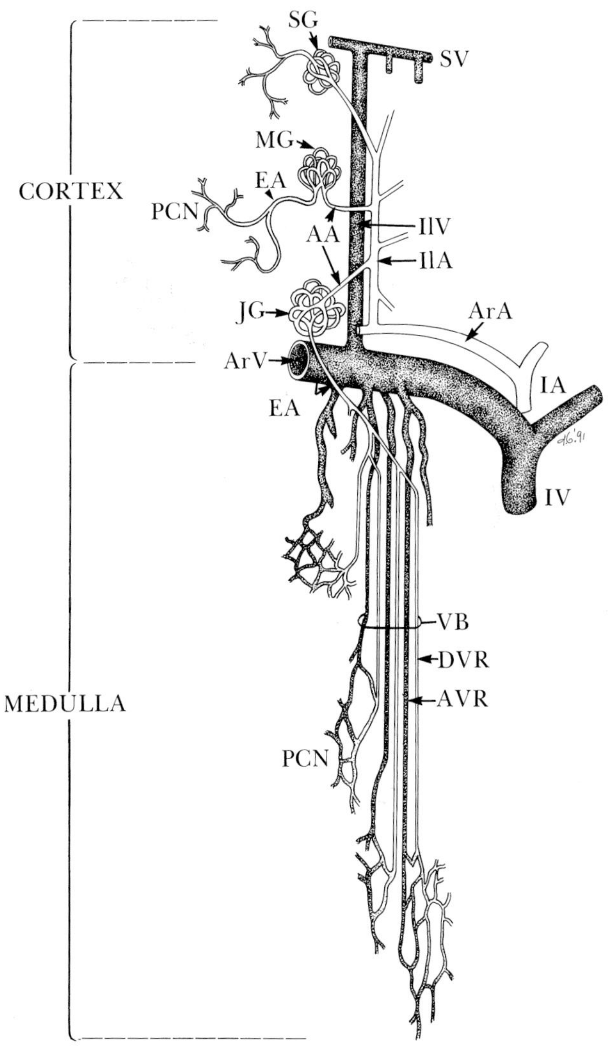

Figure 11.23. *Schematic drawing of the vasculature of the kidney. Arterial blood flow is through the renal artery, interlobar arteries (IA), arcuate arteries (ArA), interlobular arteries (IlA), afferent arterioles (AA), glomeruli, and efferent arterioles (EA). The efferent arterioles from the superficial glomeruli (SG) and the midcortical glomeruli (MG) supply the peritubular capillary network (PCN) in all parts of the cortex. The efferent arterioles from the juxtamedullary glomeruli (JG) supply the descending vasa recta (DVR) and all the peritubular capillary networks (PCN) of the medulla. Venous drainage of the peritubular capillary networks in the cortex involve the stellate veins (SV), the interlobular veins (IlV), and/or the arcuate veins (ArV). Venous drainage of the peritubular capillary networks in the medulla is primarily through the ascending vasa recta (AVR). The interlobular veins of the cortex and the ascending vasa recta of the medulla converge on the arcuate veins at the corticomedullary junction. The arcuate veins are drained by the interlobar veins (IV), which empty into the renal vein. The descending and ascending vasa recta often form vascular bundles (VB). (Redrawn from Koushanpour E, Kriz W. Renal physiology. Principles, structure and function. New York: Springer-Verlag, 1986.)*

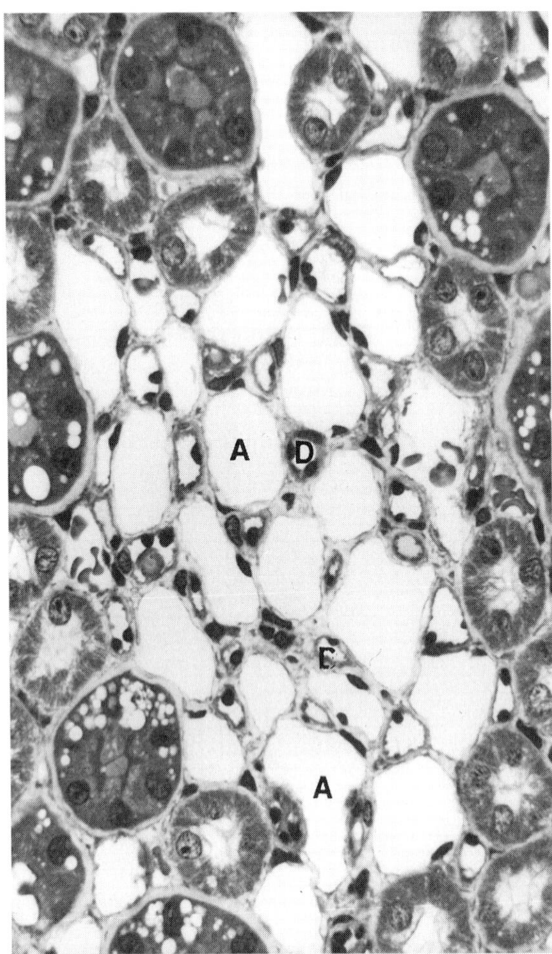

Figure 11.24. *Vascular bundle in outer medulla (dog). The descending vasa recta (D) are the small, round arterioles in the vascular bundle, and the ascending vasa recta (A) are the large, irregularly shaped, venous capillaries in the bundle. These vessels are the primary supply and drainage of the medulla. JB-4 plastic. Hematoxylin and eosin and phloxine (×530).*

kidney. The arcuate arteries do not send vessels directly to the medulla. The **interlobular arteries** course peripherally within the cortical labyrinth and give rise to the **afferent arterioles** that supply the glomeruli. The glomerular tufts of capillaries are drained by **efferent arterioles**. Efferent arterioles from glomeruli located in the superficial or middle cortex distribute to peritubular capillary networks of the cortical labyrinth and medullary rays. Efferent arterioles from glomeruli located in the juxtamedullary region supply the entire medulla. These efferent arterioles descend into the medulla to divide, within the outer stripe, into straight vessels called **descending vasa recta**. The descending vasa recta supply adjacent peritubular capillary networks at all levels of the medulla. The capillaries drain into straight vessels, which ascend in the medulla. These vessels are called **ascending vasa recta**. The descending vasa recta are arterioles, whereas the ascending vasa recta are venules with a fenestrated endothelium. Many of the descending and ascending vasa recta come together to form vascular bundles that are evenly distributed throughout the medulla (Fig. 11.24). The arrangement of medullary vessels provides an appropriate pattern for the countercurrent exchange system described later in this chapter. All peritubular capillaries in both the cortex and medulla are fenestrated.

The veins most often accompany and have names identical to the arteries. Venous drainage of the medulla is accomplished by the ascending vasa recta that enter the arcuate veins or, on occasion, the interlobular veins. Venous drainage of the cortex is primarily from the peritubular capillaries into the **stellate veins**, **interlobular veins**, or **arcuate veins**. After draining the cortex and medulla, the arcuate veins empty into the **interlobar veins**, which coalesce to form a single renal vein that leaves the hilus to enter the caudal vena cava. In carnivores, a system of superficial and deep cortical veins connects the capillaries of the superficial and deep cortical regions, respectively, to the larger veins. The superficial cortical veins carry blood toward the surface and empty into the stellate veins, whereas the deep cortical veins carry blood in the opposite direction to empty into the arcuate veins. The stellate veins are large in carnivores. In dogs, they are embedded in the cortical tissue near the surface of the kidney, whereas in cats, they are at the surface of the kidney and are referred to as capsular veins (see Fig. 11.2). The stellate veins in dogs, as in most species, empty into the interlobular veins; in contrast, the capsular veins in cats converge on the hilus of the kidney to join directly to the renal vein.

The arrangement of the intrarenal arteries does not provide a good collateral circulatory system. As a result, when a major artery becomes occluded, death of the tissue supplied by that artery quickly ensues. For example, when an arcuate artery becomes occluded, a wedge-shaped piece of the kidney, including both cortex and medulla, becomes damaged.

Lymphatics and Nerves

Lymph vessels are seen in the cortex but have not been identified with certainty in the medulla. Lymphatics are most often found in the interstitium, surrounding intrarenal arteries, and accompany arteries as they leave the kidney.

The kidney is provided with both afferent and efferent innervation; however, most of the nerves are sympathetic postganglionics. Most investigators agree that the smooth muscle of arteries, afferent and efferent arterioles, and descending vasa recta is innervated. Nerve terminals are also present on the renin-producing juxtaglomerular (JG) cells of the afferent arteriole. Some investigators have proposed direct innervation of kidney tubules; however, this is controversial.

Interstitium

The interstitium or stroma between the renal tubules and the blood vessels is normally sparse, particularly in the cortex, where the tubules and vessels are packed tightly together. More interstitium is present in the medulla and particularly in the inner medulla (Fig. 11.22). The interstitium consists of collagen fibrils and some fibrocytes. One unique cell type, especially prominent in the inner medulla, is the lipid-laden **interstitial cell**. These cells are stellate-shaped, contain varying numbers of lipid droplets, and seem to make connection between the loops of the nephron and the vasa recta.

Juxtaglomerular Apparatus

The **juxtaglomerular apparatus** is located at the vascular pole of the renal corpuscle (Fig. 11.6). Its components include the macula densa, the extraglomerular mesangial cells, and the juxtaglomerular (JG or granular) cells. The **macula densa** is a patch of densely packed epithelial cells on the renal corpuscle side of the distal straight tubule as it passes between the afferent and efferent arterioles (Figs. 11.5 and 11.25). The cells are tall and slender and are connected by complex tight junctions. Between the cells are conspicuous intercellular spaces. The bases of the cells face and are most intimately associated with the extraglomerular mesangial cells. The **extraglomerular mesangial cells** (Polkissen cells, lacis cells, Goormaghtigh cells) are found between the macula densa and the two arterioles and are continuous with the mesangial cells within the glomerulus. The cells are flattened and arranged into several layers. Gap junctions connect extraglomerular mesangial cells with each other, with intraglomerular mesangial cells, and with JG cells. They do not form junctions with the cells of the macula densa. The **JG cells** are primarily found in the media of the afferent arteriole and are derived from smooth muscle (Figs. 11.25 and 11.26). They contain specific, membrane-bound granules of irregular size and shape. The granules contain renin. Sympathetic nerve endings are found near the JG cells.

A new cell type called the **peripolar cell** has been identified recently and is believed to be part of the juxtaglomerular apparatus. The peripolar cells are located at the vascular pole of the renal corpuscle. They are found at the junction between the parietal and visceral layers of the glomerular capsule and face the urinary space. The cells contain dark-staining, membrane-bound granules. The function of these cells is uncertain.

Histophysiology of the Kidney

GENERAL FUNCTION

The basic function of the kidney is to regulate the volume and composition of body fluids by processes of conservation and elimination. The kidney conserves water, a

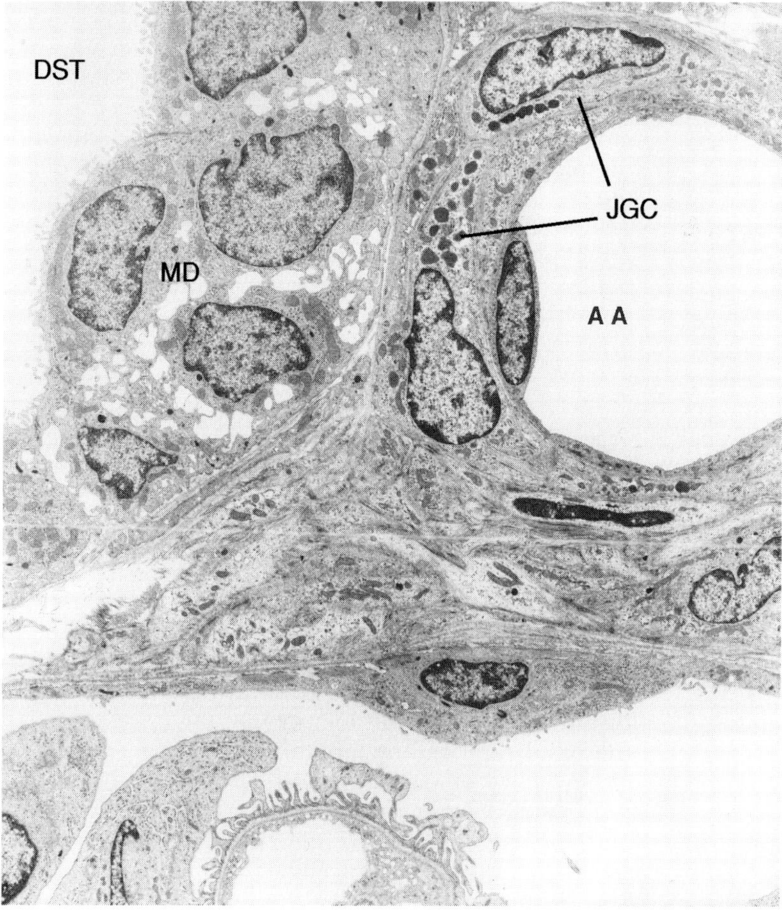

Figure 11.25. *Transmission electron micrograph of juxtaglomerular apparatus (rat). The macula densa (MD) in this section is composed of five cells with expanded intercellular spaces. The macula densa forms a portion of the wall of the distal straight tubule (DST). Two JG cells (JGC) with electron dense granules are present in the wall of the afferent arteriole (AA). A portion of a renal corpuscle is at bottom (×3700). (Courtesy of J.W. Verlander.)*

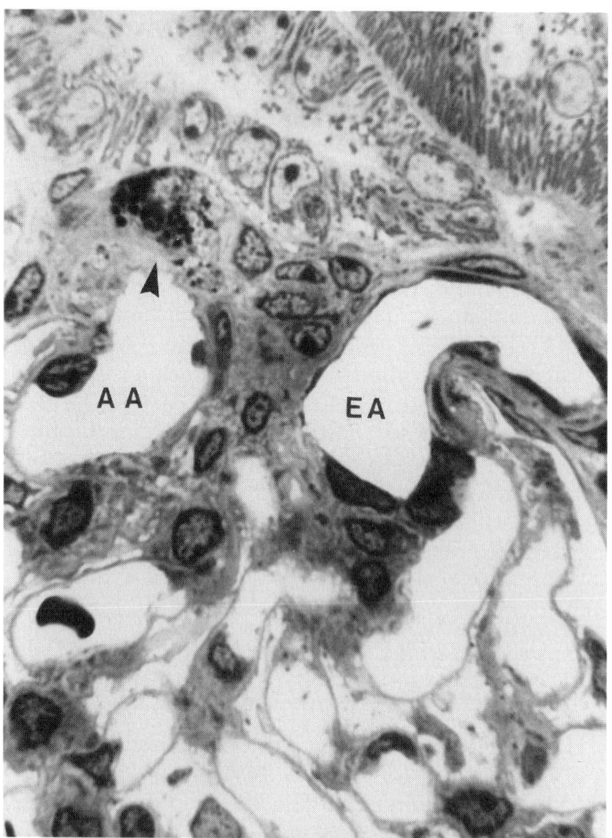

Figure 11.26. *JG cell (mouse). A juxtaglomerular cell (arrowhead) is located in the wall of the afferent arteriole (AA), whereas no JG cells are present in the wall of the efferent arteriole (EA). JG cells have dark-staining granules that contain renin. They are a component of the juxtaglomerular apparatus. A portion of a distal straight tubule is found above the JG cell and a part of a renal corpuscle is found below. Epon-Araldite. Azure II, methylene blue*

variety of solutes, and major electrolytes, such as sodium, potassium, bicarbonate, chloride, and hydrogen ions. Conversely, the kidney eliminates metabolic wastes, such as urea, uric acid, and creatinine, as well as substances that may be in excess, such as water, electrolytes, sugar, and other solutes. These functions all occur at the level of the nephron and involve three activities. First, a filtrate of the blood is formed at the glomerulus. Second, the renal tubules selectively process the filtrate by either reabsorbing substances across the epithelium and returning them to the circulatory system or secreting substances that must be eliminated from the body but which are not in high enough concentrations in the filtrate. When secretion is necessary, the tubules remove these substances from the peritubular capillaries and secrete them into the tubular lumen. Third, the renal tubules selectively conserve the water and solutes the body needs, thereby adjusting the tonicity of the final urine (Fig. 11.27).

FILTRATION

The kidneys receive a relatively large proportion (20%) of the blood pumped out of the heart. Of the amount of blood directed to the kidney, a surprising amount (20%) is pushed through the glomerular barrier to form the filtrate. As the filtrate passes along the renal tubules, 99% is reabsorbed back into the bloodstream, whereas 1% drips from the papillary ducts as urine. The capillary tuft in the glomerulus receives blood that is under considerable pressure (hydrostatic) created by the pumping action of the heart and by the resistance of the efferent arteriole. This hydrostatic pressure is apposed by colloid osmotic pressure exerted by plasma proteins and by hydrostatic pressure in the urinary space of the glomerular capsule. Both of these forces resist the movement of substances across the barrier. Much of the fluid components of the blood move through the endothelial pores of the capillary, the GBM, and the filtration slits between the foot processes of the podocytes to reach the urinary space in the glomerular capsule. The high permeability of this barrier results from the absence of any cellular layer through which to pass. The entire route is extracellular. The initial barrier is created by the endothelial pores and filters out the formed elements in the blood: the erythrocytes, leukocytes, and platelets. The more selective properties of the filtration barrier filter out macromolecules that exceed a particular size or have certain charge characteristics. The size filter is primarily located in the lamina densa of the GBM. The charge filter is created by the numerous negatively charged (anionic) molecules associated with the cell coats of the endothelial cells and podocytes, as well as with both laminae rarae of the GBM. Anionic molecules include molecules that contain heparan sulfate and sialic acid. The negatively charged components repel negatively charged molecules (anions) in the plasma and prevent them from crossing the barrier. Evidence suggests that molecules filtered out at the GBM are phagocytized by the mesangial cells, whereas molecules filtered out at the cell coat of the podocyte or at the slit membrane are phagocytized by the podocytes. In addition to their proposed phagocytic functions, the mesangial cells are also believed to control glomerular capillary perfusion through their contractile properties, to provide structural support for the glomerulus and to generate vasoactive agents.

TUBULAR PATHWAYS

From the urinary space of the glomerular capsule, the filtrate moves along the various segments of the renal tubule and is primarily reabsorbed. Reabsorption, i.e., movement of solutes and solvents across the renal tubular epithelium back into the peritubular capillaries, uses two routes: a transcellular pathway and a paracellular pathway. The transcellular pathway involves movement through the apical cell membrane, the cytoplasm, and the basolateral cell membrane. This route can involve either active or passive processes. Active solute transport, using carrier systems in the surface membranes and energy generated by mitochondria, uses this transcellular route. The paracellular pathway involves only passive movement through the junctions between epithelial cells, depending especially on the leakiness of the tight junctions, and then along the lateral intercellular spaces. This pathway is the major route for diffusion of ions. Water flows along either route but primarily along the transcellular pathway. In general, the more complex the structure of the tubular epithelial cells, the more active the processes of transport across the epithelium, e.g., the structure of the proximal and distal tubules is much more complex than that of the thin tubules or collecting ducts. Conversely, the simpler the structure, the more passive the processes. Also, the greater the membrane surface area, the greater the quantity of transport; thus, the proximal tubule, with its tall microvilli and extensive lateral interdigitations and basal infoldings, has a great transport capacity.

PROXIMAL TUBULE

In the proximal tubule, two-thirds to three quarters of the filtrate is reabsorbed. Because of the leakiness of the

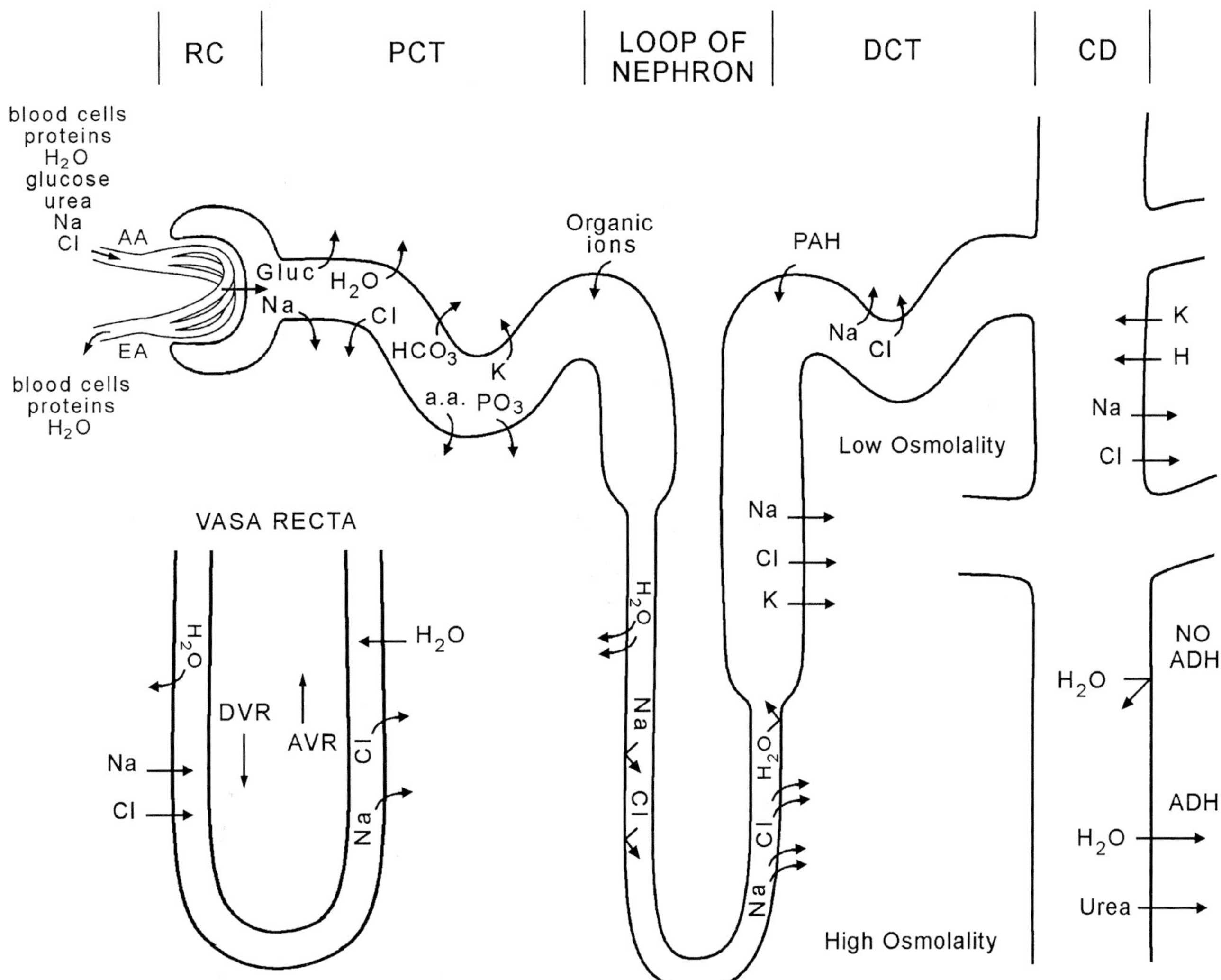

Figure 11.27. *Diagram of filtration, reabsorption, and secretion in the kidney. The first function of the nephron is to form a filtrate of the blood. Blood is brought to the renal corpuscle by the afferent arteriole (AA). The afferent arteriole breaks into numerous capillaries forming the glomerular rete. Many of the constituents of the blood cross the filtration barrier to enter the urinary space. The filtrate moves from the urinary space to the proximal convoluted tubule (PCT). Components that cannot pass through the barrier remain in the bloodstream and leave the glomerular rete in the efferent arteriole (EA). After filtration in the renal corpuscle (RC), much of the filtrate is reabsorbed in the proximal convoluted tubule (PCT). The loop of the nephron descends into the medulla, which has an interstitium of increasing osmolality. The descending thin tubule is permeable to water but impermeable to sodium and chloride. The ascending thin tubule is permeable to sodium and chloride but impermeable to water. Sodium and chloride continue to be reabsorbed along the distal tubule (DCT) and collecting duct (CD). Examples of substances secreted are organic ions, para-aminohippurate (PAH), potassium and hydrogen ions. Hormones, such as ADH, aldosterone, and ANP, have major effects on reabsorption. For example, ADH acting on the collecting duct causes water reabsorption. However, when ADH is absent, water is not reabsorbed. Urea concentration is adjusted in the collecting duct. The vascular loop in the lower left corner of the diagram represents exchanges that occur between the vasa recta and their associated capillaries) and the interstitium in the renal medulla. In the descending vasa recta (DVR), the water leaves and sodium chloride enters the vessels. In the ascending vasa recta (AVR), just the opposite occurs: the water enters and the sodium chloride leaves the vessels.*

tight junctions, much of the fluid reabsorption occurs via the paracellular pathway. Movement of most substances in the filtrate depends on the reabsorption of sodium. Much of the sodium is actively transported into the cell across the apical cell membrane and is actively transported out of the cell across the basolateral cell membrane. Normally, approximately two-thirds of the sodium is reabsorbed, in addition to the reabsorption of glucose, amino acids, bicarbonate, and some chloride. Phosphate and potassium are also reabsorbed. Fifty percent of the water is reabsorbed and follows the movement of the solutes. With the absorption of bicarbonate, hydrogen ions are secreted into the tubular lumen, thus acidifying the filtrate. Many organic ions are also secreted into the lumen of the proximal tubule. The decrease in structural complexity between the proximal convoluted and the proximal straight tubules is also reflected in reduced but similar functions. Normally, little if any protein is present in the filtrate; however, if some escapes, the extensive endocytotic lysosomal system in the proximal tubular cells will capture and metabolize these proteins. With solutes and solvent both leaving the proximal convoluted and straight tubules in similar proportions, the filtrate arrives at the thin tubule as an iso-osmotic fluid.

THIN TUBULE AND DISTAL STRAIGHT TUBULE

From the proximal straight tubule, the filtrate follows the thin tubule as it descends into the medulla and then ascends again and joins the distal straight tubule. The function of the loop can be best understood when one realizes that the interstitium increases in osmolality from the corticomedullary junction to tip of the papilla. The descending portion of the thin tubule has a high permeability to water and a low permeability to sodium and urea. Thus, as the filtrate descends into the medulla, the water moves out of the tubule while the solute remains. Consequently, the filtrate becomes increasingly concentrated as it descends into the medulla. The ascending portion of the thin tubule is impermeable to water and permeable to sodium and chloride, as well as somewhat permeable to urea. As the filtrate ascends in the medulla, it becomes less concentrated. These results are achieved primarily by passive diffusion using the transcellular pathway. This process correlates with the simple structure of the thin tubule and the complex structure of the tight junctions that do not allow leaks. The distal straight tubule has a function similar to that of the ascending portion of the thin tubule. It is impermeable to water and, although impermeable to solutes, actively transports sodium chloride, thus further reducing the tonicity of the tubular fluid and rendering the interstitium hyperosmotic. The distal straight tubule also reabsorbs calcium and magnesium. The tubular fluid always arrives at the distal convoluted tubule in a hypo-osmotic state.

DISTAL CONVOLUTED TUBULE AND COLLECTING DUCT

In the distal convoluted tubule, sodium and chloride continue to be reabsorbed. Water is also reabsorbed, however, and the tubular fluid approaches iso-osmolality. In the arched collecting ducts and the collecting ducts, sodium continues to be reabsorbed. Potassium is secreted by the principal cells. Evidence suggests that the intercalated cells secrete either hydrogen ions or bicarbonate, depending on whether they are in the protruded or retracted state, respectively. Urea flows out of the medullary collecting ducts, down its concentration gradient. The primary function of the collecting duct is to control the tonicity of the final urine. Tonicity is influenced by the presence or absence of **antidiuretic hormone** (ADH or vasopressin). In the presence of ADH, the collecting duct becomes permeable to water and water moves out into the hypertonic medullary interstitium. The resulting urine is concentrated. If ADH is absent, the collecting ducts are impermeable to water and the resulting urine is diluted. ADH also enhances the permeability of the inner medullary collecting ducts to urea.

COUNTERCURRENT MECHANISM

The kidney uses the **countercurrent mechanism** to produce a concentrated urine. A countercurrent system involves fluid flow in opposite directions in tubes that are closely apposed. The medulla of the kidney has two such systems. The first is formed by the loop of the nephron. The filtrate in the descending portion of the loop "counters" the flow of the filtrate in the ascending portion. Because of the functional properties of the cells along the loop, which include active ion transport and differential permeabilities, the interstitium becomes increasingly hypertonic toward the renal papilla. This mechanism is referred to as the **countercurrent multiplier system**. The second countercurrent system is formed by the descending and ascending vasa recta. The blood in the descending vasa recta "counters" the flow of blood in the ascending vasa recta. Substances are moved by passive diffusion down their concentration gradients, with water exiting and sodium chloride entering the descending vasa recta, while the opposite occurs in the ascending vasa recta. This vascular arrangement maintains the hyperosmolar gradient of the medulla by trapping solutes in the medullary interstitium. Any excesses of solutes and water are carried away by the blood vessels. The primary difference between the two countercurrent systems is that the loop of the nephron uses active transport mechanisms, whereas the vasa recta use passive processes to establish and maintain the osmotic gradient.

HORMONES AFFECTING RENAL FUNCTION

Several hormones alter the functions of the tubules of the kidney. ADH from the neurohypophysis causes its target, the collecting duct, to become more permeable to water, thus producing a hypertonic urine with less volume (antidiuretic effect). **Aldosterone** secreted by the adrenal cortex (zona glomerulosa) acts on the principal cells of the collecting ducts to stimulate reabsorp-

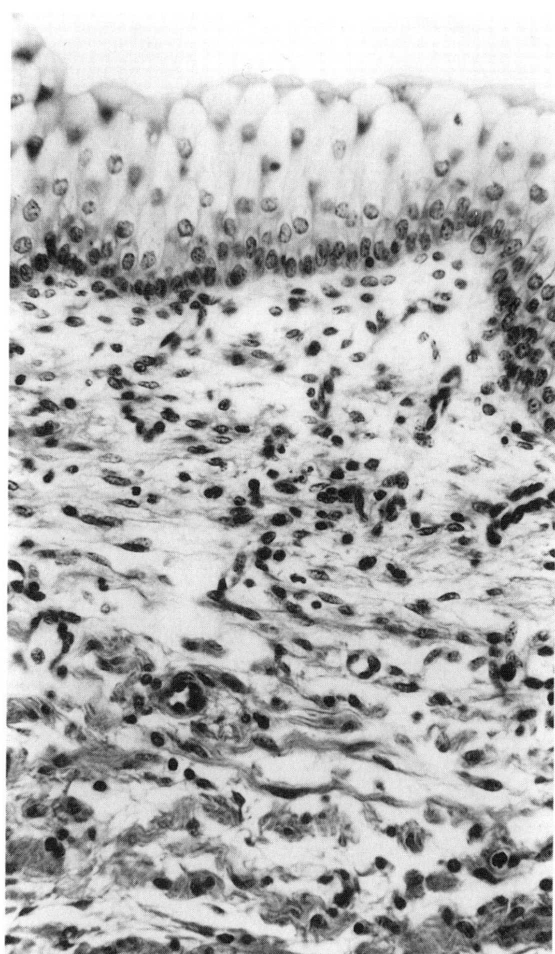

Figure 11.28. *Calyx (pig). Transitional epithelium lines the inner surface of the calyx. The propia-submucosa is a loose, irregular connective tissue layer with numerous small vessels. A few widely separated smooth muscle fibers form the tunica muscularis. Hematoxylin and eosin (×335).*

tion of sodium. Conversely, **atrial natriuretic peptide**, produced by the atria of the heart, causes the inner medullary collecting ducts to reduce reabsorption of sodium, thus leading to an increased sodium excretion in the urine (natriuresis). **Parathyroid hormone** stimulates transport and reabsorption of calcium, thus conserving calcium in the body, while also depressing tubular absorption of phosphate, thus increasing excretion of phosphate in the urine.

HORMONES PRODUCED BY THE KIDNEY

The kidney also produces several important secretions. **Erythropoietin** is produced by cells in the cortical interstitium and stimulates production and maturation of erythrocytes. 1,25-dihydroxycholecalciferol (calcitriol), the active form of vitamin D3, is produced in the proximal tubule and has a major role in regulation of plasma calcium concentration. Prostaglandins, primarily PGE2, are produced by lipid-laden interstitial cells, glomerular mesangial cells, and podocytes. Prostaglandins can effect kidney function by altering blood flow, renin release, and sodium excretion.

The JG apparatus functions to release **renin** from the JG cells in response to several separate stimuli. The JG cells may be stimulated directly by reduced renal perfusion pressure created by a decrease in circulating blood volume. The JG cells may be stimulated indirectly by sympathetic nerves responding to decreased blood pressure elsewhere in the body. Finally, the JG cells may be stimulated to release renin indirectly via the macula densa. Increases in sodium and chloride concentrations in the distal straight tubule are sensed by the extraglomerular mesangial cells across the macula densa. The extraglomerular mesangial cells stimulate renin release through their gap junctions with the JG cells. In all three instances, the released renin acts on angiotensinogen, a plasma protein, to form angiotensin I. Angiotensin I is converted to angiotensin II by the angiotensin-converting enzyme contained primarily in the lung. **Angiotensin II** causes vasoconstriction of the arterioles and stimulates secretion of aldosterone. All of these actions tend to correct the previously mentioned conditions.

URINARY PASSAGES

The urinary passages include the calyces (Fig. 11.28), the pelvis (Fig. 11.29), the ureters (Fig. 11.30), the urinary bladder (Fig. 11.31), and the urethra (Fig. 11.32). All of these structures have a similar histologic organization that includes a tunica mucosa of transitional epithelium and an underlying loose connective tissue layer (propria-submucosa); a tunica muscularis of smooth muscle forming inner longitudinal, middle circular, and outer longitudinal layers; and a tunica adventitia of loose connective tissue or a tunica serosa of mesothelium and connective tissue when a visceral peritoneal covering is present. Variations of this general pattern include the following.

1. **Calyces** and/or **pelvis**: in horses, mucous glands (simple branched tubuloalveolar glands) present in the mucosa contribute to the viscous, stringy nature of equine urine (see Fig. 11.29).
2. **Ureter**: the ureter has a narrow lumen. The mucosa is thrown into longitudinal folds, thus giving the lumen a stellate appearance. In horses, mucous glands also extend for a short distance into the proximal ureter.
3. **Urinary bladder**: the structure of the epithelium becomes increasingly flattened as the bladder fills. A lamina muscularis of small, isolated bundles of smooth muscle is present in horses, ruminants, dogs, and pigs but is absent in cats. The presence of a lamina muscularis divides the loose connective tissue layer into an inner lamina propria and an outer submucosa. The smooth muscle of the tunica muscularis, called the detrusor muscle, is not well layered but instead is composed of irregular-shaped, interweaving bundles.

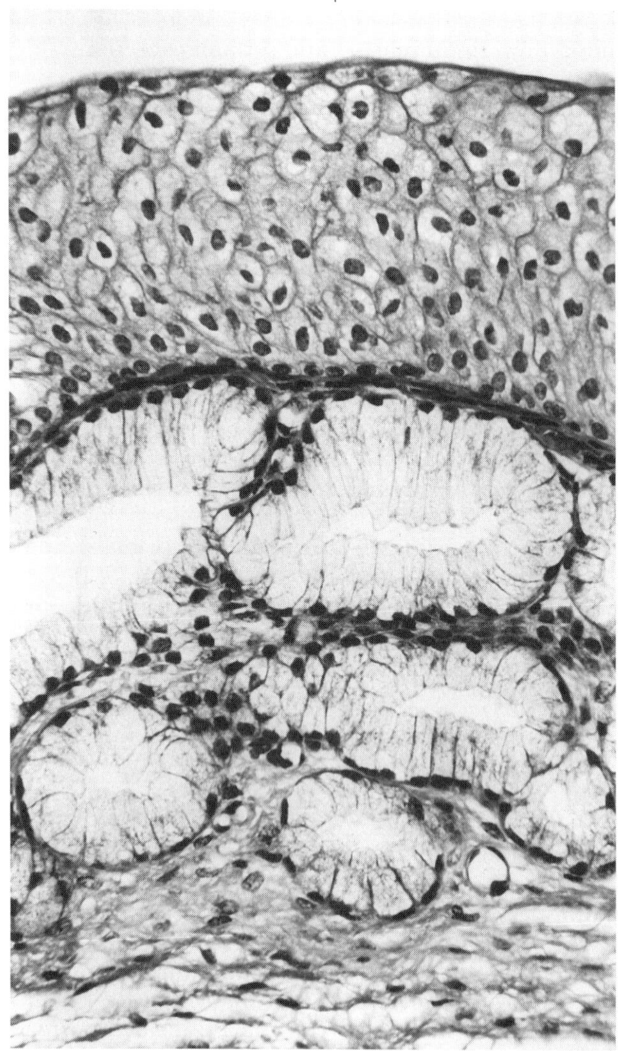

Figure 11.29. *Renal pelvis (horse). Mucous glands are found in the mucosa just beneath the transitional epithelium of the renal pelvis and the proximal part of the ureter in horses, mules, and donkeys. Ducts, not seen in this section, penetrate the overlaying epithelium and carry the secretion to the lumen, where it is added to the urine. Hematoxylin and eosin (×335).*

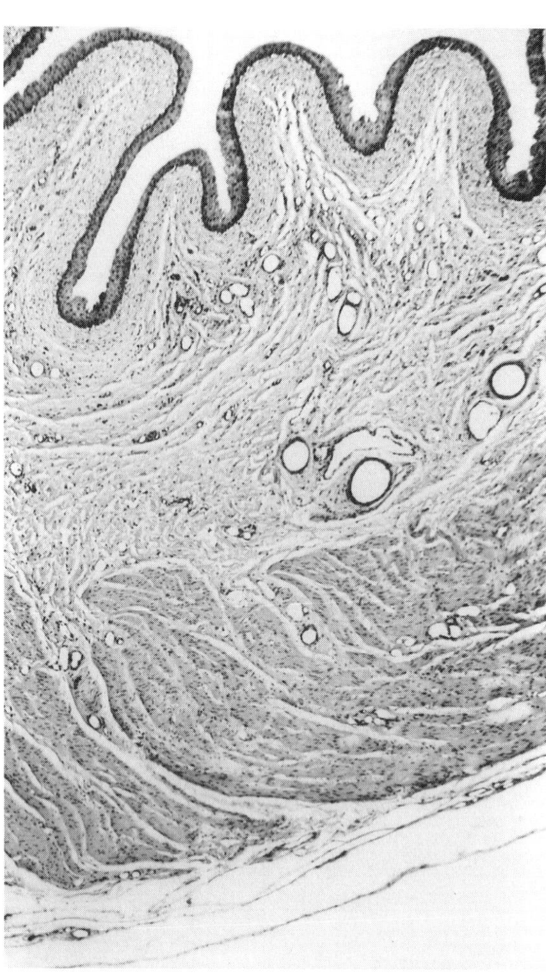

Figure 11.31. *Urinary bladder (dog). The mucosa is extensively folded and the transitional epithelium and propria-submucosa are thick. These are all characteristic features of an empty bladder. The three layers of the tunica muscularis are not separable in this section. A serosa covers the outer surface of the bladder. Hematoxylin and eosin (×50).*

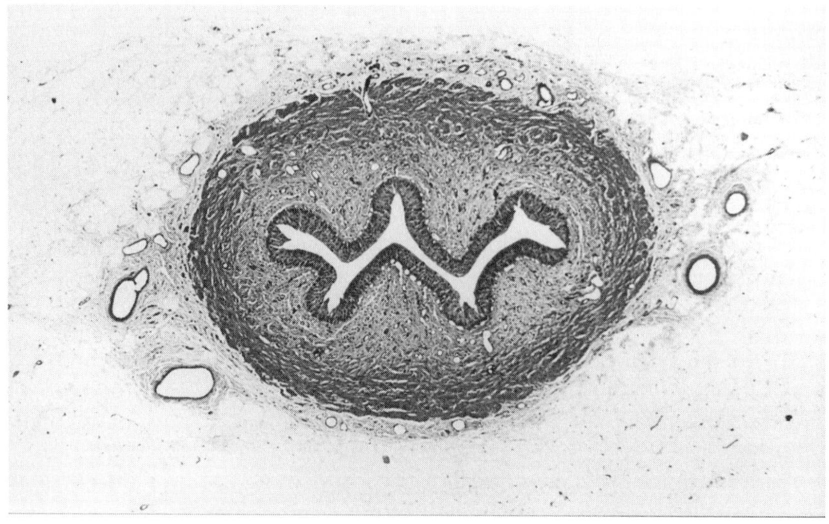

Figure 11.30. *Ureter (dog). Longitudinal mucosal folds create a stellate-shaped lumen. The epithelial connective tissue and muscular and adventitial layers are distinguishable. Hematoxylin and eosin (×50).*

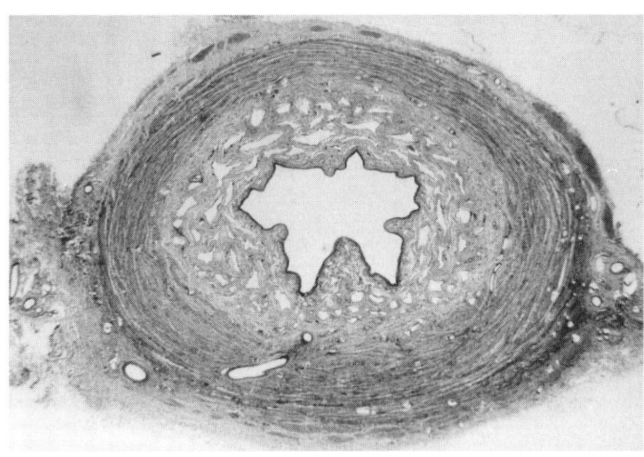

Figure 11.32. *Urethra (bitch). The mucosa has longitudinal folds. Within the loose connective tissue of the propria-submucosa are numerous irregularly shaped, cavernous spaces for blood. The tunica muscularis is made up primarily of circularly arranged smooth muscle. An adventitia of loose connective tissue surrounds the outside. Masson's trichrome (×21).*

4. **Urethra** (female): the epithelium is primarily transitional, but near the external urethral orifice, the epithelium gradually or abruptly changes to stratified squamous. Vessels that might be described as endothelial-lined cavernous spaces are scattered in the connective tissue of the lamina propria submucosa, thus giving it the appearance of erectile tissue (Fig. 11.32). The amount and distribution of these caverns along the length of the urethra are species-dependent. A few bundles of longitudinally oriented smooth muscle may form a rudimentary lamina muscularis. The arrangement of the smooth muscle in the tunica muscularis is irregular but contains both circular and longitudinal components. At the distal end of the urethra, bundles of longitudinally and circularly oriented skeletal muscle are mixed with or replace the smooth muscle in the tunica muscularis. A suburethral diverticulum lined by transitional epithelium and an underlying loose connective tissue layer is present ventral to the external urethral orifice in pigs and in ruminants. The male urethra is described in Chapter 12.

These passageways provide a conduit and storage reservoir for urine plus a mechanism for bladder filling and urine release. Urine is moved to the bladder by peristaltic contractions of the smooth muscle of the ureter. The ureters penetrate the bladder at an acute angle. This angle of entry acts as a valve that prevents the reflux of urine back into the ureter yet allows the urine to continue to enter and fill the bladder. The nervous system provides control of the muscular components of the bladder and urethra while the bladder fills and is emptied. Filling of the bladder involves *(a)* pudendal nerve stimulation of urethral skeletal muscle to close the urethral sphincter, *(b)* inhibition of parasympathetic innervation via the pelvic nerve to the detrusor muscle (the main smooth muscle mass of the bladder) to relax the bladder, and *(c)* sympathetic nerve (hypogastric nerve) stimulation of bladder neck smooth muscle (α receptors) to aid in the urethral sphincter and sympathetic nerve stimulation to the detrusor muscle (β receptors) to inhibit contraction, thus increasing relaxation of the bladder. Voiding of urine is called **micturition**. Voluntary micturition is mediated by the caudal brainstem under cortical and cerebellar control. Normal micturition involves *(a)* stimulation of the parasympathetic innervation to the detrusor muscle to contract the bladder, *(b)* inhibition of pudendal nerve innervation to urethral skeletal muscle to relax the urethral sphincter, and *(c)* inhibition of sympathetic innervation to the detrusor and bladder neck to allow contraction of the detrusor and relaxation of the bladder neck smooth muscle, respectively.

REFERENCES

Albertine KH, O'Morchoe CC. Distribution and density of the canine renal cortical lymphatic system. Kidney Int 1979;16:470.

Barger AC, Herd JA. Renal vascular anatomy and distribution of blood flow. In: Orloff J, Berliner R, Geiger S, eds. Handbook of physiology. Section 8: Renal physiology. Washington, DC: American Physiological Society, 1973:249.

Beeuwkes R. The vascular organization of the kidney. Annu Rev Physiol 1980;42:531.

Beeuwkes R, Bonventre JV. Tubular organization and vascular-tubular relations in the dog kidney. Am J Physiol 1975;229:695.

Brenner BM. The kidney. Philadelphia: WB Saunders, 1996.

Bulger RE, Cronin RE, Dobyan DC. Survey of the morphology of the dog kidney. Anat Rec 1979;194:41.

Christensen GC. Circulation of blood through the canine kidney. Am J Vet Res 1952;13:236.

Clapp WL, Madsen KM, Verlander JW, et al. Intercalated cells of the rat inner medullary collecting duct. Kidney Int 1986;31:1080.

Cullen WC, Fletcher TF, Bradley WE. Histology of the canine urethra. I. Morphology of the female urethra. Anat Rec 1981;199:177.

de Lahunta A. Veterinary neuroanatomy and clinical neurology. Philadelphia: WB Saunders, 1983.

Finco DR. Applied physiology of the kidney. In: Osborne CA, Finco DR, eds. Canine and feline nephrology and urology. Baltimore: Williams & Wilkins, 1995.

Herbert SC, Kriz W. Structural-functional relationships in the kidney. In: Schrier RW, Gottschalk CW, eds. Diseases of the kidney. Boston: Little, Brown and Co., 1993;1:3.

Koushanpour E, Kriz W. Renal physiology. Principles, structure and function. New York: Springer-Verlag, 1986.

Kriz W, Elger M, Lemley K, et al. Structure of the glomerular mesangium: a biochemical interpretation. Kidney Int 1990;38 (suppl):S2–S9.

Lacombe C, DaSilva J-L, Bruneval P, et al. Peritubular cells are the site of erythropoietin synthesis in the murine hypoxic kidney. J Clin Invest 1988;81:620.

Lemley KV, Kriz W. Anatomy of the renal interstitium. Kidney Int 1991;39:370.

Madsen KM, Clapp WL, Verlander JW. Structure and function of the inner medullary collecting duct. Kidney Int 1988;34:441.

Madsen KM, Tisher CC. Structural-functional relationships along the distal nephron. Am J Physiol 1986;250:F1–F15.

Osborne CA, Fletcher TF. Applied anatomy of the urinary system with clinicopathologic correlation. In: Osborne CA, Finco DR, eds. Canine and feline nephrology and urology. Baltimore: Williams & Wilkins, 1995:3.

Tisher CC, Brenner BM. Renal pathology with clinical and functional correlations. Philadelphia: JB Lippincott, 1994.

Yadava RP, Calhoun ML. Comparative histology of the kidney of domestic animals. Am J Vet Res 1958;19:958.

12

Male Reproductive System

KARL-HEINZ WROBEL

The male reproductive system consists of *(a)* the testes surrounded by the tunica vaginalis and the testicular envelopes, *(b)* the epididymides, *(c)* the ductus deferentes, *(d)* the accessory glands (glandular portion of the ductus deferens, vesicular and bulbourethral glands, prostate), *(e)* the urethra, and *(f)* the penis surrounded by the prepuce.

TESTIS

Stroma and Interstitium

TUNICA VAGINALIS

When the testis is removed from the scrotum, the parietal layer of the **tunica vaginalis** remains attached to the scrotum, whereas the visceral layer, the peritoneal covering of the testis (and epididymis), remains intimately associated with the underlying capsule of the testis, the tunica albuginea. The visceral layer of the tunica vaginalis consists of a mesothelium and a connective-tissue layer that blends with the tunica albuginea.

TUNICA ALBUGINEA

The **tunica albuginea** is a solid capsule of dense irregular connective tissue (Fig. 12.1). It consists predominantly of collagen fibers, a few elastic fibers, and myofibroblasts. Intratunical interstitial endocrine cells occur in the cat. Meandering branches of the testicular artery and a network of anastomosing veins constitute the vascular layer of the tunica albuginea.

SEPTULA TESTIS AND MEDIASTINUM TESTIS

The tunica albuginea is continuous with connective tissue trabeculae, the so-called **septula testis**, which converge toward the mediastinum testis. These trabeculae

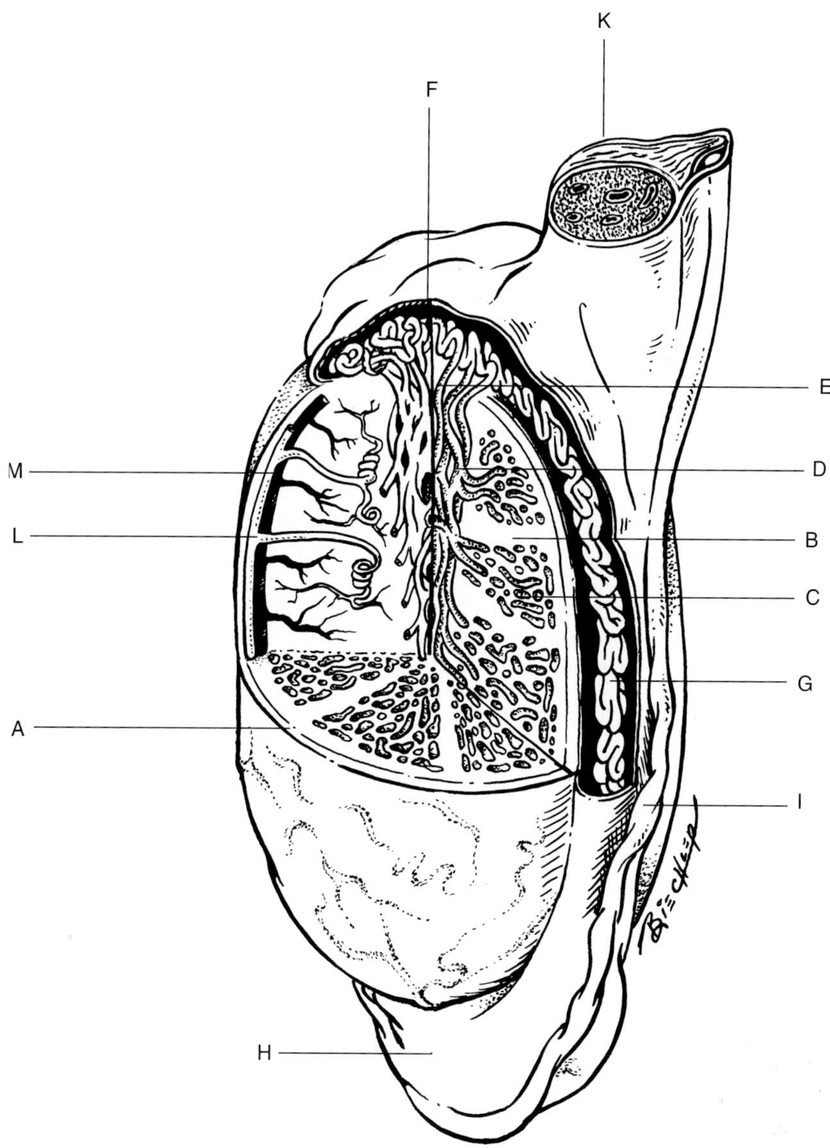

Figure 12.1. *Schematic drawing of a bovine testis, epididymis, ductus deferens, and spermatic cord. Tunica albuginea (A); interlobular septula (B); testicular lobules containing seminiferous tubules (C); rete testis (D); efferent ductules (E); head (F), body (G), and tail (H) of the epididymis; ductus deferens (I); spermatic cord (K); arteries (L) and veins (M) of the vascular stratum, the branches of which supply and drain the testicular parenchyma and stroma.*

are rather complete septa in dogs and boars, whereas in the other domestic animals, they are inconspicuous connective-tissue strands surrounding the large intratesticular vessels. The septula testis divide the testicular parenchyma into a varying number of testicular lobules, each containing one to four convoluted seminiferous tubules (Fig. 12.2). The septula testis are continuous with the mediastinum testis, a connective tissue area containing the channels of the rete testis and large blood and lymph vessels. The **mediastinum testis** of stallions, cats, and many rodents is relatively small and located in a marginal position, whereas in ruminants, pigs, and dogs, it occupies a central position along the longitudinal axis of the gonad.

INTERSTITIAL CELLS

The intertubular spaces contain loose connective tissue, blood and lymph vessels, fibrocytes, free mononuclear cells, and interstitial endocrine (Leydig) cells (Fig. 12.3). **Interstitial endocrine cells** produce testicular androgens and, in boars, large amounts of estrogen as well. Two generations of interstitial cells, fetal and pubertal, develop from mesenchymelike precursors. In some species, e.g., bovine and porcine, a third generation of interstitial cells (early postnatal) is encountered. Interstitial cells constitute approximately 1% of the entire testicular volume in adult rams, approximately 5% in bulls, and 20 to 30% in boars. In seasonally breeding males (e.g., camel), interstitial cell volume and number may change during the year. Interstitial endocrine cells occur in cords or clusters; not every cell is in close contact with a capillary. Between adjacent cells are intercellular canaliculi and gap junctions. High concentrations of steroids are found in testicular tissue and lymph.

The interstitial endocrine cells are large polymorphous cells with spherical nuclei (Fig. 12.3) and smooth endoplasmic reticulum (in bulls, an oligogranular endoplasmic reticulum is the dominating organelle in inter-

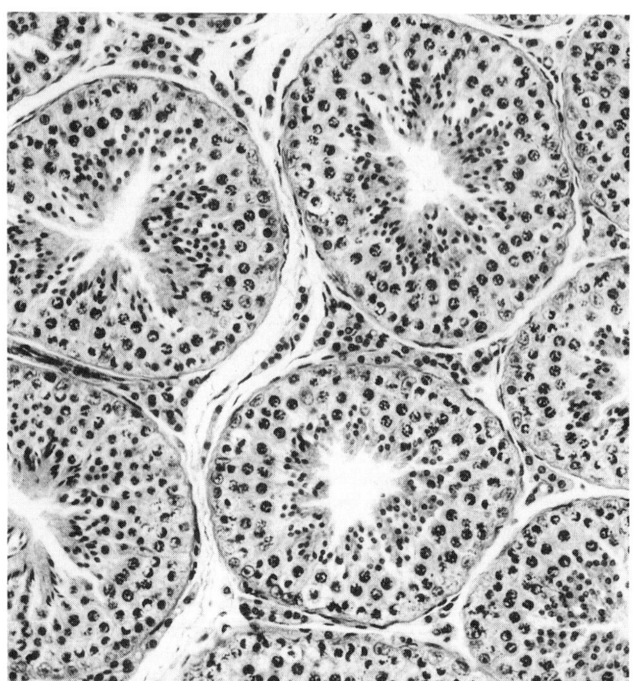

Figure 12.2. *Seminiferous tubules and intertubular tissues of the canine testis. Hematoxylin and eosin (×140).*

stitial cells). Its membranes incorporate most of the enzymes necessary for steroid biosynthesis. The mitochondria possess tubular cristae and are involved in the first step of steroid hormone production, e.g., transformation of cholesterol to pregnenolone. The relatively small Golgi complex does not participate in secretion of androgen. Release of androgen from interstitial cells is morphologically inconspicuous. Lipid inclusions are found in all species but are particularly abundant in cats.

More than 90% of all androgens in the organism are produced by the testis. Among the main functions of testosterone (to be effective, in some tissues, testosterone must be converted into dihydrotestosterone by the enzyme 5-reductase) are *(a)* promotion of normal sexual behavior (libido); *(b)* triggering of the growth and maintenance of the function of the penis, male accessory glands, and secondary sex characteristics; *(c)* control of spermatogenesis (together with follicle-stimulating hormone (FSH)); *(d)* negative feedback action on the hypophysis and hypothalamus; *(e)* general anabolic effects; and *(f)* the prenatal maintenance of the wolffian duct and its differentiation into deferent duct and epididymis.

Convoluted Seminiferous Tubules

The **convoluted seminiferous tubules** (tubuli seminiferi convoluti) in most mammals are tortuous two-ended loops with a diameter between 150 and 300 μm (see Fig. 12.1). They are lined by the stratified germinal epithelium, surrounded by a lamina propria, and connected at both ends to straight testicular tubules by a specialized terminal segment (see Fig. 12.8). The length of all seminiferous tubules in the testis of the adult bovine amounts to approximately 5000 m. Histologically, the seminiferous tubules have three components: lamina propria, sustentacular cells (somatic, supporting, or Sertoli cells), and spermatogenic cells.

LAMINA PROPRIA

The lamina propria surrounds the seminiferous tubule. Its innermost layer is a basal lamina, often with club-shaped projections into basal infoldings of sustentacular cells and spermatogonia. Some collagen and elastic fibers connect the basal lamina to the flat **peritubular cells**, which form a stratum of one to five layers, depending on species. At birth, these peritubular cells resemble mesenchymal cells, which postnatally differentiate gradually into contractile cells. In some species (e.g., boars), they acquire all features of typical smooth muscle cells; in other species (e.g., bulls), they represent myofibroblasts. The peritubular cells contain actin filament bundles arranged in circular and longitudinal directions and are responsible for tubular contractions. Thus, they participate in transport of tubular content and in spermiation, i.e., the release of spermatozoa into the tubular lumen. The outermost layer of the tubular lamina propria consists of fibrocytes and collagen fibrils. Lymphocytes and monocytes invade the lamina propria but never the intact tubular epithelium.

SUSTENTACULAR CELLS

Sustentacular cells are derived from undifferentiated supporting cells of the prepubertal gonad. These cells

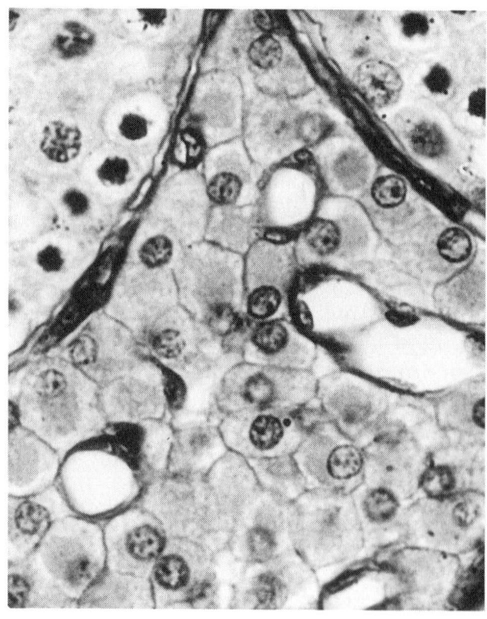

Figure 12.3. *Interstitial cells are particularly abundant in the intertubular connective tissue of the boar testis. Seminiferous tubules (st); capillaries (c). PAS (×700).*

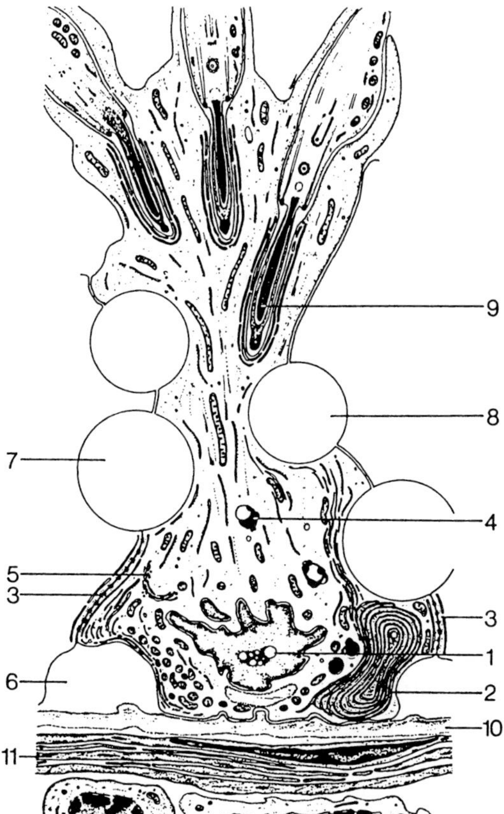

Figure 12.4. *Diagrammatic representation of sustentacular cell–germ cell interrelationships in the bull. 1 = sustentacular cell nucleus; 2 = smooth endoplasmic reticulum; 3 = tight junctions between adjacent sustentacular cells; 4 = phagolysosomes; 5 = Golgi complex; 6 = space occupied by a spermatogonium; 7 = space occupied by a primary spermatocyte; 8 = space occupied by a spherical spermatid; 9 = elongated spermatid within apical recess of sustentacular cell; 10 = basal lamina; 11 = peritubular cell (myofibroblast). (With permission from Mosimann M, Kohler T. Zytologie, Histologie und mikroskopische Anatomie der Haussäugetiere. Hamburg: Paul Parey, 1990.)*

are mitotically active, contain large amounts of rough endoplasmic reticulum, and produce the antiparamesonephric hormone, a glycoprotein that suppresses development of uterine tubes, uterus, and vagina in the male. During puberty, sustentacular cell differentiation is accompanied by a morphologic transformation and loss of mitotic capability.

The adult sustentacular cells are irregularly outlined, elongated cells. Their broad base rests on the basal lamina, and the remaining cytoplasm extends upward to the tubular lumen (Fig. 12 4). They are rather evenly spaced; approximately 20 sustentacular cells are seen in a cross section of an adult seminiferous tubule. Lateral and apical cytoplasmic processes of the sustentacular cells fill all the spaces between adjacent spermatogenic cells. The oval or pear-shaped nucleus is generally located in the broad basal portion of the cell and is often deeply infolded and contains a large nucleolus. The basal portion and the central trunk region of the sustentacular cell contain mitochondria, an inconspicuous Golgi complex, abundant sER, little rER, free ribosomes, microtubules, actin and vimentin filaments, lysosomes, and lipid inclusions. Only a few organelles are found in the lateral and apical sustentacular cell processes. The shape of the cell, the surface area, and the volume percentages of organelles (sER, nucleus, lysosomes, lipid inclusions) change in accordance with spermatogenetic events (sustentacular cell cycle). Sustentacular cells form hemidesmosomes with the basal lamina. Temporary junctions with germ cells play a part in vertical displacement and release (spermiation) of the germ cells. Adjacent sustentacular cells are joined by tight junctions associated with actin filaments and subsurface cisternae of the ER. These junctions separate a basal from an adluminal (apical) tubular compartment and constitute a diffusion barrier, also referred to as the **blood–testis barrier**. Renewal of spermatogenetic stem cells and multiplication of spermatogonia take place in the basal compartment, to which intertubular tissue fluid has relatively free access. The blood–testis barrier selectively prevents many substances from entering the adluminal compartment, where the vital processes of meiosis and spermiogenesis take place in a controlled microenvironment.

Early spermatocytes must pass through these intercellular junctions without interrupting the physiologic blood–testis barrier. Such passage is probably accomplished by a zipperlike opening of these junctions, which close again below the spermatocytes before they reach the adluminal compartment.

Sustentacular cells have nutritive, protective, and supportive functions for the spermatogenic cells. In addition, they phagocytize degenerating spermatogenic cells and detached residual bodies of spermatids. They release the spermatozoa into the lumen of the seminiferous tubules (spermiation). They mediate the action of FSH and testosterone on the germ cells, participate in the synchronization of spermatogenic events, produce an androgen-binding protein, and secrete constituents of the intratubular fluid, such as transferrin, androgen-binding protein, and inhibin. Inhibin is reabsorbed from the lumen of the efferent ductules and the initial segment of epididymis. It then reaches the bloodstream and exerts negative feedback on hypophyseal FSH secretion. Paracrine signals from sustentacular cells modulate the activity of nearby interstitial endocrine cells. Although normal sustentacular cells have only a minimal proven steroidogenic function, sustentacular cell tumors may produce large amounts of estrogen, leading to feminization of the organism.

SPERMATOGENIC CELLS

Various **spermatogenic cells**, representing different phases in the development and differentiation of the spermatozoon, are located between and above the sustentacular cells. The sequence of events in the development of spermatozoa from spermatogonia is referred to as **spermatogenesis** and is subdivided into three phases: *(a)* spermatocytogenesis, the process during which spermatogonia develop into spermatocytes; *(b)* meiosis, the maturation division of spermatocytes that results in spermatids with a reduced (haploid) number of chromosomes; and *(c)* spermiogenesis, the process of transformation of spermatids into spermatozoa. The duration of spermatogenesis is 74 days in men and approximately 50 days in bulls, rams, and stallions.

In addition to the cell population involved in spermatogenesis (cycling population), the seminiferous epithelium contains a separate stem cell and spermatogonia precursor cell line. This population can adapt to changing demands and thus guarantees uninterrupted spermatogenesis. Stem cells and spermatogonia precursor cells are morphologically similar to spermatogonia and are also located in the basal tubular compartment.

SPERMATOCYTOGENESIS

During **spermatocytogenesis**, spermatogonia multiply mitotically, resulting in A-, I- (intermediate), and B-spermatogonia and finally in preleptotene primary spermatocytes. Primary spermatocytes no longer divide mitotically but undergo two meiotic divisions, which result in a fourfold increase in the number of germ cells. Therefore, the number of spermatozoa that originate from one A-spermatogonium is decisively influenced by spermatogonial proliferation during spermatocytogenesis. In most mammals, a variable number of generations of A-spermatogonia is followed by one generation of I- (intermediate) and B-spermatogonia, respectively. In a given tubular segment, the few A-spermatogonia are irregularly distributed. Daughter cells of A- and I-mitoses drift apart to achieve an even distribution. **A-spermatogonia** are the largest spermatogonia and share an extensive contact area with the tubular basal lamina. They possess prominent nucleoli and nuclei with a pale or cloudy appearance. **B-spermatogonia** have spherical nuclei containing numerous chromatin particles and less prominent nucleoli. All B-spermatogonia of a given tubular segment form a cellular network, because they are interconnected by cytoplasmic processes. The mitotic division of B-spermatogonia results in the formation of **preleptotene primary spermatocytes**. These cells and their descendents are interconnected by true cytoplasmic bridges until shortly before spermiation. Preleptotene primary spermatocytes gradually lose contact with the basal lamina and move into the adluminal tubular compartment across the intercellular junctions between the sustentacular cells. In preleptotene primary spermatocytes, the nuclear DNA is replicated, and all chromosomes consist of two sister chromatids.

MEIOSIS

During **meiosis**, two successive nuclear divisions occur, resulting in the formation of four haploid spermatids from one primary spermatocyte. **Primary spermatocytes** are the largest spermatogenic cells in the tubular epithelium and are located in the intermediate position between spermatogonia and spermatids. Because the prophase of the first maturation division is extremely prolonged, two generations of primary spermatocytes are present in many tubular sections (Fig. 12.5). The prophase of the **first maturation division** is subdivided into the leptotene, zygotene, pachytene, diplotene, and diakinesis stages according to characteristic changes in nuclear chromatin. During the **leptotene stage**, the chromosomes become arranged in thin threadlike strands. In the **zygotene stage**, homologous chromosomes begin to pair and tetrads of four chromatids emerge. Visible evidence of pairing is the synaptonemal complexes seen with the electron microscope. Completion of pairing initiates the **pachytene phase**, during which crossing over occurs between the nonsister chromatids of the paired chromosomes. In microscopic preparations, primary spermatocytes are best identified when they are in this phase of meiosis (Fig. 12.5). During the **diplotene phase**, the paired chromosomes pull away from each other, but sister chromatids remain attached through chiasmata, i.e., sites where crossing over has occurred. During the prophase of the first meiotic division, the cells grow considerably. For instance, between preleptotene and diplotene, ovine primary spermatocytes increase in volume 4.8 times and their nuclei increase in volume 3.3 times. During **diakinesis**, the chromosomes shorten and broaden and the four separate chromatids in each chromosome are clearly evident. At the end of prophase, the nuclear membrane disappears.

The metaphase, anaphase, and telophase occur rapidly. During these phases, the paired chromosomes are first arranged at the equatorial plate. Subsequently, homologous chromosomes move to opposite poles of the cell to be distributed to the secondary spermatocytes, which possess only half the number of chromosomes but have two chromatids each (dyads). **Secondary spermatocytes** are short-lived, intermediate in size between diplotene primary spermatocytes and spherical spermatids, and occur exclusively in phase 4 of the seminiferous epithelial cycle (see Fig. 12.5).

After a short period of interphase, during which no duplication of genetic material occurs, the secondary spermatocytes undergo the **second maturation division**, with a short prophase followed by metaphase, anaphase, and telophase, which are essentially similar to those of mitotic divisions. During this division, the centromeres divide and the sister chromatids of the secondary spermatocytes separate and are distributed to each of the spermatids resulting from that division. Thus, these cells possess a haploid set of chromosomes.

SPERMIOGENESIS

The process by which interconnected clones of newly formed spermatids differentiate into individual testicular spermatozoa is referred to as **spermiogenesis**. The most important morphologic changes during spermiogenesis are formation of the acrosome, condensation of the nuclear chromatin, outgrowth of a motile tail, and loss of excess spermatid material (cytoplasm, water, organelles) not necessary for the later spermatozoon.

Spermiogenesis is divided into Golgi phase, cap

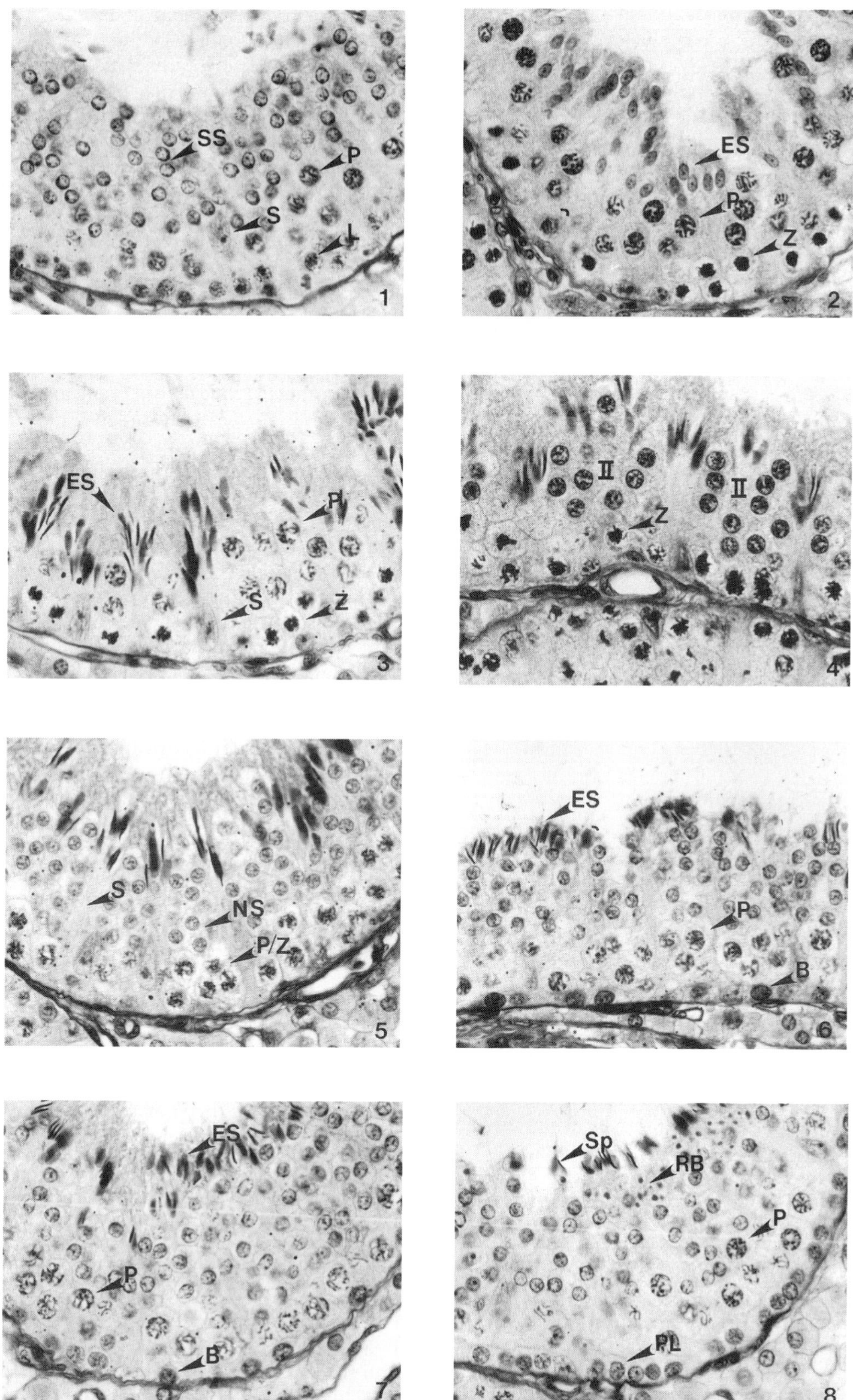

Figure 12.5. *The eight stages of the spermatogenic cycle (boar). B spermatogonia (BS); elongated spermatids (ES); leptotene primary spermatocytes (L); newly formed spermatids (NS); pachytene primary spermatocytes (P); preleptotene primary spermatocytes (PL); primary spermatocytes leaving zygotene and entering pachytene (P/Z); residual bodies (RB); sustentacular cell (S); spermatozoa in spermiation (Sp); spherical spermatids (SS); secondary spermatocytes (II). PAS (×500).*

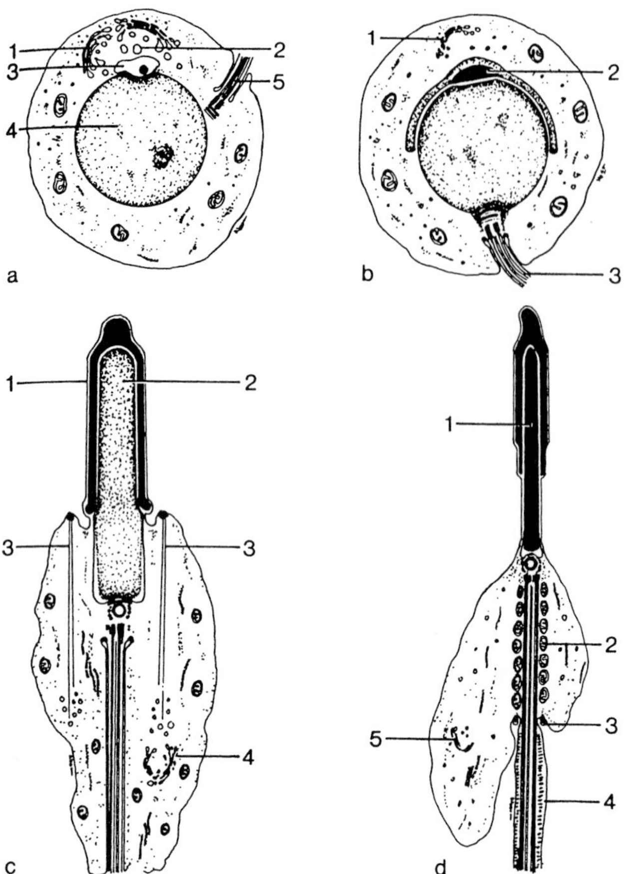

Figure 12.6. *Spermiogenesis (bull).* ***a.,*** *Spherical spermatid, Golgi phase. 1 = Golgi complex; 2 = Golgi vesicle; 3 = acrosomal vesicle containing acrosomal granule; 4 = nucleus; 5 = developing tail.* ***b.,*** *Spherical spermatid, cap phase. 1 = Golgi complex; 2 = head cap containing acrosome; 3 = developing tail.* ***c.,*** *Elongated spermatid, acrosomal phase. 1 = acrosomal cap containing acrosome; 2 = nucleus; 3 = manchette; 4 = Golgi complex.* ***d.,*** *Elongated spermatid, maturation phase. 1 = nucleus (condensation completed); 2 = middle piece with mitochondrial sheath; 3 = annulus; 4 = principal piece; 5 = Golgi complex. (With permission from Mosimann W, Kohler T. Zytologie, Histologie und mikroskopische Anatomie der Haussäugetiere. Hamburg: Paul Parey, 1990.)*

phase, acrosomal phase, and maturation phase (Fig. 12.6). In routine histologic sections, the Golgi and cap phases are characterized by spherical nuclei, whereas the acrosomal and maturation phases reveal elongated nuclei.

During the **Golgi phase**, proacrosomal granules appear in Golgi vesicles and eventually fuse to form a single acrosomal granule within a single acrosomal vesicle. Both structures make contact with an indentation of the nucleus, thus marking the anterior pole of the future sperm head.

During the **cap phase**, the acrosomal vesicle grows and forms the head cap that covers the anterior two-thirds of the nucleus. In late cap phase, the still spherical spermatid becomes polarized; nucleus and head cap are shifted to an eccentric position. The two centrioles assemble at the caudal pole of the nucleus, and the distal centriole gives rise to the outgrowing flagellum.

In the early **acrosomal phase**, the nucleus and cell body start to elongate in a craniocaudal direction. At the same time, the spermatids rotate so that the nucleus is directed toward the tubular periphery and the developing tail is directed toward the lumen. The spermatids, formerly separated by lateral sustentacular cell processes, are now embedded in apical recesses of these cells. As the nucleus begins to elongate, nuclear histones, which are responsible for the normal spatial nucleosomal arrangement of nuclear DNA, are gradually replaced by basic proteins (protamines), which allow dense packing of the chromatin. After this condensation, the DNA is transcriptionally inactive and resistant to noxious influences. During fertilization, protamines must be replaced by histones before decondensation of the chromatin. These histones are provided by the oocyte.

During the **maturation phase**, nuclear condensation is completed. In the region of the future middle piece of the spermatozoon, most of the mitochondria gather around the axoneme in a helicoidal manner. The system of the outer fibers and the fibrous sheath of the future principal piece develop. The volume of a spermatid in late maturation phase amounts to only 20 to 30% of that of a cap-phase spermatid. Autolytic processes are generally responsible for this reduction. In the bovine, sustentacular cell processes invading the spermatids participate in absorption of spermatid material. Before spermiation, the cytoplasmic bridges between maturation-phase spermatids are disconnected and excess cytoplasm is detached as residual body. Residual bodies have different fates; they may be phagocytosed by sustentacular cells, lost into the tubular lumen, or subjected to rapid autolysis when attached to the apical border of the tubular epithelium. A small remaining portion of spermatid cytoplasm, the cytoplasmic droplet of young spermatozoa, is lost during epididymal passage.

SPERMATOZOON

Spermatozoa vary in length between approximately 60 μm (boars, stallions) to 75 μm (ruminants). With the light microscope, the spermatozoon seems to consist essentially of two portions: the head and the tail. With the electron microscope, the tail is seen to be subdivided further into neck, middle piece, principal piece, and end piece (Fig. 12.7).

Head

The shape of the nucleus determines the shape of the head of the spermatozoon, which is species-dependent and subject to great variations. The anterior pole of the nucleus is covered by the acrosomal cap, with an outer and an inner acrosomal membrane that fuse at the caudal end. The acrosomal cap contains several hydrolytic and proteolytic enzymes (e.g., acrosin), which are set free during the acrosome reaction of capacitated spermatozoa in the uterine tube. Acrosomal enzymes are needed for the penetration of the zona pellucida during fertilization. The caudal region of the acrosome is characterized by a narrowing of the cap and condensation of its contents. This area is the equatorial segment of the acrosome. The base of the nucleus is surrounded by the postacrosomal sheath, which consists of fibrous proteins rich in sulfur. In dead spermatozoa, the sheath stains intensely with certain dyes, such as eosin or bromophenol blue. This reaction is used to evaluate the quality of an ejaculate. The plasma membrane of the postacrosomal head region contains receptor molecules necessary for the recognition of a homologous oocyte. At the caudal surface of the sperm head, the nuclear envelope lines an implantation groove where the tail is inserted in a joint-like manner.

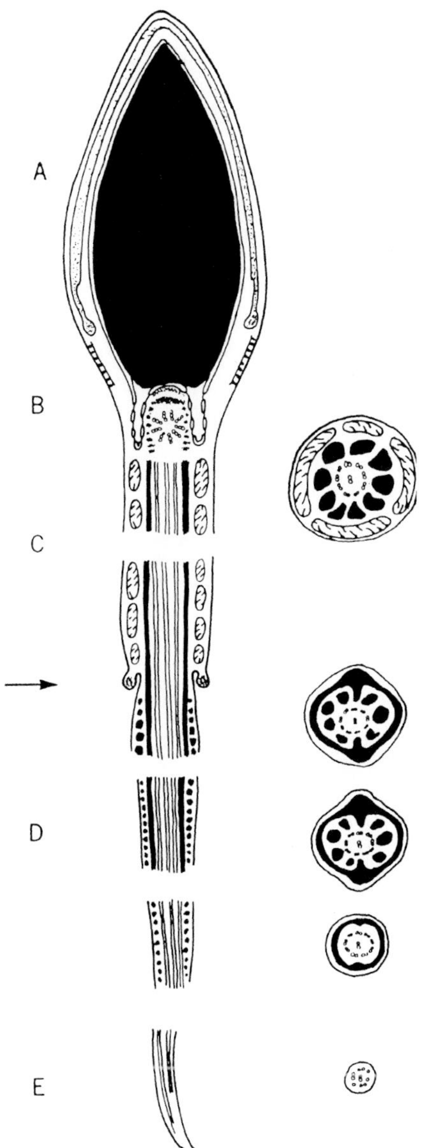

Figure 12.7. *Schematic drawing of a spermatozoon. Left: longitudinal section; right: cross sections located at the levels from which they are taken.* ***A.****, Head containing the nucleus covered by the acrosome. Note the equatorial segment of the acrosome and postacrosomal sheath.* ***B.****, Neck.* ***C.****, Middle piece with central axial filament complex, nine outer dense fibers, and the surrounding mitochondria. The middle piece terminates with the annulus (arrow).* ***D.****, Principal piece in which the outer dense fibers are surrounded by the fibrous sheath; they terminate before the end of the principal piece.* ***E.****, In the end piece, the microtubules of the axial filament complex terminate at various levels.*

Neck

The neck is a relatively short and narrow structure between the head and middle piece (connecting piece). It consists of a centrally located centriole and nine peripheral, longitudinally oriented coarse fibers continuous with the outer fibers of the middle piece.

Middle piece

The core of the middle piece has the characteristic structure of a flagellum: two central microtubules and nine peripheral doublets (microtubules) making up the axial filament complex. They are surrounded by nine longitudinally oriented, tapered outer fibers that are connected to the fibers of the connecting piece. These, in turn, are surrounded by the mitochondria in a helicoidal arrangement. In ruminants, the mitochondrial helix consists of approximately 40 turns. A ring-shaped thickening of the plasma membrane (annulus) of the middle piece marks the limit between the middle piece and the principal piece.

Principal piece

The principal piece is the longest portion of the spermatozoon. The axial filament complex has a structure identical to that of the middle piece and is surrounded by the continuing outer fibers of the middle piece. The fibers are subject to variations in size and shape and gradually taper toward the end of the principal piece. Semicircular ribs of structural proteins in a helicoidal arrangement fuse to two of the outer fibers to form the characteristic peripheral fibrous sheath of the principal piece.

End piece

The termination of the fibrous sheath marks the beginning of the end piece, which contains only the axial filament complex. Proximally, in the end piece, this complex has its characteristic nine peripheral doublets; distally, these doublets gradually become reduced to singlets and terminate at various levels.

CYCLIC EVENTS IN THE SEMINIFEROUS TUBULES

Before one spermatogenic series is completed, several (generally four) new spermatogenic series are initiated at the same level within the seminiferous tubule. As all the descendents of each B-spermatogonium develop synchronously, successive cell generations follow each other with cyclic regularity, from the periphery toward the center of the seminiferous tubule (seminiferous epithelial cycle).

Changes in the shape and stainability of the nuclei during cell division and the release of spermatozoa into the tubular lumen provide a basis for dividing the spermatogenic cycle into stages. In testes of the bulls, rams, and boars, eight stages can be identified.

Stage 1. After spermiation, spherical spermatids lie nearest to the lumen, followed basally by two generations of primary spermatocytes, i.e., old pachytenes and young preleptotenes/leptotenes (Fig. 12.5.1).

Stage 2. The spermatids and their dark-stained nuclei are elongated. The two generations of primary spermatocytes are old pachytenes and young leptotenes/zygotenes (Fig. 12.5.2).

Stage 3. Elongated spermatids are arranged in bundles and lie in deep apical recesses of the sustentacular cells (Fig. 12.5.3). The pachytenes of stage 2 have reached diplotene. A second generation of primary spermatocytes in zygotene is present in the basal region.

Stage 4. The first and second maturation divisions take place. In addition to bundles of maturing spermatids and zygotene primary spermatocytes, either diplotenes, secondary spermatocytes, or spherical spermatids are seen (Fig. 12.5.4).

Stage 5. Two generations of spermatids are present: older elongated spermatids and newly formed spherical spermatids. The zygotenes of stage 4 enter the pachytene stage and are displaced in the direction of the tubular lumen (Fig. 12.5.5).

Stage 6. The bundles of older spermatids have moved away from the vicinity of the sustentacular cell nuclei. In addition to spherical spermatids, pachytenes and numerous spermatogonia (I- or B-) are present.

Stage 7. The maturation-phase spermatids achieve a position close to the tubular lumen. All other cells as in stage 6 (Fig. 12.5.6).

Stage 8. Spermatozoa leave the tubular epithelium (spermiation) after separation from their residual bodies. Remaining within the epithelium are spherical spermatids and two generations of primary spermatocytes (older pachytenes and young preleptotenes).

In all domestic animals, not only are the descendents of one spermatogonium all more or less at the same stage of development, but identical cellular associations are found over a certain distance in cross and longitudinal sections of seminiferous tubules. These spermatogenic segments, portions with synchronized development of germ cells, are usually arranged so that one specific segment is adjacent to the preceding and following stages of the spermatogenic cycle. If stages 1 through 8 succeed each other along the length of the seminiferous tubule, the sequence is referred to as a regular spermatogenic wave, which is approximately 10 mm long in bulls. Variations, such as repetition of wave fragments (1-2-3-4-1-2-3-4) or inversions (1-2-3-4-5-4-3-2), seem to occur more frequently, however. Exactly what determines the spermatogenic cycles, segments, and waves is not known at this time.

Straight Testicular Tubules

In all domestic mammals, most of the convoluted seminiferous tubules terminate in the vicinity of the rete testis; they continue into the **straight testicular tubules** (tubuli recti), which connect them to the rete testis. Straight testicular tubules are short and have either a straight or a tortuous course. In stallions and boars, some of the convoluted seminiferous tubules terminate at the periphery of the testis and join the rete testis by long, straight testicular tubules. The terminal segment of the convoluted seminiferous tubule is lined by modified sustentacular cells that occlude the tubular lumen and project their apices into the cup-shaped initial portion of the straight testicular tubule (Fig. 12.8). All spermatozoa must pass through the narrow intercellular slits between adjacent modified sustentacular cells on their way to the straight tubule. The terminal segment may further function as a valve that prevents reflux of rete testis fluid into the seminiferous tubules.

The straight testicular tubules are lined with a simple squamous to columnar epithelium. In bulls, a simple cuboidal epithelium lines the proximal portion of the

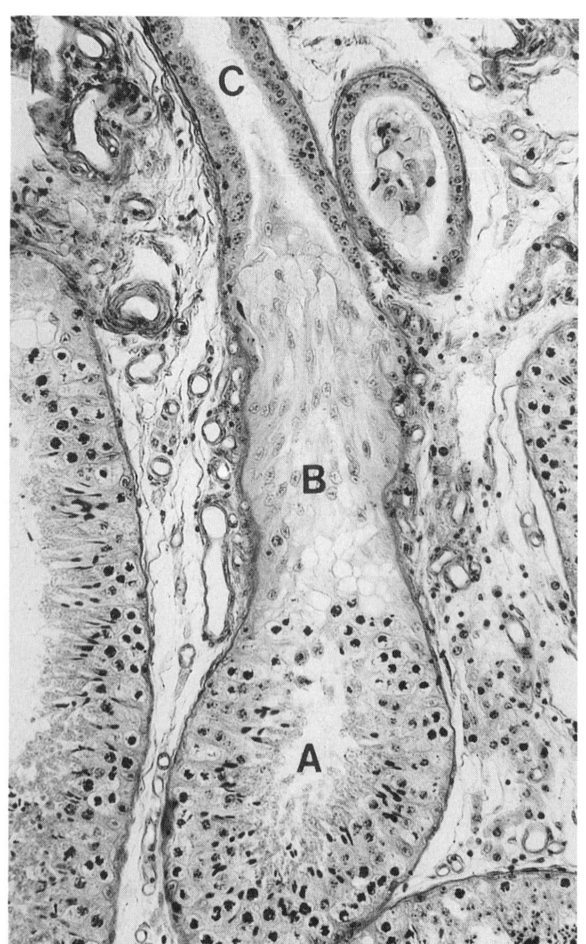

Figure 12.8. *Convoluted seminiferous tubule (A), terminal segment (B) surrounded by a vascular plexus, and straight testicular tubule (C) in the bovine testis. Iron hematoxylin (×140).*

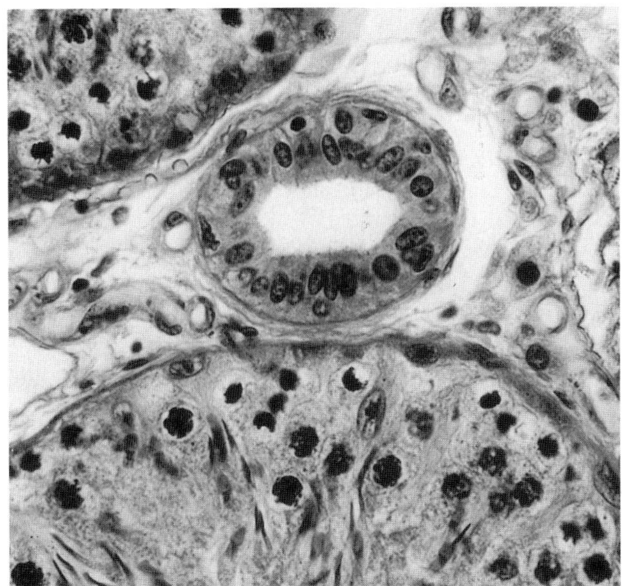

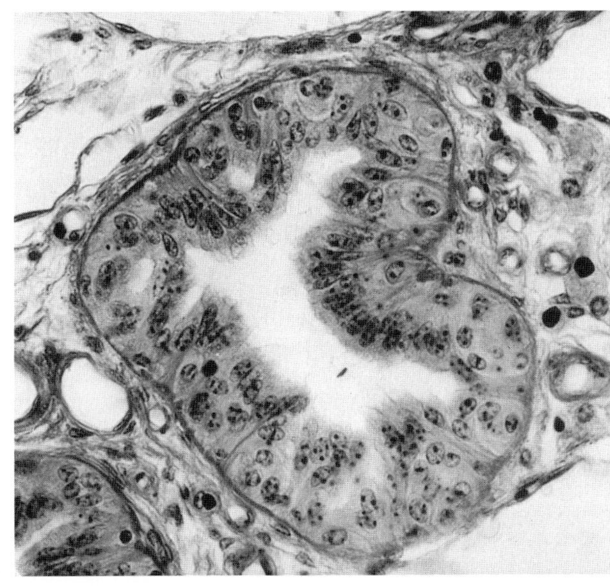

Figure 12.9. *Proximal (**A**) and distal (**B**) portion of the straight testicular tubules in the bovine testis. Note the differences in tubule diameter and the lining epithelium. Masson-Goldner (×350).*

straight tubules, and a simple columnar epithelium lines the distal portion (Fig. 12.9). This epithelium contains numerous macrophages and lymphocytes and is able to phagocytize spermatozoa.

Rete Testis

Irregularly anastomosing canals, surrounded by the loose connective tissue of the mediastinum testis, form the **rete testis** (Fig. 12.10). It is lined by simple squamous to columnar epithelium. Elastic fibers and contractile cells are present under the epithelium. Most of the testicular fluid, which is reabsorbed in the head of the epididymis, is produced in the rete testis (in the ram, approximately 40 ml/day). Rete testis fluid differs in composition from tubular seminiferous fluid, testicular lymph, and blood plasma.

Testicular Blood Supply

The testicular artery has a straight abdominal portion and becomes highly coiled after reaching the spermatic cord. Small nutritive twigs and the epididymal arteries branch from the coiled portion. As the artery reaches the testis, it courses parallel to the epididymis and is embedded in the tunica albuginea (Fig. 12.1). The testicular artery divides at the caudal testicular pole to form the arterial contributions to the vascular layer of the tunica albuginea. Within the septula testis, centripetal arteries course to the mediastinum testis, where they form heavily convoluted coils. From these convolutes, smaller centrifugal arteries return to supply the testicular parenchyma (Fig. 12.1). Most of the testicular veins empty into superficial veins situated in the tunica albuginea (Fig. 12.1). These converge at the base of the spermatic cord to form the pampiniform plexus, which completely surrounds the windings of the testicular artery. This remarkable vascular topography in the mammalian spermatic cord is believed to allow venous-arterial steroid hormone transfer and to cool the arterial blood entering the testis. Thus, testicular androgen levels are increased and testicular temperature is lowered; these are two important requirements for spermatogenesis.

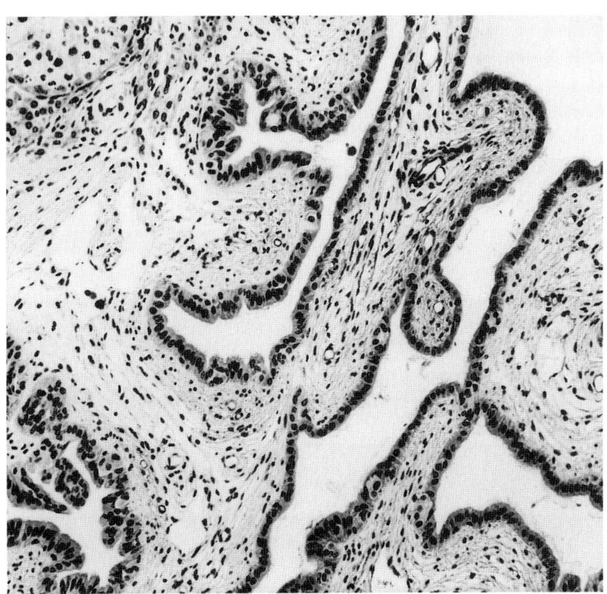

Figure 12.10. *Bovine rete testis lined with simple cuboidal epithelium and surrounded by a relatively large amount of connective tissue. Masson-Goldner (×140).*

EPIDIDYMIS

The mammalian **epididymis** is a dynamic accessory sex organ that is dependent on testicular androgens for the maintenance of a differentiated state of its epithelium. It comprises several (8 to 25) ductuli efferentes and a long, coiled ductus epididymidis. Macroscopically, the epididymis is divided into a head, body, and tail. It is surrounded by a thick tunica albuginea of dense irregular connective tissue covered by the visceral layer of the tunica vaginalis. In stallions, the tunica albuginea has a few smooth muscle cells scattered throughout the dense connective tissue.

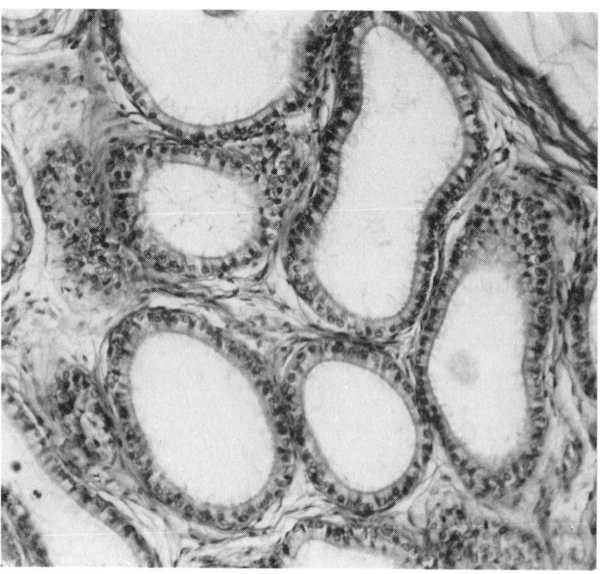

Figure 12.11. *Ductuli efferentes surrounded by highly vascularized loose connective tissue. Testis (cat). Hematoxylin and eosin (×95).*

Ductuli Efferentes

Between 8 and 25 **ductuli efferentes** connect the rete testis to the ductus epididymidis. The ductules are gathered in small lobules (coni vasculosi) with distinct boundaries of connective tissue. The epithelium of the efferent ductules is simple columnar and consists of ciliated and nonciliated cells (Figs. 12.11 and 12.12.1). Scattered lymphocytes in the basal epithelial area have been misinterpreted as a third genuine cell type. The ciliated cells (apical row of nuclei) help to move the spermatozoa toward the ductus epididymidis. The nonciliated cells (basal row of nuclei) have microvilli and morphologic characteristics of fluid-phase endocytosis, such as coated pinocytotic invaginations, coated and transport vesicles, and endosomes. Most of the nonciliated cells are involved in resorptive processes and, after resorption and digestion of ductular fluid, contain globular periodic acid-Schiff (PAS) positive residual bodies (Fig. 12.12.2); others may have a secretory activity. Intermediate forms between ciliated and nonciliated epithelial cells are occasionally observed. The ductular epithelium is surrounded by three to six loosely arranged layers of myofibroblasts and connective tissue. The ductuli efferentes and the initial portions of the ductus epididymidis constitute the head of the epididymis.

Ductus Epididymidis

The **ductus epididymidis** is extremely tortuous and coiled. The length of the duct varies considerably among species and has been estimated to be 40 m in bulls and boars and 70 m in stallions. Despite these differences, transport of sperm through the epididymis seems to require 10 to 15 days in most mammalian species.

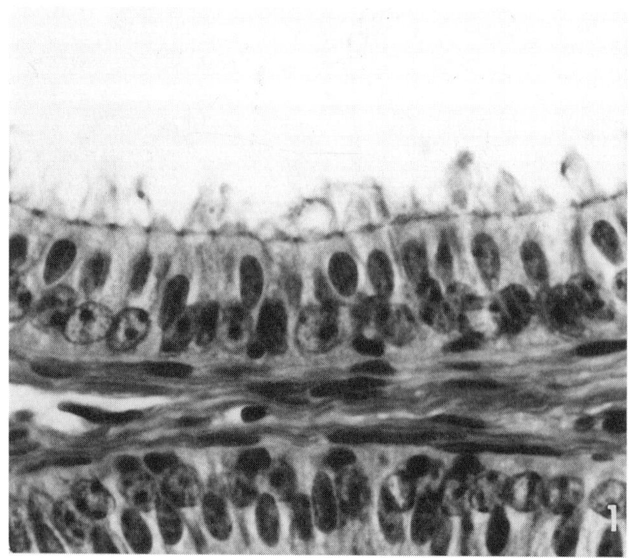

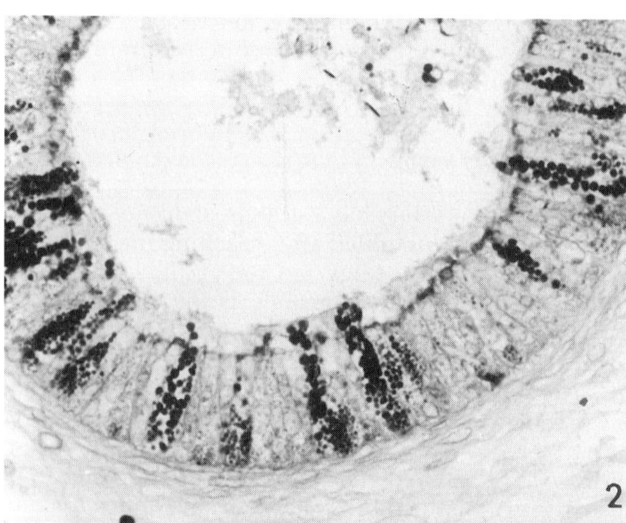

Figure 12.12. *1., The simple columnar epithelium of the efferent ductules consists of secretory and resorptive cells (light spherical nuclei) and ciliated cells (dense ovoid nuclei). Masson-Goldner-Jerusalem trichrome (×560). 2., Selective staining of nonciliated cells. PAS reaction after digestion by diastase (×350).*

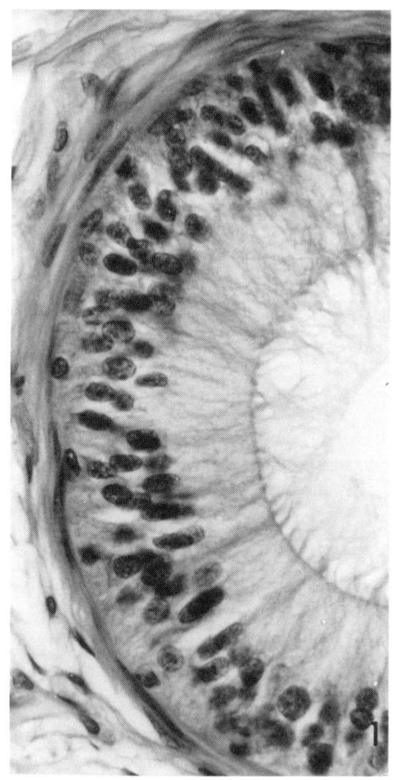

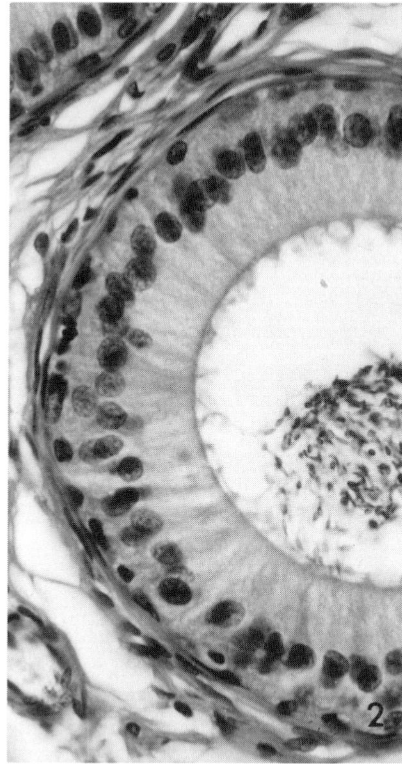

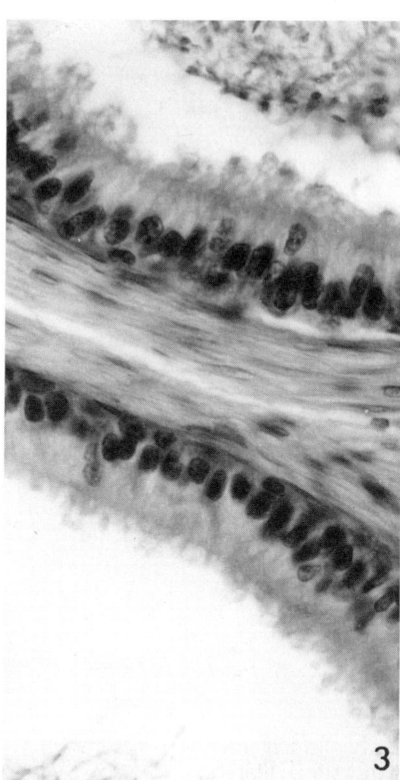

Figure 12.13. *Sections through the wall of the feline ductus epididymidis taken at the level of head (1), body (2), and tail of the epididymis (3). Note the variations in the position of the nuclei, in the height of the pseudostratified columnar epithelium, and in the length of the microvilli. Hematoxylin and eosin (×435).*

The ductus epididymidis is lined by a pseudostratified epithelium, surrounded by a small amount of loose connective tissue and circular smooth muscle fibers, the number of which increases significantly toward the tail of the epididymis. Two cell types are invariably present in the epithelium: columnar principal cells and small, polygonal basal cells (Fig. 12.13). In many species, additional cell types, such as apical cells and clear cells, are present. Macrophages and lymphocytes also occur within the epithelium.

The principal cells are generally taller in the head of the epididymis than in the remainder of the organ. The apical surfaces of the columnar cells bear long and sometimes branching microvilli (stereocilia) that become gradually shorter toward the tail. The occurrence of pinocytotic invaginations at the bases of the microvilli and the presence of coated vesicles and multivesicular bodies in the apical cytoplasm indicate that the epididymal epithelium has a high resorptive capacity. Most of the fluid (more than 90%) that leaves the testis is reabsorbed in the ductuli efferentes and the proximal part of the epididymal duct. Androgen-binding protein and inhibin produced by the sustentacular cells of the seminiferous tubules are also reabsorbed in the initial segment of the ductus epididymidis. The secretion of various substances, such as glycerophosphoryl choline, and glycoproteins, such as phosphatase and glycosidase, is also well established.

On the basis of histologic, histochemical, and ultrastructural criteria, the ductus epididymidis may be subdivided into several segments (six in bulls), the distribution and number of which are characteristic for each species (Fig. 12.13). Generally, the proximal parts of the duct (head and body) are involved in the maturation process of spermatozoa. The cauda epididymidis serves as their main storage place, e.g., 45% of bovine epididymal spermatozoa are stored here. Spermatozoa leaving the testis are both immotile and infertile, whereas spermatozoa leaving the epididymis have gained motility and fertility. During their passage through the ductus epididymidis, spermatozoa undergo a series of morphologic and functional changes that lead to the acquisition of full fertilizing capacity by the time they reach the cauda. The change in the functional status of the spermatozoa is reflected in *(a)* development of progressive motility, *(b)* modification of their metabolism, *(c)* alteration of the plasma membrane surface characteristics (activation of membrane-bound molecules necessary for recognition processes during fertilization), *(d)* stabilization of plasma membrane by oxidation of incorporated sulfhydryl groups, and *(e)* caudad movement and eventual loss of the cytoplasmic droplet, a remnant of the spermatid cytoplasm. Spermatozoa with persisting droplets are probably infertile. Once fully mature, spermatozoa can be stored in the cauda epididymidis for a remarkably long period, much longer than if they were maintained at a similar temperature in vitro.

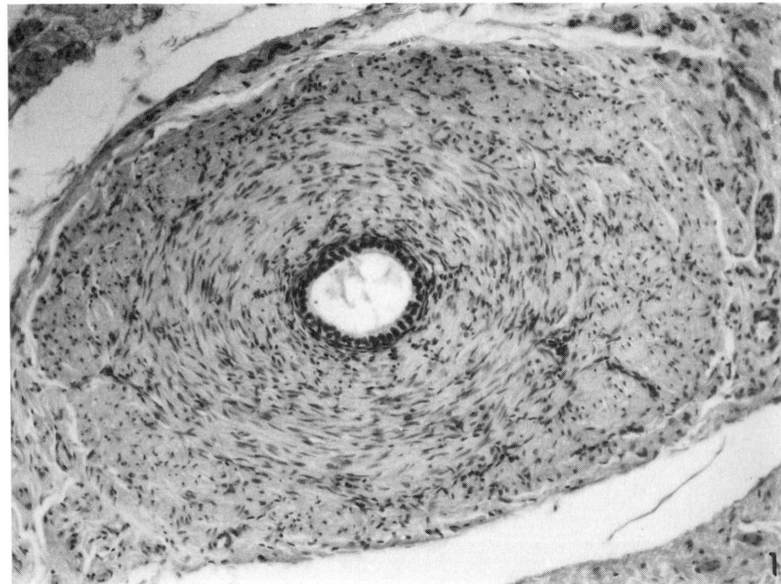

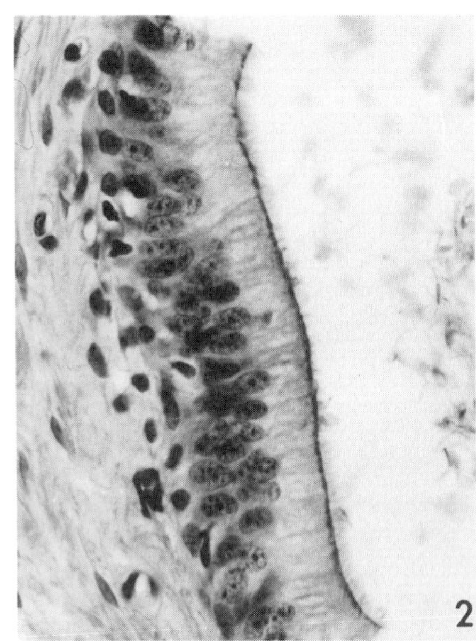

Figure 12.14. *1, Cross section through the intraabdominal portion of the feline ductus deferens. Hematoxylin and eosin (×130). 2, Pseudostratified columnar epithelium of the canine ductus deferens taken at the same level. Hematoxylin and eosin (×435).*

DUCTUS DEFERENS

The ductus epididymidis, after a sharp bend at the end of the tail, gradually straightens and acquires the histologic characteristics of the **ductus deferens**. In stallions and ruminants, the ductus deferens unites with the excretory duct of the vesicular gland to form a short ejaculatory duct, which opens at the colliculus seminalis into the urethra. The pseudostratified lining epithelium of the bovine ejaculatory duct contains engulfed spermatozoa. In boars, the ductus deferens and the excretory duct open separately into the urethra. In carnivores, the ductus deferens joins the urethra alone because the vesicular gland is absent.

The folded mucosa of the ductus deferens is lined by a pseudostratified columnar epithelium; toward the end of the duct, it may become a simple columnar epithelium (Fig. 12.14). In the proximity of the epididymis, the columnar cells possess short, branched microvilli (Fig. 12.14.2). In bulls, small lipid droplets are present in the basal cells. The loose connective tissue of the propria-submucosa is highly vascularized and rich in fibroblasts and elastic fibers. In stallions, bulls, and boars, the tunica muscularis consists of intermingled circular, longitudinal, and oblique layers; in small ruminants and carnivores (Fig. 12.14.1), an inner circular layer and an outer longitudinal layer are present. A tunica serosa with its usual components covers the organ.

The terminal portion of the ductus deferens is one of the male accessory glands, regardless of whether it forms an ampulla (stallions, ruminants, dogs) or does not (boars, cats); it contains simple branched tubuloalveolar glands in the propria-submucosa. In stallions, bulls, and rams, these glands occupy practically the entire propria-submucosa, which is rich in smooth muscle cells. In the dog and buck (Figs. 12.15.1 and 12.15.2), the glands are surrounded by periglandular connective tissue devoid of smooth muscle cells. The glands are lined by cells that vary from tall columnar cells with ovoid nuclei to cuboidal cells with spherical nuclei (Figs. 12.15.2 and 12.15.3). Apical, bleblike protrusions suggestive of secretory activity are often observed. Spherical or polyhedral basal cells are distributed irregularly between the columnar cells. In ruminants, the glandular epithelium is rich in glycogen and the basal cells contain lipid droplets of variable size. Lipid droplets are also present in the columnar cells of bulls. The lipids in bovine basal cells may coalesce, thereby giving these cells the appearance of fat cells (Fig. 12.15.3). The tunica muscularis of the terminal portion of the ductus deferens consists of variably arranged smooth muscle bundles surrounded by the highly vascularized loose connective tissue of the tunica adventitia.

The lumen of the glandular portion of the ductus deferens and the wide openings of the glands into the lumen contain a considerable number of spermatozoa in all domestic animals. In the bull, the number is sufficient for at least one normal ejaculate after recent castration or vasectomy.

ACCESSORY GLANDS

The ejaculate consists of spermatozoa and seminal plasma, which is composed of secretions from epididymis and male accessory glands. These glands are *(a)* the glandular portion of the ductus deferens, which has been described together with the ductus deferens, *(b)* the vesicular gland, *(c)* the prostate, and *(d)* the bulbourethral gland. All accessory glands are present in stallions, ruminants, and boars; the vesicular glands are absent in carnivores, and the bulbourethral gland is absent in dogs.

Vesicular Gland

The paired **vesicular gland** is a compound tubular or tubuloalveolar gland. The glandular epithelium is pseudostratified with tall columnar cells and small, spherical, often sparse basal cells (Fig. 12.16). The intralobular and main secretory ducts are lined by a simple cuboidal epithelium, or by a stratified columnar epithelium in horses.

The highly vascularized loose connective tissue of the propria submucosa is continuous with the dense connective-tissue trabeculae, which may subdivide the organ into lobes and lobules. A tunica muscularis of varying width and arrangement surrounds the organ, followed by a tunica serosa or a tunica adventitia.

SPECIES DIFFERENCES

In stallions, the vesicular glands are true vesicles, with wide central lumina (ducts) into which open the short branched tubuloalveolar glands, separated by relatively thin connective-tissue trabeculae with irregularly arranged smooth muscle cells.

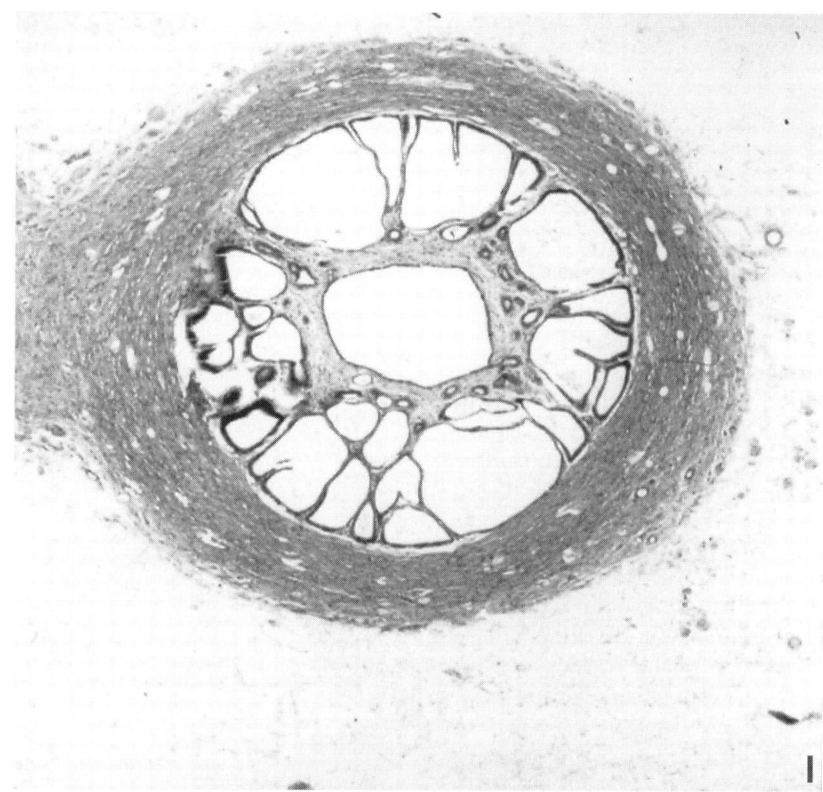

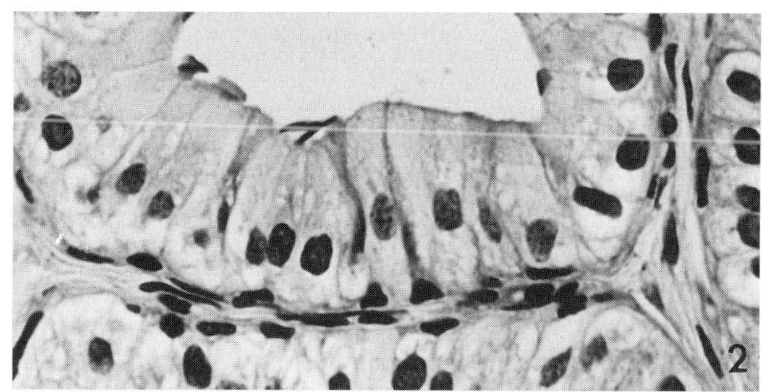

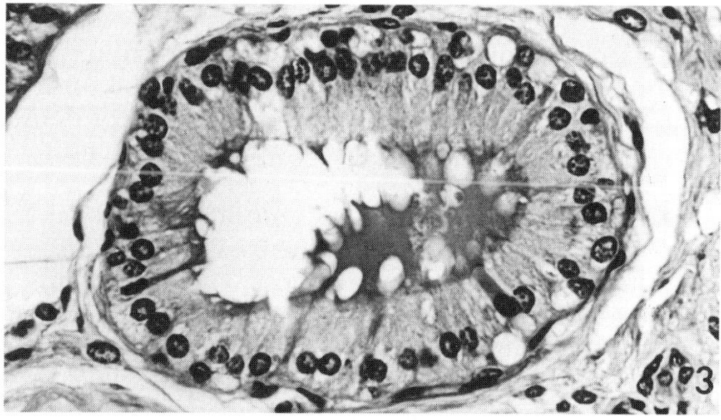

Figure 12.15. *1., Cross section through the glandular portion of the canine ductus deferens. The tunica muscularis is relatively thin . Hematoxylin and eosin (×38). 2., Part of a secretory alveolus of the glandular portion of the ductus deferens of a buck. Basal and columnar cells are present and heads of spermatozoa in the lumen. Weigert's hematoxylin (×560). 3., In this secretory alveolus of the glandular portion of the ductus deferens of a bull, some of the basal cells contain a huge lipid droplet (vacuole). Weigert's hematoxylin (×350).*

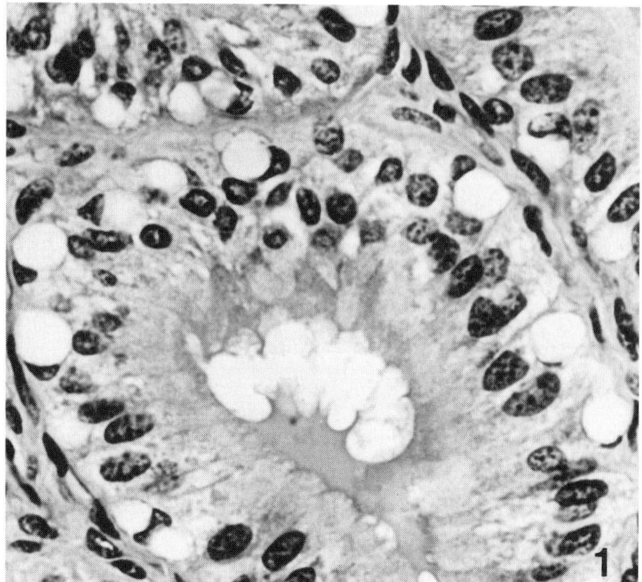

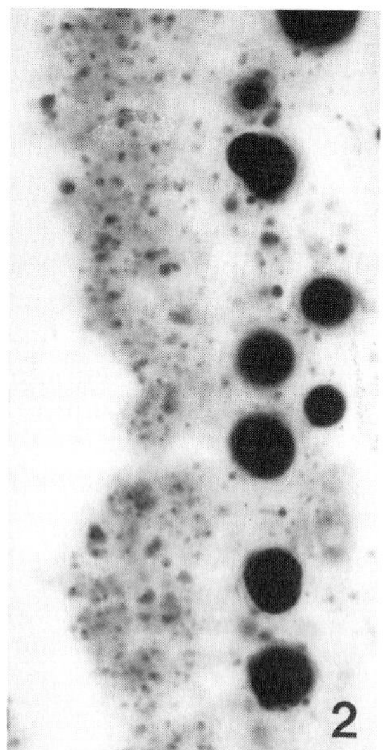

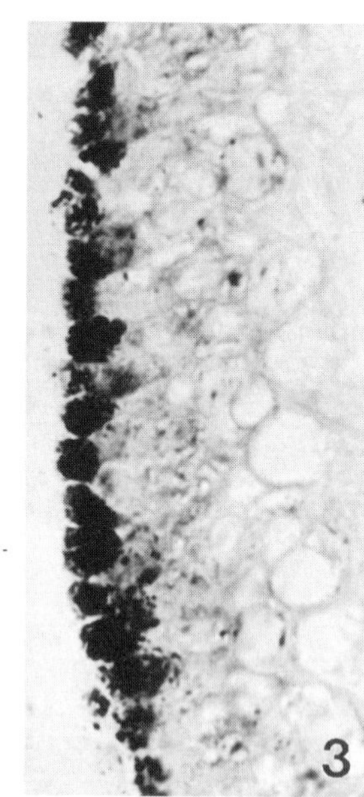

Figure 12.16. *Vesicular gland (bull).* ***1.***, *The basal cells in the pseudostratified columnar epithelial lining of the alveoli are characterized by large vacuoles containing lipid in vivo. Masson-Goldner (×560).* ***2.***, *Lipids were specifically stained with Sudan black B. Note the large lipid droplets in the basal cells and small lipid droplets in the secretory columnar cells (×560).* ***3.***, *The apices of the secretory columnar cells contain large amounts of glycogen. PAS (×560).*

In boars, the two vesicular glands possess a common connective-tissue capsule; the tunica muscularis is thin. The interlobular septa consist predominantly of connective tissue and a few small muscle cells. The tubular lumina are wide; the secretory epithelium is folded (Fig. 12.17).

In bulls, the vesicular gland is a compact, lobulated organ. Intralobular secretory ducts drain the slightly coiled tubular portions of the tubuloalveolar gland and, in turn, are drained by the main secretory duct. The secretory columnar cells have small lipid droplets and glycogen (Fig. 12.16) and give a positive alkaline phosphatase reaction. Some of the columnar cells possess light, bleblike apical projections. The basal cells are characterized by large lipid droplets, often in an infranuclear position (Fig. 12.16.2). Approximately 50% of the lipid material is cholesterol and its esters, approximately 25% is triglycerides, and approximately 10% is phospholipids. The interlobular septa are predominantly muscular, derived from the thick tunica muscularis, which is surrounded by a capsule of dense irregular connective tissue with a few smooth muscle cells.

The vesicular gland of rams and bucks is similar to that of bulls. Lipid droplets in the basal cells are absent in rams but may be present in bucks. The epithelium of the vesicular gland of bucks is considerably higher during the breeding season than during the nonbreeding season. The gelatinous, white, or yellowish-white secretory product of the vesicular gland amounts to approximately 25 to 30% of the total ejaculate in bulls, 10 to 30% in boars, and 7 to 8% in rams and bucks. It is rich in fructose, which serves as an energy source for ejaculated spermatozoa.

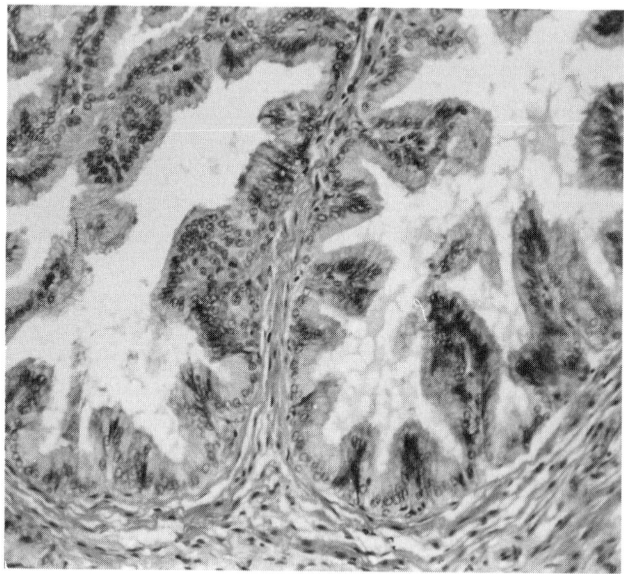

Figure 12.17. *Vesicular gland (boar). Epithelial folds project into the secretory alveoli. Hematoxylin and eosin (×130).*

Prostate Gland

The **prostate** consists of a varying number of individual tubuloalveolar glands derived from the epithelium of the pelvic urethra. Two portions may be distinguished, according more to topographic than to histologic features: the compact or external portion (corpus prostatae), and the disseminate or internal portion (pars disseminata prostatae). The external portion either entirely surrounds part of the pelvic urethra at the level of the colliculus seminalis or covers part of its dorsal aspect. The disseminate portion is located in the propria-submucosa of the pelvic urethra.

The secretory tubules, alveoli, and intraglandular ducts of the prostate gland are lined by a simple cuboidal or columnar epithelium, with occasional basal cells (Fig. 12.18). The simple epithelium changes to stratified columnar or transitional epithelium toward the terminal portions of the ducts. Some of the epithelial cells give a positive mucus reaction; most contain proteinaceous secretory granules. The tall columnar cells possess microvilli and sometimes bleblike apical protrusions. Occasionally, concentrically laminated concretions of secretory material are found in the tubules and alveoli. The duct system of the prostate possesses saccular dilatations in which secretory material may be stored.

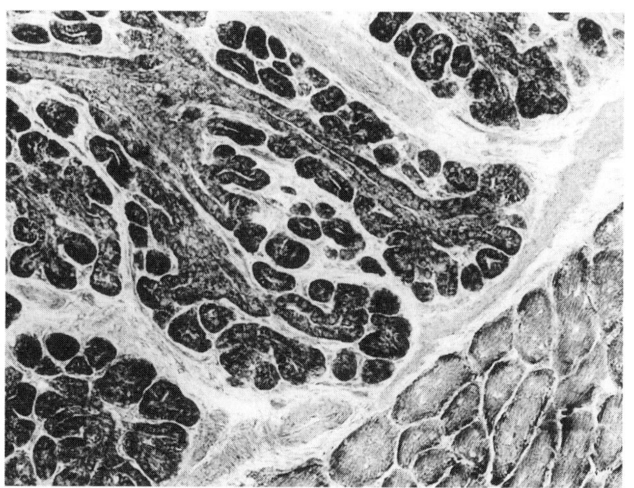

Figure 12.18. *This illustrates the general organization of the porcine disseminate prostate; smooth muscle fibers (light gray) are present in the capsule and the septa. β-D-galactosidase reaction (×100).*

The prostate is surrounded by a capsule of dense irregular connective tissue that contains many smooth muscle cells around the internal portion (Fig. 12.19), which is also surrounded by the striated urethral muscle (Figs. 12.18 and 12.20). Large trabeculae originate from the capsule and separate the external and internal portions into individual lobules. They are predominantly muscular in the external portion of the gland.

Secretory portions and ducts of the prostate gland are surrounded by loose connective tissue containing smooth muscle cells, which are particularly abundant in the external portion of the gland.

SPECIES DIFFERENCES

In carnivores, the external portion of the prostate gland is particularly well developed and separated into two distinct bilateral lobes. In dogs, these lobes completely surround the proximal portion of the pelvic urethra. In cats, they are located on the lateral and dorsal aspects of the urethra. The internal portion in dogs consists of a few glandular lobules. In cats, individual lob-

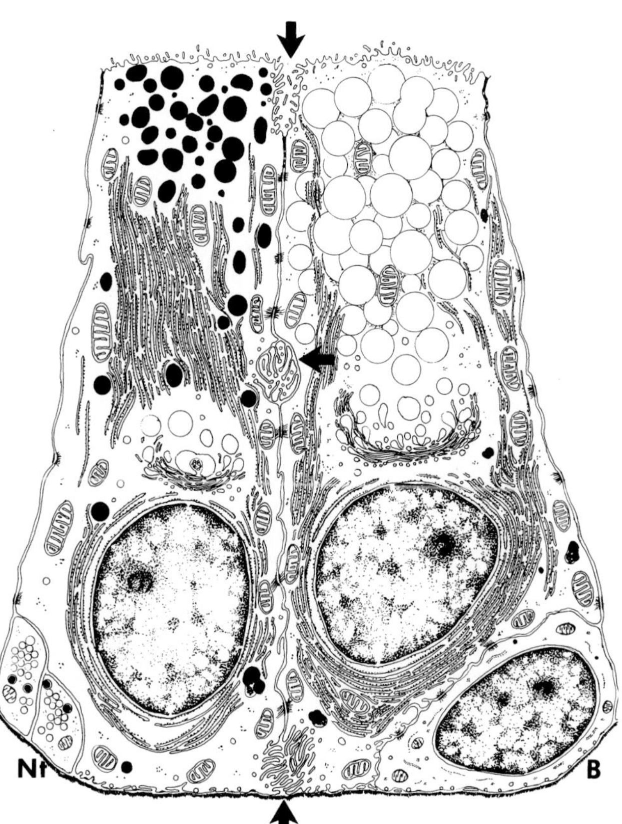

Figure 12.19. *Ruminant prostatic epithelium. The cell on the left side is a specific secretory cell containing proteinaceous granules. The cell on the right side secretes mucus. B = basal cell; Nt = intraepithelial autonomic nerve terminals. (Courtesy of A. Abou-Elmagd.)*

ules of the internal portion are found scattered between the colliculus seminalis and the bulbourethral glands. Lamellar corpuscles may be observed in the interstitium.

In stallions, only the external portion of the prostate gland is present and consists of a right and left lobe, both connected by the narrow dorsal isthmus. The individual lobes empty with 15 to 30 ducts into the pelvic urethra. The capsule, trabeculae, and interstitial connective tissue are rich in smooth muscle.

The external portion of the prostate gland of the bull is relatively inconspicuous; it is absent in small ruminants. The particularly well-developed internal portion (Fig. 12.20) encircles the urethra in bulls and bucks; in rams, it is U-shaped, and the midline of the ventral aspect of the urethra is free of glandular tissue.

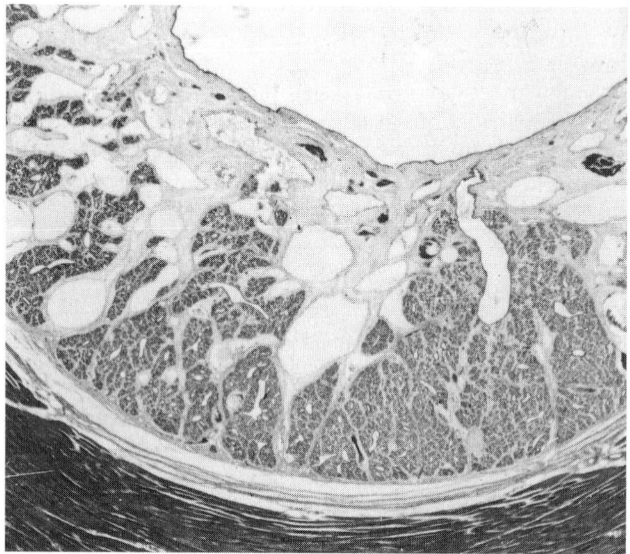

Figure 12.20. *In this cross section through part of the bovine prostatic urethra, note the large veins of the spongiose stratum and the disseminate prostate in the propria-submucosa, surrounded by the urethral muscle. Crossmon's trichrome (×11).*

In boars, the external portion of the prostate gland is a platelike organ; the internal portion (Fig. 12.18) is well developed and completely encircles the pelvic urethra.

The contribution of the prostatic secretions to the total volume of the ejaculate varies with the species. In ruminants, it is 4 to 6%; in stallions, it is 25 to 30%; and in boars, it is 35 to 60%. One of the functions of the prostate is to neutralize the seminal plasma, made acid by accumulation of metabolic carbon dioxide and lactate, and to initiate active movements of the ejaculated spermatozoa.

Bulbourethral Gland

The paired **bulbourethral gland** is located dorsolaterally from the spongiose portion of the urethra, at the bulb of the penis. It is a compound tubular (boars, cats, bucks) or tubuloalveolar (stallions, bulls, rams) gland (Fig. 12.21). It is absent in dogs.

The secretory portions of the gland are lined with a tall simple columnar epithelium and occasional basal cells. They open into collecting ducts either directly or through connecting pieces lined by simple cuboidal epithelial cells with dark cytoplasm. The collecting ducts (Fig. 12.21), lined by a simple cuboidal or columnar epithelium, unite to form larger intraglandular ducts lined by a pseudostratified columnar epithelium (Fig. 12.21). These, in turn, open into a single (or multiple) bulbourethral duct with a lining of transitional epithelium.

The gland is ensheathed by a fibroelastic capsule containing a variable amount of striated muscle cells. Trabeculae, extending from the capsule, consist of dense ir-

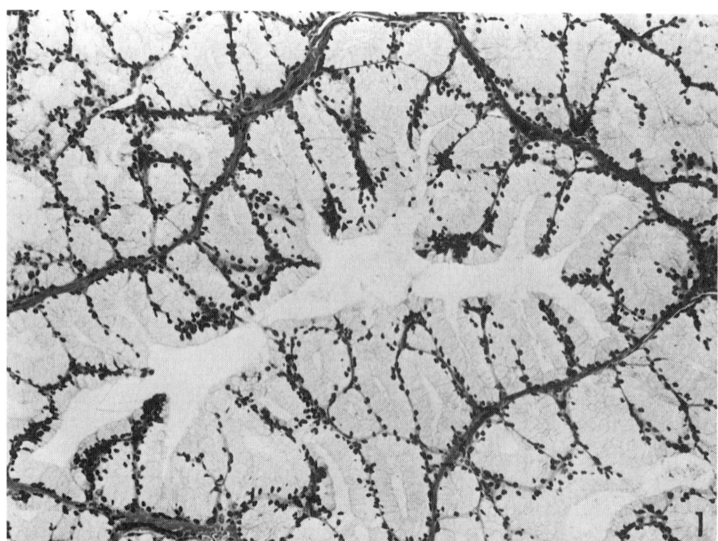

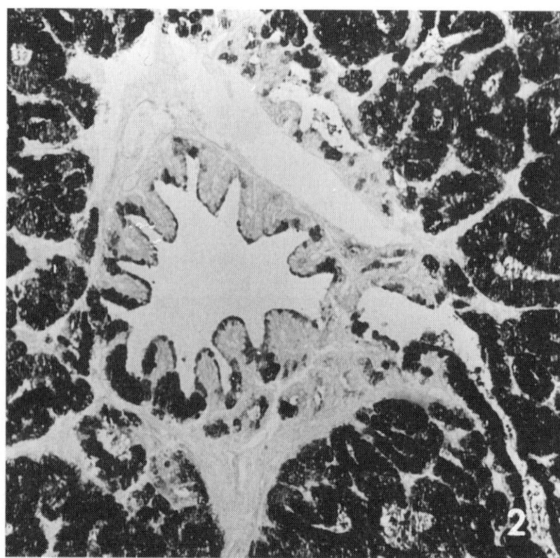

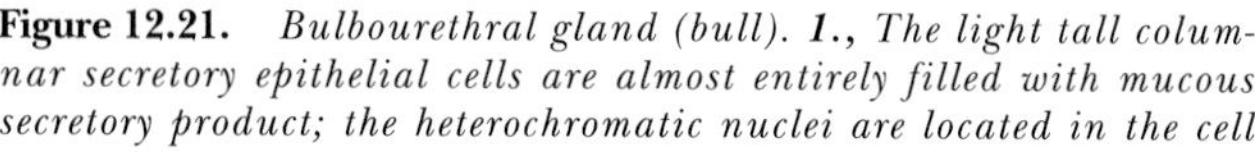

Figure 12.21. *Bulbourethral gland (bull). **1.**, The light tall columnar secretory epithelial cells are almost entirely filled with mucous secretory product; the heterochromatic nuclei are located in the cell base. Masson-Goldner-Jerusalem trichrome (×100). **2.**, Positive PAS reaction in the parenchyma and some of the lining cells of the central duct (×100).*

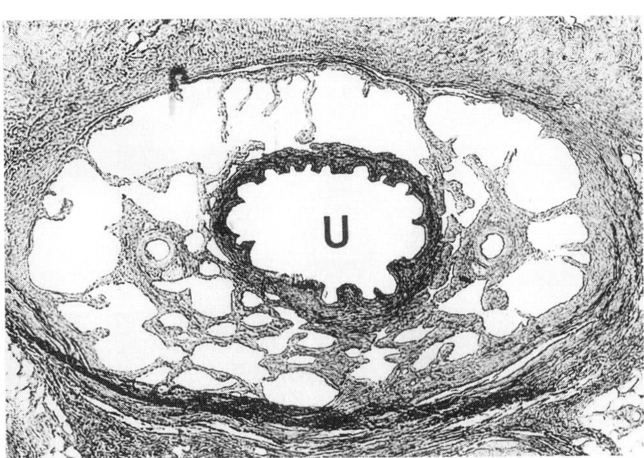

Figure 12.22. *Spongiose urethra (cat). The urethra (U) is surrounded by the cavernous spaces of the corpus spongiosum. Hematoxylin and eosin (×35).*

regular connective tissue and some smooth and striated muscle fibers. The interstitium consists of loose connective tissue and a few smooth muscle fibers.

SPECIES DIFFERENCES

In cats, the gland consists of spacious, sinuslike intraglandular ducts and short, narrow, mostly unbranched tubular end pieces. The secretory surface of the cells is increased by a well-developed system of intercellular canaliculi.

In stallions, the bulbourethral gland is completely surrounded by the bulbocavernous muscle. Three to four individual bulbourethral ducts are present.

The exceptionally large bulbourethral gland of boars is surrounded by the ischioglandular muscle. Only a few smooth muscle cells are present in the interstitium. The collecting ducts are lined by a simple columnar epithelium.

In ruminants, the gland is also surrounded by the bulbocavernous muscle. In bulls and rams, short connecting pieces link the secretory portions to the collecting ducts, which are lined by a simple cuboidal epithelium (sometimes also secretory) (Fig. 12.21.2). In bucks, the secretory portions empty directly into these ducts. Smooth muscle cells are particularly abundant within the interstitium.

The mucous and proteinaceous secretory product of the bulbourethral gland is discharged before ejaculation in ruminants, where it apparently serves to neutralize the urethral environment and to lubricate both the urethra and the vagina. In boars, the exclusively mucous secretory product, rich in sialic acid, is part of the ejaculate (15 to 30%) and possibly involved in the occlusion of the cervix to prevent loss of sperm. In cats, the secretory product is mucus and also contains glycogen. In the absence of a vesicular gland, this bulbourethral glycogen may be the source of feline seminal fructose. It may provide energy for the metabolism of the spermatozoa.

URETHRA

The male **urethra** is divided into the prostatic, membranous, and spongiose portions. The prostatic portion extends from the urinary bladder to the caudal edge of the prostate. The membranous portion begins here and terminates where the urethra enters the bulb of the penis, from which level the spongiose portion continues to the external urethral opening.

The entire urethral mucosa is thrown into longitudinal folds that flatten or disappear during erection and micturition. In the prostatic urethra, a prominent, permanent dorsomedian fold, the urethral crest, is present. It terminates as a slight enlargement, the **colliculus seminalis**. There, the following ducts open into the urethra: the ejaculatory ducts in ruminants and stallions, the ductus deferentes and the ducts of the vesicular glands in boars, and the deferent ducts in carnivores. Between these ducts, vestiges of the fused paramesonephric ducts, the uterus masculinus, may be found as either a solid epithelial cord or a short canal.

The predominant lining of the urethra is a transitional epithelium with variably sized patches of simple columnar epithelium, stratified columnar epithelium, or cuboidal epithelium. The propria submucosa consists of a loose connective tissue with many elastic fibers and smooth muscle cells and frequent diffuse lymphatic tissue or lymphatic nodules (dog). In stallions and cats, simple tubular mucous (urethral) glands are present.

Throughout the entire length of the urethra, the propria-submucosa possesses erectile properties by virtue of endothelium-lined caverns of variable size that constitute the so-called **vascular stratum** in the prostatic and membranous urethra. Around the spongiose urethra, the quantity and size of the cavernous spaces are greatly increased (Fig. 12.22); here, the vascular stratum is referred to as the **corpus spongiosum**, which begins at the ischiadic arch with a bilobed expansion, the bulb of the penis.

The tunica muscularis of the urethra consists of smooth muscle in the vicinity of the bladder or striated muscle in the remainder of the urethra. It is surrounded by a tunica adventitia of loose or dense irregular connective tissue.

In ruminants and stallions, the terminal portion of the urethra protrudes incompletely (bulls) or completely (stallions, rams, and bucks) above the glans penis to form the urethral process. The transitional or stratified squamous epithelial lining is surrounded by a corpus spongiosum containing many cavernous spaces in stallions and fewer and smaller spaces in ruminants. Two longitudinal fibrocartilaginous cords flank the urethra in bucks and rams. The urethral process is covered by a cutaneous mucous membrane.

PENIS

The penis consists essentially of *(a)* the corpora cavernosa penis, *(b)* the corpus spongiosum penis surrounding the spongiose urethra, and *(c)* the glans penis.

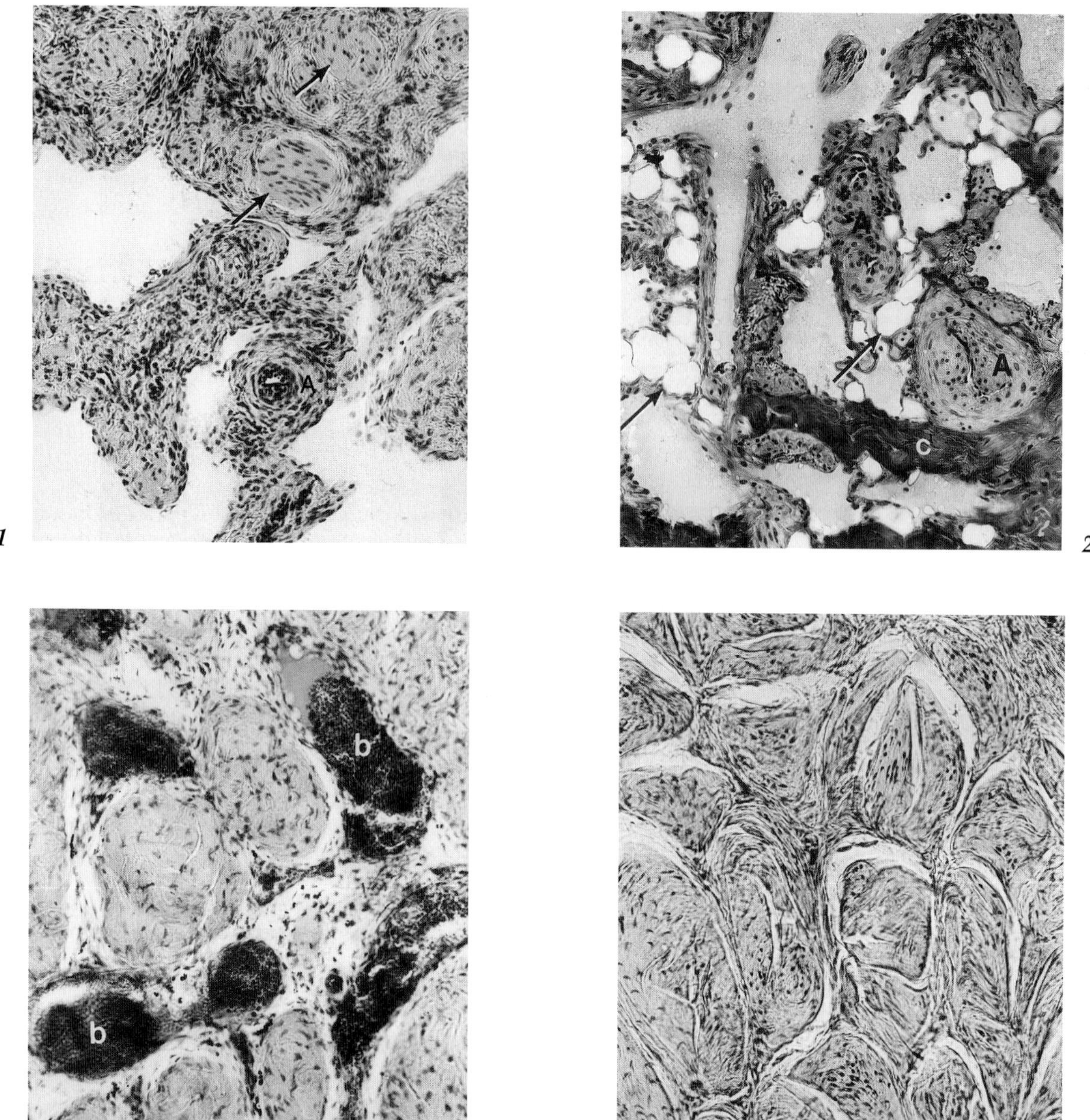

Figure 12.23. *1, Corpus cavernosum (stallion). Bundles of smooth muscle (arrows) and a helicine artery (A) are present within the connective-tissue trabeculae between the cavernous spaces. 2, Corpus cavernosum (cat). Collagen trabeculae (c) between cavernous spaces, adipose cells (arrows), and numerous helicine arteries (A). 3, Corpus cavernosum (boar). Cavernous spaces contain coagulated blood (b) between abundant connective-tissue trabeculae. 4, Corpus cavernosum (bull). Note the slitlike, empty cavernous spaces and abundant connective-tissue trabeculae (×140).*

Corpora Cavernosa Penis

The paired **corpora cavernosa penis** arise from the ischiadic tuberosities and merge to form the body of the penis. They are surrounded by the tunica albuginea, a thick layer of dense irregular connective tissue containing variable numbers of elastic fibers and smooth muscle cells. A connective-tissue septum completely (in stallions and dogs) or partially divides the corpora cavernosa penis.

The spaces between the tunica albuginea and the trabecular network arising from the tunica albuginea are filled with erectile tissue (Fig. 12.23). In stallions (Fig. 12.23.1) and carnivores (Fig. 12.23.2), this tissue consists of caverns lined by endothelium and surrounded by connective tissue, the appearance of which varies between loose and dense irregular, and by smooth muscle cells (Fig. 12.23). In stallions, these muscle bundles are oriented with the longitudinal axis of the penis, often causing a virtually complete obturation of the lumina of the cavernous spaces. Relaxation of these muscle cells causes the penis to elongate and emerge from the preputial sheath, which usually happens during micturition. In ruminants (Fig. 12.23.4) and boars (Fig.

12.23.3), the connective tissue surrounding the caverns contains few, if any, smooth muscle cells.

The cavernous spaces receive their main blood supply from arteries with a helical arrangement that are referred to as **helicine arteries** (arteriae helicinae). Characteristically, they have epithelioid smooth muscle cells in the tunica interna that protrude into the lumina of these vessels as ridges or pads, causing partial obliteration (Fig. 12.23). As the smooth muscle cells relax, the blood flow into the caverns increases considerably and causes erection. The cavernous spaces are drained by venules, several of which give origin to thick-walled veins.

The penis of stallions is classified as a vascular penis because of the predominance of caverns in the corpus cavernosum. In ruminants and boars, the caverns are less extensive and connective tissue prevails, thus the designation of the penis as fibroelastic. The penis of dogs and cats is best classified as an intermediate type.

Glans Penis

A well-developed **glans penis** is present only in stallions and dogs. It is surrounded by a tunica albuginea rich in elastic fibers. It continues into trabeculae that delineate spaces containing erectile tissue similar to that of the corpus spongiosum penis (stallions) or a plexus of large caverns (dogs) (Fig. 12.24). The glans penis is covered by the prepuce (see section later in this chapter).

Species Differences

The corpora cavernosa penis of dogs are completely separated by a connective-tissue septum and are continued cranially by the os penis, which terminates in a fibrocartilaginous tip. The glans penis consists of the bulbus glandis and the pars longa glandis. Both almost completely surround the os penis and the distal portion of the spongiose urethra and its associated corpus spongiosum. The **bulbus glandis** consists of large venous caverns separated by connective-tissue trabeculae rich in elastic fibers. The **pars longa glandis** forms the rostral portion of the glans penis; its structure (Fig. 12.24) is identical to that of the bulbus.

In cats, many adipose cells are present between the caverns of the corpus cavernosum penis. They increase in number toward the tip of the corpus cavernosum, which contains little erectile tissue. A small os penis surrounded by the corpus cavernosum of the glans is present.

The connective tissue of the corpus cavernosum of stallions contains many elastic fibers and smooth muscle cells. The glans covers the corpus cavernosum penis rostrally and possesses a long, caudally directed, dorsomedian process and an enlargement, the corona glandis, the epithelial covering of which bears cylindric papillae. An indentation of the glans, the fossa glandis, contains the slightly protruding end of the urethra (urethral process). At the level of the glans, the urethral muscle bundles are interrupted by the retractor penis muscle.

A corkscrewlike left turn characterizes approximately the cranial third of the penis of the boar. Its structure is similar to that of the penis of bulls.

The corpus cavernosum penis of bulls contains a central connective-tissue strand formed by the converging trabeculae. The tip of the penis (glans) (Fig. 12.25) consists of mesenchymal cells, adipose cells, and large intercellular spaces. An extensive erectile venous plexus is present. The penis of bucks and rams is similar to that of bulls. The glans is a large caplike enlargement that is similar to that of bulls. Two lateral outpocketings of the corpus spongiosum penis protrude from it laterally.

Mechanism of Erection

In animals with either a vascular or an intermediate type penis, erection causes an increase in size and a stiffening of the organ. In animals with a fibroelastic penis, erection results essentially in an increase in the length of the penis that emerges from the prepuce.

Relaxation of the smooth muscle cells in the helicine ar-

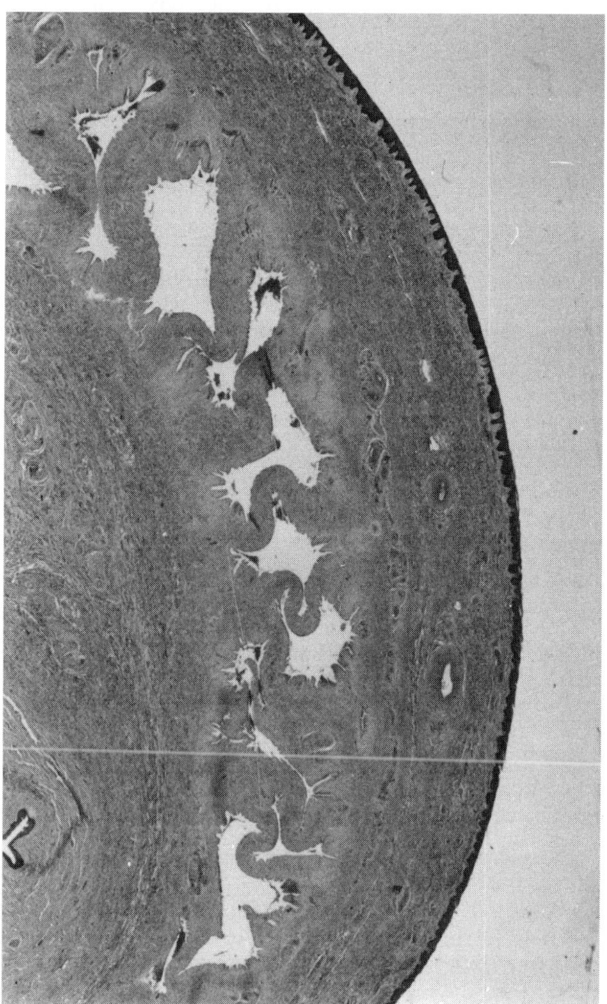

Figure 12.24. *Glans penis, pars longa (dog). Large cavernous spaces of the erectile tissue. Hematoxylin and eosin (×11).*

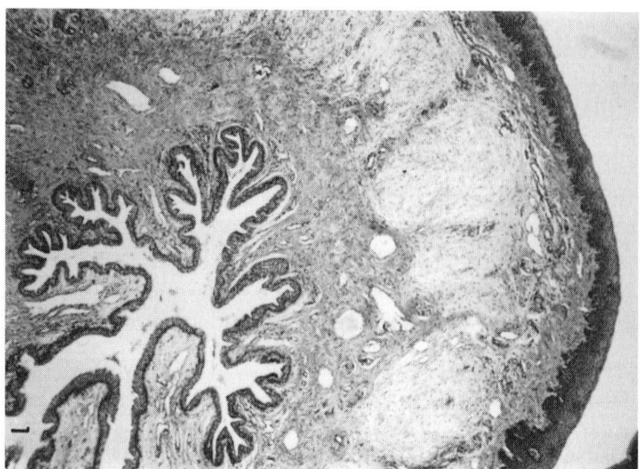

Figure 12.25. *In the bovine glans penis, the urethra is surrounded by relatively little subepithelial erectile tissue and a thick connective-tissue layer. Hematoxylin and eosin (×40).*

teries results in increased blood flow into the spaces of the corpora cavernosa. The increased blood volume compresses the veins and subsequently decreases the outflow, eventually filling the erectile tissue spaces in the corpora cavernosa and spongiosa penis and in the glans penis.

Detumescence is initiated by contraction of the musculature of the helicine arteries and thus by a decrease in arterial inflow. The contraction of the smooth muscle cells of the tunica albuginea, the trabeculae, and the erectile tissue causes the penis to return to the flaccid state. In ruminants and boars, the retractor penis muscle plays an essential role in retracting the penis into the prepuce.

During copulation, the constrictor vestibuli muscle of bitches constricts the veins that drain the entire glans and especially the bulbus glandis. This constriction causes the bulbus to enlarge to such a degree that immediate withdrawal of the penis from the vagina is impossible; consequently, coitus is prolonged.

PREPUCE

The cranial portion of the penis and the glans penis are located in a tubelike reflection of the skin, the prepuce, composed of an external and an internal layer. The external layer reflects inward at the preputial opening to form the internal layer of the prepuce. It reflects on the cranial portion of the penis and is securely attached cranially to the glans penis.

The external layer is typical skin. Numerous sebaceous glands, not always related to hairs, are present at the preputial opening. In addition, long, bristlelike hairs are found in ruminants and boars. In stallions, ruminants, boars, and dogs, fine hairs and sebaceous and sweat glands are located over a variable distance in the internal layer. In stallions, occasional hairs occur, even in the penile skin (Fig. 12.26), which is also rich in sebaceous and sweat glands. In dogs and ruminants, both the internal layer of the prepuce and the skin covering the penis contain solitary lymphatic nodules; in boars, they are present only in the internal layer. In cats, the mucosa covering the glans has numerous keratinized papillae.

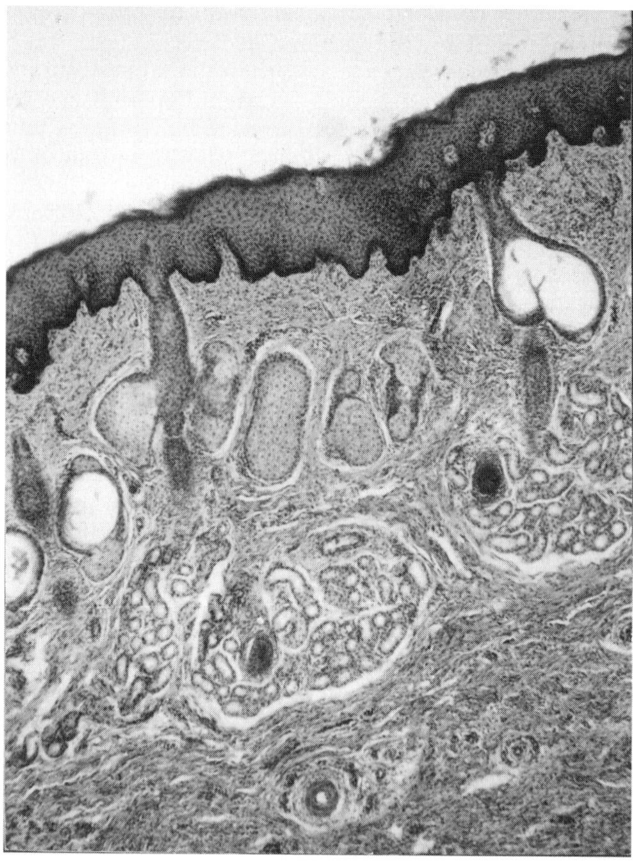

Figure 12.26. *Skin with hairs and sebaceous and sweat glands covering the corpus penis (stallion). Hematoxylin and eosin (×40).*

In boars, a dorsal evagination of the prepuce is referred to as the preputial diverticulum. It is incompletely separated into two lateral portions by a median septum. Frequently, the keratinized cutaneous mucous membrane is folded. A mixture of desquamated epithelial cells and urine forms smegma with an odor that is unpleasant to humans.

REFERENCES

Aumüller G. Prostate gland and seminal vesicles. In: Handbuch der mikroskopischen Anatomie des Menschen. Berlin: Springer-Verlag, 1979;7(6).

Cole HH, Cupps PT. Reproduction in domestic animals, 3rd ed. New York: Academic Press, 1977.

Fawcett DW, Bedford JM, eds. The spermatozoon. Maturation, motility, surface properties and comparative aspects. Baltimore: Urban and Schwarzenberg, 1979.

Guraya SS. Biology of spermatogenesis and spermatozoa in mammals. New York: Springer-Verlag, 1987.

Knobil E, Neill JD, eds. The physiology of reproduction. New York: Raven Press, 1988.

Russell LD, Griswold MD, eds. The sertoli cell. Clearwater, FL: Cache River Press, 1993.

Setchell BP. The mammalian testis. London: Paul Elek, 1978.

Steinberger A, Steinberger E. Testicular development, structure and function. New York: Raven Press, 1980.

Van Blerkom J, Motta P, eds. Ultrastructure of reproduction. Boston: M. Nijhoff, 1984.

13

Female Reproductive System

JĀNIS PRIEDKALNS
RUDOLF LEISER

The female reproductive system consists of bilateral ovaries and uterine tubes (oviducts), a usually bicornuate uterus, cervix, vagina, vestibule, vulva, and associated glands. It is concerned with the production and transport of ova, the transport of spermatozoa, fertilization, and the accommodation of the conceptus until birth.

OVARY

The ovary is a combined exocrine and endocrine gland, i.e., it produces both ova (exocrine "secretion") and ovarian hormones, chiefly estrogens and progesterone (endocrine secretion). The structure of the normal ovary varies greatly with the species, age, and phase of the sexual cycle. It is an ovoid structure divided into an outer cortex and an inner medulla (Fig. 13.1). In the mature mare, these areas become reversed, and the cortical tissue remains on the surface only in the ovulation fossa, which is the site of all ovulations.

Cortex

The cortex is a broad peripheral zone containing follicles in various stages of development and corpora lutea embedded in a loose connective tissue stroma (Fig. 13.1). It is covered by a low cuboidal surface epithelium. A thick connective tissue layer, the **tunica albuginea**, lies immediately beneath the surface epithe-

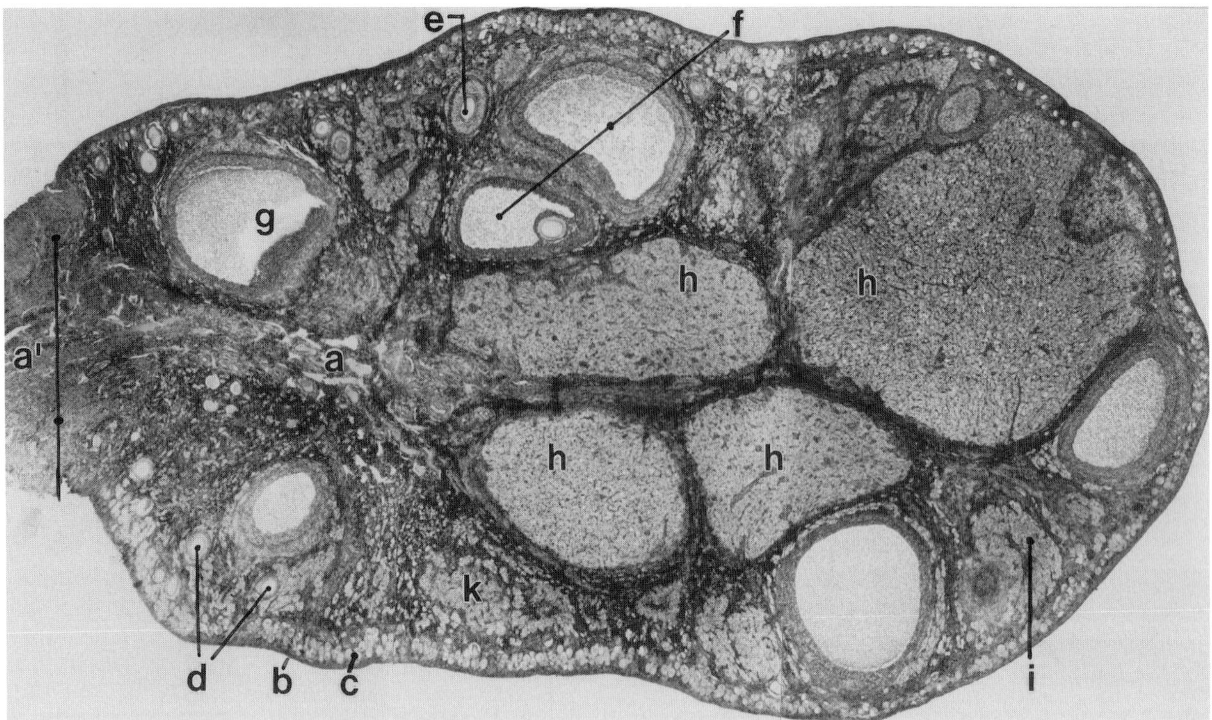

Figure 13.1. *Ovary of queen showing the development and the regression of follicles and corpora lutea in the ovarian cortex. The ovarian medulla contains blood vessels (a) that enter the ovary at the hilus and from the mesovarium (a'). Surface epithelium with adjacent tunica albuginea (b); subtunical layer with primordial follicles (c); primary follicles (d); secondary follicle (e); tertiary follicles, in one case containing an oocyte within the cumulus oophorus (f); early atretic follicle (g); corpora lutea (h); corpus regressivum (i); interstitial endocrine cells (k) (×20).*

lium. It is disrupted by the growth of ovarian follicles and corpora lutea and may be inconspicuous during increased ovarian activity. In the ovary of rodents, bitches, and queens, the cortical stroma contains cords of polyhedral interstitial endocrine cells. In the ovary of bitches, **cortical tubules** are also prominent; these are narrow channels lined by a cuboidal epithelium that, in some sites, are continuous with the surface epithelium.

FOLLICULAR DEVELOPMENT

An **ovarian follicle** is a structure composed of an oocyte surrounded by specialized epithelial cells; during follicular development, the epithelial cells become surrounded by specialized stroma cells and a fluid-filled cavity develops among the epithelial cells.

Primordial (unilaminar, preantral, resting) follicles are composed of a **primary oocyte** surrounded by a **simple squamous** epithelium of **follicular cells** (Figs. 13.1 and 13.2). Primordial follicles arise prenatally by mitotic proliferation of **internal epithelial cell masses** in the ovarian cortex. In some species, e.g., bitches, they may arise also postnatally. The internal epithelial cell masses are believed to arise after interaction of cortical stroma, ovarian surface epithelium, or **rete ovarii** with **primordial germ cells (PGCs)**; the PGCs arrive in the gonadal ridge from the entoderm of the yolk sac. During proliferation, the internal epithelial cell masses become separated into cell clusters. The central cell of a cluster becomes the **oogonium**. The oogonia enlarge, enter the prophase of the first meiotic division, and are then termed **primary oocytes**, approximately 20 μm in diameter in most species. The primary oocytes then go through the leptotene, zygotene, pachytene, and diplotene stages and then remain in the dictyotene stage. As the primary oocyte forms, the surrounding cells form a single layer of flat follicular cells resting on a basal lamina. Together, these **components** constitute the primordial follicle, approximately 40 μm in diameter. Primordial follicles are located mainly in the outer cortex. They are evenly distributed in ruminants and the sow and occur in clusters in carnivores.

Primary (unilaminar, preantral, growing) follicles are composed of a **primary oocyte** surrounded by a **simple cuboidal** epithelium of **follicular cells** (Fig. 13.2). The primary oocytes begin the first meiotic division before birth, but the completion of prophase does not occur until the time of ovulation. The primary oocytes thus remain in suspended prophase (dictyotene stage) until after puberty. Several hundred thousand to 1,000,000 potential oocytes may be present at birth in a single ovary in various species. Most of these regress before or after birth, and only several hundred ovulate during a normal lifetime. The processes involved in the selection of follicles for growth from a pool of nonproliferating primordial follicles are poorly understood.

Secondary (multilaminar, preantral, growing) follicles are composed of a **primary oocyte** surrounded by a

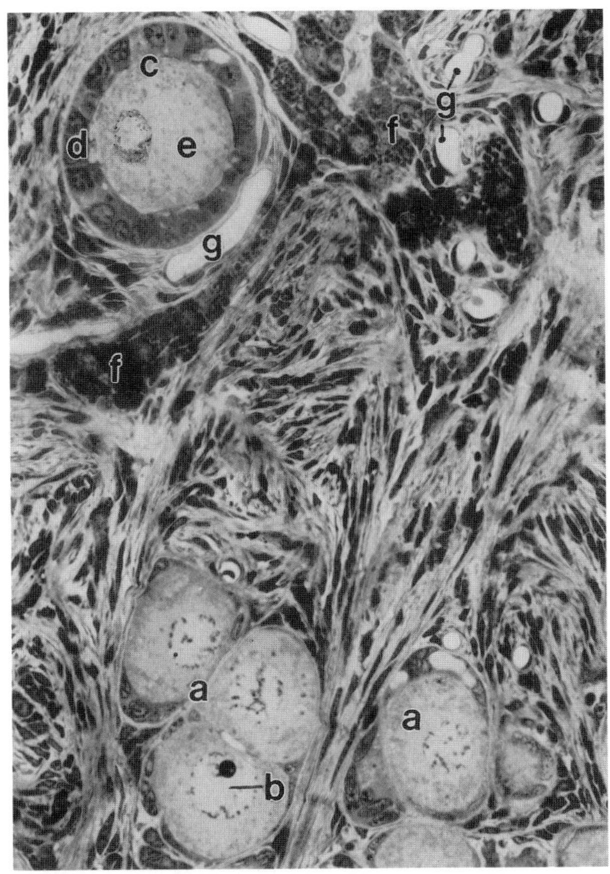

Figure 13.2. *Ovary of queen showing primordial follicles (a), which consist of primary oocytes surrounded by a simple squamous epithelium. Nucleus with nucleolus (b). Primary follicle (c), in which a cuboidal epithelium (d) encloses an enlarged primary oocyte (e). Interstitial endocrine cells containing granules (f) are seen near capillaries (g) (×460).*

stratified epithelium of **polyhedral follicular cells**, termed **granulosa cells** (Fig. 13.3). The multilaminar stratum of granulosa cells arises from proliferating follicular cells of the primary follicle. In carnivores, sows, and ewes, polyovular follicles, which contain several oocytes, may develop. In cows, the late secondary follicle is approximately 120 μm in diameter and contains an oocyte approximately 80 μm in diameter. Secondary follicles are marked by the development of a 3- to 5-μm-thick glycoprotein layer, the **zona pellucida**, around the plasma membrane of the oocyte. The zona pellucida is secreted by the granulosa cells immediately surrounding the oocyte and, in part, by the oocyte itself. There is partial penetration of this zone by the oocyte microvilli. Cytoplasmic extensions of the granulosa cells situated around the oocyte penetrate the zona pellucida and associate closely with these microvilli (Fig. 13.4). As follicular development continues, small fluid-filled clefts are formed among the granulosa cells. A vascularized multilaminar layer of spindle-shaped stroma cells, termed **theca cells**, begins to form around the granulosa cell layer in late secondary follicles.

Tertiary (multilaminar, antral, growing) follicles, also termed **vesicular** or **Graafian follicles**, are composed of a **primary oocyte** (or a **secondary oocyte** immediately before ovulation in most species) surrounded by a stratified epithelium of **granulosa cells**; the granulosa cells are surrounded by a multilaminar layer of specialized stroma cells, termed the **theca**, and a fluid-filled cavity, the **antrum**, develops among the granulosa cells (Fig. 13.5). The antrum, which characterizes tertiary follicles, is formed when the small, fluid-filled clefts among the granulosa cells of secondary follicles coalesce to form a single large cavity containing **liquor folliculi**. Late tertiary follicles, just before ovulation, are termed **mature follicles** (Fig. 13.6A). In mature follicles, before or just after ovulation, depending on the species, the primary oocyte completes the first meiotic division, thereby giving rise to a secondary oocyte and the **first polar body**.

The primary oocyte in tertiary follicles measures 150 to 300 μm in diameter, depending on the species. It has a spherical, centrally located nucleus with a sparse chromatin network and a prominent nucleolus. The Golgi complex, initially dispersed in the cytoplasm, becomes concentrated near the plasma membrane. Lipid granules and lipochrome pigment occur in the cytoplasm. As the antrum enlarges through the accumulation of liquor folliculi, the oocyte is displaced eccentrically, usually in a part of the follicle nearest to the center of the ovary (Fig. 13.6B). The oocyte then lies in an accumulation of granulosa cells, the **cumulus oophorus**. In large tertiary follicles, the granulosa cells immediately surrounding the oocyte become columnar and radially disposed; they are termed the **corona radiata** (Figs. 13.4A and 13.6B). The corona radiata cells are believed to provide nutrient support for the oocyte. They are lost at the time of ovulation in ruminants but generally persist until just before fertilization in other species.

In tertiary follicles, the granulosa cells form the pari-

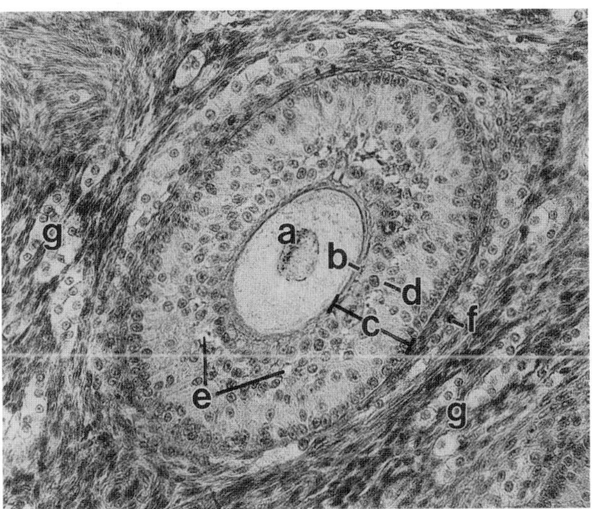

Figure 13.3. *Ovary of queen showing a secondary follicle, in which the primary oocyte (a) is surrounded by a thin (initially) zona pellucida (b) and a stratified epithelium of polyhedral cells (c), of which the inner cell layer forms the corona radiata (d). Call-Exner bodies (e). The connective tissue cells that surround the follicle will form the theca interna (f). Interstitial endocrine cells (g) (×230).*

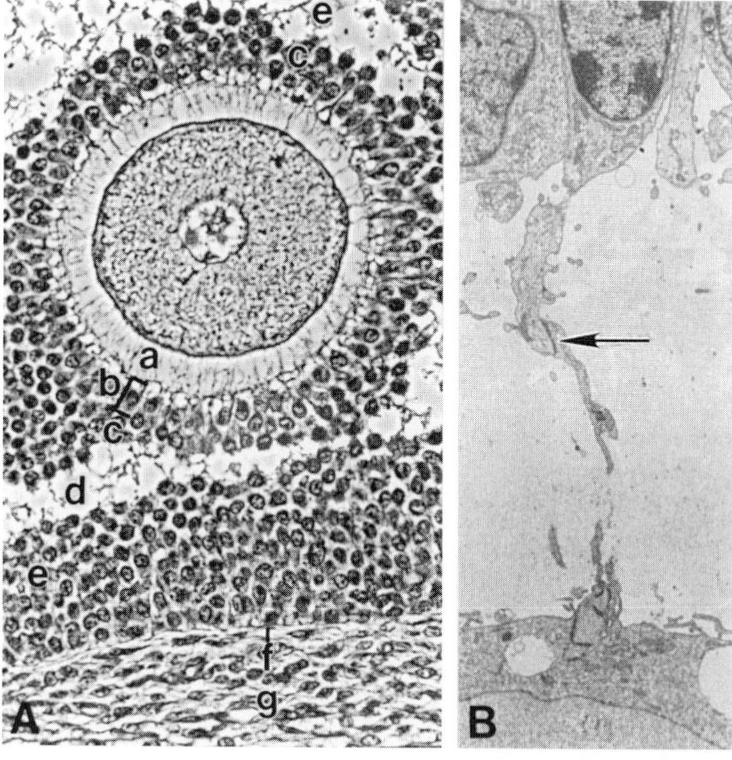

Figure 13.4. *A., A bovine oocyte, surrounded by a zona pellucida (a), a corona radiata (b), and cells of the cumulus oophorus (c), is separated from the stratum granulosum of the follicular wall (e) by a gap (d) that developed during oocyte detachment from the follicle wall during the beginning stages of ovulation. Basal lamina of stratum granulosum (f), theca interna (g) (×640).* ***B.****, An electron micrograph from the bovine ovary showing projections of a corona radiata cell (top) and of an oocyte (bottom), traversing a homogeneous zona pellucida, being in gap-junctional contact (arrow) with each other (×9000). (Courtesy of P. Hyttel. From Leiser R. Weibliche geschlechtsorgane. In: Mosimann W, Kohler T, eds. Zytologie, histologie und mikroskopische anatomie der haussugetiere. Berlin: Verlag Paul Parey, 1990:232.)*

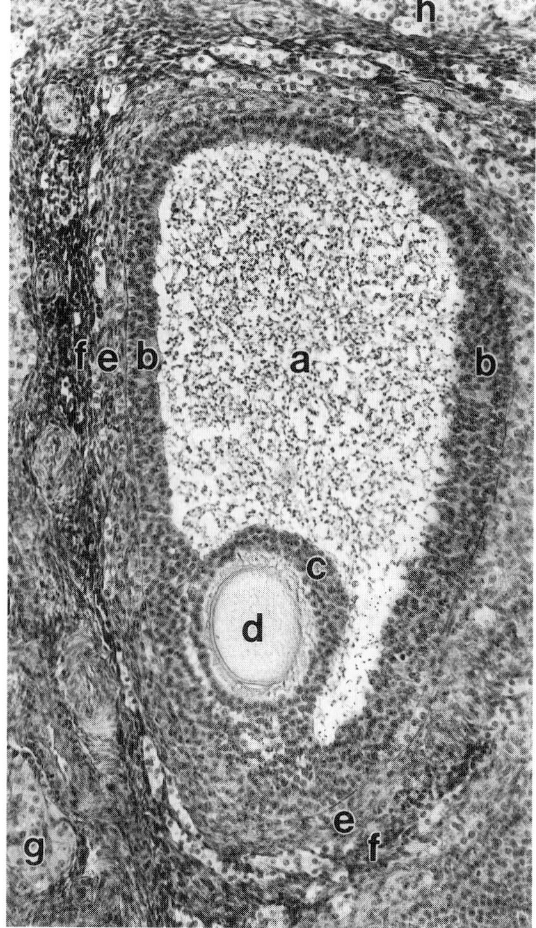

Figure 13.5. *Ovary of queen showing a tertiary follicle, which contains an antrum (a) and a multilayered epithelium called the stratum granulosum (b), which forms a cumulus oophorus (c) enclosing the primary oocyte (d). The antrum contains a flocculent liquor folliculi. A connective tissue layer, called the theca, which surrounds the follicle, can be divided into an inner theca interna, with light voluminous cells (e), and an outer theca externa, with dark fibrocytes (f). Marginal cells of the corpus luteum (g) have features of interstitial endocrine cells (h) (×150).*

etal follicular lining, the **stratum granulosum**. Most of the parietal granulosa cells are polyhedral, but the basal layer may be columnar. Some of the granulosa cells may contain large periodic acid-Schiff (PAS) positive inclusions, the Call-Exner bodies, which represent intracellular precursors of liquor folliculi. In the large tertiary follicle, the granulosa cells have the fine structural characteristics of protein-secreting cells, notably an extensive granular endoplasmic reticulum (ER). Before ovulation, the granulosa cells of the mature follicle assume the characteristics of steroid-secreting cells, especially an agranular ER and mitochondria with tubular cristae.

The stratum granulosum is surrounded by the theca, which in tertiary follicles differentiates into two layers: an inner vascular **theca interna** and an outer supportive **theca externa** (Fig. 13.5). The **theca interna** cells are spindle-shaped in early tertiary follicles and located in a delicate reticular fiber network. An extensive blood and lymph capillary network is present in the theca interna, but it does not penetrate the stratum granulosum. Sympathetic nerve endings are present around the larger follicles. In mature follicles, many of the spindle-shaped theca interna cells adjacent to the stratum granulosum increase in size and become polyhedral and epithelioid. The nuclei of the epithelioid cells have a lighter chromatin pattern and more distinct nucleoli than those of the spindle-shaped cells. Cytoplasmic organelles in the epithelioid cells become typical of steroid-secreting cells: the mitochondria have tubular cristae and agranular tubular ER, and lipid inclusions are present. The epithelioid cells are abundant in mature follicles during proestrus and estrus and during their early regression.

The **theca externa** consists of a thin layer of loose connective tissue with fibrocytes arranged concentrically around the theca interna. Blood vessels of the theca externa supply capillaries to the theca interna.

One or more mature follicles reach maximal development near the time of ovulation. The primary oocyte in these follicles completes the first meiotic division to become a secondary oocyte. During the first meiotic division, chromosome pairs are established and a mixture of parental genetic material occurs. Separation of the pairs and the production of the secondary oocyte and the first polar body (with little cytoplasm) follow at the completion of the division. In domestic animals, the first meiotic division is completed shortly before ovulation, except in the bitch and the mare, in which it is completed shortly after ovulation, i.e., a primary oocyte is ovulated in the bitch and the mare. The second meiotic division begins immediately after the first meiotic division but is arrested in metaphase; it is not completed unless fertilization occurs. At fertilization, the secondary oocyte becomes an **ovum** and the **second polar body** (with little cytoplasm) is given off. The ovum becomes a **zygote** when the male and female pronuclei in the ovum fuse.

OVULATION

When the follicle is fully developed, it protrudes from the surface of the ovary. Abundant blood and lymph vessel networks surround the follicle and an increased rate of secretion of a thin liquor folliculi occurs. The increased secretion rate is facilitated by increases in the follicular blood capillary pressure and permeability during proestrus and

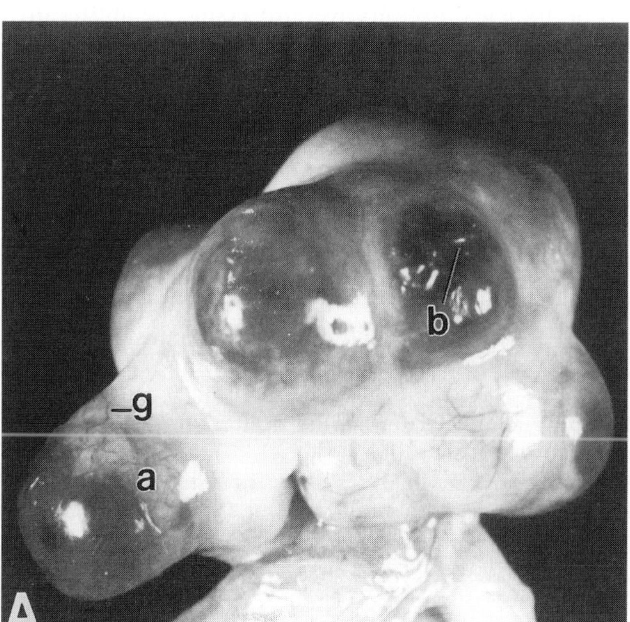

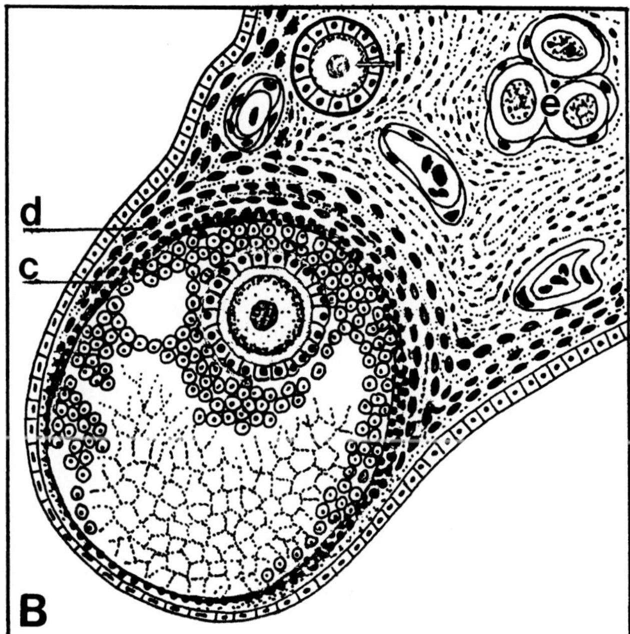

Figure 13.6. ***A.***, *Ovary of sow with mature tertiary follicles immediately before ovulation (a) and one just ovulated as indicated by the stigma in the dark area (b) (×2.7).* ***B.***, *A schematic drawing of the follicle in* ***A*** *(left) shows the oocyte ready to disengage itself from the stratum granulosum at a site opposite the thinned, protruding follicular wall where the ovulation site, the stigma, will soon occur. Theca interna (c) and theca externa (d). Primordial (e) and primary (f) follicles. A subepithelial vein (g) is also visible in* ***A***.

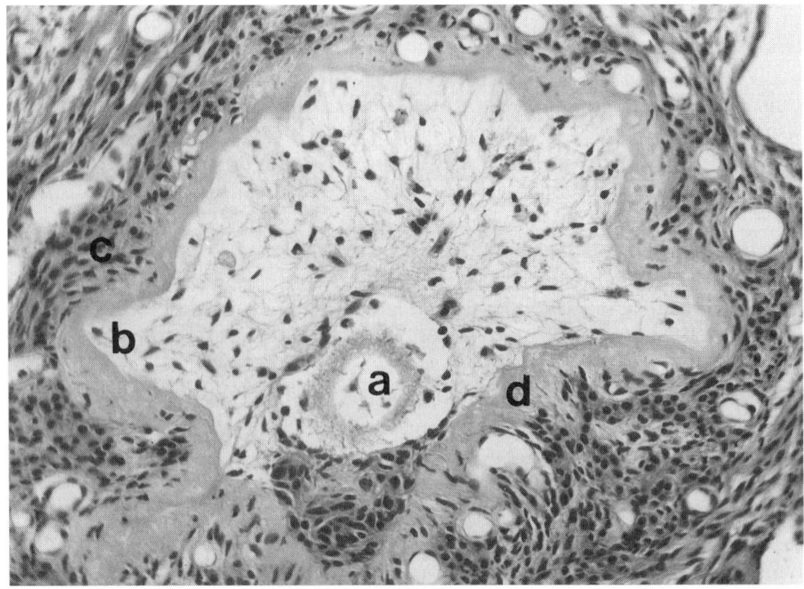

Figure 13.7. *Atretic tertiary follicle (mature bitch). The oocyte (a) and granulosa layer (b) have degenerated, and the theca layer (c) has fibrosed. "Glassy membrane" (d) (×170). (With permission from Adam WS, Calhoun ML, Smith EM, et al. Microscopic anatomy of the dog: a photographic atlas. Springfield, IL: Charles C. Thomas, 1970.)*

estrus. The increased accumulation of liquor folliculi causes the follicles to swell, but intrafollicular pressure does not significantly increase. Small hemorrhages occur in the follicular wall. The follicular wall becomes thin and transparent at the future site of follicular rupture, the **stigma**. The mature ovulatory follicles attain a size of 15 to 20 mm in cows; 50 to 70 mm in mares; approximately 10 mm in ewes, goats, and sows (Fig. 13.6A); and approximately 2 mm in bitches and queens.

Changes in the wall of the follicle preceding rupture are caused by the release of collagenases. Luteinizing hormone (LH) stimulates the production of prostaglandins (PG) F_2 and E_2. PGF_2 is believed to release collagenases from follicular cells, causing digestion of the follicular wall and its distension at the stigma. The process of digestion also releases proteins that provoke an inflammatory response with leukocytic infiltration and the release of histamine. All of these processes degrade the connective tissue of the follicular wall and the ground substance of the cumulus oophorus, so that the follicle ultimately ruptures at the stigma and the oocyte is released. The oocyte, usually surrounded by the corona radiata, escapes into the peritoneal cavity, from which it is swept directly into the infundibulum of the uterine tube. On rare occasions, an oocyte may fail to enter the uterine tube and, if fertilized, may establish ectopic pregnancy. In most species, the corona radiata cells disperse in the uterine tube in the presence of spermatozoa; in ruminants, they already are lost at the time of ovulation. The oocyte generally remains fertilizable for less than 1 day; when not fertilized, it degenerates and is resorbed. Most domestic animals ovulate spontaneously, but ovulation in queens is induced by a copulatory stimulus.

FOLLICULAR ATRESIA AND INTERSTITIAL ENDOCRINE CELLS

Most follicles regress at some time during their development, and only a small percentage of all potential oocytes is ovulated from the ovary. This regression is called **atresia**; many more follicles become atretic than ever attain maturity. Prominent signs of atresia in follicular wall cells are nuclear pyknosis and chromatolysis. During atresia, the basal lamina of the granulosa layer may fold, thicken, and hyalinize; it is then called the **glassy membrane** (Fig. 13.7). Eventually, atretic follicles are resorbed, except that small fibrous tissue scars may remain after atresia of mature follicles.

In cows, in atresia of primary and secondary follicles, the oocyte commonly degenerates before the follicular wall, whereas in tertiary follicles, the reverse is true. Atretic changes in bovine tertiary follicles may result in the formation of two different morphologic types of atretic follicles: obliterative and cystic. In **obliterative atresia,** the granulosa and theca layers both infold, hypertrophy, and extend inward to occupy the antrum. In **cystic atresia,** both the granulosa and theca layers may atrophy, or only the granulosa layer may atrophy and the theca layer may luteinize, become fibrotic, or hyalinize around the antrum (Fig. 13.8). In cystic atretic follicles, the theca interna cells containing LH receptors may continue to synthesize androgens after the regression of the granulosa cells, which converted the androgens to estrogens.

In the ovaries of the bitch, the queen, and rodents, **interstitial endocrine cells** are prominent; they arise chiefly from the epithelioid theca interna cells of atretic antral follicles or from hypertrophied granulosa cells of atretic preantral follicles (Fig. 13.5). They are usually absent from the ovaries of other adult domestic animals. The interstitial endocrine cells are polyhedral and epithelioid and contain lipid droplets. In species such as rabbits and hares, they show an abundance of steroid-synthesizing organelles.

CORPUS LUTEUM

At ovulation, the follicle ruptures, collapses, and shrinks as the liquor pressure is reduced. Folding of the follicular wall is extensive. The ruptured follicle is referred to as a **corpus hemorrhagicum** because of the blood that may fill the antrum. Bleeding after rupture in mares, cows, and sows is greater than that in carnivores and small ruminants. Immediately before ovulation, some cells of the stratum granulosum exhibit signs of pyknosis. After ovulation, the stratum becomes vascularized by an extensive capillary network originating from blood vessels in the theca interna. The granulosa cells enlarge, luteinize, and contribute to the **large luteal (lutein) cell** population of the corpus luteum. Simultaneously, folding of the follicular wall results in the incorporation of the theca interna into the corpus luteum, and in most species, the theca interna cells contribute initially to the **small luteal (lutein) cell** population of the corpus luteum.

Luteinization is the process by which the granulosa and theca cells transform into luteal cells. It includes hypertrophy and hyperplasia of both cell types. A yellow pigment, lutein, appears in the luteal cells in cows, mares, and carnivores; it is absent in ewes, goats, and sows. A black pigment has been observed in the luteal cells of mares. In cows, postovulatory mitosis lasts for approximately 40 hours in the granulosa luteal cells and for approximately 80 hours in the theca luteal cells. The increase in size of the corpus luteum, after the period of mitotic activity, results mainly from hypertrophy of the large luteal cells. The small luteal cells make up a minor part of the corpus luteum and occupy mainly trabecular and peripheral areas.

The large luteal cells are polygonal, measure approximately 40 μm in diameter, and have a large spherical vesicular nucleus. They contain numerous metabolic lipid inclusions (Fig. 13.9). During metestrus and diestrus, the cells contain organelles characteristic of steroid-synthesizing cells, such as mitochondria with tubular cristae and abundant tubular agranular ER (Fig. 13.10). The small luteal cells have more lipids but have fewer steroid-synthesizing types of organelles than do the large luteal cells (Fig. 13.9A-B). The two luteal cell types eventually become mixed in the corpus luteum and are then difficult to distinguish. They both produce progesterone. In cows, the corpus luteum is fully developed and vascularized 9 days after ovulation but continues to grow until day 12, when it attains a diameter of approximately 25 mm.

The first sign of luteal regression is seen in late diestrus and involves the condensation of lutein pigment, which then appears reddish, followed by fibrosis and resorption of most of the corpus luteum. In cows,

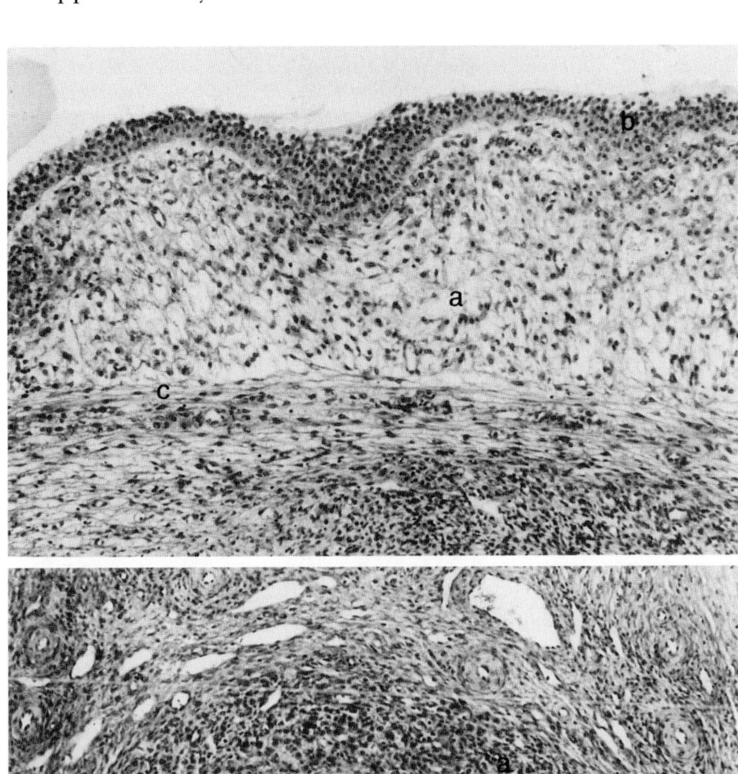

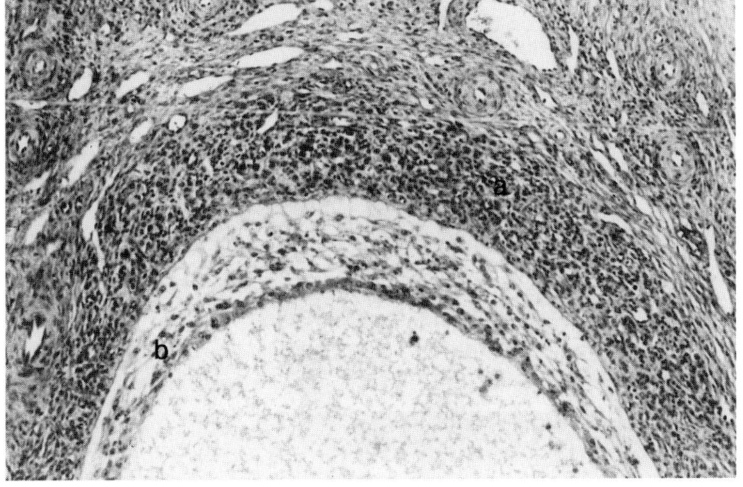

Figure 13.8. *Atresia of a large tertiary ovarian follicle (cow). Top: Extensive hyalinization of theca interna (a) and loss or pyknosis of granulosa cells (b). Theca externa (c) (×100). Bottom: Fibrosis of theca interna (a). Granulosa cell remnants (b) (×125). (From Priedkalns J. Effect of melengestrol acetate on the bovine ovary. Z Zellforsch 1971;122:85.)*

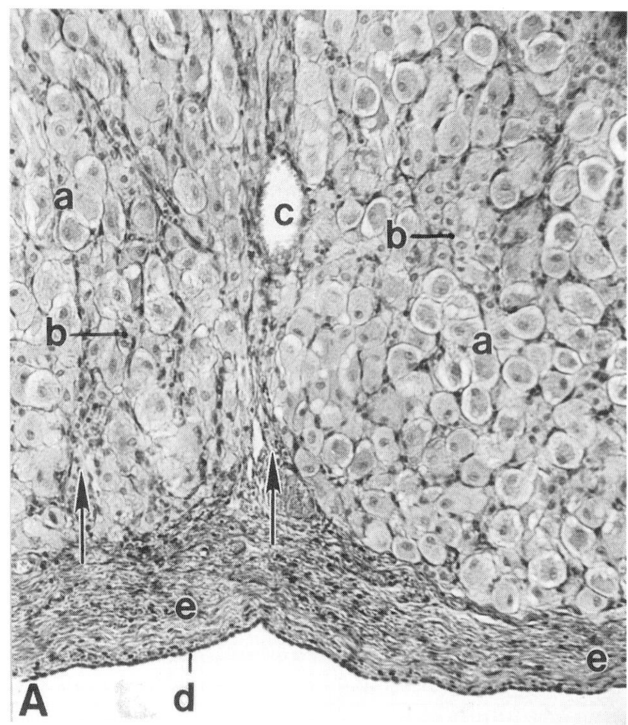

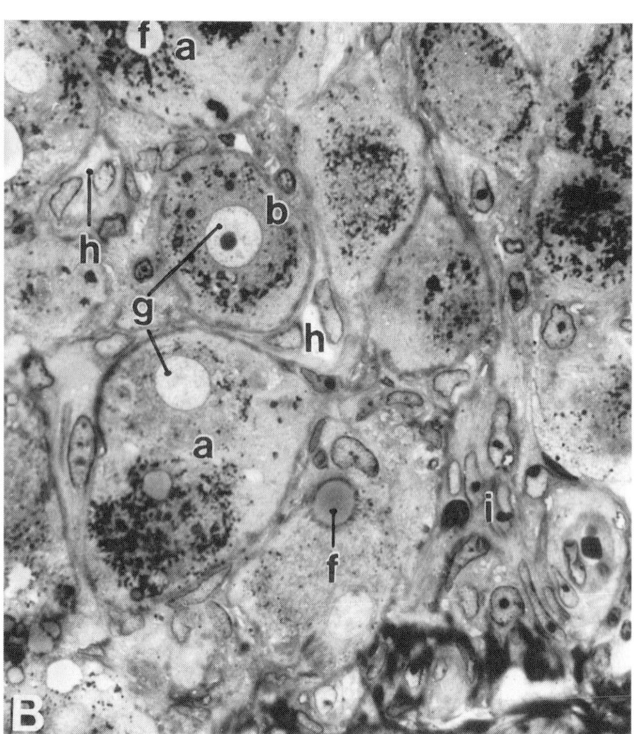

Figure 13.9. *A., Part of a mature corpus luteum (sow). The corpus luteum consists of large luteal cells (a) intermingling with groups of small luteal cells (b). The corpus luteum is supplied with blood vessels (c) entering from the periphery and the trabeculae (arrows). Ovarian epithelium (d) and adjacent tunica albuginea (e) (×160). **B.**, Enlarged segment of **A** showing large (a) and small (b) luteal cells containing fine granular inclusions and lipid droplets (f). Nuclei (g). Capillaries (h). Strand of connective tissue (I) (×830).*

Figure 13.10. *Large luteal cell from a cyclic corpus luteum from the same ovary of a sow as in Figure 13.9. Nucleus (a); granular endoplasmic reticulum (b); tubular and smooth endoplasmic reticulum (c); Golgi complex (d); secretory granules (e); mitochondria with tubular cristae (f) (×15,700).*

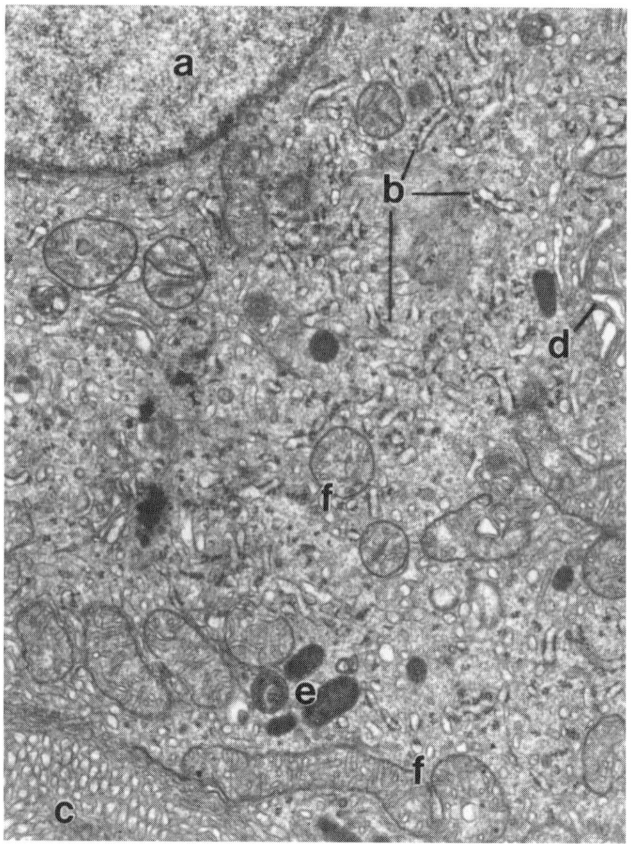

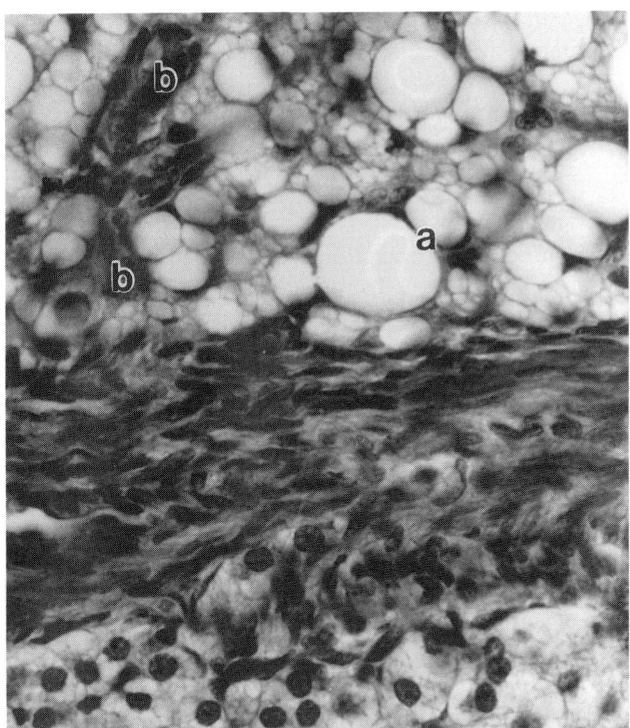

Figure 13.11. *Bovine corpus luteum in regression on day 19 of the estrous cycle (top) with adjacent connective tissue of theca origin (middle area) and ovarian interstitial endocrine cells (bottom). Lipid droplets of varying sizes (a) are typical of regressing luteal cells. Connective tissue cells in the corpus regressivum (b) (×820).*

these signs are first observed 15 days after ovulation; further shrinkage of the corpus luteum occurs rapidly after day 18, and regression is complete 1 to 2 days after estrus. Large lipid droplets and crystalloid inclusions are typical of regressing luteal cells (Figs. 13.11 and 13.12). The vascular connective tissues of the corpus luteum become conspicuous in regression, with the muscle cells of the walls of luteal arteries transformed by cellular hypertrophy and sclerosis. The connective-tissue scar remaining after luteal regression is called the **corpus albicans**. In older ovaries, there is an abundance of such scars.

Medulla

The medulla is the inner area of the ovary containing nerves, many large and coiled blood vessels, and lymph vessels (Fig. 13.1). It consists of loose connective tissue and strands of smooth muscle continuous with those in the mesovarium. Retia ovarii are located in the medulla; they are networks of irregular channels lined by a cuboidal epithelium or solid cellular cords. They are prominent in carnivores and ruminants. It is claimed that the rete may differentiate into follicular cells when in juxtaposition to an oocyte.

Blood Vessels, Lymphatics, and Nerves

Arteries enter the ovary at the hilus. In the medulla, they form plexuses and give off branches to the follicular thecae, corpora lutea, and stromal tissue. Around the larger follicles, the branches form a capillary wreath. During cyclic regression of the corpora lutea and the follicles, muscle hypertrophy and sclerosis occur in the walls of the arteries supplying these structures. The venous return is parallel to the arterial supply. Lymph capillaries accompany blood vessels in the follicular thecae and in the corpus luteum.

The nerves that supply the ovary are generally nonmyelinated. They are vasomotor in nature but include some sensory fibers. The nerves follow blood vessels and terminate in the walls of the vessels and around the follicles, in the corpora lutea, and in the tunica albuginea. They are derived mainly from the sympathetic system through renal and aortic plexuses, but vagal supply of the ovary also has been claimed.

UTERINE TUBE (OVIDUCT)

The uterine tubes are bilateral, tortuous structures that extend from the region of the ovary to the uterine horns and convey ova, spermatozoa, and zygotes. Three segments of the uterine tube can be distinguished: *(a)* the **infundibulum**, a large funnel-shaped portion (Fig. 13.13); *(b)* the **ampulla**, a thin-walled section extending caudally from the infundibulum (Fig. 13. 14A); and (c) the **isthmus**, a narrow muscular segment joining the uterus (Fig. 13.14B).

Histologic Structure

The epithelium is simple columnar or pseudostratified columnar with motile cilia on most cells (Fig. 13.13). Both ciliated and nonciliated cell types possess

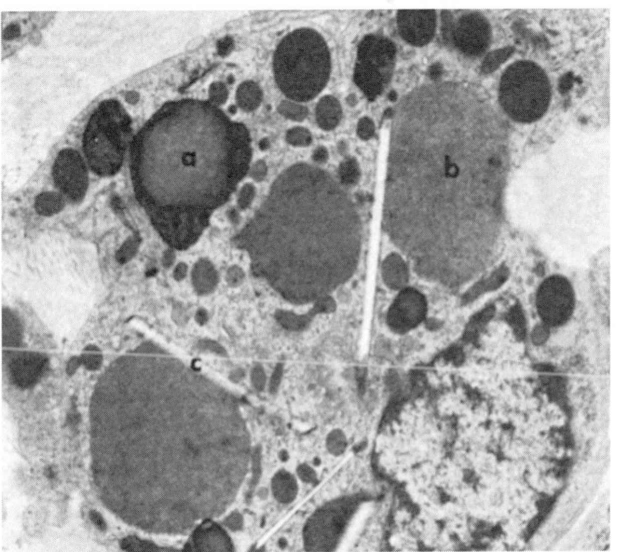

Figure 13.12. *Electron micrograph of a regressed luteal cell, ovary (cow). Note the characteristic large remnant lipid droplets (a), granular bodies (b), and crystalloid inclusions (c) (×8725). (From Priedkalns J, Weber AF. Ultrastructural studies of the bovine Graafian follicle and corpus luteum. Z Zellforsch 1968;91:554.)*

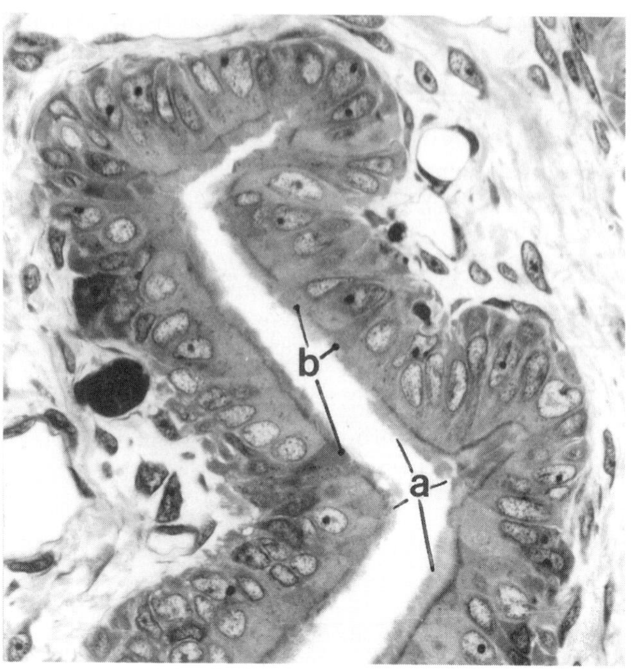

Figure 13.13. *Columnar epithelium of the infundibulum of the uterine tube (queen) in estrus. Ciliated cells (a) are more numerous than dark cells with microvilli (b) (×610).*

microvilli. Morphologic signs of secretory activity are evident only in the nonciliated cells. Ciliated and secretory cells occur more commonly in the cranial end of the uterine tube, and in cows, many of these cells are seen at estrus. During the luteal phase, the secretory cells become taller than the ciliated cells. Their secretion provides the ovum and zygote with the necessary nutrients.

The mucosa is continuous with the submucosa in the female reproductive tract because the lamina muscularis is absent. In the uterine tube, the propria-submucosa consists of loose connective tissue with many plasma cells, mast cells, and eosinophils. The tunica mucosa-submucosa of the ampulla is highly folded, especially in sows and mares. In cows, approximately 40 primary longitudinal folds are present in the ampulla, each with secondary and tertiary folds (Fig. 13.14A). With increasing distance from the ampulla, secondary and tertiary folds gradually disappear, and at the isthmus–uterus junction, where the isthmus is embedded in the uterine wall, only four to eight primary folds and no secondary or tertiary folds are present.

The tunica muscularis consists chiefly of circular smooth muscle bundles, but isolated longitudinal and oblique bundles also occur. The muscle layer gives off radial strands into the mucosa. In the infundibulum and

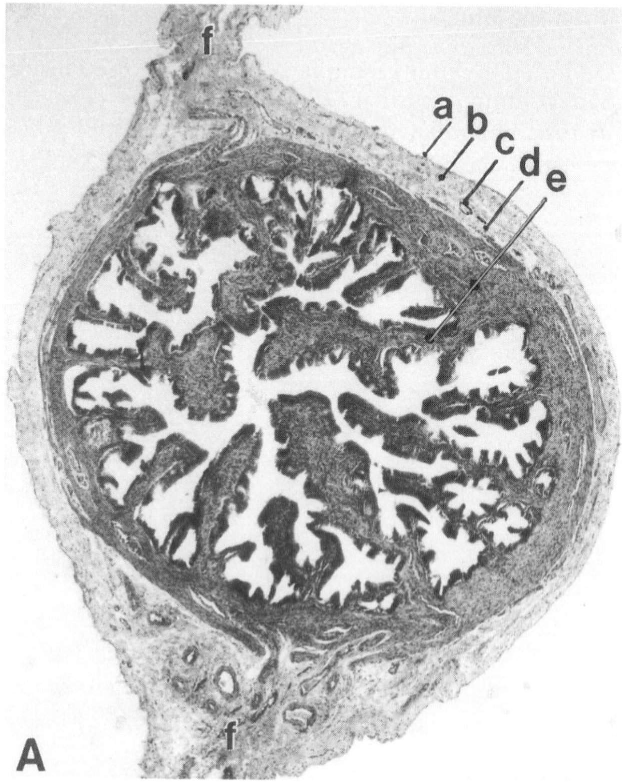

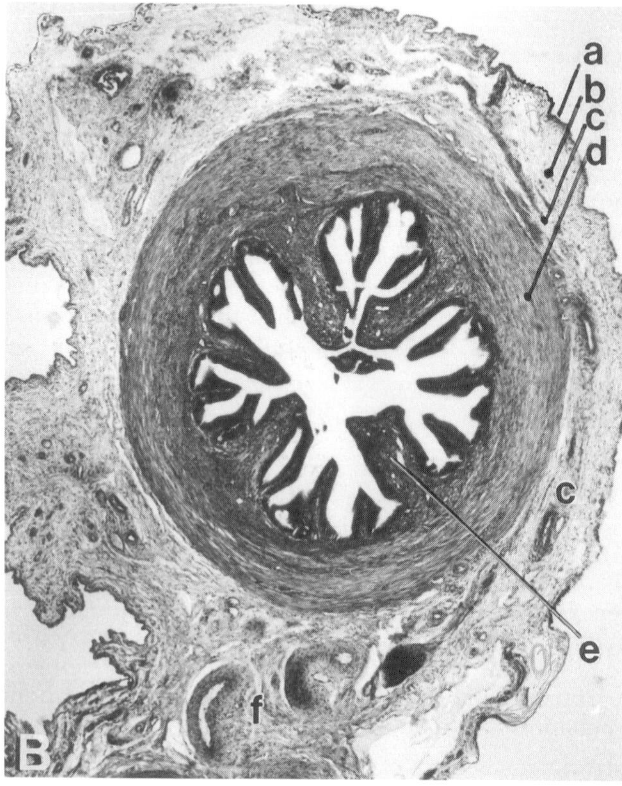

Figure 13.14. *Cross sections of the ampulla* **(A)** *and isthmus* **(B)** *of the uterine tube (cow). Tunica serosa (a); longitudinal muscle layer (b); stratum vasculare (c); circular muscle layer (d); mucosal-submucosal folds (e); mesosalpinx with blood vessels (f) (×42).*

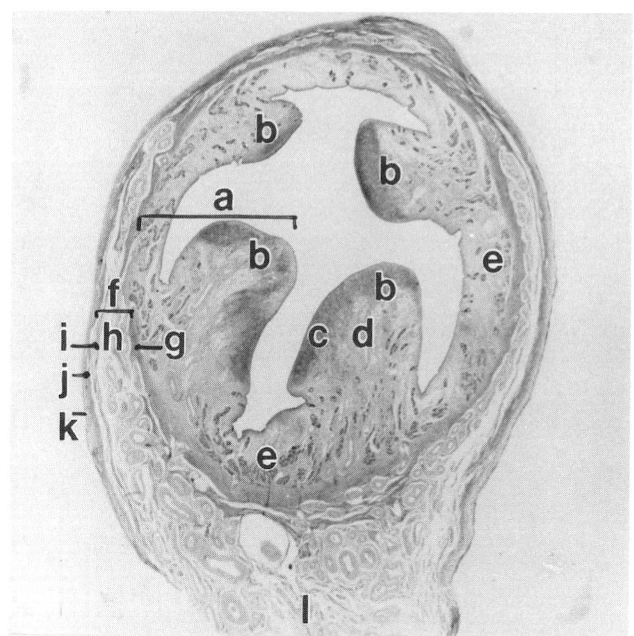

Figure 13.15. *Cross section through the uterine horn (prepuberal cow). Endometrium (a) forms four caruncles (b) with a distinct (dark) stratum cellulare (c) and a (clear) stratum reticulare (d). Glands (e) are present between the caruncles. Myometrium (f) consists of an inner muscle layer (g), a stratum vasculare (h), and an outer muscle layer (i) Perimetrium or serosal layer (j); mesothelium (k); mesometrium (l) (×6). (From Leiser R. Weibliche Geschlechtsorgane. In: Mosimann W, Kohler T, eds. Zytologie, histologie und mikroskopische anatomie der Haussäugetiere. Berlin: Verlag Paul Parey, 1990:232A.)*

ampulla, the tunica muscularis is thin and composed of an inner circular layer and a few outer longitudinal bundles of smooth muscle (Fig. 13.14A). In the isthmus, the inner muscle layer is prominent and blends with the uterine circular muscle (Fig. 13.14B).

A tunica serosa is present and contains many blood vessels and nerves.

Blood Vessels, Lymphatics, and Nerves

The blood vessels form subepithelial vascular plexuses and proliferate during pregnancy. Lymph vessels have capillary networks in the mucosal and serosal layers and drain into the lumbar lymph nodes.

Both myelinated and nonmyelinated nerve fibers with many subepithelial branches are present. They are derived mainly from the sympathetic system.

Histophysiology

The infundibulum secures oocytes extruded from the ovary. It is enclosed in the ovarian bursa or, in species without a definite ovarian bursa (e.g., the mare), it is applied partly around the ovary at estrus. It has fingerlike projections called **fimbriae**. At the time of ovulation in most species, blood vessels in the fimbriae become engorged. The turgid fimbriae move over the surface of the ovary as a result of rhythmic smooth muscle contractions. At the same time, cilia of the infundibular epithelial cells, mostly beating toward the uterus, transport the egg into the ampulla.

The caudal ampulla is the site of fertilization. In the ampulla, ciliary activity is the primary force propelling the egg toward the isthmus, but in some species, muscle contractility is also involved. In the isthmus, muscle contractility is the primary force propelling the zygote toward the uterus, with ciliary activity involved in some species. The directionality of isthmus contractions varies according to the phase of the estrous cycle. In the follicular phase, antiperistaltic contractions tend to move the luminal contents toward the ampulla, whereas in the luteal phase, segmental contractions gradually propel the zygote toward the uterus. Zygotes require 4 to 5 days to traverse the isthmus. This length of time is independent of the isthmus length or of the gestation time among species.

The passage of spermatozoa to the ampulla is accounted for by muscular contractions of the uterine and tubal walls. Inert particles and nonmotile spermatozoa can ascend the uterine tube at the same speed as motile spermatozoa, suggesting that the ascent of spermatozoa is not primarily the result of their innate motility. In cows, spermatozoa can reach the ampulla within 5 minutes after mating. Ascent at this rate is too fast to be accounted for by the motility of spermatozoa and/or by the ciliary movement of tubal cells.

Although spermatozoa develop in the male reproductive tract, their ability to fertilize is attained in domestic animals only after **capacitation** in the uterine tube.

UTERUS

The uterus is the site of implantation of the conceptus. It undergoes a definite sequence of changes during the estrous and reproductive cycles. In most species, it consists of bilateral horns (cornua) connected to the uterine tubes and an unpaired body (corpus) and a neck (cervix), which joins the vagina. The cervix is considered separately in this chapter. In primates, the entire uterus is a single tube, called the uterus simplex.

Histologic Structure

The uterine wall consists of three layers (Fig. 13.15): *(a)* the mucosa-submucosa or **endometrium**, *(b)* the muscularis or **myometrium**, and *(c)* the serosa or **perimetrium.** The perimetrium, the longitudinal layer of the myometrium, and the vascular layer of the myometrium are all continuous with corresponding structures in the broad ligament of the uterus (Fig. 13.16A).

ENDOMETRIUM

The endometrium is composed of two zones that differ in structure and function. The superficial layer, called the **functional zone**, degenerates partially or fully

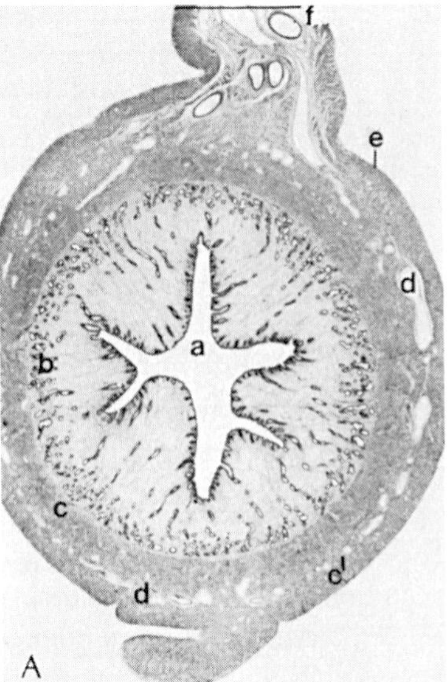

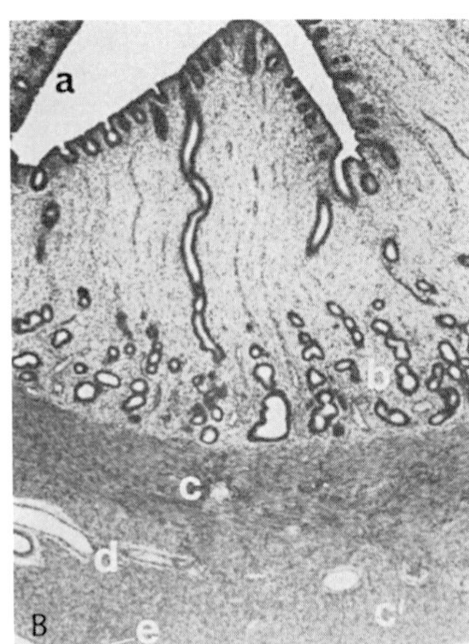

Figure 13.16. *Sections through the uterine horn (bitch) in estrus.* ***A.,*** *Uterine lumen (a); uterine glands (b); circular muscle layer (c), longitudinal muscle layer (c'); vascular layer (d); tunica serosa (e); broad ligament of the uterus (f) (×10).* ***B.,*** *Note (a) to (e) as in* ***A*** *(×38).*

after pregnancy or after estrus. A thin deep layer, the **basal zone**, persists after these events, and the functional zone is restored from this layer (Fig. 13.17).

The surface epithelium of the functional zone is simple columnar in the mare, the bitch, and the queen. It is pseudostratified columnar and/or simple columnar in sows and ruminants. In isolated areas, the epithelium may be simple cuboidal. The height and structure of the epithelial cells are related to the secretion of ovarian hormones throughout the cycle. The subepithelial, superficial part of the functional zone consists of a richly vascular, loose connective tissue with many fibrocytes, macrophages, and mast cells. Neutrophils, eosinophils, lymphocytes, and plasma cells are also present; melanophores are present in sheep. The deep part of the functional zone consists of loose connective tissue that is less cellular than that of the superficial part. In ruminants, during estrus, large irregular fluid-filled tissue spaces are present in the functional zone; this is termed **endometrial edema**.

Simple coiled, branched tubular glands are present throughout the endometrium in most species (Fig. 13.18). The glands are absent from the caruncles of ruminants (Fig. 13.15). The simple columnar glandular epithelium comprises secretory and nonsecretory ciliated cells (Fig. 13.18). Rising estrogen levels stimulate the growth and branching of the glands, but coiling and copious secretion of the glands generally do not occur until progesterone stimulation occurs. The branching and coiling of the glands are extensive in mares, whereas less branching is seen in carnivores (Fig. 13.16B). **Endometrial cups** occur in mares in early pregnancy after endometrial invasion by fetal cells (see Chapter 14).

In ruminants, circumscribed thickenings of the endometrium, known as **caruncles**, are present (Figs. 13.15 and 13.19). They are rich in fibrocytes and have an extensive blood supply. Approximately 15 caruncles in each of four rows are present in each uterine horn in ruminants. They are dome-shaped in cows and cup-shaped

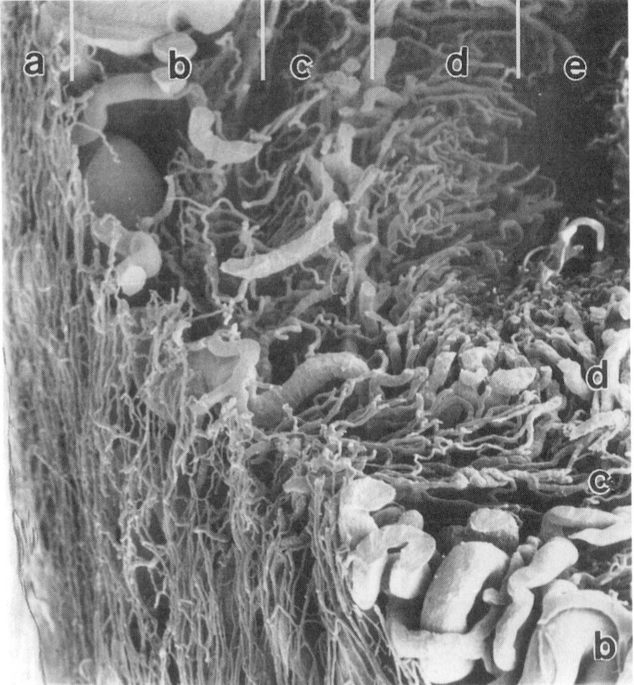

Figure 13.17. *Section through a blood vascular corrosion cast of the uterus (queen). Outer muscle layer (a); vascular layer (b); inner muscle layer (c); endometrium (d); uterine lumen (e) (×275).*

(i.e., a dome with a central depression) in ewes. Caruncles are the sites of attachment of the maternal (endometrial) placenta to the corresponding sites of the fetal placenta, the cotyledons (see Chapter 14).

MYOMETRIUM

The myometrium consists of a thick inner layer, which is mostly circular, and an outer longitudinal layer of smooth muscle cells that increase in number and size

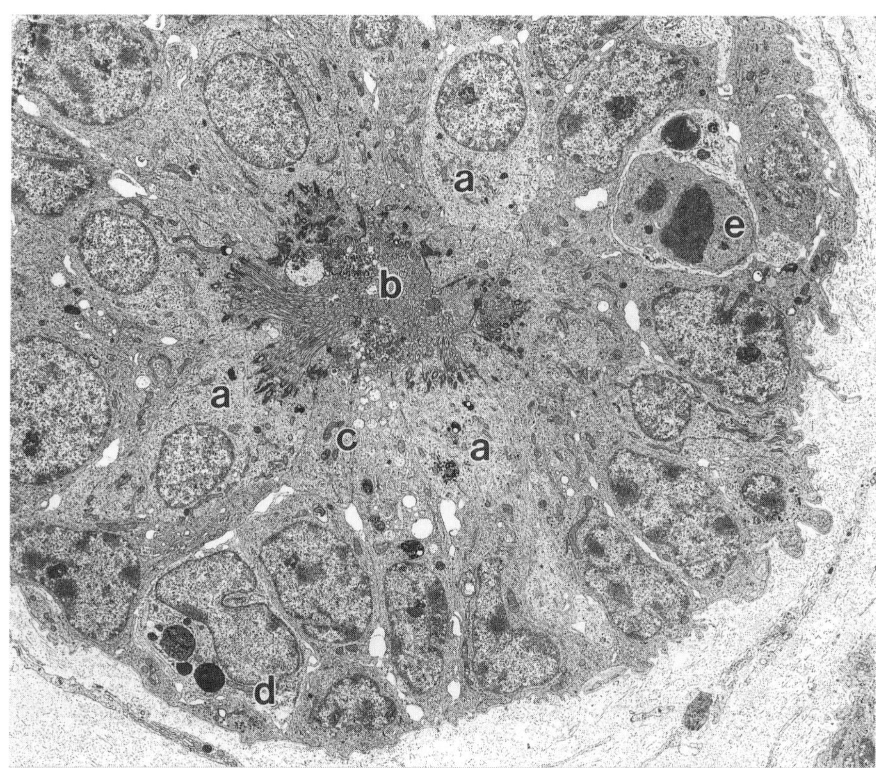

Figure 13.18. *Electron micrograph of a section through a uterine gland (sow) in estrus. Columnar cells (pale appearance) (a) are ciliated with the cilia filling the gland lumen (b). Dark cells with microvilli and containing secretory granules (c). Macrophage (d); mitosis (e) (×2700).*

during pregnancy. Between the two layers, or deep in the inner layer, is a vascular layer consisting of large arteries, veins, and lymph vessels (Figs. 13.16 and 13.19).

PERIMETRIUM

The perimetrium, or the tunica serosa, consists of loose connective tissue covered by the peritoneal mesothelium. Smooth muscle cells occur in the perimetrium. Numerous lymph and blood vessels and nerve fibers are present in this layer.

Blood Vessels, Lymphatics, and Nerves

Between the inner and outer layers of the myometrium, or deep in the inner layer, is a vascular layer consisting of large arteries, veins, and lymph vessels (Figs. 13.16, 13.17, and 13.19). These vessels supply the endometrium. They are especially large in the caruncular regions in ruminants. Numerous lymph and blood vessels and nerve fibers are present in the perimetrium.

The nerves are derived mainly from the sympathetic system through the uterine and pelvic plexuses. They branch in all of the tunics. Parasympathetic supply from the sacral segments reaches the uterus through the pelvic plexus.

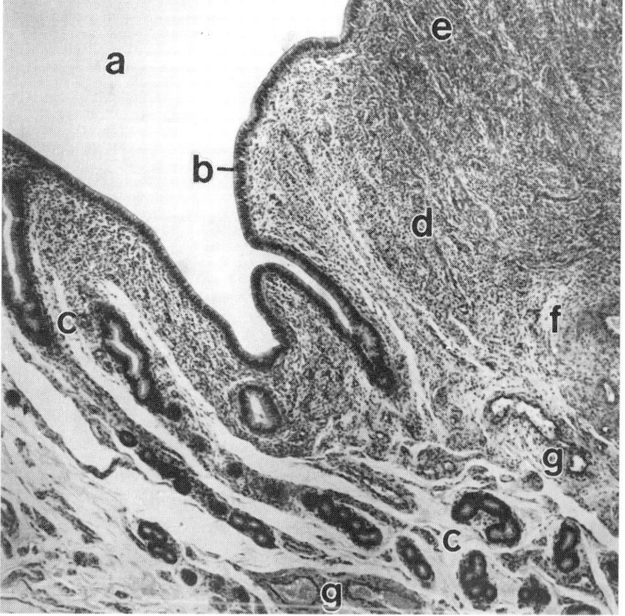

Figure 13.19. *Endometrium (cow), 10 days postestrum. Uterine lumen (a); pseudostratified columnar epithelium (b); tubular uterine glands (c); caruncle (d) with a stratum cellulare (e) and a stratum reticulare (f); blood vessels (g) (×55).*

CERVIX

The cervix or neck of the uterus is thick-walled, muscular, and rich in elastic fibers. The mucosa-submucosa forms high primary folds with secondary and tertiary folds. In cows, four large circular and 15 to 25 longitudinal primary folds, each with many secondary and tertiary folds, are present (Fig. 13.20A). The folding may give a false impression of glandular structure. Uterine

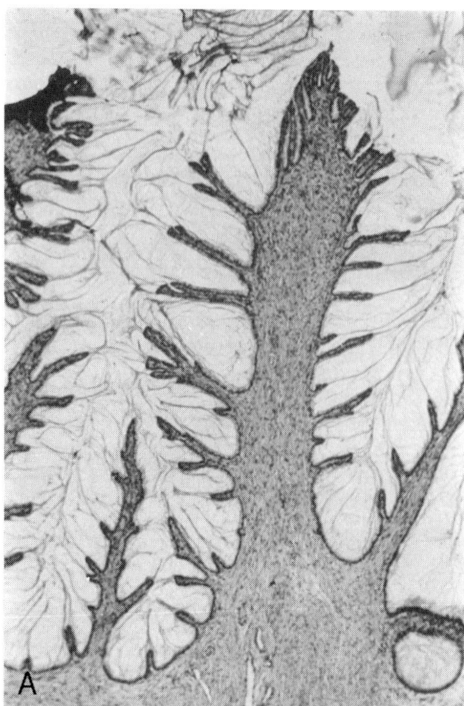

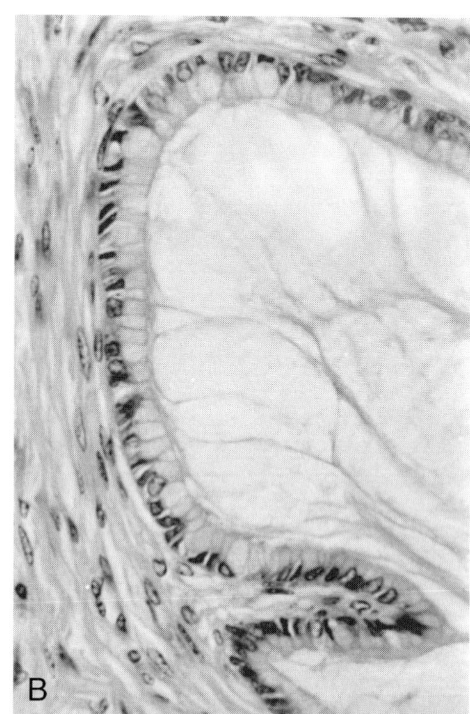

Figure 13.20. *Cervix uteri (cow). **A.**, Section of a large primary mucosal-submucosal fold with small secondary and tertiary folds projecting into the cervical lumen in which fine strands of coagulated mucus are present (×39). **B.**, Note the mucous secretory activity of the epithelial cells and the coagulated mucus in the cervical lumen (×360).*

glands do not extend into the cervix, and the glandular elements present in the cervix are mostly mucigenous (Fig. 13.20B).

Histologic Structure

In most species, the epithelium is of the simple columnar type with many mucigenous cells, including goblet cells. Increasing quantities of mucus are secreted during estrus and pregnancy, and much of the mucus passes to the vagina. In pregnancy, the mucus thickens to form the cervical seal. A small proportion of the epithelial cells is ciliated in some species. Intraepithelial and simple tubular glands may be present in ruminants. In sows, more than 90% of the cervix may have a vaginal type of mucosa with stratified squamous epithelium that undergoes cyclic alterations as in the vagina. These features and alterations have relevance for the porcine copulatory mechanism.

The propria-submucosa consists of dense irregular connective tissue, which becomes edematous and assumes a loose areolar structure during estrus. In mares and bitches, venous plexuses are present in the deep part of the propria-submucosa.

The tunica muscularis consists of inner circular and outer longitudinal smooth muscle layers. Elastic fibers are prominent in the circular layer. Both muscle and elastic fibers are important in reestablishing cervical structure after parturition. The muscle layers of the cervix are continuous with those of the body of the uterus and the vagina. The cervical circular muscle layer is variously modified in different species. Thickening and infolding of the circular layer occurs in the region of the circular folds or prominences in the small ruminants and sows. In mares and cows, the thickened circular layer forms the body of the intravaginal portion of the cervix. The orifice of the intravaginal portion of the cervix in bitches is surrounded by a loop of the vaginal muscle.

The tunica serosa of the cervix consists of loose connective tissue. A longitudinal duct of the epoophoron (Gartner's duct) may be present in this layer on one or both sides.

VAGINA

The vagina is a muscular tube extending from the cervix to the vestibule. Flat longitudinal mucosal-submucosal folds extend throughout the length of the vagina. In cows, prominent circular folds are also present in the cranial portion of the vagina. Cyclic variations occur in epithelial height and structure. Intraepithelial glands are present in some species. The increased amounts of vaginal mucus during estrus originate mainly in the cervix.

Histologic Structure

The vaginal mucosa is lined mostly by stratified squamous epithelium that increases in thickness during proestrus and estrus (Fig. 13.21). In the cranial part of the bovine vagina, a surface layer of columnar and goblet cells containing PAS-positive mucosubstances is present on the stratified squamous epithelium. In mares, the epithelial cells are generally polyhedral, with a few layers of flattened cells on the surface. The propria-submucosa consists of loose or dense irregular connective tissue, containing lymphatic nodules in the caudal part of the vagina.

The tunica muscularis consists of two or three layers. A thick inner circular smooth muscle layer is separated into bundles by connective tissue and is surrounded by a thin outer longitudinal smooth muscle layer. In sows and bitches, and to a small extent in queens, an additional thin layer of longitudinal muscle is present inside the circular layer.

The tunica adventitia or, cranially, the tunica serosa consists of loose connective tissue and contains large blood vessels, nerves, and ganglia. A thin outer longitudinal smooth muscle layer may be present in the tunica serosa and is referred to as **muscularis serosae**.

Blood Vessels, Lymphatics, and Nerves

Extensive venous and lymph plexuses are present in the tunica serosa or adventitia and in the connective tissue joining the vagina to the surrounding structures. Numerous nerve bundles and ganglia occur in the tunica serosa or adventitia. The innervation is primarily sympathetic, derived from the pelvic plexus.

VESTIBULE, CLITORIS, AND VULVA

The wall of the **vestibule** is similar to that of the caudal portion of the vagina, except for the presence of more subepithelial lymphatic nodules, especially in the region of the clitoris. Blood vessels, erectile cavernous tissue, venous plexuses, and small lymph vessels are abundant in the vestibular wall. They become congested during estrus. An erectile corpus cavernosum, called the **bulbus vestibuli**, is present beneath the vestibular mucosa in the mare and the bitch. It resembles the corpus spongiosum penis.

Major vestibular glands are bilateral compound tubuloacinar mucous glands located in the deep part of the propria-submucosa. They occur in ruminants and queens. The terminal secretory acini contain large mucigenous cells. The small ducts draining the acini are lined by columnar mucous cells, with isolated areas of goblet cells. The large ducts leading to the vestibule are lined by a thick stratified squamous epithelium. Individual or aggregated lymphatic nodules may surround the large ducts.

The glands provide mucous lubrication of the vestibule. They may be compressed during coitus and secrete mucus, thereby providing mucous lubrication also of the caudal vagina. They are homologous with the male bulbourethral glands.

Minor vestibular glands are bilateral small, branched, tubular mucous glands scattered in the vestibular mucosa in most domestic animals. They are homologous with the male urethral glands.

The **clitoris** consists of paired, joined erectile corpora cavernosa clitoridis, a rudimentary glans clitoridis, and a preputium clitoridis. The corpus cavernosum clitoridis, homolog of the corpus cavernosum penis, is well developed in mares. The glans clitoridis, homolog of the glans penis, is functionally erectile only in mares. A nonerectile fibroelastic tissue cover replaces the glans in queens, sows, and ewes; in ewes, the cover contains a venous plexus. The clitoris contains many lymphatic nodules and is richly supplied with sensory and autonomic nerve endings.

The **vulva** is formed by the labia vulvae, which are covered by skin that is richly supplied with apocrine and sebaceous glands. Striated muscle fibers of the constrictor vulvae are found in the hypodermis. The labia are well supplied with small blood and lymph vessels, which become congested during estrus, especially in sows and bitches.

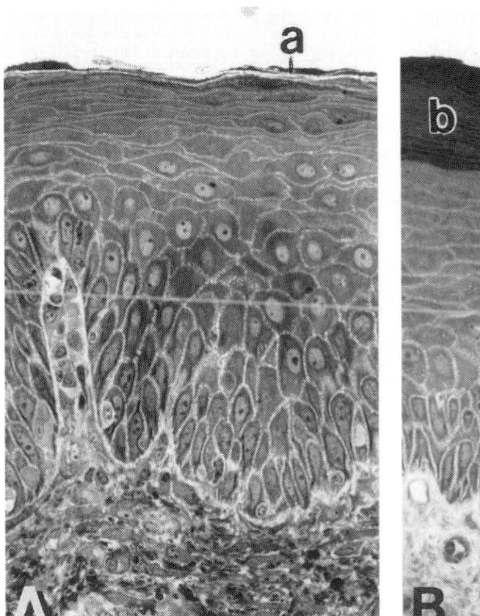

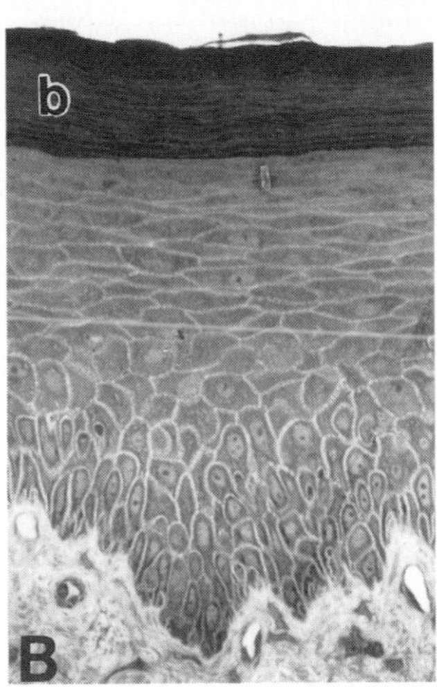

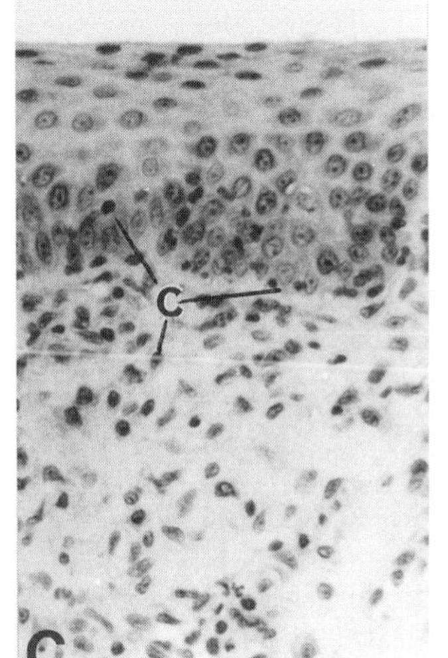

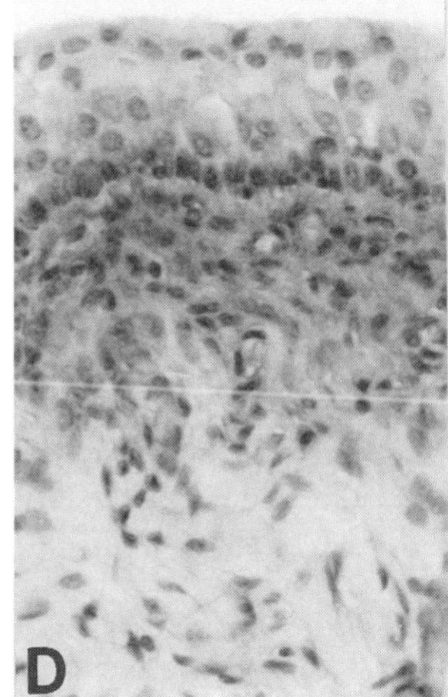

Figure 13.21. *Stratified squamous epithelium of the vagina in the bitch. Proestrus (**A**): the epithelium has a thin layer of keratinized cells (a). Early estrus (**B**): a thick layer of keratinized cells is present. Metestrus (**C**): the epithelium is nonkeratizinized and leukocytes (c) are present within the relatively thin epithelium. Diestrus/anestrus (**D**): the epithelium comprises only a few layers of epithelial cells (×240).*

THE ESTROUS CYCLE

Hormones of the Ovary

The ovary has important endocrine functions. It secretes the female sex hormones, mainly estrogens and progesterone. **Estrogens** are produced primarily during estrus by the granulosa cells, which convert androgens, secreted by the theca interna cells, to estrogens. **Progesterone** is produced primarily by the large luteal cells during metestrus, diestrus, and pregnancy and by the placenta. In certain species, the interstitial endocrine cells secrete large amounts of steroid sex hormones. Estrogen induces the growth and development of the female reproductive tract and estrous behavior. Progesterone stimulates the development of uterine glands, induces them to secrete, and renders the endometrium receptive to the implantation of the blastocyst. It also prevents follicular maturation and estrus and promotes behavior appropriate to pregnancy. Estrogens and progesterone promote development of the mammary gland.

The growth and maturation of ovarian follicles and their estrogen secretion are controlled by pituitary **gonadotropins.** Both the granulosa and theca cells of late secondary or early tertiary follicles become responsive to gonadotropic hormones. The granulosa cells develop follicle-stimulating hormone (FSH) receptors, and the theca cells develop LH receptors. In mature tertiary follicles, the granulosa cells are induced by FSH also to develop LH receptors.

In tertiary follicles, LH interacts with receptors on the theca interna cells to stimulate the production of androgens and small amounts of estradiol. The androgens either are secreted into capillaries or traverse the basal lamina to reach the granulosa cell layer. Receptors on the granulosa cells interact with FSH to activate the aromatase enzyme system, which converts the thecal androgens (testosterone, androstenedione) to estrogens (estradiol-17, estrone). Granulosa cells themselves are unable to produce the androgens. The estrogens are secreted into the follicular fluid and also enter capillaries. The antral concentration of estradiol-17 is some 1000 times greater than that of the bloodstream. The high local concentration of estrogens maintains a favorable environment for follicular maturation. The action of FSH, as well as of LH, on follicular cells is mediated by an increased production of cyclic adenosine-3′,5′-monophosphate (cAMP), which acts as an intracellular "second messenger."

Immediately before ovulation, the ovulatory surge of LH interacts with the LH receptors on the granulosa cells to induce events leading to ovulation. In addition, the LH surge seems to inhibit the aromatase activity of granulosa cells and thus to diminish estrogen secretion. In the mature preovulatory follicle, LH is involved also in the induction of oocyte maturation, i.e., the completion of the first meiotic division. Several other physiologically active substances accumulate in the fluid of the mature preovulatory follicle, including inhibin, a large protein that selectively suppresses pituitary FSH secretion.

Ovarian secretion of estrogen triggers the release of an ovulatory surge of LH, usually on the day of estrus, thereby inducing the processes leading to ovulation. The peak level of FSH occurs on the day before estrus; the peak level of LH, like estrogens, occurs on the day of estrus. Pituitary LH also initiates the formation of the corpus luteum. LH interacts with receptors on the cells of the ruptured follicular wall to initiate luteinization and progesterone secretion. In some species, such as rats and mice, luteotropic hormone (LTH) is needed to maintain the corpus luteum and its progesterone secretion.

Luteal cells produce progesterone during late metestrus and most of diestrus. Secretion peaks in late diestrus shortly before luteal regression sets in. They also secrete estrogens and relaxin. In cells of the developing and mature corpus luteum, the lipids are mostly phospholipids with traces of triglycerides and cholesterol and its esters. During regression, cholesterol accumulates in the luteal cells, thus suggesting decreased cholesterol utilization for steroid hormone synthesis. In active luteal cells, the lipid droplets are small and even in size and distribution, whereas during regression, they are large and unevenly distributed. With the light microscope, they appear as large vacuoles (Fig. 13.11). Regression of the corpus luteum may follow withdrawal of LH, luteotropic hormone, or both, or may be caused by a uterine luteolytic factor reaching the ovary by local blood supply in the ewe, the cow, and the sow. The main luteolytic factor is PGF_2. If pregnancy occurs, the corpus luteum persists as the corpus luteum of pregnancy for different periods of time in various species. In cows and does, progesterone production by the corpus luteum continues throughout gestation. The corpus luteum of pregnancy is supported by luteotropic hormones from the pituitary as well as from the placenta. The embryo in ewes provides, in addition to luteotropic hormones, an antiluteolytic factor that overcomes the luteolytic effect of the uterus. In later stages of pregnancy in most species, the corpus luteum is not important because the placenta secretes the progesterone required for the successful maintenance of pregnancy. Ovarian and placental steroid hormones in turn influence pituitary gonadotropin secretion by a feedback effect on the hypothalamus, regulating mainly the release of the hypothalamic gonadotropin-releasing hormones. Other diencephalic structures, such as the pineal gland, also influence gonadotropic functions.

Phases of the Estrous Cycle

The estrous cycle is regulated by an intrinsic hypothalamo-hypophysial-ovarian rhythm that is modulated by environmental and internal neuroendocrine factors. In domestic animals, the estrous cycle is generally divided into the following sequential phases.

1. **Proestrus** is the phase of follicular maturation and endometrial proliferation after regression of the corpus luteum of the previous cycle. During this phase, the progesterone level falls, thus

allowing release of FSH. Rising estrogen levels lead to estrus.

2. **Estrus** is the phase of sexual receptiveness, during which ovulation occurs in most species. Ovulation is preceded by a surge of LH. At the end of estrus, estrogen levels decline.
3. **Metestrus** is the phase of corpus luteum development and initial progesterone secretion.
4. **Diestrus** is the phase of the active corpus luteum in which the influence of luteal progesterone on accessory sex structures predominates. Endometrial glandular hyperplasia and secretion are maximal during diestrus. Toward the end of diestrus, however, the corpus luteum regresses and endometrial involution, including glandular regression, sets in. Diestrus can be prolonged into pseudopregnancy or gestational and lactational diestrus.
5. **Anestrus** is the prolonged period of sexual inactivity.

The average duration (in days) of the phases of the estrous cycle in cows and sows, respectively, is as follows: proestrus — 3, 3; estrus — 1, 2; metestrus — 3,3; diestrus — 14,12. Thus, during proestrus and estrus, large ovarian follicles produce estrogens, whereas during metestrus and diestrus, the corpus luteum produces mainly progesterone.

Cyclic Changes of the Endometrium

The cyclic changes in the endometrium (Fig. 13.22) are, to a large extent, caused by the ovarian hormones estrogen and progesterone. During pregnancy, these hormones are produced chiefly by the placenta.

Some animals, e.g., bitches and queens, are **monestrous** and have one or two estrous cycles per year, followed by a long anestrous period. Continuously cycling animals, without an anestrous period (e.g., cows and sows), or seasonally cycling animals (e.g., mares, ewes, and goats) are **polyestrous**. The endometrium of monestrous animals degenerates and regenerates to a much greater extent than that of polyestrous animals. The immediate factor precipitating uterine degenerative changes is probably local ischemia. Uterine regenerative changes are induced by estradiol and continued by progesterone, which induces glandular secretory activity and causes the endometrium to produce a maternal placenta when stimulated by the presence of the blastocyst. A detailed description of the cyclic changes in the cow and bitch follows.

COW

In the cow, the estrous cycle lasts 21 days (Fig. 13.23). Ovulation occurs on the day after estrus, or approximately 30 hours after the onset of estrus. The day of estrus may be called "day 0" or "day 21" of the cycle, and the last day of proestrus may be referred to as "day 20." During the last 3 to 4 days of **diestrus**, the endometrial stroma shrinks and the epithelium becomes lower. The glands become shorter, their epithelium becomes lower, and their secretions cease. During **proestrus**, under the influence of estrogens, the endometrium is restored; the mucosa becomes thickened, congested, and edematous with a predominance of mucin-filled epithelial cells. Glandular proliferation, however, is limited to straight lumen growth without significant branching or coiling. During **estrus**, endometrial edema and hyperemia are maximal. During **metestrus**, the edema lessens, and a breakdown occurs in some of the congested endometrial blood vessels. With the onset of **diestrus**, under the influence of progesterone, the endometrium transforms from a proliferative to a secretory type, with glandular epithelial growth and glandular branching, coiling, and secretion. During the first 11 days of diestrus, endometrial glandular secretion is greatest. If pregnancy does not occur, the glands again regress along with the corpus luteum during the last 3 days of diestrus.

Mitotic activity begins in the surface and glandular epithelia and in the interstitial elements during estrus and continues for approximately 6 days after estrus. Heterophils invade the lamina propria, epithelia, and uterine lumen from late proestrus to approximately day 3 or 4 after estrus. An invasion of agranulocytes, mainly lym-

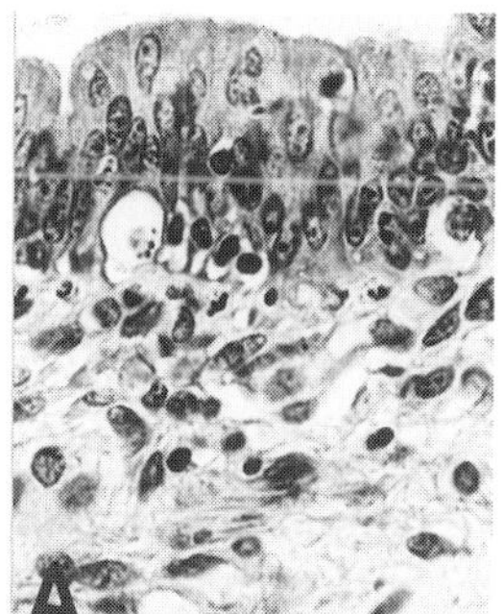

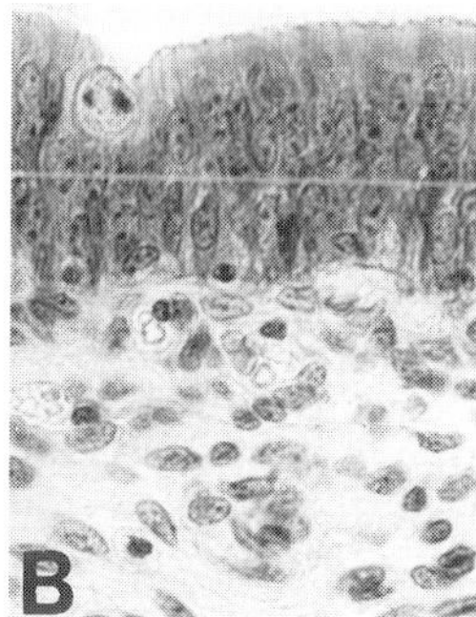

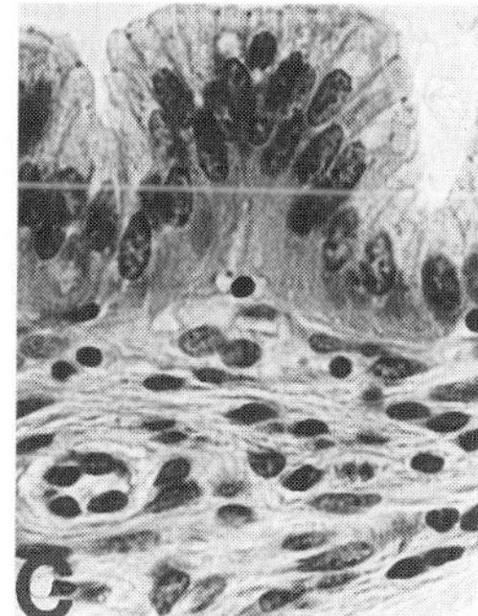

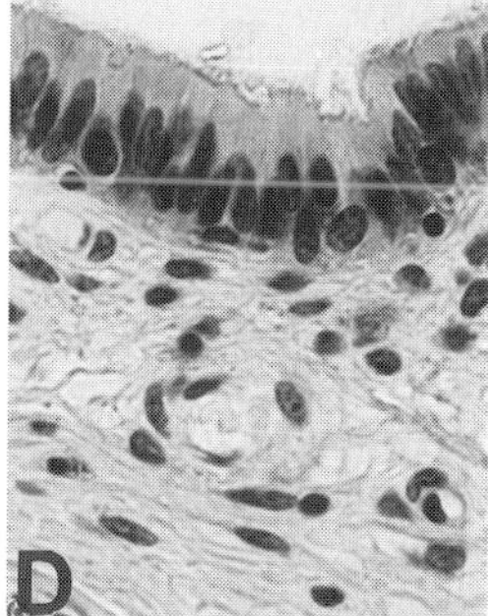

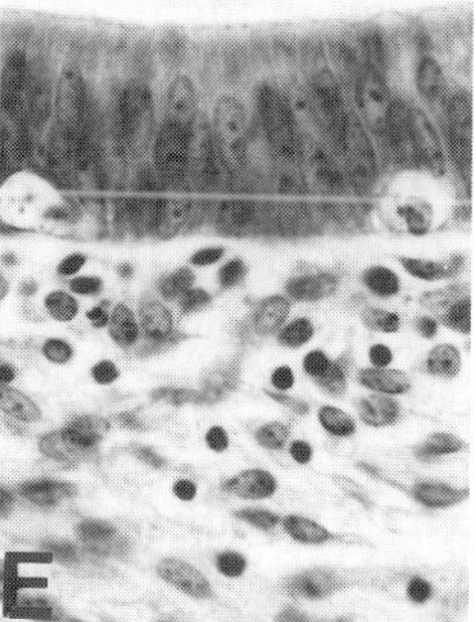

Figure 13.22. *Endometrial epithelium through the estrous cycle, sow. Estrus **(A)**; metestrus **(B)**; early diestrus **(C)**; late diestrus **(D)**; proestrus **(E)** (×250).*

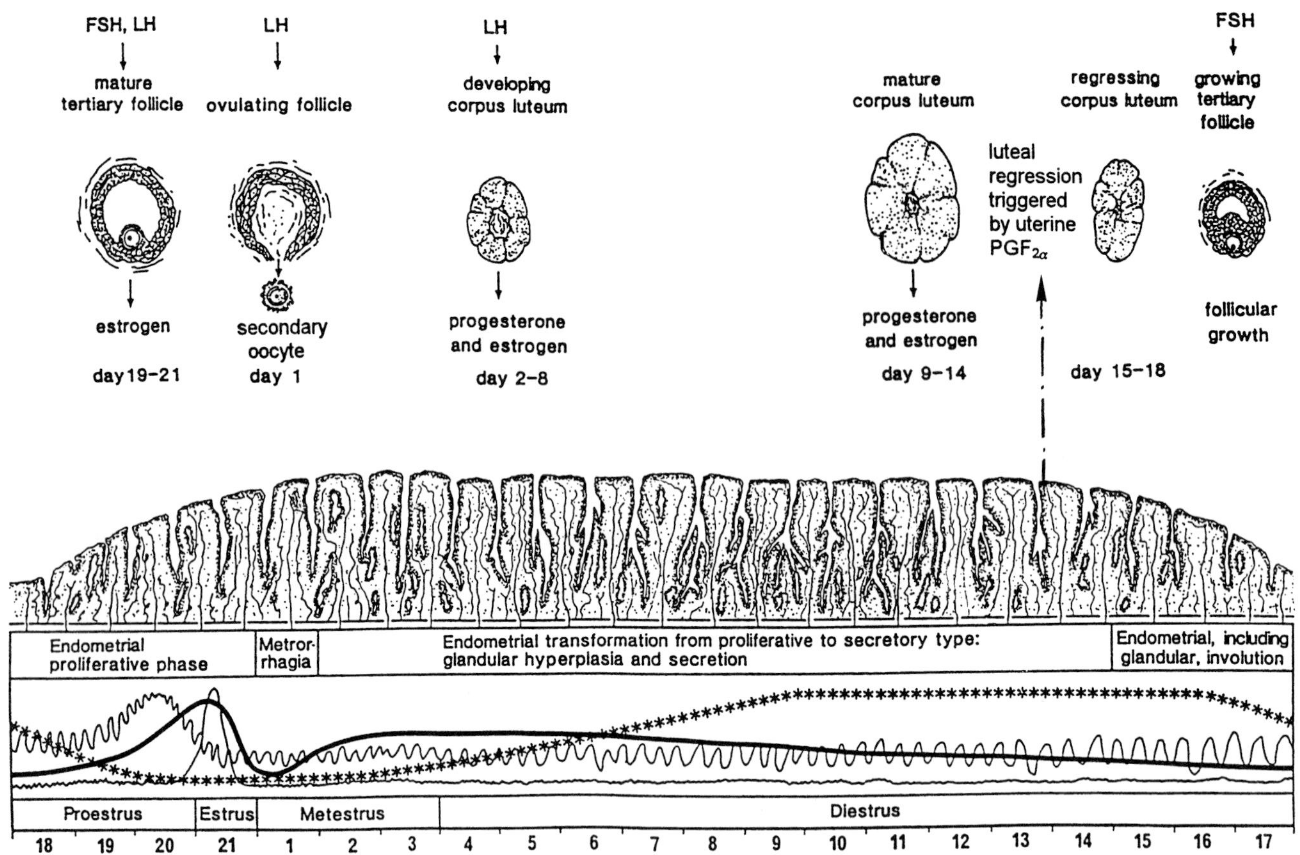

Figure 13.23. *The ovarian and uterine changes during the estrous cycle in the cow are shown schematically. The ovarian follicular (days 15–21) and luteal (days 1–14) phases and the endometrial proliferative and secretory phases, with maximal glandular branching and activity on days 8–12, and endometrial involution (triggered by local prostaglandin F_2) are indicated. The relative blood levels of the following hormones are shown:*

********** *progesterone*
—— *estrogens*
∿∿∿ *follicle-stimulationg hormone (FSH)*
—∿— *luteinizing hormone (LH)*
The scale indicates days 1–21 of the estrous cycle.

phocytes, occurs from day 3 to 5 after estrus. These cells are especially abundant in the basal zone of the endometrium. An eosinophilic invasion may occur from estrus to midcycle. Mast cells increase in number at the time of maximal edema, especially in the caruncular areas. **Metrorrhagia** refers to the microscopic hemorrhages in the functional zone of the endometrium that begin shortly before the time of ovulation in the cow. At ovulation, metrorrhagia becomes widespread and is prominent in the pitted central areas of the caruncles. Metrorrhagia is greatest immediately after maximal endometrial edema. Capillaries rupture in the mucosa and blood accumulates in "blisters" beneath the surface epithelium. The blisters rupture, and blood and shreds of mucosa are liberated into the uterine lumen. Blood in the caruncular areas is mainly phagocytized and resorbed and generally does not reach the uterine lumen. Tissue fluid, as well as blood, may be lost at points of rupture in the intercaruncular areas. Metrorrhagia ends abruptly near the end of day 2 after estrus. A bloody vulvar discharge occurs at this time.

BITCH

Proestrus and estrus each lasts approximately 1 to 2 weeks in the bitch. If pregnancy does not follow estrus, pseudopregnancy and anestrus ensue. Endometrial edema, congestion, and hemorrhages occur during proestrus. Ovulation occurs soon after the onset of estrus. On approximately day 6 of estrus, corpora lutea become functional, and uterine glands and interstitial elements begin to proliferate. The glandular epithelium becomes high columnar, and the glands become coiled. In the nonpregnant state, involution of the endometrial glands and stroma begins approximately 20 to 30 days after the onset of estrus. During anestrus, the endometrium is thin and regressed, and the epithelium is mainly cuboidal. A prolonged and incomplete endometrial regression may occasionally result in pyometra.

PRIMATES

Menstruation in primates is an entirely different phenomenon from the uterine bleeding seen in the bovine and the canine species. The uterine hemorrhages in the cow and the bitch occur during a **regenerative phase** of the endometrium near estrus.

Menstruation, on the other hand, occurs during a **degenerative phase** of the endometrium, precipitated by the withdrawal of estrogens and, more importantly, withdrawal of progesterone after the involution of the corpus luteum. The occurrence of hemorrhage in primates has been related to special coiled arteries in the endometrial functional zone that periodically constrict and dilate as the support of progesterone and estrogens wanes. The arterial constriction causes ischemia and necrosis of tissue, and the dilatation that follows leads to the rupture of the blood vessels, hemorrhage, and loss of tissues of the functional zone.

In certain animal species, the period most analogous to the period of human menstrual regression is the termination of pseudopregnancy. In bitches, pseudopregnancy invariably follows estrus and spontaneous ovulation if the animal has not become pregnant. In other animals, pseudopregnancy follows estrus and ovulation only if a mating stimulus resulting in a corpus luteum of pseudopregnancy has occurred, i.e., a corpus luteum of prolonged and sometimes greater activity than that of the corpus luteum of diestrus. Pseudopregnancy is terminated by a cessation of hypophysial luteotropic stimulation. Such a halt results in regression of the corpus luteum, decrease of the progesterone and estrogen supply, and consequent regression of the endometrium and the termination of pseudopregnancy. Although no external bleeding occurs in bitches at this time, microscopic hemorrhages of the endometrium have been observed.

Cyclic Changes of the Vaginal Epithelium

COW

The epithelium varies with the site and hormonal status of the animal. Under the influence of **progesterone**, the epithelium in the cranial part of the vagina consists of approximately three layers of cells and increases to approximately 10 layers in the caudal part.

Under the influence of **estrogens**, the rate of epithelial cell proliferation is increased throughout the vagina and the epithelium thickens. In early estrus, the superficial layer of columnar and goblet cells in the cranial part of the vagina attains maximal height as a result of stored mucus. The epithelium of the caudal part is at maximal height from 2 days after estrus until midcycle, during which period the surface cells are more squamous than at other times and desquamation occurs. True keratinization (cornification) of the superficial epithelial cells is not observed, however.

Heterophils invade the vaginal epithelium from estrus until 2 days after estrus. Lymphocytes and plasma cells are more common under the influence of progesterone. (Attempts to identify the stage of the estrous cycle by the vaginal smear method are not as successful as in the bitch.)

BITCH

Cyclic cellular changes that occur in the vaginal epithelium of the bitch are clinically useful and important for estimating the times of estrus and breeding (Fig. 13.24). The assessment of cellular changes by the vaginal smear method is widely used. After staining, vaginal smears appear as follows.

1. **Proestrus** (approximately 9 days in duration). Numerous erythrocytes (of uterine origin) and many large flat keratinized cells are present.
2. **Estrus** (approximately 9 days in duration). Some erythrocytes and numerous keratinized cells are present. As estrus progresses, the keratinized cells become wrinkled and distorted and are frequently invaded by bacteria.
3. **Metestrus-diestrus** (approximately 3 months in duration). Epithelial cells are less keratinized and appear more like unstained living cells. Heterophils are numerous on day 3 of metestrus and gradually disappear until day 10 to 20 of metestrus.
4. **Anestrus** (approximately 2 months in duration). Numerous unstained nonkeratinized epithelial cells, a few large stained cells with pyknotic nuclei, and a few heterophils and lymphocytes are present.

The cyclic histologic changes in the vaginal epithelium in the bitch are shown in Fig. 13.21. Although the epithelial lining of the vagina is thin in anestrus, with only approximately two to three layers of cells, it proliferates during proestrus and may be 12 to 20 cells thick at the beginning of estrus, with keratinization of the surface layers (Fig. 13.25). By late estrus, desquamation of the keratinized layers begins (Fig. 13.26). Intraepithelial glands are common during estrus.

AVIAN FEMALE REPRODUCTIVE SYSTEM

Ovary

In adult birds, only the left ovary is present. The ovarian cortex and medulla are distorted by the presence of large "follicles" in various stages of development or atresia. Each is attached to the ovarian stalk by a peduncle. True follicles are not present in the avian ovary because a fluid-filled follicular antrum does not develop. In the follicle, the oocyte is surrounded by one or several layers of granulosa cells. The granulosa cells are sur-

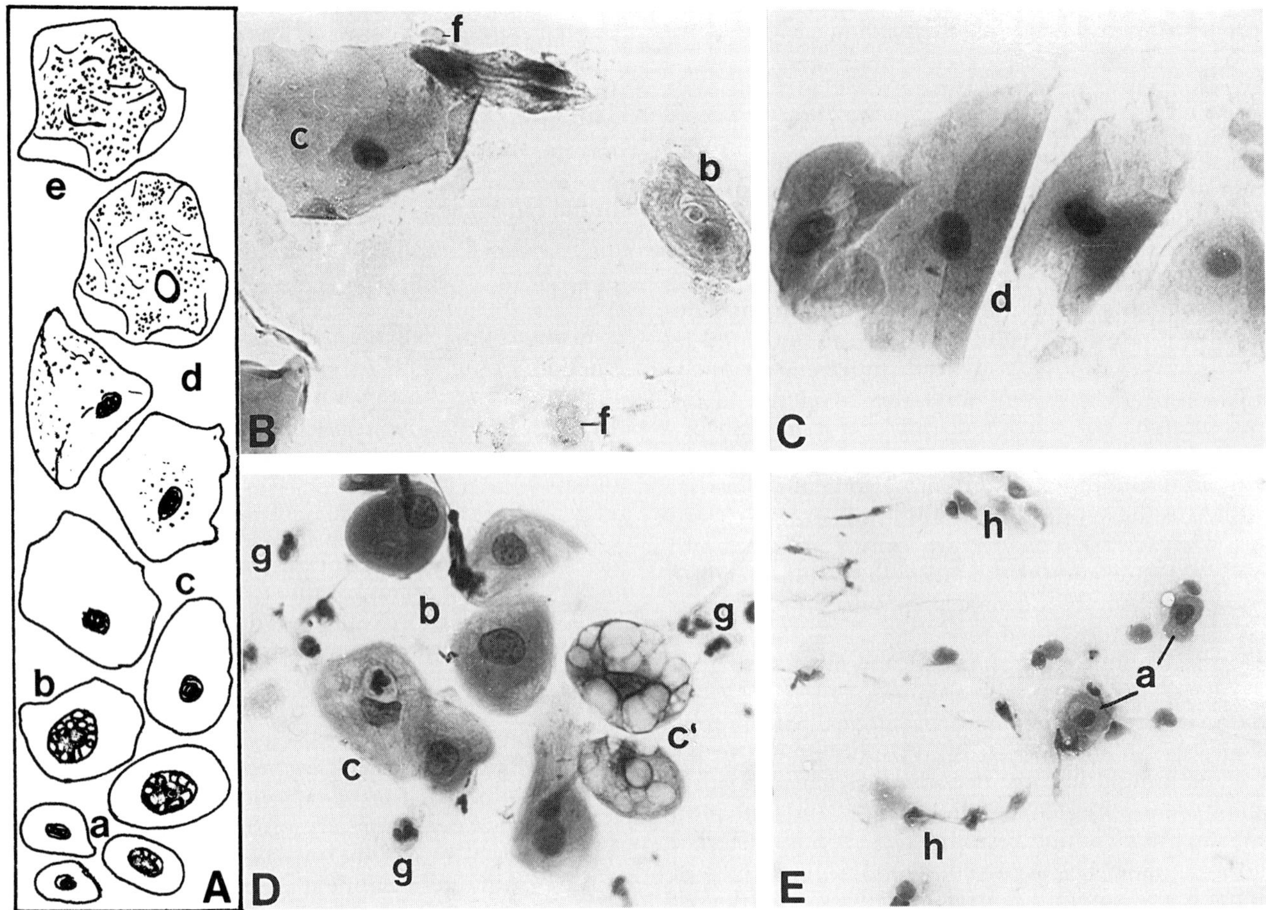

Figure 13.24. *Cyclic cellular changes of the vaginal epithelium in the bitch illustrated by a scheme of epithelial cells* ***(A)*** *and vaginal smears (epithelial and blood cells)* ***(B, C, D, E)****. Parabasal cells (a); small intermediate cells (b); large intermediate cells (c); superficial cells (d); keratinized cells (e, without nuclei); erythrocytes (f); leukocytes (g).* ***B.****, Proestrus; note small intermediate cells (b), large intermediate cells (c, centrally keratinized), and erythrocytes.* ***C.****, Estrus; note superficial cells (d, keratinized, pyknotic nuclei).* ***D.****, Metestrus, note small intermediate cells (b), large intermediate cells (c) undergoing disintegration (c'), and granulocytes (g).* ***E.****, Anestrus, note parabasal cells (a), and cell debris (h) (×680).*

rounded by cells of the theca interna and theca externa. The granulosa cells are shed with the oocyte at ovulation, whereas the theca cells remain to form a transient corpus luteum. Interstitial endocrine cells are found at the periphery of the ovary.

Formation of follicles usually begins in the post-hatching period, during which time the oogonia enlarge and become primary oocytes surrounded by follicular cells. The primary oocytes then enter the first meiotic division. At the time of sexual maturity (5 to 6 months in hens), secondary oocytes are ovulated. The second meiotic division is completed at fertilization, and an ovum, then a zygote, results. Although the primary oocyte is primarily protoplasmic, the secondary oocyte contains mainly yolk. Abundant yolk is accumulated at one end of the cell; the nucleus is at the other end. The secondary oocyte and ovum are thus termed **macrolecithal, telolecithal cells**. The yolk contains lipids, such as lecithin, cholesterol, and carotene, arranged in concentric layers. The oocyte is surrounded by a plasma membrane, termed the **vitelline membrane**. After ovulation, other layers are added to the outside of the egg cell during passage through the female reproductive tract.

Oviduct

The term **oviduct** in the bird is used to describe the entire reproductive duct. It is present in the adult only on the left side. The left oviduct consists of the **infundibulum**, **magnum**, **isthmus**, **uterus**, and **vagina** (Fig. 13.27). Although each of these divisions has special structural and functional features, they all have two morphologic elements essential for egg formation: *(a)* a muscle layer, which supports the oviduct and propels the egg, and *(b)* a glandular epithelial lining, which secretes all the parts of the egg outside the yolk-filled oocyte/zygote. Moreover, the mucous membrane produces a slimy secretion that forms a soft resilient cushion for the egg as it passes through the oviduct.

The following secretions of the oviduct are added onto the oocyte/zygote:

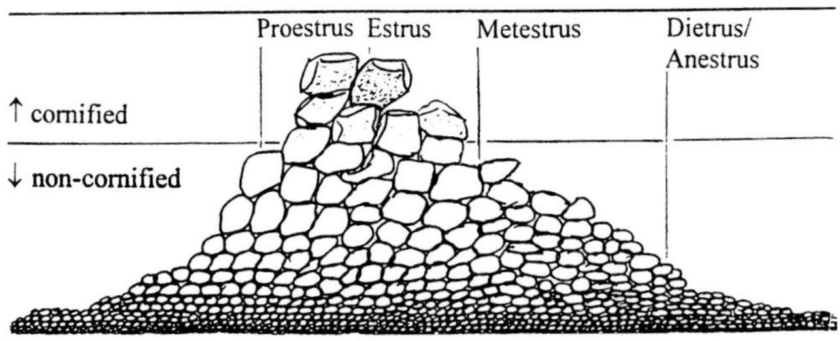

Figure 13.25. *Schematic drawing of the cyclic changes of the vaginal epithelium in the bitch. (Modified from Tammer I, Blendinger K, Sobiraj A, et al. über den Einsatz der exfoliativen Vaginalzytologie im Rahmen der gynækologischen Befunderhebung bei der Hündin. Tierärztl: Praxis 1994;22:199.)*

1. Four layers of albumen are added in the magnum (the cranial part of the oviduct).
2. A shell membrane, consisting of a thin inner and a thick outer layer of protein (mainly keratin) filaments, is added in the isthmus; the two layers are separated in the air chamber at the blunt end of the egg.
3. A porous shell is formed in the uterus. This shell consists of an inner layer of conical calcareous masses, surrounded by a spongy organic layer, and an outer shell cuticle. An organic pigment layer may be added externally in some breeds.

INFUNDIBULUM

The cranial extremity of the infundibulum is dilated and has long fimbriae that grasp the egg cell as it is released from the ovary. The infundibulum is the usual site of **fertilization**. The mucosa-submucosa is thrown into low longitudinal ridges or primary folds; in addition, secondary mucosal-submucosal folds are present in the caudal infundibulum. The egg remains in the infundibulum for approximately 25 minutes.

The epithelium is ciliated pseudostratified columnar. It contains occasional goblet cells, except at the bottom of the folds, where the epithelium is nonciliated simple columnar. Toward the caudal portion of the infundibulum, glandular cells increase in number and become aggregated in **glandular grooves** that resemble the tubular glands of the magnum.

The propria-submucosa consists of loose connective tissue containing many lymphocytes and plasma cells. The tunica muscularis is composed of scattered bundles of longitudinal smooth muscle. The tunica serosa consists of loose connective tissueand mesothelium.

MAGNUM

The magnum has a thick wall and tall thick longitudinal primary and secondary mucosal-submucosal folds. **Albumen** is added to the egg in the magnum. The egg remains in the magnum for approximately 3 hours.

The epithelium of the magnum is simple columnar with close to equal numbers of ciliated cells and goblet cells. The loose connective tissue of the propria-submucosa is packed with many long, branched, coiled tubular glands. The cells are pyramidal and contain coarse basophilic granules. An inner circular and an outer longitudinal smooth muscle layer are present. A thin tunica serosa consists of loose connective tissue and mesothelium. The magnum is sharply divided from the next portion of the oviduct, the isthmus, by a 1- to 3-mm segment devoid of glands.

ISTHMUS

The isthmus has pronounced longitudinal ridges. The egg remains in the isthmus for approximately 1 hour. The **shell membranes** are formed in this region.

The epithelium is simple columnar with close to equal numbers of ciliated and goblet cells.

The lamina propria tunica submucosa is filled with distended branched tubular glands. The glands are lined by pyramidal cells with cytoplasm that contains many acidophilic secretory granules. The tunica muscularis consists of circular and longitudinal smooth muscle layers. The tunica serosa consists of loose connective tissue and mesothelium.

UTERUS

The uterus, or **shell gland**, is thick-walled, saclike, and distensible. Primary and secondary longitudinal folds are obscured by a series of primary and secondary circular folds. Rotation of the egg, associated with twisting of the chalazia, occurs here. The egg remains in the uterus for approximately 20 hours. Shell components, such as organic matrix, shell cuticle, and inorganic material, are formed here.

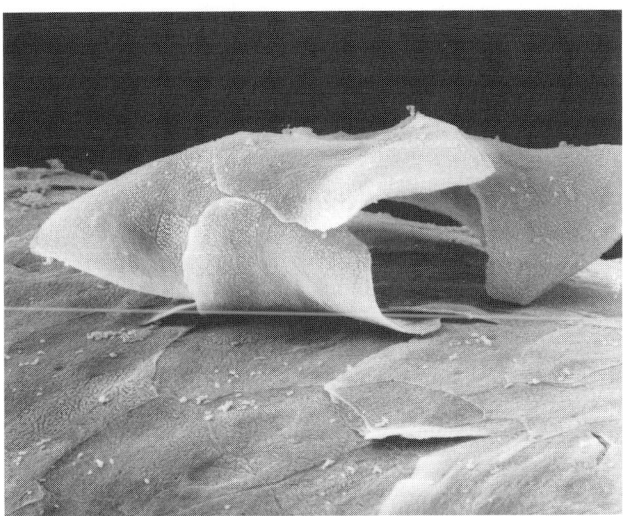

Figure 13.26. *Scanning electron micrograph showing the desquamation of keratinized superficial cells from the vaginal epithelium in the bitch in estrus (×650).*

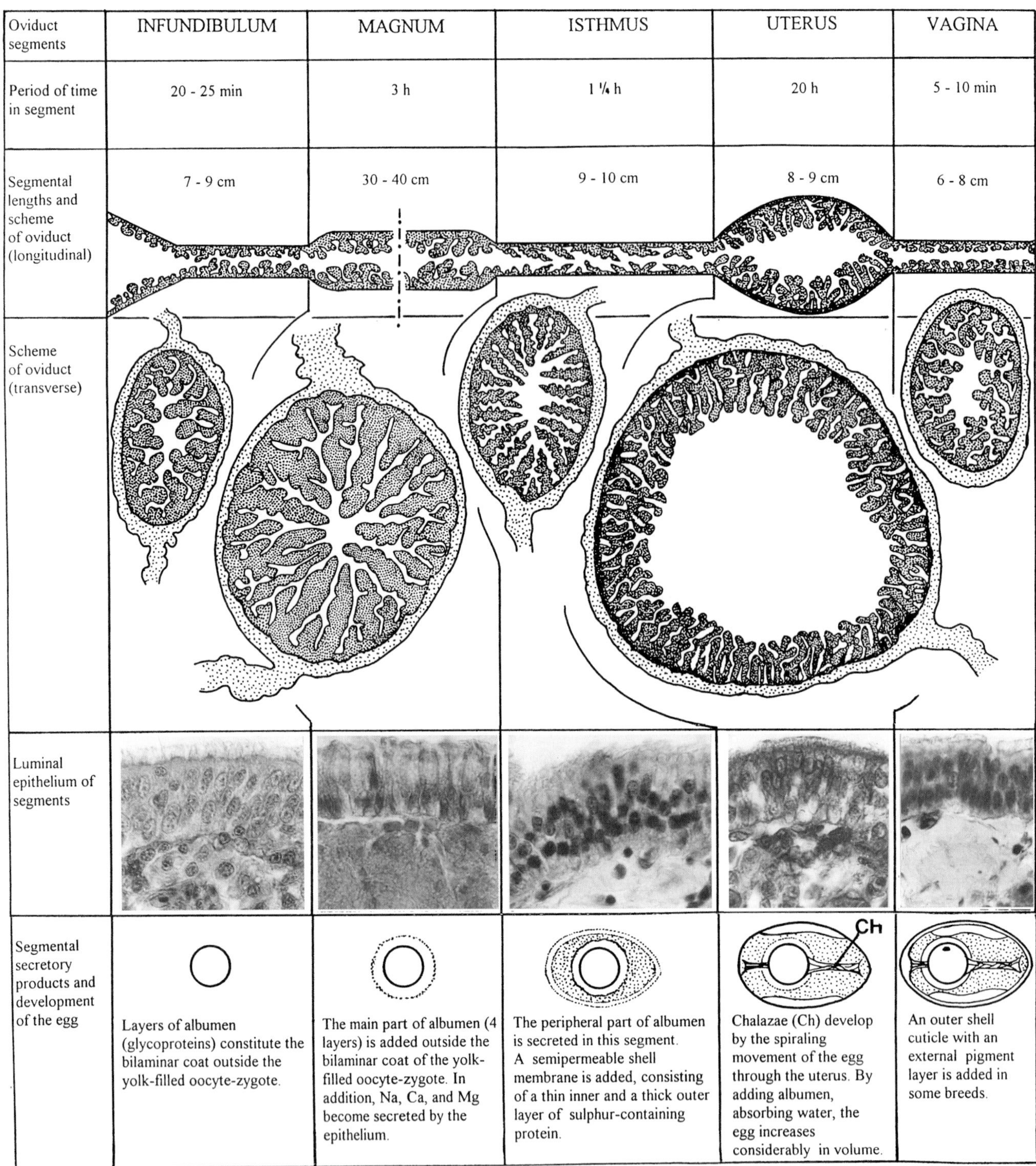

Figure 13.27. *Egg development in the laying domestic hen: structural changes of the egg in the various segments of the oviduct. Luminal epithelium of oviduct segments (×560). (Modified from Salomon F-V. Weibliches Geschlechtssystem. In: Lehrbuch der Geflügelanatomie. Stuttgart: Verlag, 1993:197.)*

The epithelium is ciliated pseudostratified columnar. The propria-submucosa contains branched, coiled tubular glands. The cells of these glands are pyramidal and have a diffusely granular and vacuolated cytoplasm. Loose connective tissue is sparse between the glands. The tunica muscularis consists of two layers of smooth muscle. The inner circular layer is thick and forms a sphincter at the boundary with the vagina. The tunica serosa consists of loose connective tissue and mesothelium.

VAGINA

The vaginal wall is thick and has low primary and secondary longitudinal folds. The egg remains in the vagina for a short time, and the vagina does not participate in the formation of the egg. It is glandless, except for the so-called **sperm-host glands** at the uterovaginal junction that are used for the storage of spermatozoa.

The epithelium is ciliated pseudostratified columnar with few goblet cells. The lamina propria/tunica submucosa is loose connective tissue that frequently contains lymphocytes, plasma cells, and granulocytes. The tunica muscularis is functional in expelling the egg and consists of a thick inner circular layer and an outer longitudinal layer. The tunica serosa consists of loose connective tissue and mesothelium.

Cloaca

The vagina, colon, and ureters open into the cloaca. The epithelium of the cloaca is simple columnar and contains many goblet cells.

REFERENCES

Baker TG. Oogenesis and ovulation. In: Austin CR, Short RV, eds. Reproduction in mammals, 2nd ed. Cambridge: Cambridge University Press, 1982:17.

Baird DT. The ovary. In: Austin CR, Short RV, eds. Reproduction in mammals, 2nd ed. Cambridge: Cambridge University Press, 1984:91.

Blandau RJ, Bourdage R, Halbert S. Tubal transport. In: Beller FK, Schumacher GFB, eds. The biology of the fluids of the female genital tract. North Holland: Elsevier, 1979:319.

Byskov AGS. Primordial germ cells and regulation of meiosis. In: Austin CR, Short RV, eds. Reproduction in mammals, 2nd ed. Cambridge: Cambridge University Press, 1982:1.

Goodman RL, Karsch FJ. The hypothalamic pulse generator: a key determinant of reproductive cycles in sheep. In: Follett BK, Follett DE, eds. Biological clocks and seasonal reproductive cycles. Colston Papers No. 32. Bristol: John Wright, 1981:223.

Guraya S. Biology of ovarian follicles in mammals. Berlin: Springer Verlag, 1985.

Leiser R. Weibliche Geschlechtsorgane. In: Mosimann W, Kohler T, eds. Zytologie, Histologie und mikroskopische Anatomie der Haustiere. Berlin: Verlag Paul Parey, 1990:232.

Liggins GC. The fetus and birth. In: Austin CR, Short RV, eds. Reproduction in mammals, 2nd ed. Cambridge: Cambridge University Press, 1983:114.

Knobil E, Neill JD. The physiology of reproduction, 2nd ed. New York: Raven Press, 1994;II.

Lincoln GA, Short RV. Seasonal breeding: nature's contraceptive. Recent Prog Horm Res 1980;36:1.

Mastroianni L Jr, Go KJ. Tubal secretions. In: Beller FK, Schumacher GFB, eds. The biology of the fluids of the female genital tract. North Holland: Elsevier, 1979:335.

McDonald LE. Veterinary endocrinology and reproduction, 3rd ed. Philadelphia: Lea & Febiger, 1982.

Moore RM. Seamark RF. Cell signaling, permeability and microvascularity changes during antral follicle development in mammals. J Dairy Sci 1986;69:927.

Pauerstein CJ, Eddy CA. Morphology of the fallopian tube. In: Beller FK, Schumacher GFB, eds. The biology of the fluids of the female genital tract. North Holland: Elsevier, 1979:299.

Priedkalns J. Pregnancy and the central nervous system. In: Steven DH, ed. Comparative placentation: essays in structure and function. London: Academic Press, 1975:189.

Priedkalns J, Weber AF, Zemjanis R. Qualitative and quantitative morphological studies of the cells of the membrana granulosa, theca interna, and corpus luteum of the bovine ovary. Z Zellforsch 1968;85:501.

Rajakoski E. The ovarian follicular system in sexually mature heifers with special reference to seasonal, cyclical and left-right variations. Acta Endocrinol (Kbh.) 1960;34 (Suppl 52):1.

Salomon F-V. Geschlechtssystem. In: Lehrbuch der Geflügelanatomie. Jena: Gustav Fischer Verlag, 1993:197.

Van Blerkom J, Bell H, Weipz D. Cellular and developmental biological aspects of bovine meiotic maturation, fertilization and preimplantation embryogenesis in vitro. J Electron Microsc Tech 1990;16:298.

Wassarman P. The mammalian ovum. In: Knobil E, Neill J, eds. The physiology of reproduction. New York: Raven Press, 1988;I:69.

Wrobel K-H, Laun G, Hees H, et al. Histologische und ultrastrukturelle Untersuchungen am Vaginalepithel des Rindes. Anat Histol Embryol 1986;15:303.

14

Placentation

VIBEKE DANTZER
RUDOLF LEISER

EMBRYOLOGY

The fusion of a female and male gamete results in a **zygote**. After repeated cleavage during the transport through the uterine tube to the uterine cavity in higher mammals (Eutheria), it develops into a fluid-filled vesicle, a **blastocyst**, with a wall of simple epithelium, a **trophoblast**, and an eccentrically located **inner cell mass**. The free-living blastocyst is nourished by secretion from endometrial glands (uterine milk). Because the increasing demand from the growing embryo necessitates a more efficient nutritive arrangement, i.e., a vascular transport system, the embryo produces membranes that, in a process called **implantation,** gradually attach to the endometrium and thereby establish a close relationship between fetal and maternal circulatory systems for physiologic exchange. As a result, a combined organ, the **placenta**, is formed. In this bimodal structure, a **fetal placenta** (placenta fetalis) and a **maternal placenta** (placenta materna) are recognized. The fetus and fetal membranes, including the fetal placenta, are known as the **conceptus**. The manner of attachment and of formation of the placenta is termed **placentation**.

The first events in placentation occur in the blastocyst stage. The trophoblast is essential for the transfer of nourishment to the offspring during intrauterine life but has no function after birth of the young and is expelled with the afterbirth (secundinae). The inner cell mass differentiates into three germ layers in two stages, forming first **ectoderm** and **endoderm** and then, between them, the **mesoderm**. These layers form the embryo, but they also participate in the formation of the fetal membranes. The ectoderm forms a vesicle enclosing the embryo, the **amnion**. It provides buoyancy and freedom of development to the embryo. The endoderm gives rise to the **yolk sac**, communicating with the midgut, and the **allantois**, a diverticulum from the hindgut (Fig. 14.1).

The further development of the fetal membranes is directed by the mesoderm. The lateral mesoderm splits into a somatic and a splanchnic layer. The resulting intramesodermal cleft gives rise to the body cavity (intraembryonic coelom), which, at this stage, has an extension to extraembryonic location, **exocoelom**. The somatic mesoderm combines with trophoblast to form the **chorion** or with the ectoderm of the amnion. These membranes constitute the extraembryonic **somatopleure**. The splanchnic mesoderm fuses with the endoderm of the yolk sac and the allantois, and together they form the extraembryonic **splanchnopleure**.

The somatic mesoderm, and hence the chorion, is initially avascular. The blood islands and vessels first arise in the splanchnic mesoderm of the yolk sac and later in the mesoderm of the allantois. Eventually, the avascular

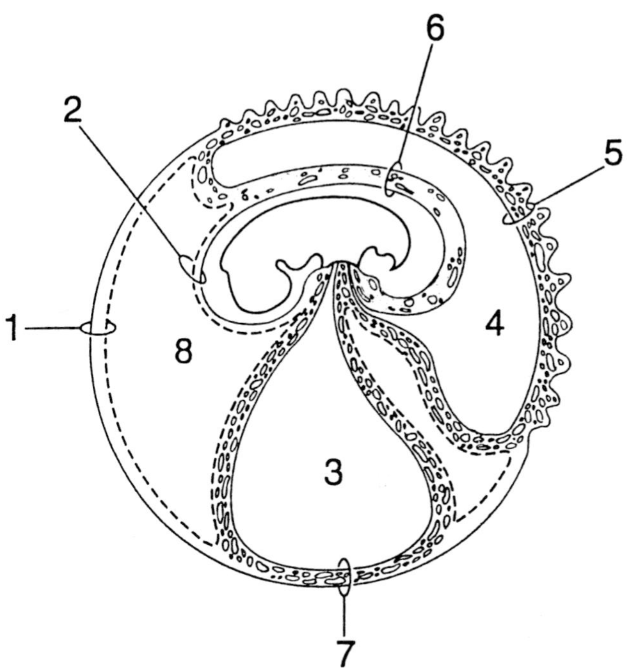

Figure 14.1. *Diagram of fetal membranes. The arrangement is subject to wide variation in different species. Chorion (1); amnion enclosing the amniotic cavity with the embryo (2); yolk sac cavity lined by yolk sac endoderm and associated vascular mesoderm (3); allantois with allantoic cavity lined by allantoic endoderm and vascular mesoderm (4); chorioallantoic placenta (5); allantoamnion (6); choriovitelline placenta (7); exocoelom (8). (From Dellmann H-D, Carithers JR. Cytology and microscopic anatomy. Philadelphia: Williams & Wilkins, 1996.)*

mesoderm of the chorion fuses with the mesoderm of the allantois and then becomes vascularized. The placental vessels, together with the vitelline and allantoic ducts, are contained in the **body stalk** and later develop into the **umbilical cord** (see Fig. 14.10A).

CLASSIFICATION

The placenta is subject to great species-dependent variations. These variations have given rise to many different systems of classification. The following classification is based on five main criteria: *(a)* fetal extraembryonic membrane contributions, *(b)* macroscopic structure of the placenta, *(c)* three-dimensional structure of the maternal–fetal interface, *(d)* tissue layers of the fetal–maternal interhemal barrier, and *(e)* degree of fetal–maternal anchoring and fate at birth.

Fetal Extraembryonic Membrane Contributions

Two types of placentae occur in domestic mammals: the choriovitelline placenta (omphaloid or yolk sac) and the chorioallantoic placenta. The yolk sac, and hence the choriovitelline placenta, develops before the allantois and the chorioallantoic placenta. Early during gestation, the choriovitelline and chorioallantoic placentae coexist temporarily, and then the choriovitelline placenta regresses.

CHORIOVITELLINE PLACENTA

The **choriovitelline** or **yolk sac placenta** is formed when the yolk sac wall (omphalopleure) combines with the chorion and then contacts the endometrium. It may be fully or partially vascularized by the omphalomesenteric artery and vein (Figs. 14.1 and 14.16). In sows and ruminants, the yolk sac wall is simply apposed to the uterine epithelium, and the yolk sac begins its involution 3 to 4 weeks after conception. However, in carnivores and mares, it is well developed early in gestation and the yolk sac persists throughout gestation. In carnivores, a temporary lamellar choriovitelline placenta develops (see Fig. 14.16). In all domestic mammals, the choriovitelline placenta is of minor importance in physiologic fetal–maternal exchange.

In the **inverted yolk sac placenta**, the endoderm of the yolk sac is directly exposed to the uterine luminal content. It occurs in mice, rats, rabbits, and guinea pigs and participates in selective absorption and transmission of maternal immunoglobulins for fetal immunoprotection.

CHORIOALLANTOIC PLACENTA

When the allantois fuses with the chorion, an **allantochorion** is formed (Fig. 14.1), resulting in a **chorioallantoic placenta**. This organ is the most efficient for mediating physiologic exchange between mother and offspring. It is very well vascularized by umbilical arteries and vein.

The principle of providing a vast fetal–maternal area of interchange determines the placental structure at the gross and microscopic anatomical levels. The structural variations of the placenta are immense. Intermediate forms exist, and the placenta also changes its internal structure during the period of gestation.

Macroscopic Structure of the Placenta

The part of the chorion where folds, lamellae, or villi increase its surface is called **frondose chorion** (chorion frondosum), and the smooth part, without projections, is the **smooth chorion** (chorion laeve). Three types of placentae, comprising the frondose chorion and its uterine counterpart, are recognized macroscopically in domestic mammals namely diffuse, cotyledonary, and zonary (Fig. 14.2), whereas in humans and some other species, the discoid type develops.

In the **diffuse placenta** (placenta diffusa), most of the chorionic sac forms a frondose chorion attached to the endometrial epithelium (sows, mares, camels) (see Figs. 14.5 and 14.11A).

In the **cotyledonary placenta** (placenta multiplex), tufts of chorionic protrusions (cotyledons) attach to preformed endometrial prominences (caruncles). Cotyledons and caruncles combine to form **placentomes**. In the intercaruncular area, a smooth chorion is apposed to the endometrial epithelium (ruminants) (see Fig. 14.13).

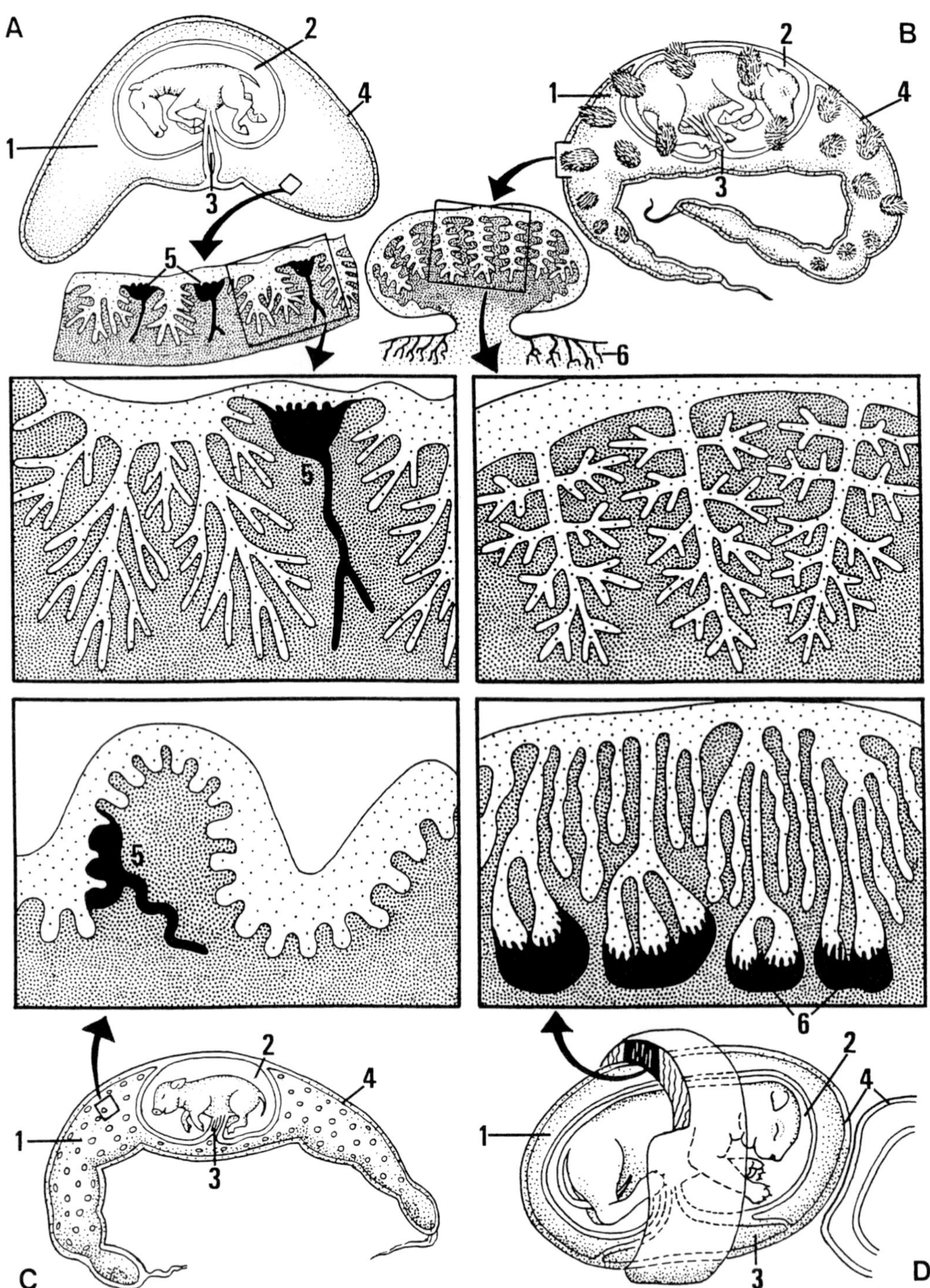

Figure 14.2. *Schematic drawings of the fetus in the fetal membranes to show differences in placental shape and internal structure among species. Horse with a diffuse villous (microcotyledonary) placenta* ***(A)****; ruminants (cow), with a cotyledonary villous placenta* ***(B)****; pig with a diffuse folded placenta provided with macroscopically visible areolae* ***(C)****; carnivores, here cat, with a zonary (girdle) lamellar or tightly folded placenta* ***(D)****. Allantoic cavity (1); amnionic cavity (2); yolk sac (3); allantochorion (4). In the higher magnification views, the maternal side is dark, the fetal side is bright, and the areola–gland complex (5) in horse and pig and the endometrial glands (6) in bovine and cat are black.*

In the **zonary placenta** (placenta zonaria), the frondose chorion forms a band or girdle around the equator of the chorionic sac. Outside the girdle, the smooth chorion apposes to the endometrial epithelium (carnivores, minks) (see Figs 14.16 and 14.17).

In the **discoid placenta** (placenta discoidalis), the frondose chorion forms a disc-shaped area of fusion with the endometrium (e.g., humans, apes, mice, rats, rabbits, guinea pigs).

Three-Dimensional Structure of the Interface Between the Maternal and Fetal Tissues

The capacity for exchange between maternal and fetal tissues is enhanced by the increased surface area of a folded, villous, or labyrinthine interface (Fig. 14.2). This vast fetal–maternal contact area is further increased by microvilli on both trophoblast and endometrial surface epithelial cells or by an irregular cell surface (see Figs. 14.8, 14.9, and 14.12B).

In the **folded placenta**, enlargement of the fetal–maternal contact surface takes place by vascularized macroscopic folds (**plicae**) of varying magnitude and by microscopic ridges (**rugae**) of varying height (sows) (see Figs. 14.5 through 14.7) or by lamellae (carnivores) (see Figs. 14.17 and 14.18).

In the **villous placenta**, the allantochorion forms **cotyledons**, i.e., arborizing **chorionic villi** with vascular mesenchymal cores that fit into corresponding **caruncular crypts**. Together, they form macroscopic (ruminants) or microscopic placentomes (mares) (see Figs. 14.11 through 14.13), or the villous tree is bathed in the maternal intervillous blood space (humans).

In **labyrinthine placentation**, the trophoblast of the allantochorion forms an intercommunicating network that envelopes the endothelium of maternal blood vessels, as seen in carnivores, or it is in direct contact with maternal blood in trophoblast-lined vascular channels (rats, mice, rabbits).

Tissue Layers of the Fetal–Maternal Interhemal Barrier

The fetal and maternal placental circulations are separated by tissue layers that form the placental or fetal–maternal interhemal barrier, which is a highly selective transport avenue in the fetal–maternal exchange (Fig. 14.3). The fetal component of this barrier is chorionic tissue vascularized by allantoic vessels and consists of three tissue layers: endothelium, mesenchyme, and trophoblast. The maternal counterpart consists basically of three corresponding layers in reverse order: endometrial surface epithelium, connective tissue, and endothelium.

Although constant in the fetal placental membrane, the number of tissue layers of the maternal component varies with the species. Therefore, placentae are classified on the basis of the number of uterine tissue layers:

In the **epitheliochorial placenta** (placenta epitheliochorialis), all three layers of the maternal component are present. This type of placenta occurs in sows, mares (see Figs. 14.8 and 14.12A), and ruminants (see Fig. 14.15). In ruminants, however, binucleated trophoblast cells migrate and fuse with the endometrial surface epithelium, and the placenta is designated as **synepitheliochorial**.

In the **endotheliochorial placenta** (placenta endotheliochorialis), the endometrial surface epithelium and the connective tissue are absent, and endothelium alone, lined by an interstitial layer, separates the maternal blood from the trophoblast. This type of placenta is primarily present in carnivores and minks (see Fig. 14.18B).

In the **hemochorial placenta** (placenta hemochorialis), all three maternal layers are absent, rendering the trophoblast freely exposed to maternal blood. Up to three layers of trophoblast may be present (hemotrichorial), of which at least one is syncytiotrophoblast (fusion of trophoblast cells into a symplasm, syncytic trophoblast). This type of placenta is present in humans, rats, mice, rabbits, and guinea pigs.

Fetal–Maternal Anchoring and Fate at Birth

The degree to which the endometrium is changed and the fetal membranes are anchored into the maternal tissue determines the amount of uterine tissue lost at parturition. On this basis, two types of chorioallantoic placentations, nondeciduate and deciduate, are recognized (Fig 14.3).

In the **nondeciduate placenta**, the fetal components interlock with relatively intact uterine tissue, from which they separate without much loss of endometrium, as in epitheliochorial placentae (ungulates).

In **deciduate placentae**, the transformed part of the endometrial stroma, the **decidua**, is shed with the fetal membranes after parturition.

NOURISHMENT OF THE EMBRYO BEFORE IMPLANTATION

The main physiologic principle of the chorioallantoic placenta is the substantial exchange between maternal and fetal blood. The substance that nourishes the offspring is termed **embryotrophe**. It comes from both maternal blood, the **hemotrophe**, and uterine glandular secretions and cell fragments, the **histiotrophe**. Both are taken up by the trophoblast. Histiotrophe and uterine epithelial cell fragments nourish the offspring before implantation. During gestation, it is present in **areolae**, which are indentations of the chorion opposite the openings of endometrial glands. The areolae are scattered in the diffuse placenta of pigs and mares or located in the smooth chorion of the ruminant placentae. In the carnivore placenta, histiotrophe is found in the junctional zone. It is typically seen as the areola–gland complex in the diffuse placenta as well as in relation to the smooth chorion in the cotyledonary placenta (Fig. 14.2).

PLACENTAL VASCULARITY AND CIRCULATION

After successful implantation, the embryo is nourished by hemotrophe, metabolites that cross the placental barrier from maternal circulation. The two blood cir-

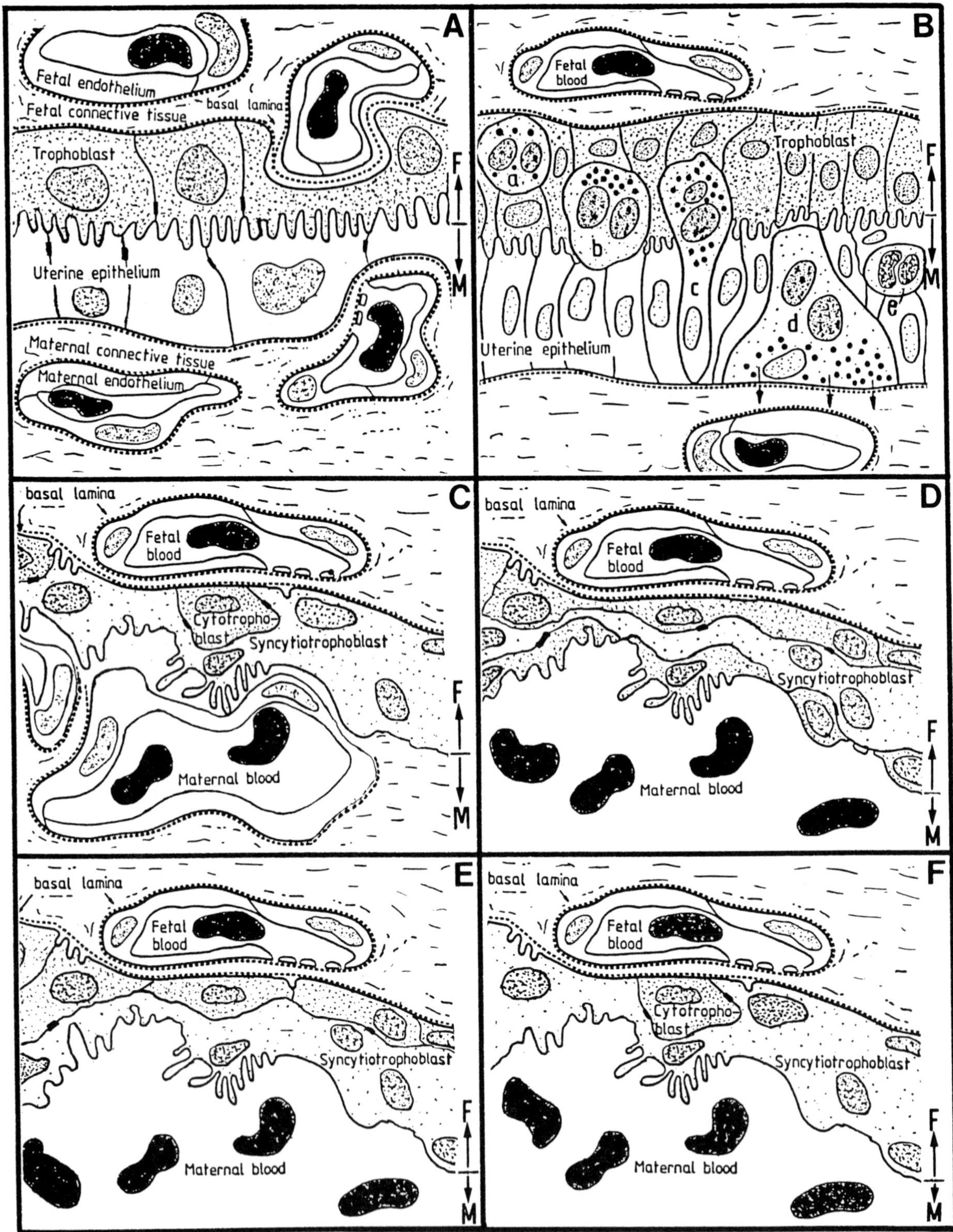

Figure 14.3. *Schematic drawings of the tissue layers of the fetal–maternal interhemal barrier of placenta, including fetal components of the allantochorion (F) and maternal components (M). Dependent on species a reduction of the maternal components takes place, illustrated here by steps (**A–F**) until the trophoblast of the chorion comes into direct contact with maternal blood. Species differences in the trophoblast are also shown. The different placental types and corresponding species are: **A.**, epitheliochorial — sow, mare; **B.**, synepitheliochorial — ruminants (a–e show migration of binucleate trophoblast cells [a,b], fusion of binucleate cell with uterine epithelial cell [c], maternal-fetal hybrid cell which secretes granular content (arrow) into maternal stroma [d], degenerating hybrid cell [e]); **C.**, endotheliochorial — carnivores (bitch, queen); **D.**, hemotrichorial — rat, mouse; **E.**, hemodichorial — rabbit; **F.**, hemomonochorial — man, guinea pig. (Modified from Leiser R, Kaufmann P. Placental structure: in a comparative aspect. Exp Clin Endocrinol 1994;102:122–134.)*

culatory systems always remain morphologically separated by a varying number of tissue layers, depending on the species, as classified above. The fetal capillaries have smaller lumina than the maternal ones, and both are partially fenestrated and are surrounded by basal laminae (Figs. 14.3, 14.4 and 14.18B).

In the maternal placenta, the blood is either contained in vessels or bathes the trophoblast directly. Uterine vessels also become leaky by local degeneration of endometrial tissue, forming **placental hematomata**, which are deposits of stagnant maternal blood between endometrial epithelium and trophoblast in carnivores and ruminants (Fig. 14.17). In hemochorial placentae, the uterine vessels are absent from the placental barrier, and the blood flows through trophoblastic tubules or intervillous spaces (lacunae). Regardless of the type of chorioallantoic placentation, however, trophoblast and fetal endothelium are always present in the placental interhemal barrier (Fig. 14.3).

The supply of oxygenated blood to the placenta is derived from the uterine artery and anastomoses from the ovarian and vaginal arteries. The arteries are enlarged during pregnancy, and their placental capillaries develop into a species-specific architecture (Figs. 14.4 and 14.11B) reflecting the internal three-dimensional structure of the placenta; in hemochorial placentation, they lose their endothelium and form blood spaces. The uterine placenta is drained by veins.

The fetal placenta is vascularized for the uptake of oxygen and nutrients and for delivery of waste products. To facilitate exchange, the different placental circulatory systems perform multivillous, crosscurrent, or countercurrent flows between allantoic and uterine vessels; although the least efficient, the concurrent exchange system is only theoretical (Fig. 14.4). It is also noteworthy that the fetal veins leave the placenta apposed to the origin of uterine arterioles, thus enhancing the capability of exchange. The capillaries underlying maternal epithelium and trophoblast bend and dilate (Figs. 14.4 and 14.8). The bending of the vessels provides a flow stress that enhances vascular growth through interaction with hormones and cytokines. Dilation of blood vessels slows blood flow, enhancing the possibility for the active exchange of nutrients.

The yolk sac placenta, when present, receives blood from the omphalomesenteric or vitelline arteries, which arise from the abdominal aorta. The oxygenated blood is returned to the heart by the omphalomesenteric veins.

The chorioallantoic placenta receives blood from the paired umbilical arteries, which originate from the caudal aorta, and returns oxygenated blood through the umbilical veins. The left umbilical vein carries blood to the heart via the liver and the caudal vena cava, whereas the right vein undergoes involution within the fetus.

SPECIALIZED CELLS OF THE PLACENTA

Decidual cells are specialized cells derived from fibroblasts in the endometrium. They may develop in the placenta of carnivores (Fig. 14.18A) and are always present in hemochorial placentae. Decidual cells are enlarged rounded or polyhedral and are subject to considerable species variations in size, contents (lipid, glycogen, hormones and growth factors), and structure.

The trophoblast performs many different functions (absorption, exchange of metabolites, hormone synthesis, as well as other signal transmitter substances). This diversity is reflected in the complex structure of individual cells and the cell types developed by differentiation (see sow placenta below, as a species example). The discrete trophoblast cell is termed a **cytotrophoblast**. Another form of differentiation is the binucleate trophoblast cell or **giant cell** found in ruminants (see Figs. 14.14 and 14.15). If multiple trophoblast cells fuse, they form a **syncytiotrophoblast** (Figs. 14.3 and 14.18). When both cytotrophoblasts and syncytiotrophoblasts are present, as in carnivores, the cellular form is primitive whereas the syncytial form is more differentiated with respect to the development of organelles. The presence of binuclear or multinuclear trophoblast cells corresponds to increasing invasion of the endometrium. In ruminants and mares, a relatively low degree of invasion occurs in the presence of binucleate cells, compared to the extensive endometrial invasion of multinucleated syncytiotrophoblasts in carnivores, rodents, and primates.

CHANGES DURING PLACENTATION

The placenta continuously changes in size, shape, and internal structure throughout gestation. After implantation, it grows at a rapid, although gradually decreasing, rate and may be subject to minor involution before term. Rearrangements at the cellular level are reflected in apoptosis (regulated cell death) and mitotic activity. In addition, the physical barrier between the maternal and fetal circulatory systems progressively attenuates with time (for details see function–structure relationships below).

FUNCTION–STRUCTURE RELATIONSHIPS

Structural differences in the various placenta types do not necessarily reflect their function. The transfer mechanism of the respiratory gases, i.e., oxygen and carbon dioxide under gradient pressure is essentially simple diffusion. Therefore, the diffusion distance across the interhemal barrier is of major importance.

Capillaries from both fetal and uterine sides of the placenta approach and indent the respective epithelia during gestation (Figs. 14.3 and 14.8). Consequently, the diffusion barrier thins and, despite a varying number of layers in the interhemal barrier, the diffusion distance becomes almost similar for all species, namely 2 μm.

An important structure in cellular transport is the plasma membrane with its variety of receptors, because it regulates the cellular uptake and transfer of nutrients as well as export of unusable metabolic components. Therefore, placental selective barrier and transport functions are critically dependent on the number and activity of plasma membranes to be traversed. As parts of the placental barrier, the plasma membranes are present only in epithelium and endothelium. To traverse a

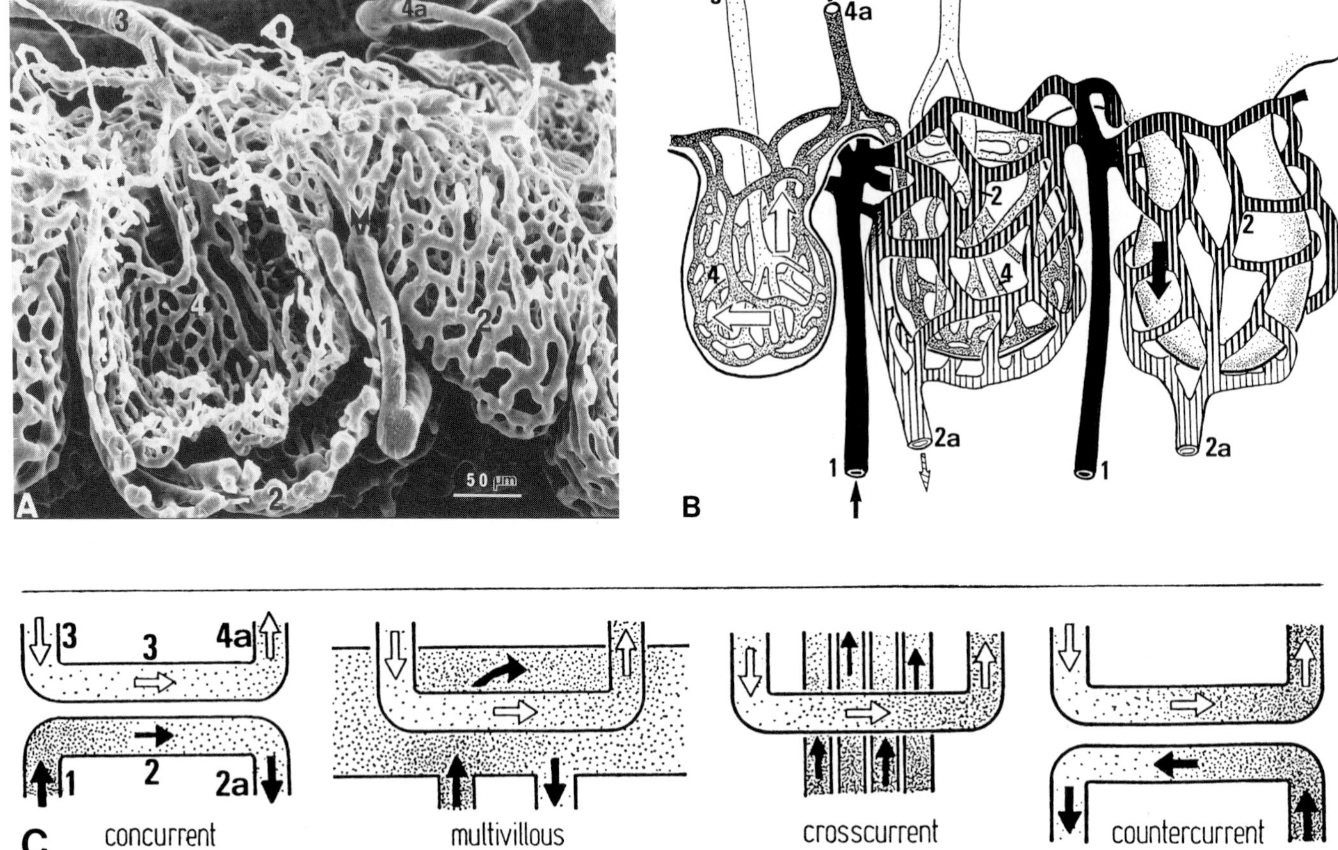

Figure 14.4. *Combined maternal and fetal vascular cast* ***(A)*** *and corresponding scheme from the placenta of the pig at day 99 of pregnancy* ***(B)****, and idealized arrangement of placental blood flows* ***(C)****. The maternal arterioles (1) run to the top of maternal ridges, where they branch into the maternal capillary networks (2), which are drained by venules (2a). The fetal arterioles (3) can be followed into the fetal capillary networks (4), which have outlets through the fetal venules (4a). The large arrows in* ***B*** *demonstrate a mixture of crosscurrent (black/vertical versus white/horizontal arrows) and countercurrent (black/vertical versus white/vertical arrows) maternal-fetal blood flow interrelationship in the pig. The schematic* ***C*** *demonstrates, from left to right, bloodstreams of four different placental exchange types linked to typical species, like concurrent (theoretical), multivillous (man), crosscurrent (queen), countercurrent (guinea pig). The density of dots in the fetal venules (4a) illustrates the efficiency of the various exchangers in diffusional exchange (for example oxygen).* ***A****: ×260. (****C****: From Dantzer V, Leiser R, Kaufmann P, et al. Comparative morphological aspects of placental vascularization. Trophoblast Res 1988;3:235.)*

cell (or syncytium), a substance must pass both the apical and basal plasma membrane.

Among important inorganic elements, e.g., calcium, phosphorus, iodine, and iron, a directional preference from mother to fetus generally exists. This characteristic is especially true of iron, as no retrograde transfer of iron from fetus to mother occurs. In different species, however, the iron transfer takes place by different mechanisms. In carnivores and to a lesser extent in ruminants, iron is absorbed from blood hemoglobin in maternal hemorrhages, whereas in the sow and horse and also to some extent in ruminants, the source is a glycoprotein with iron secreted by the endometrial glands (Fig 14.2). In hemochorial placentation, the trophoblast takes up iron from circulating maternal transferrin. Calcium is transferred in different regions of the fetal membranes, depending on the species. In sows, the transfer occurs across the folded interhemal barrier of the interareolar region, whereas in cows, it occurs at the intercotyledonary region.

The hemoglobin of the growing offspring contains different types of polypeptide chains during different phases of development. The earliest (nucleated) erythrocytes from the yolk sac mesoderm contain embryonic hemoglobin. Later, in intrauterine life, hepatic and splenic erythrocytes carry fetal hemoglobin, and near the time of birth, a gradual change in bone marrow cells with adult hemoglobin takes place. Embryonic and fetal hemoglobin have a higher affinity for oxygen than does the adult form, and thus, they are able to extract oxygen diffusing across the placental barrier more efficiently than can adult hemoglobin. This difference is an adaptation for intrauterine life with low oxygen pressure.

Proteins of high molecular weight of maternal origin, like immunoglobulins (IgGs), which protect newborns against infectious diseases, do sufficiently bypass the placental barrier in endotheliochorial placentae with hematomas and hemochorial placentae but do not in epitheliochorial placentae, although some may be transferred at hematomas in ruminants. The latter are therefore totally dependent on the immunoglobulins in the colostrum immediately after parturition, when the epithelium in the intestinal tract is temporarily permeable for these large molecules.

The placental trophoblast secretes hormones, e.g., chorionic gonadotropin (mares), placental lactogen (ruminants), estrogens, and progesterone. During pregnancy, the placenta also produces a wide spectrum of other factors for the regulation of metabolic activity, growth, and structural changes (paracrine factors). These factors are used differently among species to regulate gestation and complete successful placentation.

SPECIES DIFFERENCES

The beginning of placentation and length of gestation vary considerably in different species (Table 14.1).

Sow

In early stages, the yolk sac is unusually large and well vascularized; its maximal development occurs at approximately day 20. A choriovitelline placenta of insignificant extent is formed but disappears as the yolk sac rapidly decreases in size.

The chorioallantoic placenta is diffuse, folded, epitheliochorial, and nondeciduate. The fusiform chorionic sac adheres to the endometrium over its entire area, except at the avascular extremities and over the uterine gland openings, where **areola–gland complexes** are formed (Figs. 14.2, 14.6, and 14.7).

The blastocyst undergoes extremely rapid elongation from day 10 to day 12. It changes from a sphere of approximately 2 mm in diameter to a membranous hollow "thread" approximately 100 cm in length. At days 12 to 14, the migration of the blastocysts is fulfilled and they are evenly distributed in both uterine horns along the mesometrial side. Placentation begins close to the embryo, where the endometrium forms epithelial proliferations covered with corresponding caplike formations of the chorion at days 13 to 14, thus giving an anchoring effect until interdigitating microvilli begin to develop between uterine epithelium and trophoblast at day 15.

The chorionic–endometrial contact area is increased approximately three times by macroscopic primary and split circular folds (plicae). The folds are stable on the maternal side but unstable on the fetal side as they passively follow the existing endometrial folds (Figs. 14.2C and 14.5). When the whole chorionic sac is spread out, it measures approximately three times the length of the corresponding permanently folded endometrium. The microscopic folds form rugae separated by fossae that are permanent on both maternal and fetal sides. They are first irregular and later develop into more regular circular rugae (Figs. 14.5 through 14.7), which become further subdivided, thereby changing the fetal rugae into bulbous protrusions in late gestational stages. The microscopic foldings increase the exchange area approximately four times.

Table 14.1.
Implantation and Gestation in Domestic Animals

	Beginning of Implantation (day)	*Gestation Time (days)*
Bitch	17–18	58–63
Queen	12.5–14	63–65
Mare	35–40	329–345
Sow	13–14	112–115
Cow	16–18	279–285
Ewe	15–20	144–152

The epithelial cells differentiate as the trophoblast lining the chorionic fossae forms arcades of high columnar epithelium, which are apposed to the low columnar epithelium of the summit of the endometrial rugae. The remaining chorionic and uterine epithelia are cuboidal or flattened (Fig. 14.8).

As gestation proceeds, allantoic and uterine capillaries indent those parts of the respective rugae where the trophoblast and endometrial epithelium are low. Thus, the connective tissue interposed between the capillaries and epithelia is reduced to basal laminae (Figs. 14.3A and 14.9). In advanced stages, the thickness of the interhemal membrane can be less than 2 μm, consisting of six layers, four of which are cellular (Figs. 14.3 and 14.8).

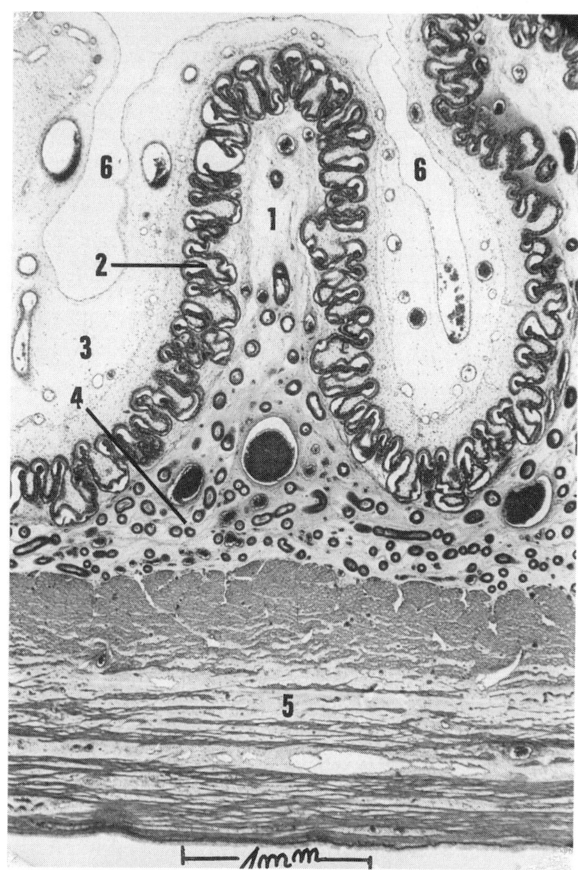

Figure 14.5. *Longitudinal section of uterine horn with placenta (sow), late midpregnancy. Primary fold (1); rugae (2); allantochorion (3); endometrium with glands (4); myometrium (5); allantoic cavity (6) (×20). (Courtesy of A. Hansen.)*

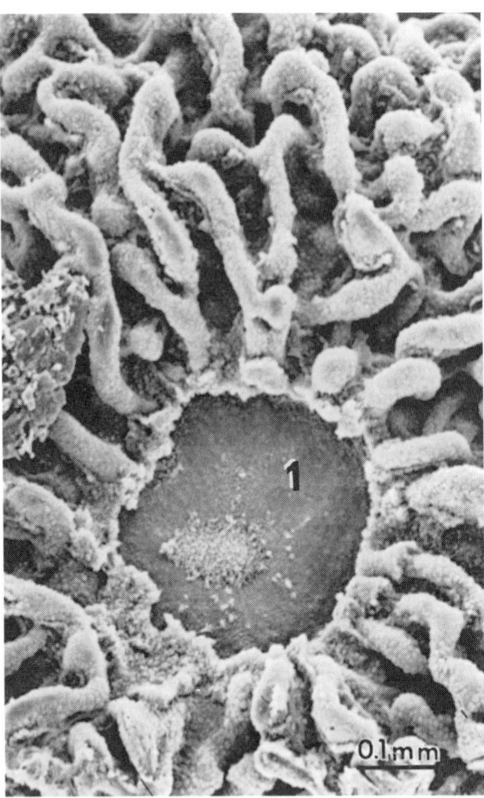

Figure 14.6. *Maternal part of porcine placenta from midgestation after separation from the fetal side to illustrate the maternal side of an areola (1) with some accumulation of uterine milk covering the opening of the uterine gland. The maternal rugae radiate around the areola and the parallel arrangement can be discerned at the top of the picture. These rugae are complementary to the fetal fossae between the fetal rugae (see Fig. 14.7) (×90). (From Dantzer V. Scanning electron microscopy of exposed surfaces of the porcine placenta. Acta Anat 1984;118:96.)*

The trophoblastic and uterine epithelial cells are provided with interdigitating microvilli, thereby increasing the area of exchange additionally by a factor of approximately 10 (Fig. 14.9).

The uterine epithelial cells contain spherical nuclei with small nucleoli. The ER is mainly of the rough type. The Golgi complex is extensive, and small mitochondria are scattered in the cytoplasm (Fig. 14.9). Numerous lysosomes are characteristic for the maternal epithelial cells. The trophoblast cells have rounded nuclei with distinct nucleoli. The composition of the ER varies. The rER occurs mainly in the basal part of the cells intermingled with electron-dense, periodic acid-Schiff (PAS) positive bodies and lysosomes, indicating a high metabolic and secretory activity. Soon after day 80, aggregations of smooth endoplasmic reticulum (sER) are also seen basally and laterally in the cells, and their occurrence is correlated with high estrogen synthesis. Evidence of high endocytic activity is indicated by the presence of mitochondria located apically in the cells among coated pits and vesicles, tubular endosomes, and multivesicular bodies (Fig. 14.9).

The placental subunit, the areola–gland complex, is macroscopically visible as small opalescent vesicles, the areolae, which contain uterine milk or histiotrophe (see Figs. 14.2C, 14.6, and 14.7). The maternal areolae are smooth-surfaced shallow cups surrounding the openings of uterine glands. The fetal areolae are rosettelike structures composed of villi (Fig. 14.7). Histiotrophe, composed of secretory products and degenerating cell material, accumulates in the areolae between the uterine and fetal epithelia in the intermicrovillous space. The main transfer of iron from mother to fetus takes place via the areola–gland complex. The uterine glands of the complex secrete an iron-containing glycoprotein, uteroferrin, which is subsequently taken up by the areolar trophoblast and transferred to the underlying fetal capillary network. The areola–gland complexes also participate in the transfer of vitamin A (retinoids).

The blood-flow relationship between maternal and fetal circulation in the sow is a mixture of crosscurrent and countercurrent (Fig. 14.4). Exchange across the porcine placental barrier is midrange in efficiency compared to other species described in this text.

Mare

A large yolk sac is present 3 weeks after insemination and becomes an important fetal–maternal interchange medium, temporarily composed of an avascular yolk sac

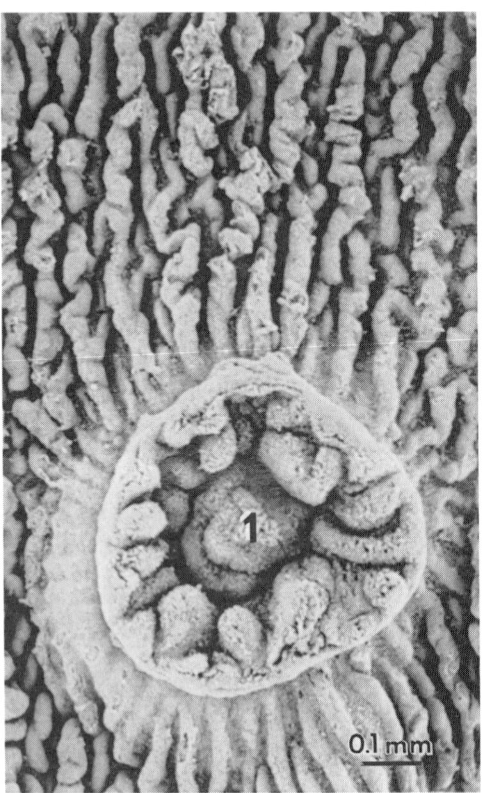

Figure 14.7. *Complementary surface to Figure 14.6 of the porcine allantochorion from midgestation with a medium-sized fetal areola (1) with villi. The chorionic rugae radiating from its periphery fuse with parallel chorionic rugae after a short distance (×50). (From Dantzer V. Scanning electron microscopy of exposed surfaces of the porcine placenta. Acta Anat 1984;118:96.)*

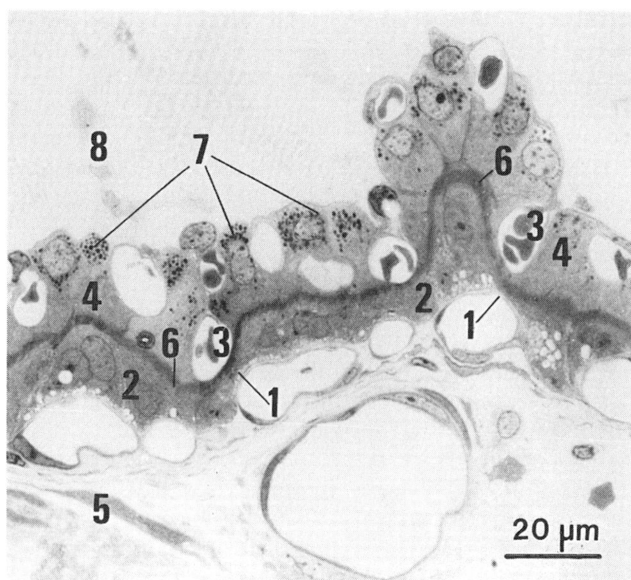

Figure 14.8. *Detail of placental fold (sow) day 99 of pregnancy, perfusion fixation from maternal side. The distance of the placental barrier is shortened by endometrial capillaries (1) indenting the uterine epithelium (2) and fetal capillaries (3) indenting the trophoblast (4). Uterine connective tissue (5); border of interdigitating microvilli (6); characteristic dense bodies in trophoblast cells (7); fetal mesenchyme (8). Epon section, perfusion-fixed from the maternal side (×660).*

wall and, in a marginal zone, a choriovitelline placenta. About the end of week 6, the change from the vitelline to the allantoic circulation is effected, and the yolk sac, although persisting until term, undergoes gradual involution (Fig 14.10A).

The chorioallantoic placenta of the mare is diffuse, villous, epitheliochorial, and nondeciduate. The embryo emerges from the zona pellucida at days 8 to 9 and then becomes completely encapsulated in an acellular glycoprotein capsule, which persists until at least day 21.

Although the equine blastocyst becomes fixed in position in the uterus at approximately day 16, the allantochorionic villi are not aggregated into tufts, called **microcotyledons**, until approximately day 60. The conceptus thus remains spherical and lies unattached in the uterine lumen, held in place merely by a pronounced increase in uterine tone until day 50.

At the junction of the developing allantochorion and the regressing yolk sac, the chorion forms an annulate **chorionic girdle** consisting of projections of rapidly proliferating trophoblast cells. Between days 36 and 38, the trophoblast cells of the girdle become binucleate and begin to invade the endometrium by ameboid movements. They destroy the uterine epithelium almost completely and implant themselves in the endometrial stroma, where they form **endometrial cups** (Fig. 14.10). The cups measure a few millimeters to approximately 5 cm in diameter. The endometrial epithelium regenerates quickly. The cup cells become densely packed and intermingled with uterine glands. They grow to large polyhedral cells with two nuclei and rER as the dominating cytoplasmic organelle. The cup cells elaborate equine chorionic gonadotropin (eCG), which helps to stabilize the hormonal function of the corpora lutea and can be used in diagnosis of pregnancy.

The endometrial cups eventually become surrounded by leukocytes, which invade and destroy the cup cells as they begin to degenerate after approximately 80 days of gestation. From days 120 to 150, their remnants are rejected. This process coincides with regression of the primary and secondary corpora lutea (formed concurrently with the cup formation), whereafter the placenta takes over the production of progesterone at a reduced level. After detachment, the cups are encapsulated by chorionic folds and form allantochorionic pouches. Also, flattened oval bodies of disputed origin, **hippomanes**, float freely in the allantoic fluid.

Fetal allantochorionic tufts and complementary

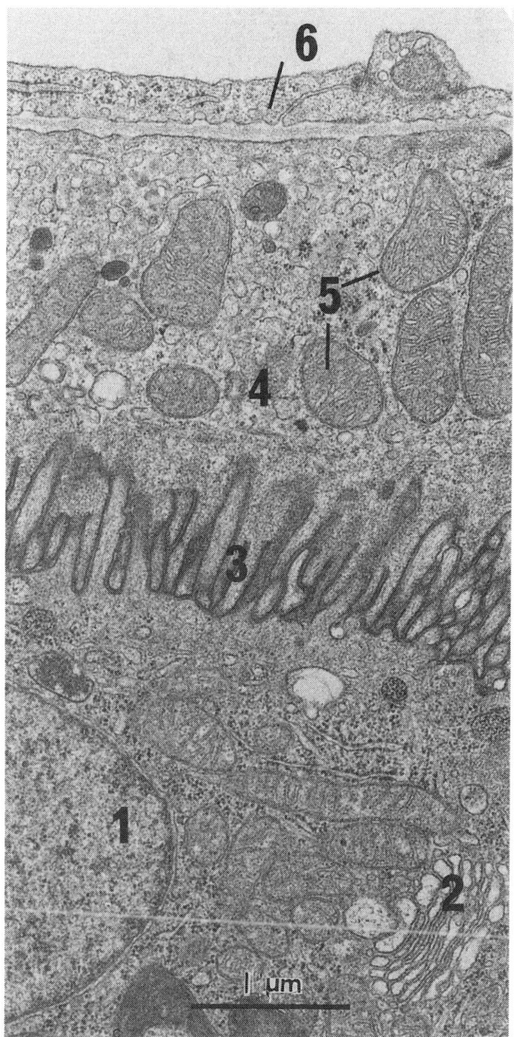

Figure 14.9. *Transmission electron micrograph from the placenta of the sow illustrates the interdigitating microvilli between the maternal epithelium and the trophoblast, as well as the accumulation of mitochondria in the trophoblast close to the apical exchange area. Nucleus of the maternal epithelium (1); Golgi complex (2); interdigitating microvilli (3); trophoblast (4); mitochondria (5); endothelium of fetal capillary (6) (×21,000).*

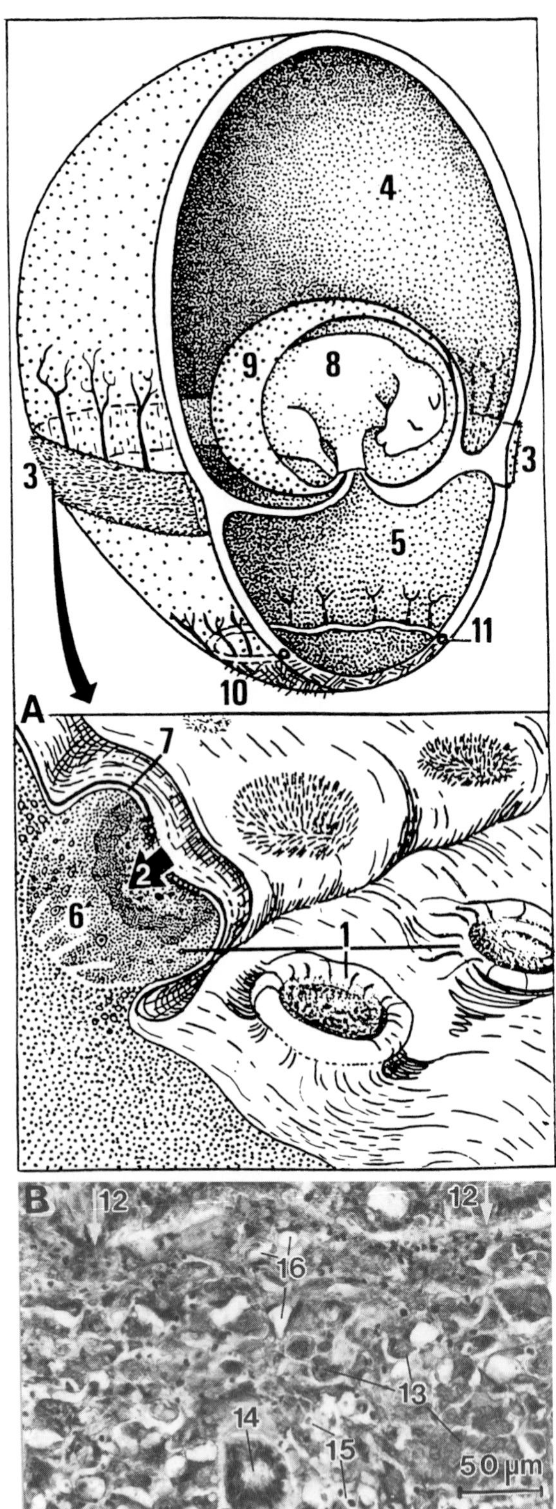

Figure 14.10. *Endometrial cups (mare) 50 days of pregnancy.* ***A.****, Schematic overview drawings of conceptus with its chorionic girdle (top) and detail with the chorion partly separated from the endometrium (bottom). Formation of endometrial cups (1) is due to trophoblast cell migration (2) from the chorionic girdle (3) — located between allantois (4) and yolk sac (5) — into the endometrial stroma (6). Uterine lumen (7); young fetus (8); amnion (9); choriovitelline placenta (10) bordered by sinus terminalis (11).* ***B.****, Histologic section from the region 2 in* ***A*** *shows the chorion in loose contact with the surface of endometrial cup (12, small arrows); large epithelioid (trophoblastogenic) cup cells (13); endometrial gland (14); leukocytes (15); uterine capillaries (16) (×220).*

maternal endometrial crypts develop after the initiation of endometrial cups (days 38 to 40), and at approximately day 150, the typical microcotyledonary placenta has been formed over the entire surface of the endometrium (Figs. 14.2A and 14.11). The fetal tufts, which are provided by a dense capillary system (Fig 14B), and corresponding crypts form placental units, **microplacentomes** (Fig. 14.11). Between these microplacentomes, the areola–gland complexes are located, with the areolae surrounding the fetal base of the microplacentomes. Uterine glandular secretory products are released into the areolar cavity between simple cuboidal endometrial luminal epithelium and columnar trophoblast lining the areolar villi; consequently, these epithelia are not in close contact (Fig. 14.11A).

In the microcotyledons, the fetal villi consist of vascular mesenchyme covered with trophoblast. The villi fit into crypts lined with simple uterine epithelium of varying height. The crypts are separated by septa consisting of vascular uterine connective tissue. Indentations of capillaries into the trophoblast and maternal epithelium are seen in later pregnancy (Fig. 14.12A).

Uterine cryptal epithelial cells are light staining. The trophoblast cells are slightly darker and have a more compact rER. In both epithelia but most prominent in the trophoblast, the sER is well developed, reflecting the high synthesis of steroids, especially estrogens and progesterone. The apical surface of the trophoblast and the uterine epithelium bear microvilli that interdigitate and form a dark border as seen with light and electron microscopy (Fig. 14.12). In the later stages of gestation before placental detachment after delivery, local apoptosis of trophoblast and cryptal epithelium is indicated by dark-staining epithelial cytoplasm and the presence of cellular debris.

Cow

The yolk sac at first has a rather large vascular area and forms a functional choriovitelline placenta. The yolk sac is rapidly outgrown by the allantois, and after 3 weeks, it begins to degenerate.

The chorioallantoic placenta is cotyledonary, villous, epitheliochorial of the subtype synepitheliochorial, and nondeciduate. The elongated blastocyst implants close to the embryo at day 18 to 19 and gradually proceeds peripherally. In the intercotyledonary areas, the trophoblast develops papillae that extend into the uterine gland openings, possibly also functioning as an anchor. They occur until day 21. At day 22, the blastocyst extends equally into both uterine horns, and by day 27, an overall intimate contact between trophoblast and maternal epithelium by interdigitating microvilli is established. A firm fetal–maternal connection is initiated at days 32 to 34. Simple villi develop from areas of the chorionic sac in contact with elevated, convex structures of the maternal endometrium (caruncles). The simple chorionic villi project into the caruncles and ramify to form branching cotyledons. The anchoring stalk of the

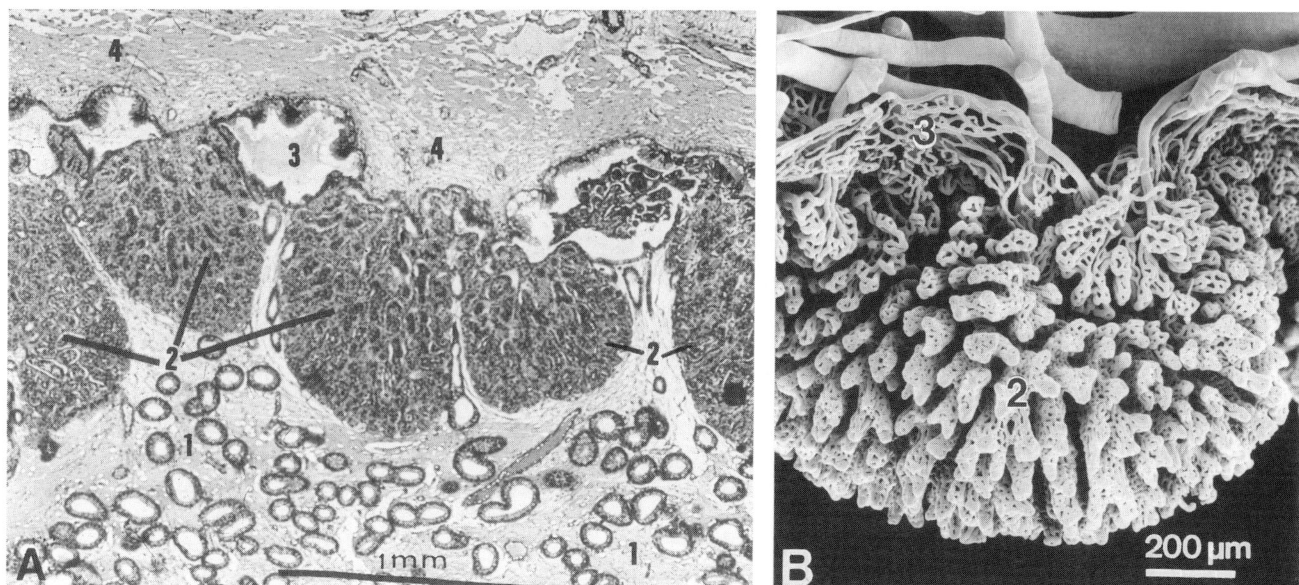

Figure 14.11. *Histologic cross section of mare placenta **(A)** and scanning electron microscopy of corresponding vascular cast showing the fetal capillary network of a microcotyledon **(B)**. **A.**, Endometrium with uterine glands (1); microplacentomes (2); areolae (3); chorionic mesenchyme (4). **B.**, The fine capillary network of the fetal villi of a microcotyledon (2) and the more loose network at the fetal areola (3). **A**: ×40; **B**: ×60. (**A**: From Björkman N. An atlas of placental fine structure. London: Baillière, Tindall & Cassell, 1970; **B**: from Dantzer V, Leiser R. Areola-gland subunits in the epitheliochorial types of placentae from horse and pig. Micron Microscopa Acta 1992;23:79–80.)*

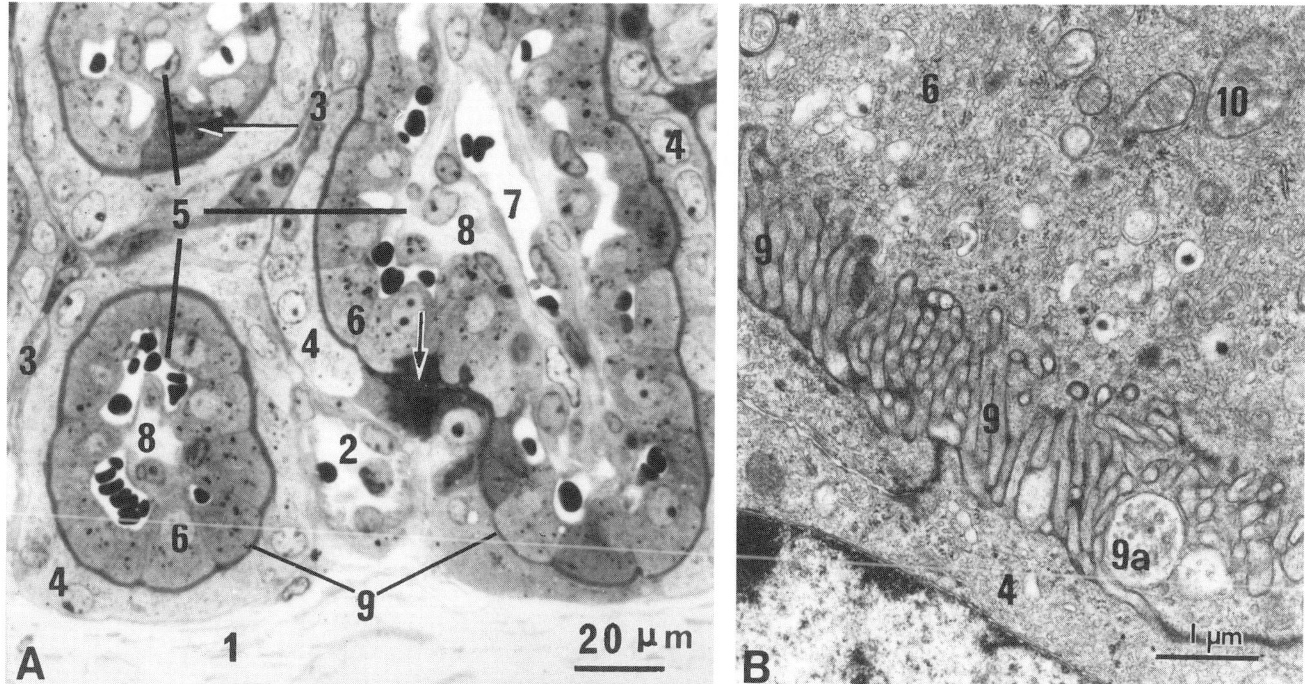

Figure 14.12. *Light microscopy of epon section of microplacentome **(A)** and transmission electron microscopy **(B)** of interhemal barrier (mare). **A.**, Endometrial connective tissue (1); maternal capillaries (2); maternal septum (3); uterine epithelium (4); chorionic villi (5); trophoblast (6); fetal capillaries (7); fetal mesenchyme (8); border of microvilli (9). The dark parts of trophoblast and uterine epithelium (arrows) are apparently undergoing apoptosis. **B.**, Detail of the uterine epithelium (4) and trophoblast (6) showing the complementary interdigitating microvilli (9) closely associated to a multivesicular body (9a); in the trophoblast, many signs of high endocytic activity, coated pits, endosomes, and multivesicular bodies and mitochondria (10). **A**: ×630; **B**: ×15,000. (**B**: From Björkman N. An atlas of placental fine structure. London: Baillière, Tindall & Cassell, 1970.)*

caruncle contains maternal blood vessels (Fig. 14.13). No uterine glands open at the caruncle (Fig. 14.12B). Together, the fetal cotyledon and maternal caruncle form the collective structure, the placentome. During gestation, the placentomes grow approximately 5000-fold, but undergo a slight involution toward term.

The bovine placentome is a slightly elongated convex structure provided with a stalk containing maternal vessels (Fig. 14.13). A chorionic villus consists of a main stem that ramifies progressively into villi of higher orders. The villi generally fit into corresponding crypts, where main septa give off septa of secondary and higher orders to form the complementary maternal constituent.

The chorionic villi of the cotyledon consist of vascular mesenchyme covered with a simple layer of trophoblast. The trophoblast is composed of mononuclear columnar or irregularly shaped cells and large binucleate cells (giant cells) (Fig. 14.14). The mononuclear cells have rounded or irregularly shaped nuclei with large nucleoli. They have a sparse rER. Relatively numerous mitochondria occur mainly in the apical portion of the cells.

Binucleate cells have spherical, separated nuclei with conspicuous nucleoli, and the cytoplasm is voluminous. At the ultrastructural level, the cell surface lacks microvilli. The cytoplasm contains a great diversity of organelles and inclusions. The Golgi complex is well developed and mitochondria are numerous but moderate in size. The cells synthesize progesterone, prostaglandin, and placental lactogen. In contrast to the mononuclear cells, giant cells show no morphologic evidence of absorption. Furthermore, the binucleate cells lack desmosomes and are mobile within the chorionic epithelium. They migrate into the cryptal epithelium, where they fuse with uterine epithelial cells to form trinucleate hybrid cells, thus transferring hormone-containing granules from the fetal to the maternal compartment (Figs. 14.3B and 14.14).

The cryptal epithelium of the caruncle is cuboidal or flattened (Fig. 14.14). The cells have spherical nuclei with distinct nucleoli. Among them are cryptal giant cells with three or more nuclei, generated by hybridization with trophoblast binucleate cells (see above and Fig. 14.14). The apical surfaces of both cell types have microvilli.

The apical borders of the trophoblast and the cryptal epithelial cells have interdigitating microvilli that are more irregular in cows than in mares or sows. The narrow space between the microvilli contains a dense granular material. Most uterine epithelial cells contain lipid inclusions in the infranuclear region.

Regressive changes occur frequently in the placentome. Both trophoblast cells and cryptal epithelial hybrid cells undergo apoptosis. In the latter case, functionally insignificant, small areas of temporary syndesmochorial placenta are formed.

Hematomata develop at the base of the chorionic villi

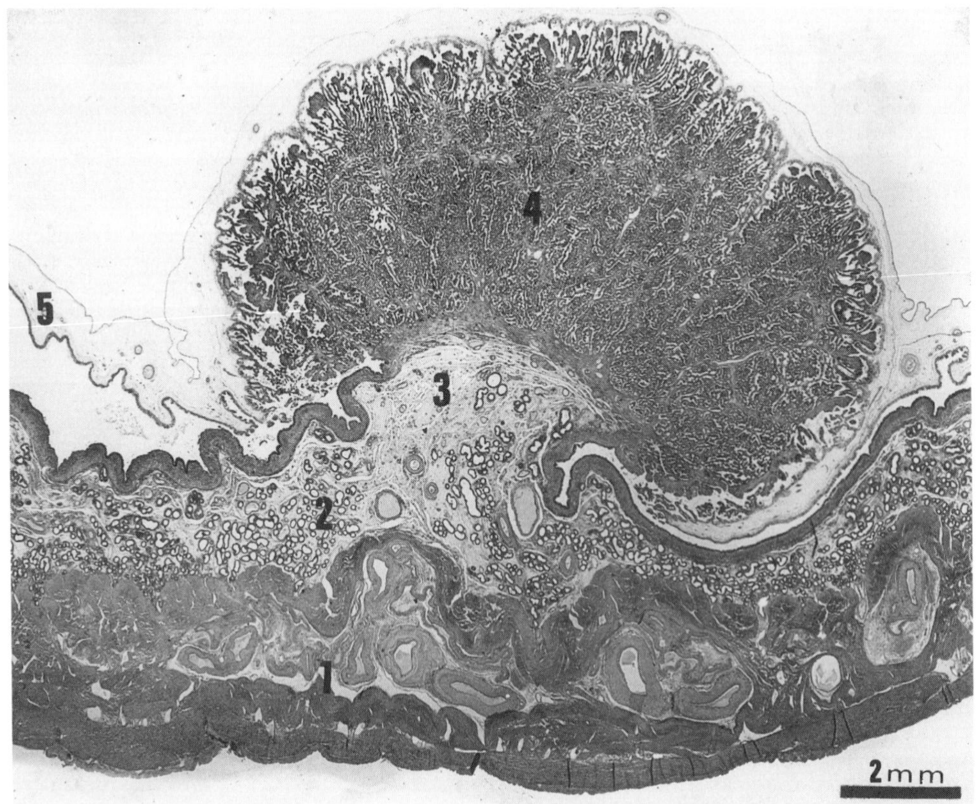

Figure 14.13. *Cross section of placentome (cow) midpregnancy. Myometrium separated into two layers by uterine vessels (1); endometrium with glands (2); stalk of placentome (3); placentome (4); chorion laeve (5) (×8). (Courtesy of A. Hansen.)*

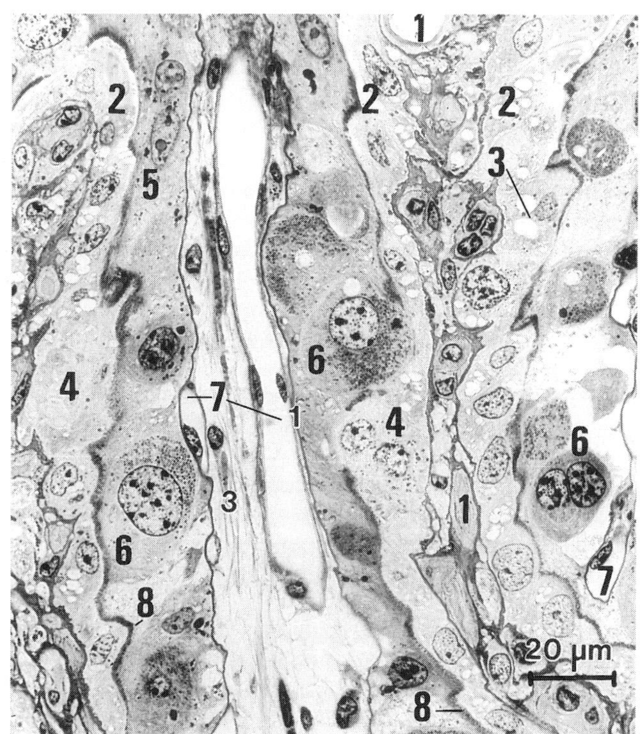

Figure 14.14. *Detail of placentome (cow) midpregnancy (compare to Figure 14.3B). Maternal septal stroma with capillaries (1); uterine epithelial cells (2), lipid droplets (3); trophoblast-uterine epithelial hybrid cells (4); mononuclear trophoblast cells (5); binuclear trophoblast giant cells with granules (6); fetal capillaries (7); maternal-fetal contact line (8) (×560).*

in the later part of gestation. Blood collects in the fetal tissues surrounding leaky vessels. Erythrocytes are phagocytized by trophoblast cells and broken down by lysosomes. Hemoglobin from the erythrocytes is digested and iron is released. These areas may be subject to bacterial infections during pregnancy.

After parturition, the chorionic villi are pulled out of the crypts. Normally, the separation occurs at the line of interdigitating microvilli, and the trophoblast and cryptal epithelium remain intact. A common complication of parturition in cattle, however, is **retained afterbirth** (retentio secundinarum), in which the villi are trapped in the crypts and the adhesiveness between the fetal and maternal tissues remains high.

In the intercotyledonary area, a smooth chorion adheres to the endometrium, except over the glandular openings, where areolae are formed. The simple columnar trophoblast and the simple uterine epithelium are both provided with interlocking brush borders (microvilli). Interdigitations are tight during early pregnancy and become less pronounced as pregnancy advances. In the intercotyledonary area, binucleate trophoblast cells are also frequent.

Amniotic plaques are yellow irregular elevations of stratified ectodermal epithelium on the inner surface of the amnion. They measure from a fraction of a millimeter to a few millimeters and contain large quantities of glycogen.

The interrelationship of the maternal and fetal capillary system is predominately countercurrent with some crosscurrent flow, making it the most efficient system of species described in this text.

Ewe and Goat

The placentae of ewes and goats are similar to bovine placentae but differ in some respects. Implantation, occurring as in cows, begins at days 14 to 15, with development of interdigitating microvilli between trophoblast and maternal epithelium at days 16 to 18. Chorionic villi are seen from day 13 to day 20. Grossly, the placentome has a concave surface. The placentome of goats is flatter than that of ewes but has a similar internal structure.

Microscopically, the villi are more irregular (Fig. 14.15). The cryptal lining consists mainly of multinucleated cell masses, symplasm, or syncytium, which has been generated by fusion of trophoblast binucleate cells (hybridization), after migration across the fetal–maternal microvillous junction (Fig. 14.3B). Here, in contrast to the bovine, this hybridization is much more active. The trophoblast also has mononuclear cells, which gives rise to the typical ovoid binucleate cells.

Hematomata are more pronounced and are located in the central concave area of the placentome. They occur earlier than in cows. Amniotic plaques are also present in ewes.

Bitch, Queen, and Mink

The yolk sac forms a choriovitelline placenta, with trophoblastic villi invading eroded uterine mucosa. This transient lamellar placenta is originally extensive (Fig. 14.16) but eventually disappears. The yolk sac, however, persists until term.

The chorioallantoic placenta is zonary, lamellar, endotheliochorial, and deciduate. Implantation occurs at day 17 in bitches, whereas it is delayed in minks. Here, the conceptus development may be arrested for more than 1 month before implantation. Implantation in queens begins at day 13 with the formation of gap junctions between trophoblast and maternal epithelium. At day 14, the trophoblast of the girdle area has intruded into the endometrium, thereby forming an endotheliochorial placenta with syncytiotrophoblast and cytotrophoblast. Here, the frondose chorion and uterine capillaries form tightly arranged lamellae (Fig. 14.2 and 14.18A), which are localized in a girdle around the equator of the chorionic sac. In the girdle, located beneath the lamellar zone is a **junctional zone** containing terminal parts of placental lamellae, maternal vessels, cell debris, and glandular secretions. The junctional zone is specifically enlarged in bitches and this layer is connected with the **glandular zone**, which is formed by the dilated upper parts of the uterine glands. In the late stages of gestation, the invasion into the glandular zone has progressed almost to the deep end of the glands, where histiotrophe and cell debris are accumulated, leaving remnants of the glandular zone at parturition

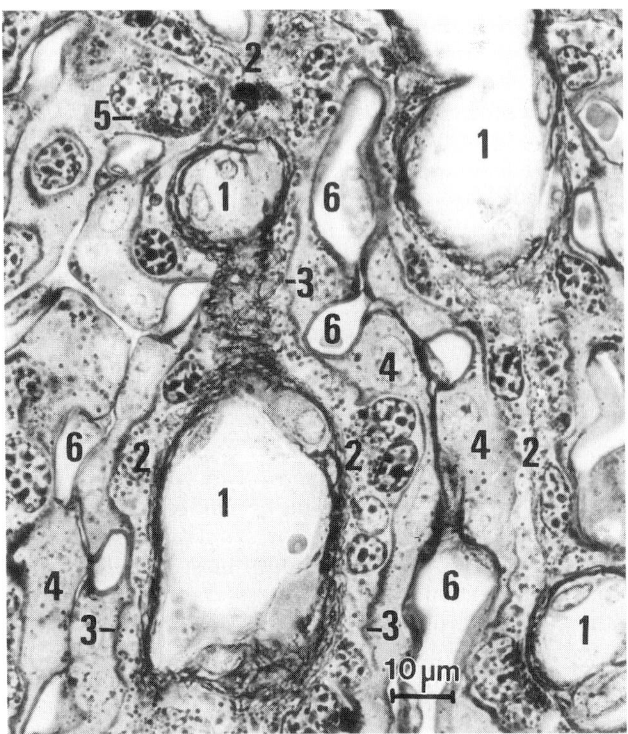

Figure 14.15. *Section of placentome (ewe) midpregnancy. Maternal capillaries (1); maternal syncytium of trophoblast-uterine epithelial hybrid cells (2); maternal-fetal contact border of microvilli (3); trophoblast (4) with a binucleate cell with typical granules (5); fetal capillaries which often deeply indent the trophoblast (6). Silver staining (×810).*

(Fig. 14.2D). Outside the girdle, a chorion laeve is apposed to the uterine surface epithelium.

Hemorrhage of uterine blood within and outside the placental girdle gives rise to hematomas. In bitches, distinct **marginal hematomas** with large blood compartments are formed (Fig. 14.17). In queens, smaller hemorrhages occur in irregular positions in the placental girdle and between the smooth chorion and the endometrium along the girdle. In minks, the hematoma is located centrally and antimesometrially. The columnar trophoblast lining of the hematomal compartments has phagocytic characteristics and is believed to be involved in the absorption of large molecules and iron from destroyed maternal erythrocytes. After breakdown of the blood, the hematomas become brown or green (in bitches) because of degradation of the hemoglobin.

The fetal part of the placenta is composed of trophoblast-covered mesenchymal lamellae, which contain small thin-walled capillaries. In bitches, the lamellae are branched, whereas in queens, the lamellae are more regularly stacked (Figs. 14.17 and 14.18), and in minks, they are rigorously twisted giving a labyrinthine appearance. Relatively wide and thick-walled maternal capillaries are enclosed by trophoblast and surrounded by a mesh of fetal capillaries (Fig. 14.18A), which gives a labyrinthine appearance in histologic sections. The maternal capillaries are surrounded by a thick, basal laminalike amorphous layer, the interstitial layer, which is especially irregular in queens (Figs. 14.3C and 14.18B). The maternal endothelial cells are prominent. Giant de-

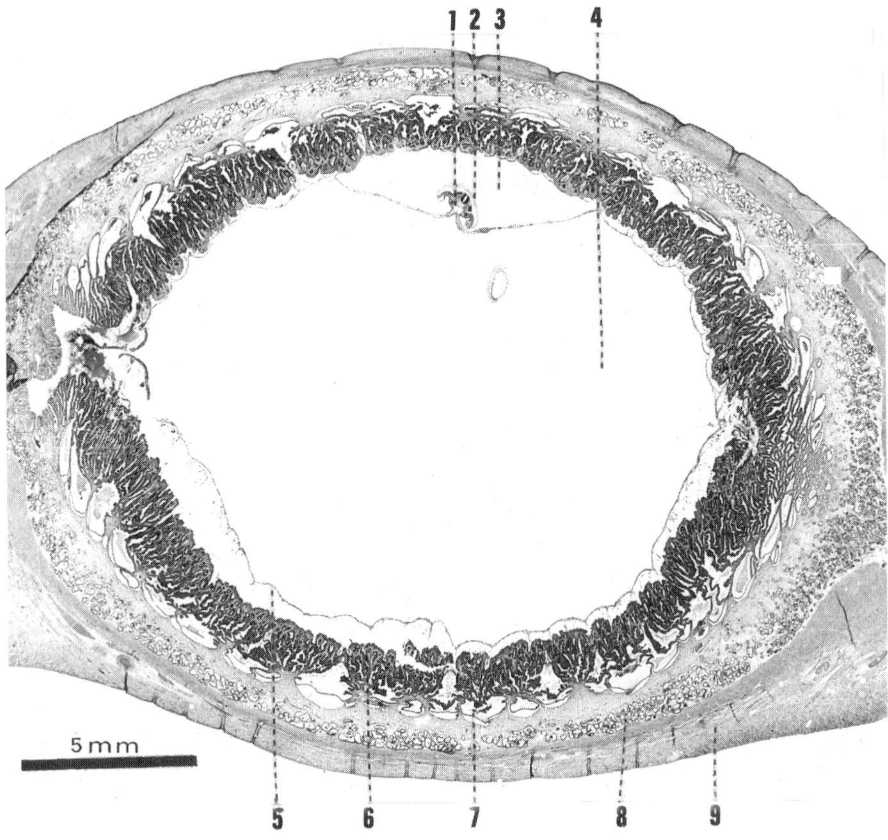

Figure 14.16. *Cross section of a uterine horn (bitch) 3 weeks pregnant. Embryo (1); amnion (2); exocoelom (3); yolk sac cavity (4); yolk sac wall (omphalopleure (5); hypertrophied epithelial surface of the endometrium containing chorionic villi (choriovitelline placenta) (6); junctional zone (7); glandular zone (8); myometrium (9) (×5). (Courtesy of A. Hansen.)*

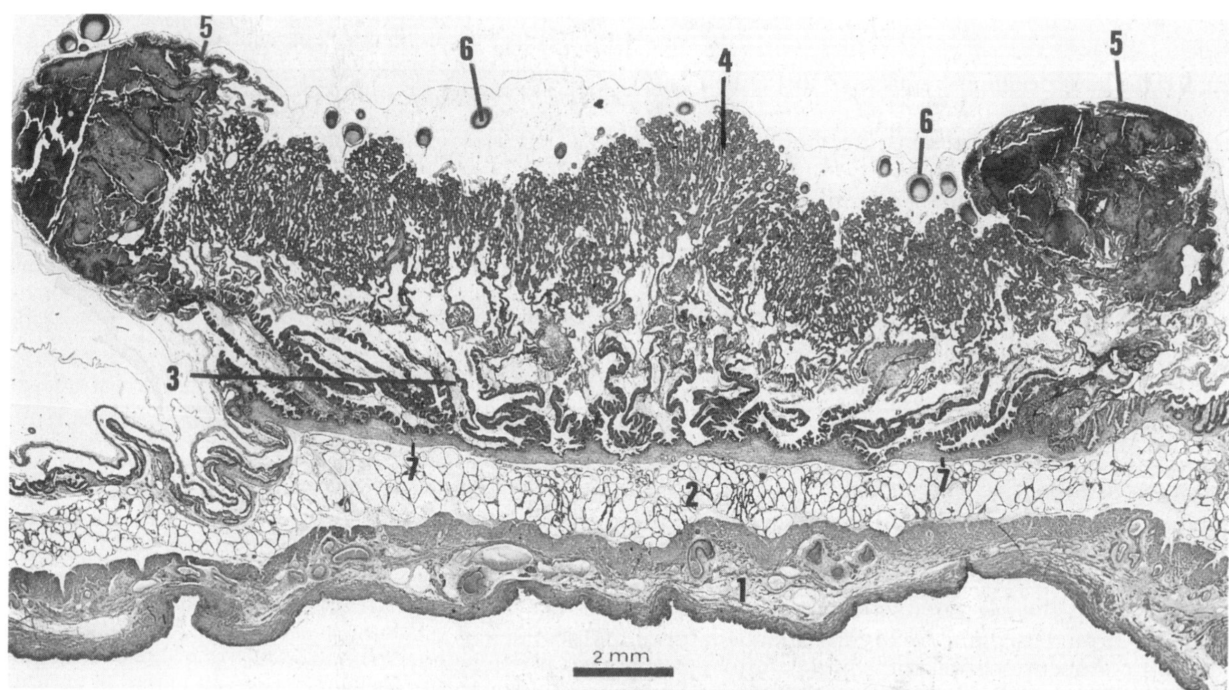

Figure 14.17. *Cross section of placental girdle (bitch) midpregnancy. Myometrium (1); glandular zone (2); junctional zone (3); placental lamellae (4); marginal hematomas (5); fetal vessels in mesenchyme (6); the supraglandular layer (7) above which the placenta is separated from the endometrium at parturition (×2.7). (Courtesy of A. Hansen.)*

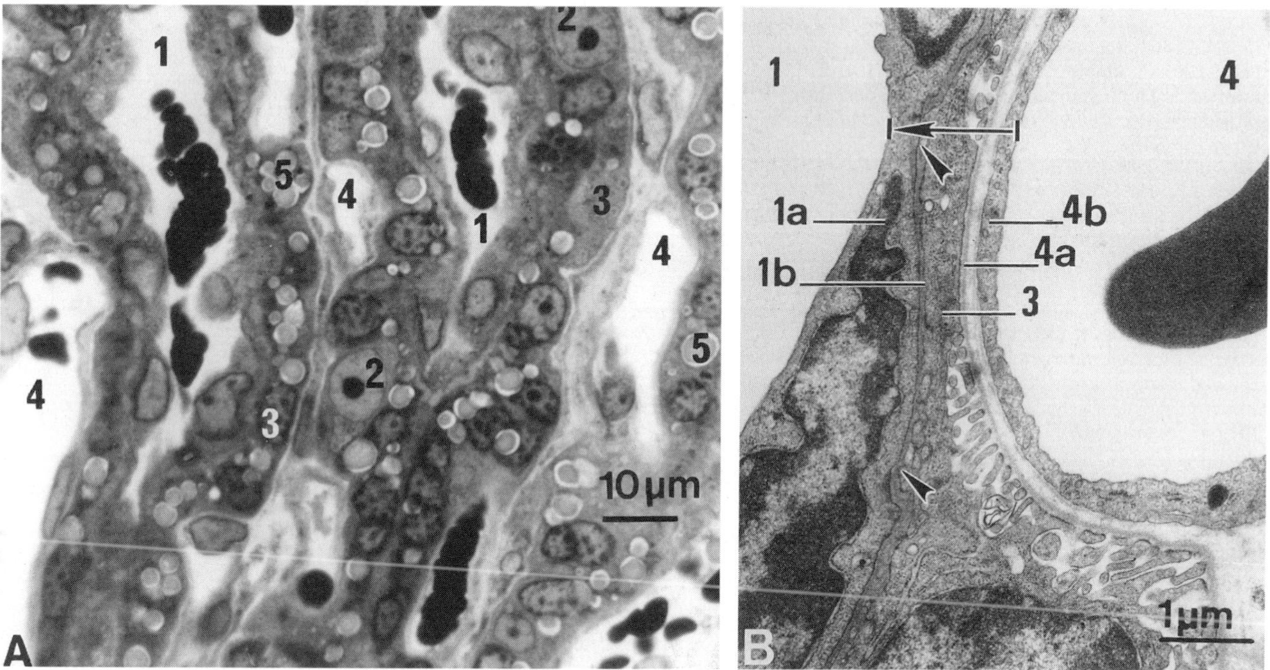

Figure 14.18. *Histology of placental lamellae (**A**) and transmission electron microscopy of interhemal barrier (**B**) (queen) late pregnancy. Maternal capillaries (1); maternal endothelium (1a), maternal interstitial layer (1b); decidual cells (2); syncytiotrophoblast (3); fetal capillaries (4); fetal basal lamina (4a), fetal endothelium (4b); lipid droplets (5), endotheliochorial contact (arrowheads); minimal interhemal distance of about 1.5 µm (arrow). **A**: ×1,000; **B**: ×12,500. (**B**: from Leiser R, Koob B. Development and characteristics of placentation in a carnivore, the domestic cat. J Exp Zool 1993;266:642–656.)*

cidual cells occur in queens (Fig. 14.18) and, less frequently, in bitches.

The trophoblast originally consists of discrete cells. A syncytium is formed by the coalescence of some cells. Thus, the trophoblast includes cytotrophoblast and syncytiotrophoblast. The syncytium constitutes the major part of the lamellae and forms a continuous interhemal barrier. The cytotrophoblast is discontinuous, and the cells occur mainly along the mesenchymal parts of the lamellae (Figs. 14.3C and 14.18A). The discrete cells contain free ribosomes and a poorly developed ER. The syncytium possesses a conspicuous ER, numerous mitochondria, and dense bodies, apparently lysosomes. In queens, the syncytium contains numerous lipid droplets (Fig. 14.18A).

In queens, in the placental girdle, the maternal and fetal capillary system meet in a simple crosscurrent blood flow interrelation. This classifies this species into a rather low efficient type of transplacental diffusion among the species described here.

At parturition, the placenta separates from the endometrium through the junctional zone above a layer of condensed connective tissue, the supraglandular layer (Fig. 14.17).

REFERENCES

Abdel Naeim MM, Saber AS, Abou EL-Magd A, et al. Scanning electron microscopical study on the microvascular development of the Dromedary maternal placenta. Placenta 1997 (in press).

Allen WR. Immunological aspects of the endometrial cup reaction and the effect of xenogeneic pregnancy in horses and donkeys. J Reprod Fertil 1982;31(Suppl):57.

Amoroso EC. The mammalian placenta. In: Parkes AS, ed. Marshall's physiology of reproduction, 3rd ed. London: Longmans, Green and Co., 1952;II:138.

Anderson JW. Ultrastructure of the placenta and fetal membranes of the dog. 1. The placental labyrinth. Anat Rec 1969;165:15.

Björkman N. An atlas of placental fine structure. London: Baillière, Tindall & Cassell, 1970.

Björkman N, Dantzer V, Leiser R. Comparative placentation in laboratory animals. A review. Scand J Lab Anim Sci 1989;16:129.

Burton GJ. Review article. Placental uptake of maternal erythrocytes: a comparative study. Placenta 1982;3:407.

Dantzer V. Electron microscopy of the initial stages of placentation in the pig. Anat Embryol 1985;172:281.

Dantzer V. An extensive lysosomal system in the maternal epithelium of the porcine placenta. Placenta 1984;5:117.

Dantzer V, Leiser R. Areola-gland subunits in the epitheliochorial types of placentae from horse and pig. Micron Microscop Acta 1992;23:79.

Dantzer V, Björkman N, Hasselager E. An electron microscopic study of histiotrophe in the interareolar part of the porcine placenta. Placenta 1981;2:19.

Dantzer V, Leiser R, Kaufmann P, et al. Comparative morphological aspects of placental vascularization. Trophoblast Res 1988;3:235.

Dantzer V, Svenstrup B. Relationship between ultrastructure and oestrogen levels in the porcine placenta. Anim Reprod Sci 1986;11:139.

Dellmann H-D, Carithers JR. Cytology and microscopic anatomy. Media: Williams & Wilkins, 1996.

Enders AC, Liu IKM. Trophoblast-uterine interactions during equine chorionic girdle cell maturation, migration and transformation. Am J Anat 1991;192:366.

Friess AE, Sinowatz F, Skolek-Winnisch R, et al. The placenta of the pig. II. The ultrastructure of the areolae. Anat Embryol *163*:43, 1981.

Friess AE, Sinowatz F, Skolek-Winnisch R, et al. The placenta of the pig. Anat Embryol 1980;158:179.

Guillomot M, Fléchon J-E, Wintenberger-Torres S. Conceptus attachment in the ewe: an ultrastructural study. Placenta 1981;2:169.

Guillomot M, Guay P. Ultrastructural features of the cell surfaces of uterine and trophoblastic epithelia during embryo attachment in the cow. Anat Rec 1982;204:315.

King BF, Enders AC. Comparative development of mammalian yolk sac. In: Nogales FF, ed. The human yolk sac and yolk sac tumors. Heidelberg: Springer-Verlag, 1993:1.

King GJ, Atkinson BA, Robertson HA. Implantation and early placentation in domestic ungulates. J Reprod Fertil 1982;31(Suppl):17.

Krebs C, Winther H, Dantzer V, et al. Vascular interrelationship of near term mink placenta: light microscopy combined with scanning electron microscopy of corrosion casts. Microscop Res Tech 1997 (in press).

Leiser R, Kaufmann P. Placental structure: in a comparative aspect. Exp Clin Endocrinol 1994;102:122.

Leiser R, Koob B. Development and characteristics of placentation in a carnivore, the domestic cat. J Exp Zool 1993;266:642.

Leiser R, Koob B. Structural and functional aspects of placental microvasculature studies from corrosion casts. In: Motta PM, Murakami T, Fujita H, eds. Scanning electron microscopy of vascular casts: methods and applications. Boston: Kluwer Academic Publishers, 1992:261.

Leiser R, Dantzer V. Structural and functional aspects of porcine placental microvasculature. Anat Embryol 1988;177:409.

Lennard SN, Stewart F, Allen WR, et al. Growth factor production in pregnant equine uterus. Biol Reprod Mono 1995;1:161.

Morgan G, Wooding FBP, Care AD, et al. Genetic regulation of placental function: a quantitative in situ hybridization study of calcium binding protein (Calbindin-D_{9k}) and calcium ATPase mRNA in sheep placenta. Placenta 1997;18:211.

Morgan G, Whyte A, Wooding FBP. Characterization of the synthetic capacities of isolated placental binucleate cells from sheep and goats. Anat Rec 1990;226:27.

Mossman HW. Vertebrate fetal membranes: comparative ontogeny and morphology, evolution, phylogenetic significance, basic functions, research opportunities. New York: Macmillan Press, 1987.

Ramsey EM. The placenta. Human and animal. New York: Praeger Publishers, 1982.

Reimers TJ, Ullmann MB, Hansel W. Progesterone and prostanoid production by bovine binucleate trophoblastic cells. Biol Reprod 1985;33:1227.

Steven DH. Comparative placentation. New York: Academic Press, 1975.

Stewart F. Roles of mesenchymal-epithelial interactions and hepatocyte growth factor-scatter factor (HGF-SF) in placental development. Rev Reprod 1996;1:144.

Stroband HWJ, Van der Lende T. Embryonic and uterine development during early pregnancy in pigs. J Reprod Fertil 1990;40(Suppl):261.

Wooding FBP. Frequency and localization of binucleate cells in placentomes of ruminants. Placenta 1983;4:527.

Wooding FBP. The synepitheliochorial placenta of ruminants: binucleate cell fusions and hormone production. Placenta 1992;13:101.

Wooding FBP, Flint APF. Placentation. In: Lamming GE, ed. Marshall's physiology of reproduction, 4th ed. London: Chapman and Hall, 1994;III:233.

15

Endocrine System

H. DIETER DELLMANN

The endocrine system is characterized by parenchymal cells that release their secretory products, the hormones, directly into the intercellular or perivascular connective-tissue spaces whereby they reach the circulatory system. The circulating hormones regulate the functions of cells in general or of specific tissues or organs, referred to as **target organs**. The endocrine system, together with the nervous system, participates in the maintenance of a steady physiologic state, called **homeostasis**. The functions of the endocrine and nervous systems are intimately linked, coordinated, and sometimes even integrated, e.g., in the hypothalamo-hypophysial systems.

The endocrine system comprises the endocrine organs proper and cell groups and single cells that are part of nonendocrine organs. Endocrine cells are usually large epithelioid cells in intimate contact with a sinusoidal blood capillary. The capillary network of the endocrine organs and cell groups is among the densest in the organism and reflects both the high metabolic activity and the route of secretion.

The **endocrine organs** include the hypophysis, pineal gland, thyroid gland, parathyroid glands, and adrenal glands.

Endocrine cell groups within nonendocrine organs are hypothalamic neurosecretory neurons, the pancreatic islets, theca interna, granulosa, interstitial and corpus luteum cells in the ovary, interstitial cells in the testis, and atrial cardiac myocytes.

Single cells with endocrine functions are scattered among the epithelium of the gastrointestinal and respiratory systems.

ENDOCRINE ORGANS

Hypophysis

The hypophysis has two portions, the **adenohypophysis** and the **neurohypophysis**. During ontogenetic de-

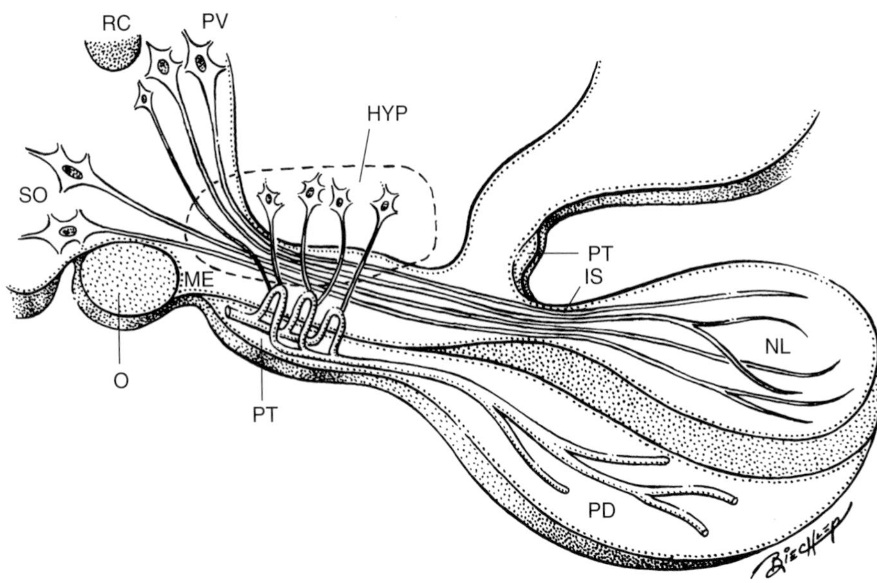

Figure 15.1. *Schematic drawing of the hypothalamo-adenohypophysial and the hypothalamo-neurohypophysial systems. Optic chiasm (O); rostral commissure (RC). Hypophysiotropic area of the hypothalamus (HYP) delineated by a dotted line; axons from the parvicellular neurons of this region terminate in contact with the primary capillaries of the hypophysial portal system in the external zone of the median eminence, into which they release their releasing or inhibitory hormones. These hormones are conveyed to the pars distalis (PD) through the hypophysial portal venules and gain access to the cells of the pars distalis via secondary capillaries. Pars intermedia (PI); pars tuberalis (PT). Axons originating from the magnocellular hypothalamic supraoptic (SO) and paraventricular nuclei (PV) course through the median eminence (ME) and the infundibular stalk (IS) to terminate in the neural lobe (NL), where oxytocin and vasopressin are stored and released.*

velopment, the adenohypophysis originates as a dorsal evagination of the epithelial roof of the embryonic pharynx (Rathke's pouch), which establishes contact with the neurohypophysis and then becomes disconnected from the pharynx. The neurohypophysis is a ventral outgrowth of the hypothalamus. This development results in intimate neural and vascular relationships between the hypothalamus and hypophysis. Consequently, the functions of the hypophysis are tightly controlled by the hypothalamus.

The glandular adenohypophysis consists of three parts (Figs. 15.1 and 15.2). The **pars distalis** (anterior lobe) constitutes the bulk of the gland, the **pars intermedia** (intermediate lobe) is closely apposed to the neural lobe, and the **pars tuberalis** forms a sleeve around the median eminence. The neurohypophysis consists of the **median eminence**, which is continuous with the hypothalamus proximally, the **infundibular stalk**, which is the distal continuation of the median eminence, and the **neural lobe (lobus nervosus)**.

The neural lobe, pars intermedia, and pars distalis are surrounded by a common capsule of dense irregular connective tissue of variable thickness that blends dorsally with the diaphragm of the sella turcica.

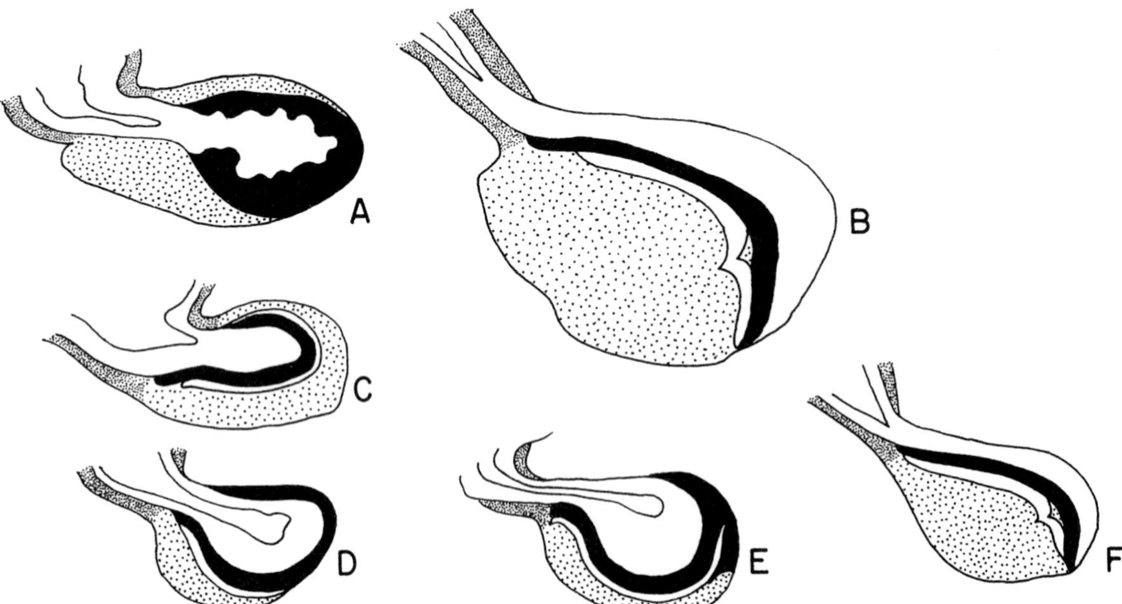

Figure 15.2. *Schematic drawing of a midline sagittal section through the hypophysis of horse* **(A)**; *large ruminant* **(B)**; *dog* **(C)**; *pig* **(D)**; *cat* **(E)**; *small ruminant (sheep)* **(F)**. *White: neurohypophysis with hypophysial cavity; small dots: pars tuberalis of the adenohypophysis; large dots: pars distalis of the adenohypophysis; black: pars intermedia of the adenohypophysis. (From Dellmann HD. Veterinary histology: an outline text–atlas. Philadelphia: Lea & Febiger, 1971.)*

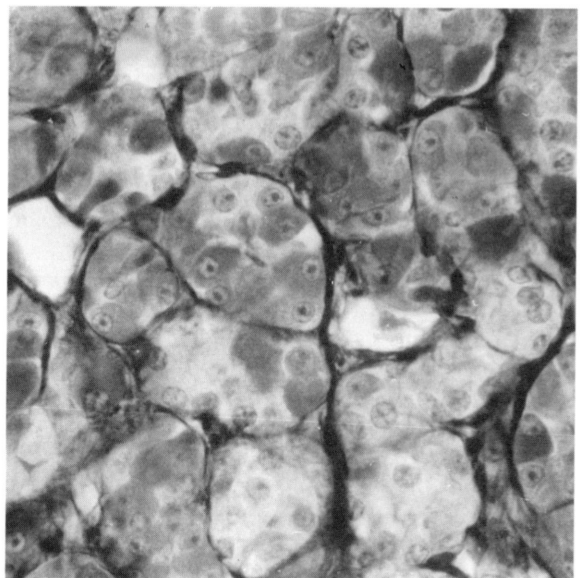

Figure 15.3. *Pars distalis of the bovine adenohypophysis with groups of dark-staining basophils and light-staining acidophils. Azan (×500).*

ADENOHYPOPHYSIS

Structure

PARS DISTALIS. The pars distalis consists of clusters and cords of cells in close apposition to a dense network of sinusoidal capillaries. The classic tinctorial distinction and classification of the various cell types according to the staining affinity of their secretory granules into acidophils, basophils, and chromophobes is useful for routine examinations of the pars distalis (Fig. 15.3). Unequivocal identification of specific, functionally distinct cell types in a given species is not a routine matter; because of species-specific staining affinities, it is subject to wide variations. With immunohistochemical methods, however, the various adenohypophysial cells can be identified with certainty in all domestic mammalian species according to the hormone (or hormones) they contain. The following hormones are synthesized by the pars distalis: growth hormone or somatotropin (STH); prolactin; thyrotropin (thyroid-stimulating hormone [TSH]); gonadotropins, follicle-stimulating hormone (FSH), and luteinizing hormone (LH); and procorticolipotropin that is cleaved into adrenocorticotropin (adrenocorticotropic hormone [ACTH]) and β-lipotropin (β-LPH).

The fine structural characteristics of the cells of the pars distalis are those typical of protein-secreting cells (Fig. 15.4). The secretory granules differ in size, num-

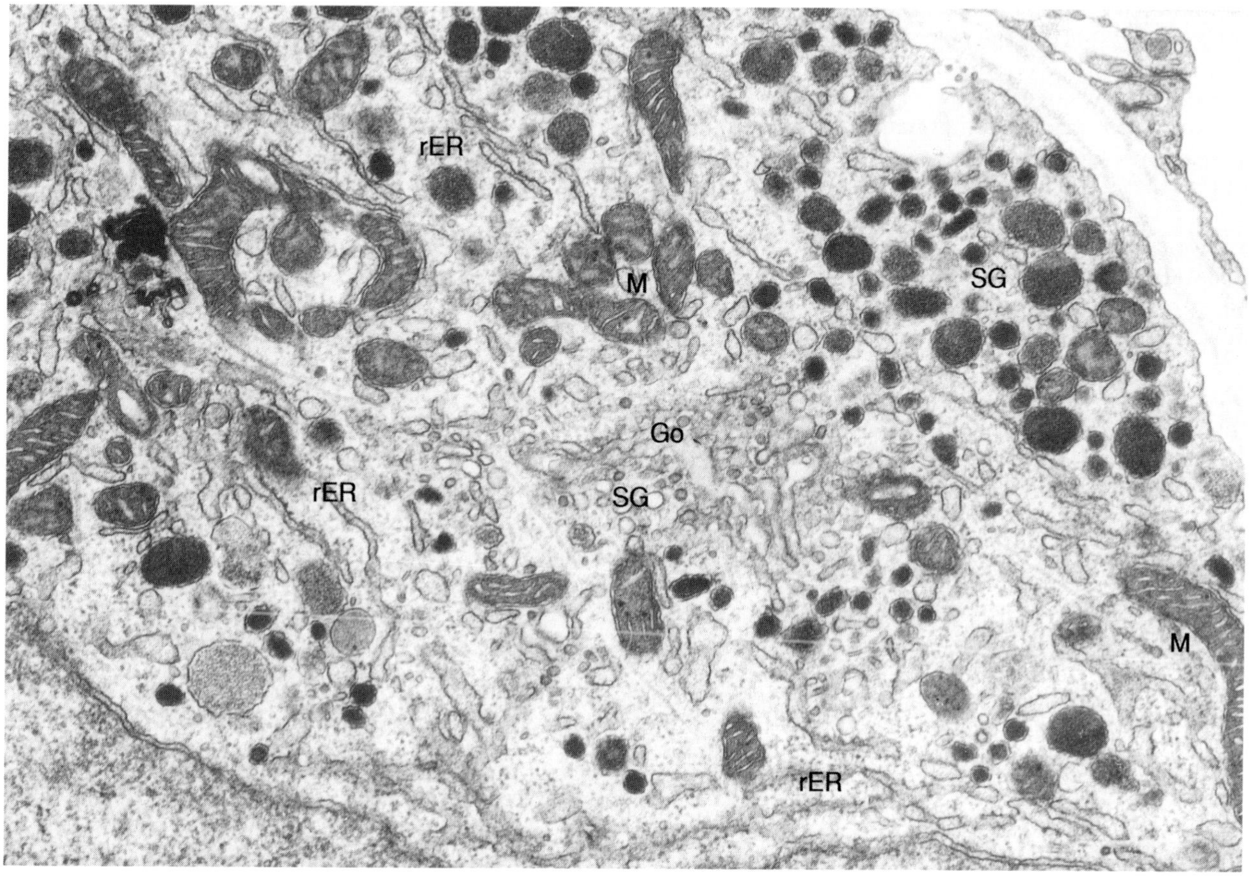

Figure 15.4. *Organelles typical of an adenohypophysial cell are depicted in this electron micrograph. Rough endoplasmic reticulum (rER); flat section through the trans Golgi network (Go); mitochondria (M); secretory granules (SG) of varying sizes and maturational stages (×28,000).*

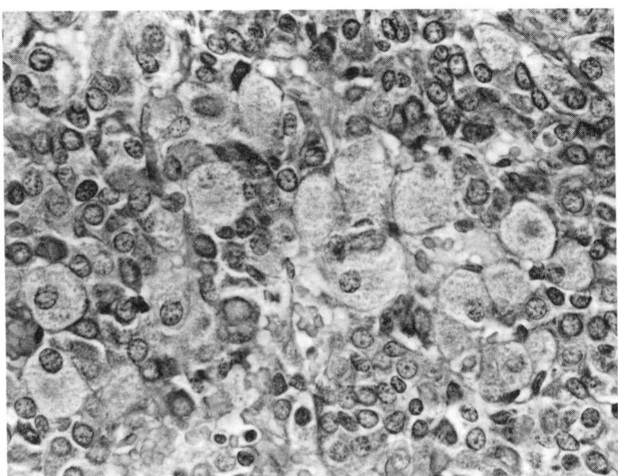

Figure 15.5. *In this pars distalis of a castrated cat, enlarged gonadotropes (castrations cells) are present. Hematoxylin and eosin (×450).*

ber, and intracellular location and permit identification of various cell types. Significant changes may be observed in the number and size of a given cell type and in its fine structural as well as light microscopic morphology. These changes are related to gender, age, physiologic (e.g., gravidity, lactation) and pathologic conditions, and experimental or surgical interventions. Many of these changes reflect the negative feedback of the target organs on the cells of the pars distalis. Affected cells often enlarge considerably and their hormone content increases, as, for example, in gonadal deficiencies or after castration (Fig. 15.5).

Acidophils. The granules of acidophils are eosinophilic. Two types of acidophils are distinguished using immunohistochemistry or electron microscopy.

Somatotropes predominate in the lateral portions of the pars distalis; their abundant secretory granules immunostain for STH, stain with orange G, and measure 300 to 400 nm in diameter.

Lactotropes or prolactin cells give a positive immunohistochemical reaction for prolactin and stain faintly and erratically with erythrosin and carmoisin in normal animals. Their staining affinity increases when the cells are hypertrophied and contain many secretory granules, as in pregnancy and during lactation. An extensive Golgi complex, long endoplasmic reticulum (ER) cisternae and lysosomes, and large granules (up to 800 nm in diameter) also characterize these cells.

Basophils. All basophilic cells give a strong periodic acid-Schiff (PAS) reaction owing to the presence of glycoprotein hormones. Furthermore, all basophil secretory granules have some degree of affinity for alcian blue. The use of immunohistochemistry and electron microscopy has identified the basophilic cell types as thyrotropes, gonadotropes, and corticotropes.

Thyrotropes predominate in the midventral region of the pars distalis; they are irregularly shaped or angular cells that are immunoreactive for TSH (Fig. 15.6) and stain with aldehyde-fuchsin. Their secretory granules are the smallest among all adenohypophysial cells (maximum diameter of 150 nm).

Gonadotropes are relatively small cells that are not always readily identified with routine histologic methods. They are immunoreactive for FSH and/or LH and stain with alcian blue and aldehyde-thionine. The rough endoplasmic reticulum (rER) of these cells is extensive, and its cisternae are sometimes dilated. Granules measure approximately 200 nm in diameter.

Corticotropes are dispersed throughout the pars distalis and are usually difficult to identify with the light microscope. The cells may be spherical, ovoid, or stellate, depending on the species. Their granules stain immunohistochemically for ACTH and β-LPH; they average 150 to 200 nm in diameter and frequently are located peripherally.

Chromophobes. The chromophobes comprise three cell types. Most chromophobic cells vary widely in shape and size, contain a few specific secretory granules, and are considered to be temporarily **resting degranulated chromophils**. The other two types do not contain any secretory granules. They are **follicular cells** that line follicles of unknown significance and **stellate cells** that are interspersed between the other cells of the pars distalis.

PARS INTERMEDIA. In most domestic mammals, the pars intermedia almost completely invests the neural lobe and is widely separated from the pars distalis by the hypophysial cleft (Fig. 15.2). Pars intermedia cells may invade the neural lobe; hypothalamic axons innervating the pars intermedia include dopaminergic axons that mediate tonic inhibitory action and serotoninergic, adrenergic, and γ-aminobutyric acid (GABA)-ergic axons with a modulatory function. Capillaries and interstitial connective tissue are generally sparse (Fig. 15.7).

In all domestic mammalian species, **melanotropes** are most abundant. They are large cells that may surround colloid-filled follicles (Fig. 15.8). Their granules stain

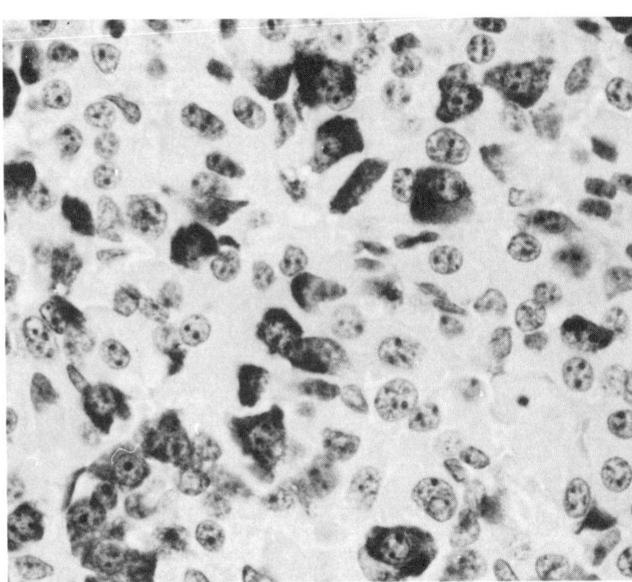

Figure 15.6. *Thyrotropes in the ovine pars distalis. Thyrotropin immunostaining (×650). (Preparation courtesy of B.D. Stahl.)*

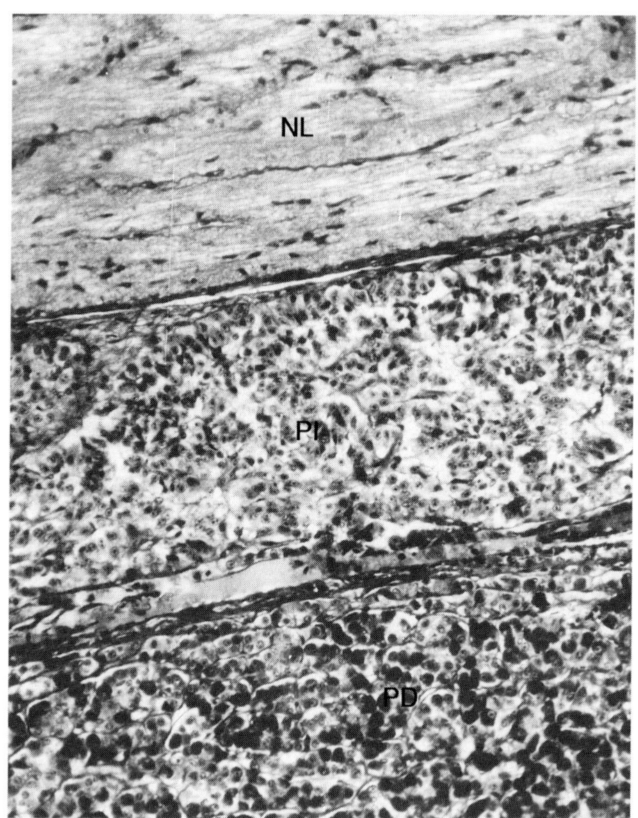

Figure 15.7. *Hypophysis (large ruminant). Neural lobe (NL), pars intermedia (PI), and pars distalis (PD) of the adenohypophysis. Azan (×170).*

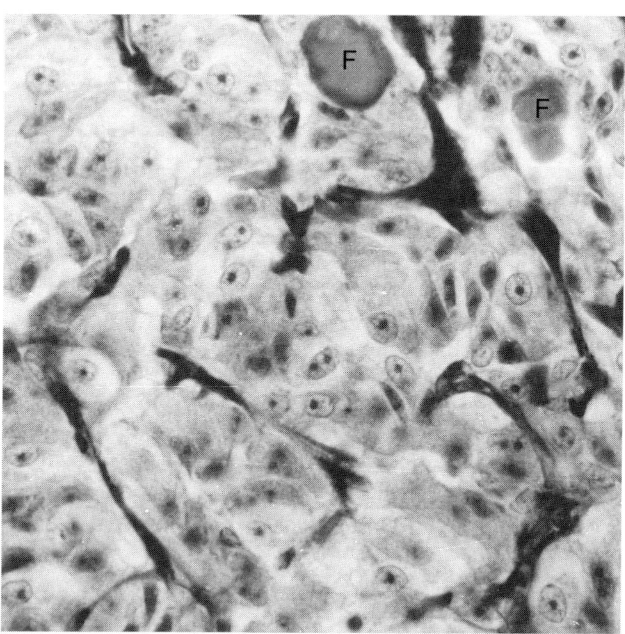

Figure 15.8. *Pars intermedia of the adenohypophysis (large ruminant). The large parenchymal cells are melanotropes, that also surround colloid-filled follicles (F). The relatively abundant connective tissue strands are characteristic of large ruminants. Azan (×550).*

immunohistochemically for melanocyte-stimulating hormone (MSH) and, in some species, for β-LPH.

Other cell types are subject to great species variation and include typical pars distalis cells (especially ACTH cells), follicular cells, stellate cells, and low cuboidal epithelial cells that line the hypophysial cleft.

PARS TUBERALIS. The pars tuberalis surrounds the median eminence like a sleeve (Fig. 15.9) and consists of clusters of epithelial cells often forming small follicles. It is traversed longitudinally by the wide hypophysial portal venules that receive tributaries mainly from the primary capillary plexus in the median eminence.

Pars tuberalis-specific secretory cells are most numerous. They possess morphologic characteristics of peptide-secreting cells that are subject to seasonal variations. They also have a high density of melatonin receptors. These cells are believed to play a role in the seasonal reproductive cycle of some domestic mammals. In addition, a few gonadotropes and thyrotropes and follicular cells are present.

Hypothalamic control of the adenohypophysis — the hypothalamo-adenohypophysial system

COMPONENTS. Most of the adenohypophysial functions are tightly controlled by the hypothalamus, which, to-

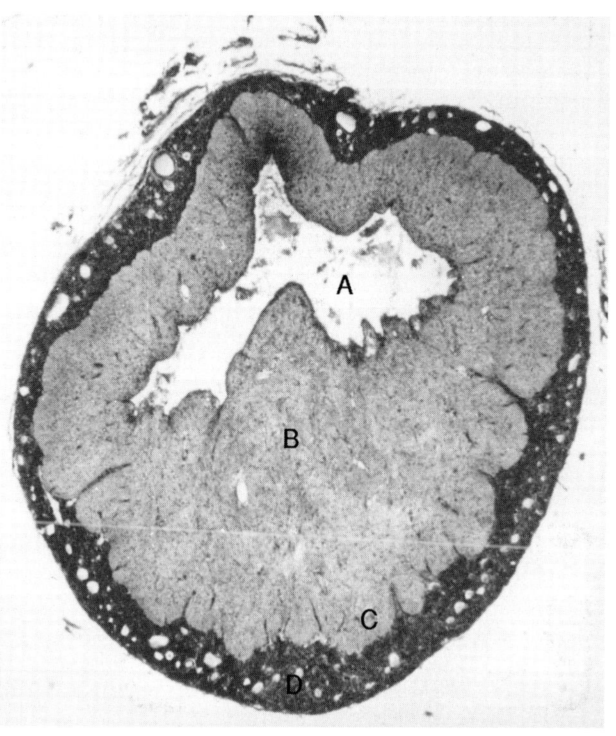

Figure 15.9. *Horizontal section through the median eminence (large ruminant). Hypophysial cavity (A); internal zone (B); external zone (C); pars tuberalis of the adenohypophysis with numerous portal venules (D). Masson's trichrome (×24).*

gether with the adenohypophysis, forms a functional unit, the hypothalamo-adenohypophysial system. This system comprises a hypothalamic neuronal component, a vascular component, and an adenohypophysial component.

Neuroendocrine cells located within the hypophysiotropic area of the basal hypothalamus (Fig. 15.1) synthesize hormones or factors that are transported intra-axonally to the external zone of the median eminence, where they are released into the primary capillaries of the **hypophysial portal system** (Figs. 15.1 and 15.9). The substances released at the axon terminals reach the **cells of the pars distalis** through this system. The hypophysial portal system consists of *(a)* a primary capillary plexus of short and long capillary loops in the median eminence, *(b)* a secondary capillary plexus in the pars distalis, and *(c)* connecting portal venules in the pars tuberalis (Figs. 15.1 and 15.9).

The functions of the pars intermedia are controlled by direct innervation and not via the hypophysial portal system.

Functions

The **hypothalamic neurohormones** or **factors** stimulate or inhibit the release of specific adenohypophysial hormones; therefore, they are called releasing hormones (RH), releasing factors (RF), or inhibitory factors (IF). They include the following: somatotropin-releasing hormone (SRH), somatostatin (SST; inhibits the release of growth hormone), prolactin-releasing factor (PRF), prolactin-inhibiting factor (PIF), thyrotropin-releasing hormone (TRH), gonadotropin-releasing hormone (GnRH, for LH and FSH), corticotropin-releasing hormone (CRH), and melanotropin-inhibiting factor (MIF).

Somatotropic hormone (STH; growth hormone, somatotropin) is a protein that promotes growth after birth. Hyposecretion of somatotropin results in dwarfism; hypersecretion leads to gigantism in young animals and acromegaly in adult animals.

Prolactin is also a protein that induces secretion in the mammary gland (lactogenic activity), stimulates growth and secretory activity of the pigeon crop sacs (crop-stimulating activity), activates the corpus luteum in some mammalian species (e.g., rat), and, finally, has prelactational mammogenic activity. Prolactin secretion is predominantly under inhibitory hypothalamic control through PIF.

Thyroid-stimulating hormone (TSH; thyrotropic hormone, thyrotropin) is a glycoprotein that acts almost exclusively on the thyroid gland, inducing the synthesis and release of thyroxine.

In female animals, **follicle-stimulating hormone** (FSH) stimulates the growth of primary and older ovarian follicles. **Luteinizing hormone** (LH) is required for the follicle to reach full size and to secrete estrogen. LH, in conjunction with FSH, causes ovulation and is necessary for the subsequent development of a corpus luteum and the secretion of progesterone.

In male animals, **FSH** stimulates the growth of the seminiferous tubules and promotes the first phases of spermatogenesis. The late phases of spermatogenesis (spermiogenesis), as well as the full development of the testis and the synthesis and release of androgens, depend on the presence of **LH**.

Adrenocorticotropic hormone (ACTH; adrenocorticotropin) affects primarily the adrenal cortex by stimulating growth of the zonae fasciculata and reticularis and by regulating their secretory activity, i.e., the secretion of glucocorticoids. In the pars distalis corticotropes, the preprohormone proopiomelanocortin (POMC) is cleaved into ACTH and β-LPH. In the pars intermedia, ACTH is further cleaved to α-MSH (melanotropin) and CLIP (corticotropin-like intermediate lobe peptide). In both lobes, β-LPH is further cleaved to γ-LPH and β-endorphin. MSH causes dispersion of melanophores in amphibians and promotes melanization of growing hair in some mammals. Evidence reveals its participation in learning, memory control, and fetal growth. LPH, in some species, causes liberation of fatty acids from adipocytes. β-endorphin action is similar to that of morphine.

NEUROHYPOPHYSIS AND THE HYPOTHALAMO-NEUROHYPOPHYSIAL SYSTEM

Structure

Embryologically, the neurohypophysis is a derivative of the ventral hypothalamus, with which it remains connected both morphologically and functionally. The hypothalamo-neurohypophysial system encompasses both the hypothalamic and neurohypophysial components.

The hypothalamic component is composed of the magnocellular hypothalamic **supraoptic** and **paraventricular nuclei**. These nuclei are characterized by large neuronal cell bodies with a positive immunohistochemical reaction for either antidiuretic hormone (ADH; also called vasopressin) or oxytocin (Fig. 15.10). Both

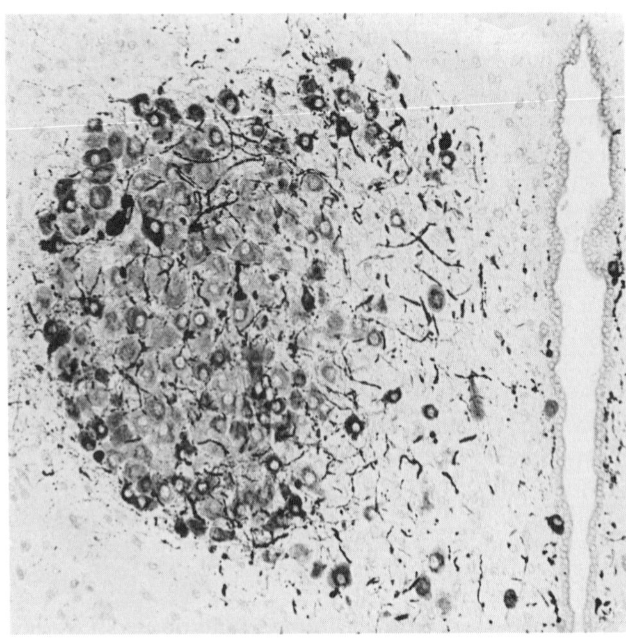

Figure 15.10. *Neurosecretory cells in the hypothalamic paraventricular nuclei have a positive staining reaction for antidiuretic hormone (ADH) (×270).*

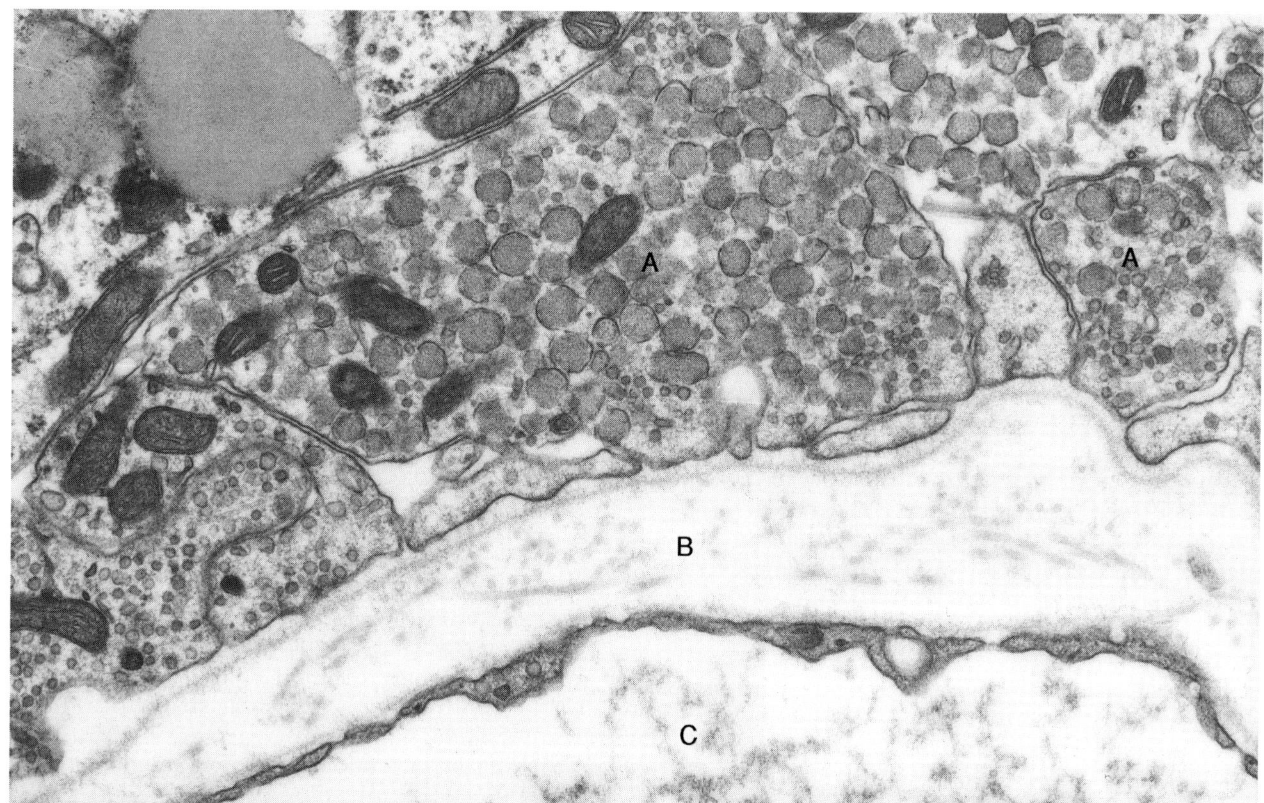

Figure 15.11. *Neurosecretory axons (A) terminate at the outer basal lamina of the connective tissue space (B) surrounding a fenestrated capillary (C) in the neural lobe. In these axon terminals, large electron-dense, hormone-containing neurosecretory vesicles are stored and their contents are released by exocytosis. The large lipid inclusions in the upper left corner of the illustration are in a pituicyte (×31,500).*

hormones are contained within secretory vesicles, referred to as neurosecretory granules, that are transported to the neural lobe within the axons of the hypothalamo-neurohypophysial tract (Fig. 15.11).

The neurohypophysial component comprises the median eminence, infundibular stalk, and neural lobe (Fig. 15.1). The hypothalamo-neurohypophysial tract courses through the internal zone of the **median eminence** and the **infundibular stalk** before its axons branch repeatedly into numerous collaterals in the **neural lobe**. Along the entire length of the tract, large axon dilatations occur, containing neurosecretory granules and other organelles in varying quantities that are considered places of storage and lysosomal degradation of ADH and oxytocin. In the neural lobe, axon terminals abut the perivascular spaces of sinusoidal capillaries; they store and release neurosecretory granules (Fig. 15.11). When many of these granules are present, they can be seen at the light microscopic (LM) level when stained immunohistochemically for the hormones they contain or with certain dyes, such as aldehyde-fuchsin (Fig. 15.12).

The glial cells of the neurohypophysis are primarily modified astrocytes and are referred to as **pituicytes**. They form an extensive, three-dimensional framework among axons and capillaries, especially in the neural lobe. In addition, microglial cells are present.

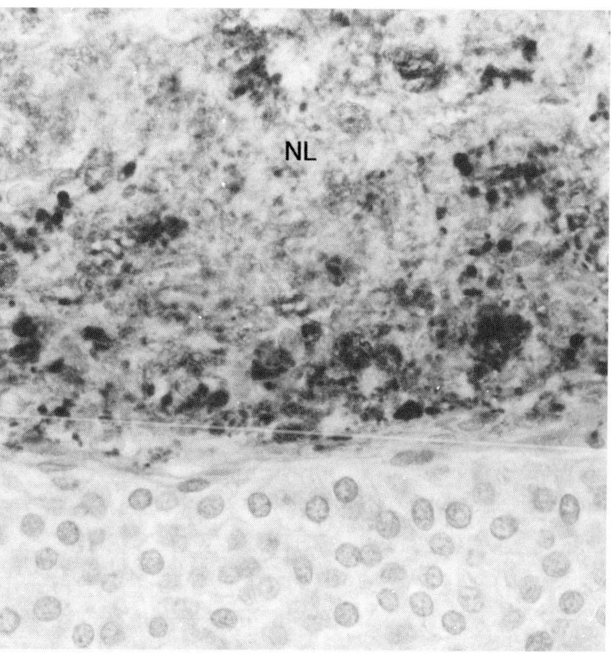

Figure 15.12. *The dark staining reaction in the neural lobe (NL) is caused by accumulations of neurosecretory granules. Pars intermedia of the adenohypophysis (PI). Aldehyde-fuchsin (×540).*

Functions

The major hormones of the hypothalamo-neurohypophysial system are ADH and oxytocin, which are synthesized as part of a larger precursor molecule in separate hypothalamic neurons. During their axonal transport, the precursor molecules are enzymatically cleaved to yield the active hormones and neurophysins, all of which are released by exocytosis of the neurosecretory granules. With immunocytochemical methods, a variety of biogenic amines, acetylcholine, GABA, enkephalin, dynorphin, and other peptides have been found in neural lobe axon terminals, either coexisting with ADH and oxytocin or in independent neural systems. Evidence shows that these substances modulate the release of ADH or oxytocin.

ADH is released in response to varying stimuli, e.g., increased plasma osmolality or hypovolemia, and acts specifically on the lining epithelium of the collecting ducts of the kidney, rendering them permeable to water. Absence or failure of release of ADH causes diabetes insipidus, characterized by increased urine output (polyuria), decreased urine osmolarity, and increased water consumption (polydipsia).

Oxytocin is released by hypothalamic neurosecretory cells in response to afferent impulses generated by mechanical stimulation of the teat. This release causes the myoepithelial cells of the mammary gland to contract, thereby resulting in ejection of milk. Oxytocin is also released during parturition, which causes the uterine musculature to contract. The functional significance of neurophysins is unknown.

Pineal Gland

STRUCTURE

The mammalian pineal gland or epiphysis cerebri is an outgrowth of the roof of the diencephalon, to which it is attached by a stalk. It is surrounded by a thin layer of pial connective tissue, from which originate connective-tissue septae and trabeculae. These structures partition the organ into irregular lobules, composed of parenchymal cell cords and follicles. The parenchyma consists mainly of pinealocytes and glial cells (Fig. 15.13).

Stellate **pinealocytes** (pineal endocrine cells) predominate in the mammalian pineal gland. Their processes establish contact with other pinealocytes or pericapillary spaces. Synaptic contacts on pinealocytes are exclusively by postganglionic nerve fibers from the cranial cervical ganglia. Glial cells are predominantly **astrocytes** with characteristics similar to those in the remainder of the central nervous system. **Ependymal cells** line the pineal recess, an extension of the third cerebral ventricle. Intercellular calcium deposits (brain sand, corpora arenacea) occur frequently. The pineal gland is permeated by a sinusoidal capillary network into which pinealocytes release their secretory products.

FUNCTIONS

The main secretory product of the pinealocytes is melatonin, the secretion of which is driven by the dark phase of the photoperiod. Information from the retina reaches the pineal via the hypothalamic suprachiasmatic nucleus, midbrain tegmentum, cervical spinal cord, and cranial cervical ganglion. The reported actions of melatonin include direct or indirect involvement in daily and seasonal photoperiodically induced rhythms, in sexual behavior and reproduction, and in thermoregulation.

Thyroid Gland

STRUCTURE

The thyroid gland is surrounded by a thin **capsule** of dense irregular connective tissue from which septa extend into the parenchyma, subdividing it into lobules. These lobules comprise thyroid follicles, parafollicular cells, sparse interstitial loose connective tissue, and dense networks of sinusoidal and lymph capillaries.

Thyroid follicles (Fig. 15.14) (20 to 500 μm in diameter) are vesicles that are lined by follicular cells and usually filled with colloid. Follicular structure reflects various physiologic conditions. When resting, the simple epithelium is low cuboidal or even squamous, and the colloid appears dense and uniformly stained. When stimulated, the cells become cuboidal or columnar, and the colloid is nonuniformly stained and often contains peripheral vacuoles.

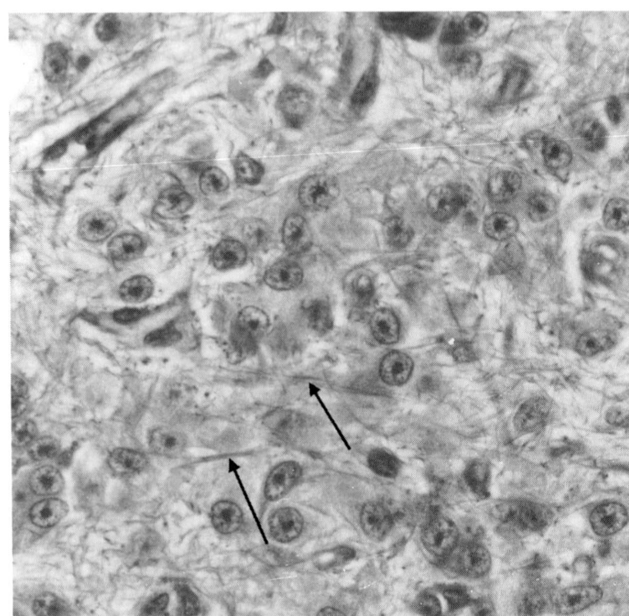

Figure 15.13. *In this section from a bovine pineal gland, the spherical nuclei with distinct nucleoli belong to pinealocytes, the cytoplasm of which has little staining affinity. Numerous delicate astrocyte processes are present (arrows). Azan (×560). (From Dellmann H-D. Veterinary histology: an outline text–atlas. Philadelphia: Lea & Febiger, 1971.)*

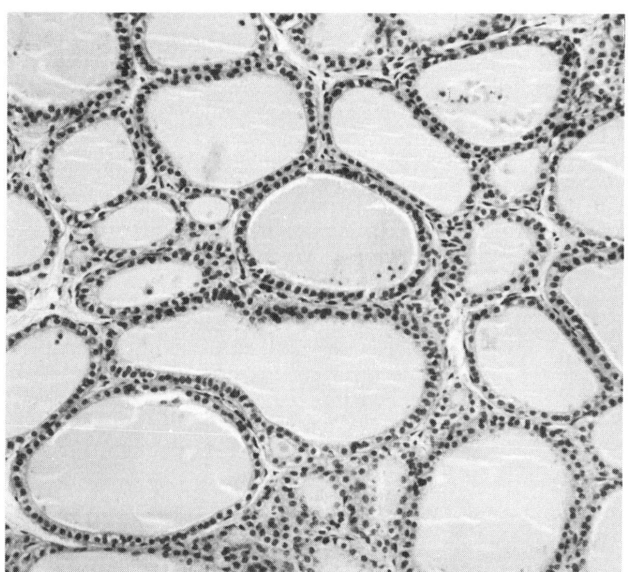

Figure 15.14. *Thyroid follicles of varying sizes and shapes are filled with colloid and lined with a simple cuboidal follicular epithelium (×145).*

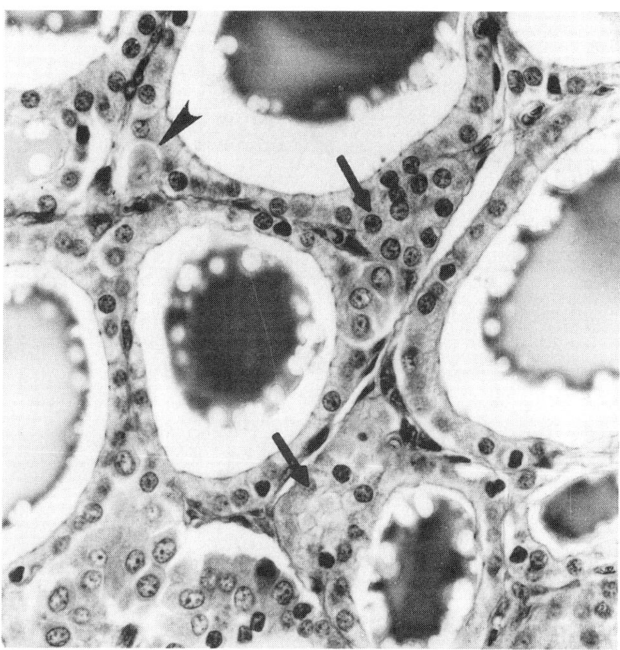

Figure 15.15. *Parafollicular cells in the dog thyroid gland occur as single cells (arrow head) but frequently form relatively large clusters (arrows). Trichrome (×270).*

The follicular colloid stains with either acid or basic dyes; it is PAS-positive because of its content of thyroglobulin, an iodinated glycoprotein, which is the storage form of thyroxine.

Active **follicular cells** have a distinct structural polarity. The nucleus is located in the cell base. Mitochondria, rER, ribosomes, and polysomes are distributed throughout the cytoplasm. The Golgi complex lies between the nucleus and the microvillous apical cell surface. The apical cytoplasm also contains condensing vacuoles, which originate from the Golgi complex and contain thyroglobulin, which is secreted by exocytosis into the follicular lumen. In addition, large, membrane-bound colloid droplets, lysosomes, and phagolysosomes are present.

Parafollicular or **C cells** derive from the neural crest. They belong to the APUD (**a**mine **p**recursor **u**ptake and **d**ecarboxylation) system of endocrine cells (see p. 302). They usually occur as single cells enclosed within the basal lamina of the follicles but may also form groups in the same location or outside the follicles (Figs. 15.15 and 15.16), especially in dogs. C cells are characterized by light-staining cytoplasm, little ER, abundant Golgi complex, many mitochondria, and especially numerous, small secretory granules (Fig. 15.16). They secrete calcitonin (thyrocalcitonin).

FUNCTIONS

Thyroid hormone biosynthesis and secretion are regulated by adenohypophysial TSH and occur simultaneously in active follicles, so that hormone release is a continuous process. Biosynthesis begins with the formation of thyroglobulin in the usual rER–Golgi complex sequence followed by secretion, via secretory vesicles, into the follicular lumen (Fig. 15.17). By way of the same synthetic steps and very likely the same route, thyroperoxidase is synthesized, packaged, and released into the follicular lumen, where it is responsible for the iodination of thyroglobulin, i.e., the attachment of iodine to the tyrosyl radicals of thyroglobulin. Pseudopods form at the luminal surface of follicular cells and initiate endocytosis of the stored thyroglobulin, resulting in large colloid droplets. These droplets merge with lysosomes to form phagolysosomes, in which thyroglobulin is broken down by proteolytic digestion to yield the active hormones (thyroxine [T_4] and triiodothyronine [T_3]) that diffuse into the cytosol and out of the cell base into the pericapillary space.

The cellular actions of thyroid hormones and their physiologic and metabolic functions, as well as their morphologic effects, are too varied and numerous to be enumerated here. The reader is referred to specialized texts.

The C cells secrete primarily calcitonin, which lowers the blood calcium level by suppressing bone resorption. In addition, serotonin, somatostatin, and a variety of other substances characteristic of APUD cells are present; their functions remain to be elucidated.

Parathyroid Gland

STRUCTURE

The parathyroid gland is surrounded by a capsule of dense irregular connective tissue. Delicate septa are present in most domestic mammalian species.

The highly vascularized parenchyma is generally arranged in clusters, strands, or cords and contains mainly

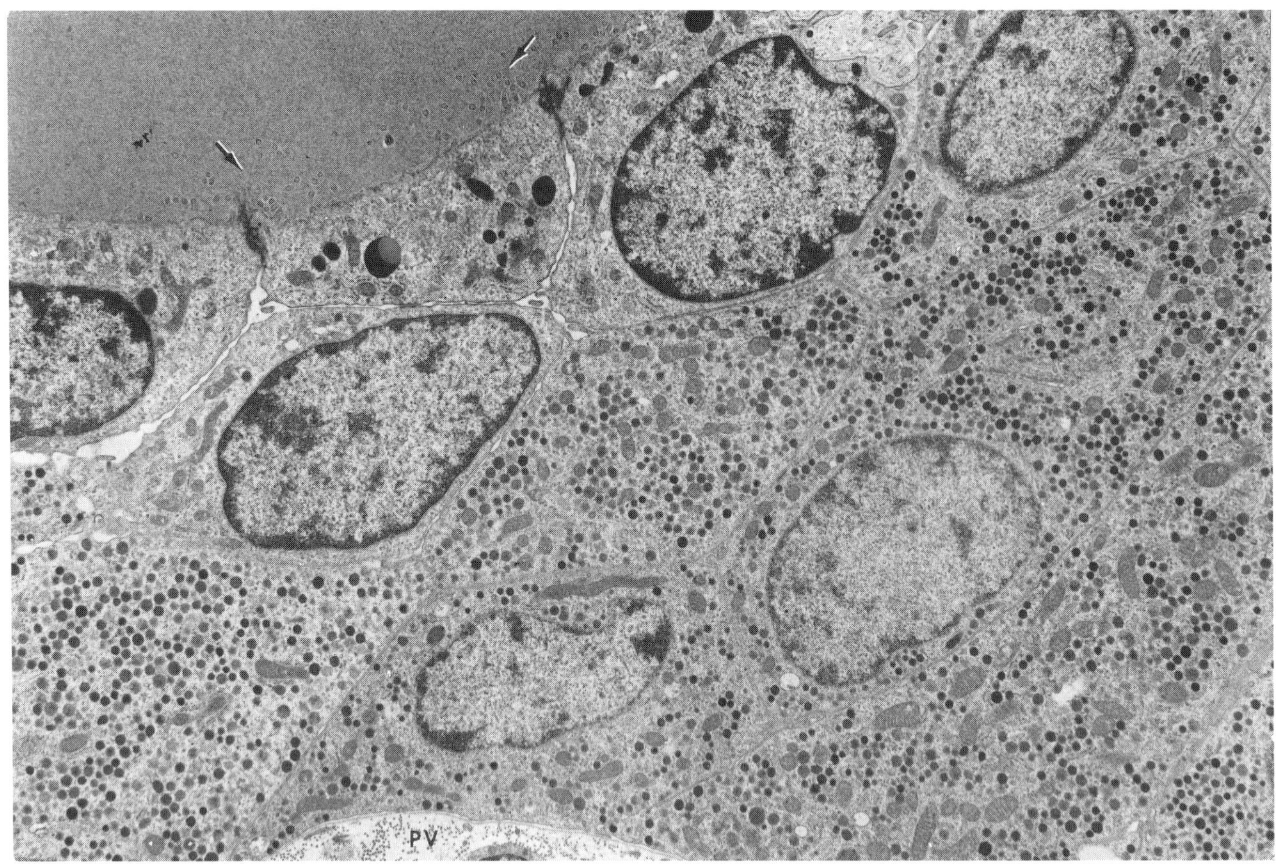

Figure 15.16. *This electron micrograph illustrates follicular cells with microvilli (arrows) projecting into the follicular colloid and a cluster of parafollicular cells abutting a pericapillary space (PV)(×7900). (Courtesy of K.R. Moore and S.L. Teitelbaum.)*

a single basic cell type, the principal cell (Fig. 15.18.1). Principal cells are in various stages of secretory activity and designated as inactive (light) and active (dark) principal cells.

The **inactive** (light) **principal cells** usually are the most frequent cell type (Fig. 15.18.2). They are considered to be in a resting stage or at the end of a secretory cycle. They are relatively large, acidophilic cells. The Golgi complex is inconspicuous, the rER is concentrated in small areas, and secretory granules are occasionally present; lipid droplets and lipofuscin inclusions (cattle) or glycogen (cats) may be present.

In **active** (dark) **principal cells** (Fig. 15.18.2), the cytoplasm appears dark and contains an extensive Golgi complex, abundant rER, and numerous mitochondria and secretory granules. The entire appearance is that of a stimulated cell.

In addition, a second cell type, the **oxyphil cell**, is present rather regularly in horses and large ruminants but is rare in other domestic mammals. These large cells (up to 27 μm in diameter in horses) occur either singly or in clusters (Fig. 15.19). They possess a small heterochromatic nucleus and a light-staining cytoplasm, which is literally filled with mitochondria. Golgi complex, rER, and secretory granules are scarce, suggesting an inactive stage of secretion. The functional significance of oxyphil cells is unknown.

A **transitional cell** type with structural characteristics intermediate between those of principal and oxyphil cells, i.e., with many mitochondria, relatively abundant rER, Golgi complex, and secretory granules, is likewise present.

In goats and sheep, the periphery of the gland is occupied by light principal cells, and the dark principal cells are in the center. In all other domestic mammals, the dark and light principal cells are distributed randomly with one or the other form prevailing, depending on the functional phase of the glands. Colloidal cysts with ciliated lining cells are frequent.

In dogs and sometimes in horses, the parenchymal cells form a simple pericapillary epithelial layer with occasional rosettelike formations (Fig. 15.18.1).

FUNCTIONS

The parathyroid glands produce parathormone, principal role of which is to maintain normal levels of calcium and phosphorus in the blood. It does so by inducing an increased absorption of calcium from the

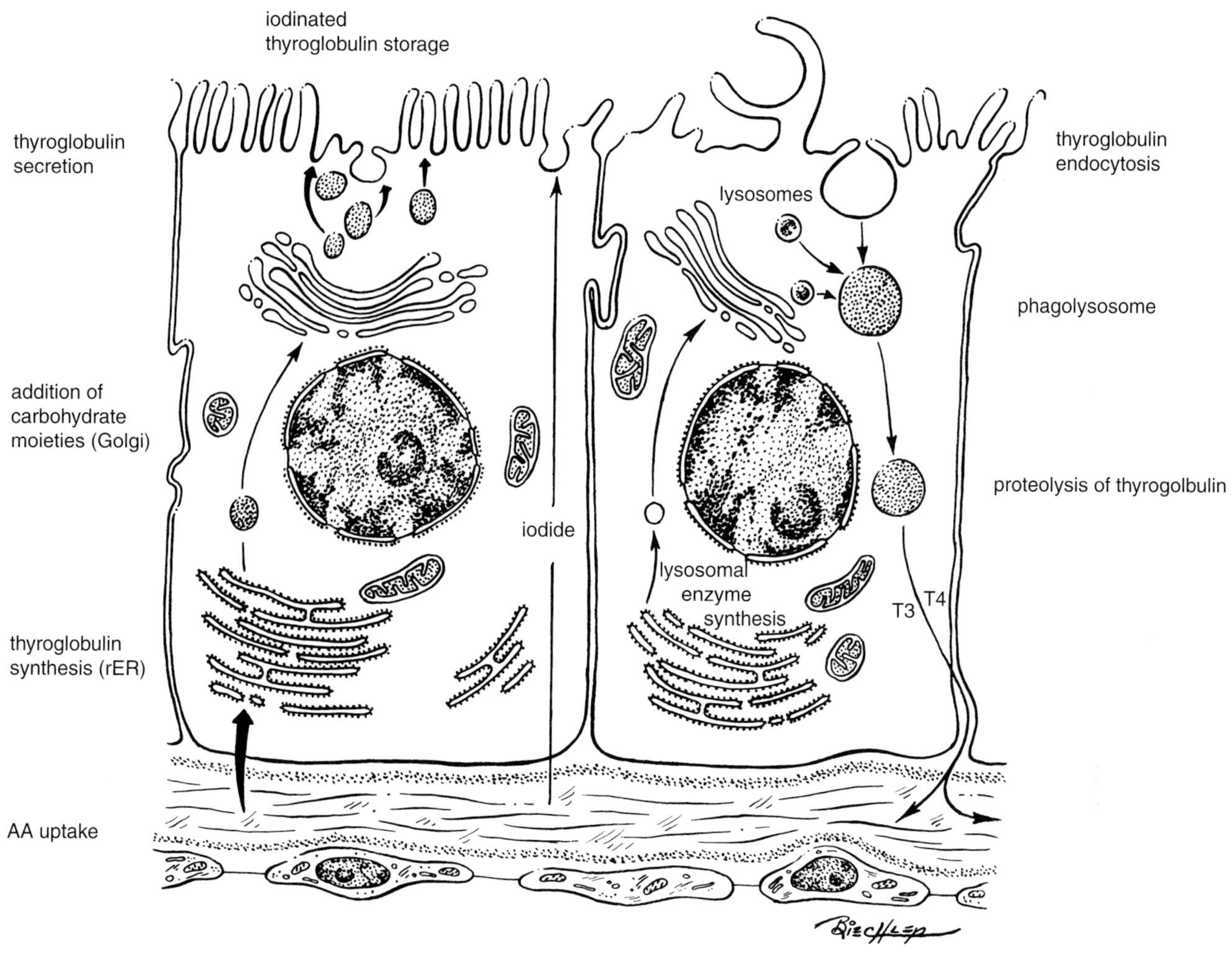

Figure 15.17. *Schematic drawing of the biosynthesis of thyroglobulin (left) and its resorption and proteolysis (right). For didactic purposes, events are depicted in two cells but they do occur in the same cell.*

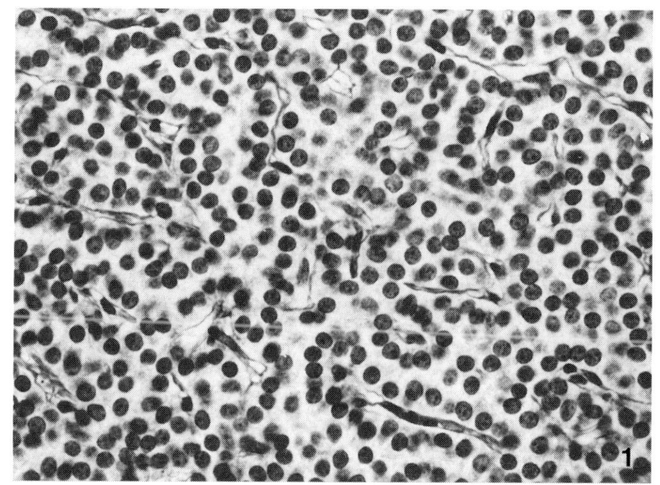

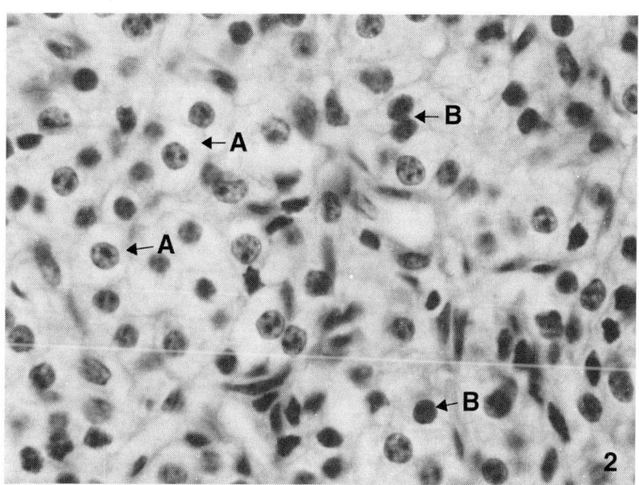

Figure 15.18. *1., In the canine parathyroid gland, cells are arranged in strands along capillaries. Hematoxylin and eosin (×690). 2., Inactive parathyroid cells (A) are characterized by light-staining cytoplasm whereas that of active cells (B) is much darker. Hematoxylin and eosin (×940). (From Dellmann H-D. Veterinary histology: an outline text–atlas. Philadelphia: Lea & Febiger, 1971.)*

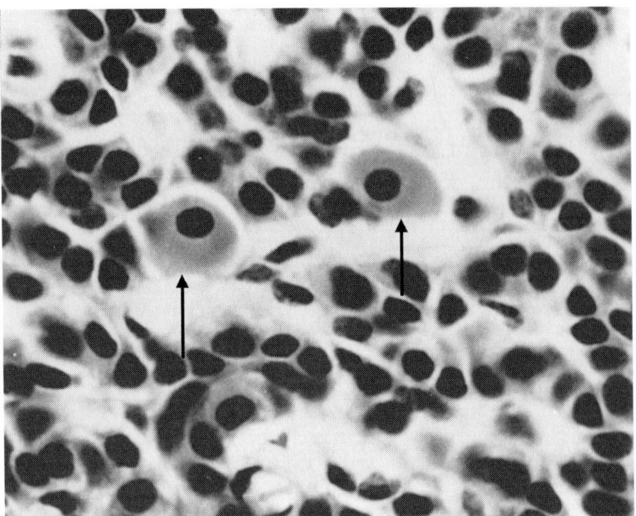

Figure 15.19. *Two large oxyphil cells (arrows) in an equine parathyroid gland. Hematoxylin and eosin (×925).*

intestine, a resorption of calcium from bones (activation of osteoclasts), and a decreased loss of calcium in the urine. Parathyroid hormone acts directly on the proximal tubules of the kidney to inhibit the reabsorption of phosphate and to promote the reabsorption of calcium.

In severe parathyroid hormone deficiencies (e.g., after parathyroidectomy), the decreased blood calcium level causes fibrillary twitching in various muscles (increase in neuromuscular irritability), followed by clonic movements of the limbs and, finally, by rigid spasms (tetany) and death.

Adrenal Gland

STRUCTURE

The adrenal gland comprises an outer cortex of mesodermal origin and an inner medulla, derived from neuroectoderm. It is surrounded by a common thin capsule of dense irregular connective tissue that contains occasional smooth muscle fibers (Fig. 15.20). Thin trabeculae originate from the capsule and penetrate the cortex but rarely enter the medulla. Clusters of cells, considered to be undifferentiated cells that later become the cells of the zona glomerulosa, are seen in the capsule (Fig. 15.21).

Cortex

The adrenal cortex is subdivided into three distinct zones (Fig. 15.20): *(a)* the outermost zona glomerulosa, followed by *(b)* the zona fasciculata and *(c)* the zona reticularis, which lies adjacent to the medulla.

The **zona glomerulosa** in ruminants (Fig. 15.22A) is formed of irregular clusters and cords of cells. In horses, donkeys (Fig. 15 22B), carnivores, and pigs, this zone is called the **zona arcuata** because the cells are arranged in arcs, with their convexity directed toward the periphery.

In horses and donkeys, the cells are tall columnar cells (Fig. 15.22B); they are spherical in the other domestic mammals (Fig. 15.22A). Their fine structural characteristics are those of steroid-secreting cells, i.e., abundant sER, tubular-type mitochondria, little rER, a multilocular

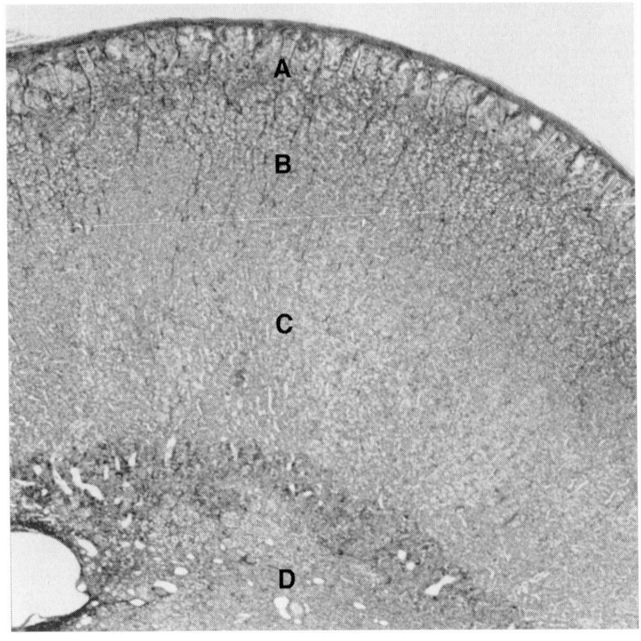

Figure 15.20. *In this equine adrenal gland, the three zones of the cortex, the zona glomerulosa (arcuata) (A), zona fasciculata (B), and zona reticularis (C), as well as the highly vascularized medulla (D) are readily distinguished. Hematoxylin and eosin (×20). (From Dellmann H-D. Veterinary histology: an outline text–atlas. Philadelphia: Lea & Febiger, 1971.)*

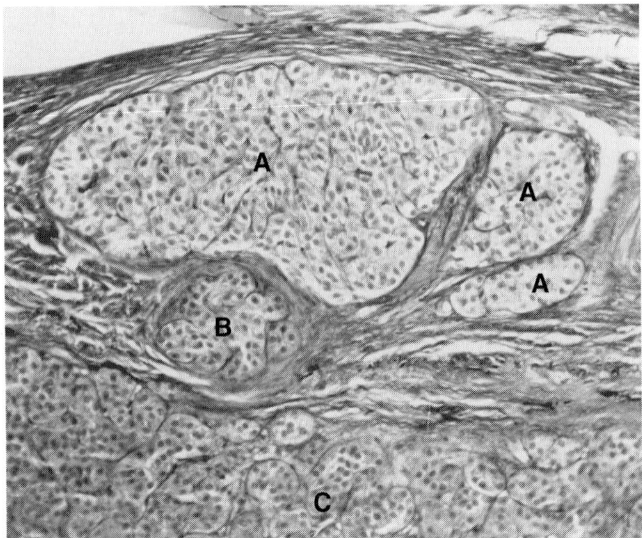

Figure 15.21. *Clusters (A) of light staining undifferentiated cells within the capsule of a bovine adrenal gland. Note that the cells in the small, slightly deeper cluster (B) resemble those of the zona glomerulosa (C). Hematoxylin and eosin (×175). (From Dellmann H-D. Veterinary histology: an outline text–atlas. Philadelphia: Lea & Febiger, 1971.)*

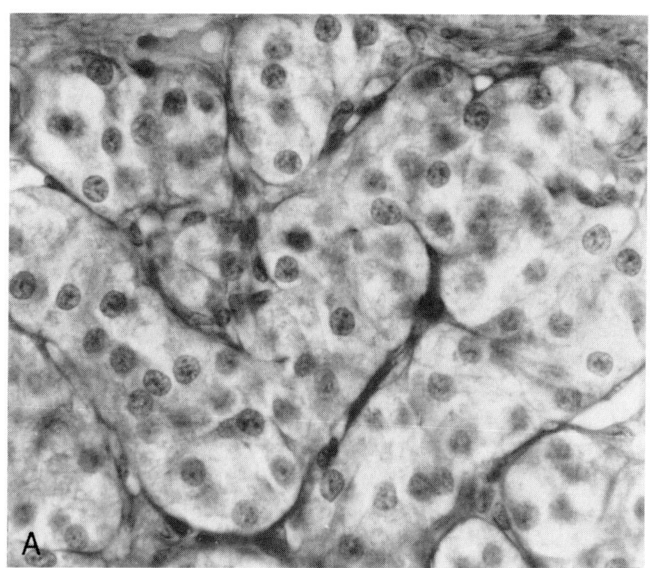

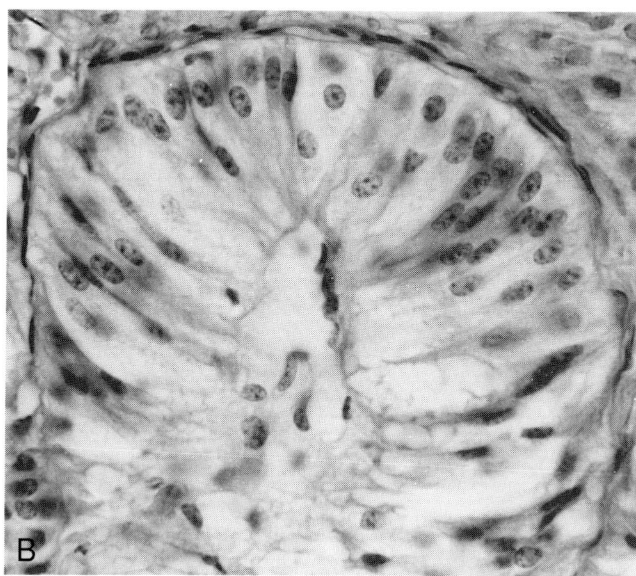

Figure 15.22. *In the bovine adrenal gland (**A**), the outermost cortical zone is formed of cell clusters or irregular cords, whereas in the donkey (**B**), the cells are arranged in arcs. Hematoxylin and eosin (×570). (From Dellmann H-D. Veterinary histology: an outline text–atlas. Philadelphia: Lea & Febiger, 1971.)*

Golgi complex usually in the vicinity of the nucleus, and a few lipid droplets. Acidophilic granules of unknown significance are present in the bovine zona glomerulosa.

A **zona intermedia** occurs in horses, carnivores, and to a lesser degree, in ruminants. This zone of small undifferentiated cells is transitional between the zona glomerulosa and the zona fasciculata.

The **zona fasciculata** consists of radially arranged cords of cuboidal or columnar cells usually one cell layer in thickness (Fig. 15.23). The fine structural characteristics of the cells are similar to those of the zona glomerulosa, except for quantitative differences; additionally, in most cells, a large number of lipid droplets is present. During routine tissue processing, these droplets are dissolved and the resulting vacuoles confer a foamy appearance to the cells, which are therefore referred to as **spongiocytes**.

The **zona reticularis** is an irregular network of anastomosing cell cords (Fig. 15.24). The cells are polyhedral and have morphologic features similar to those of the zona fasciculata. They contain fewer lipid droplets and more lipofuscin, however, and their nuclei are generally heterochromatic and often pyknotic.

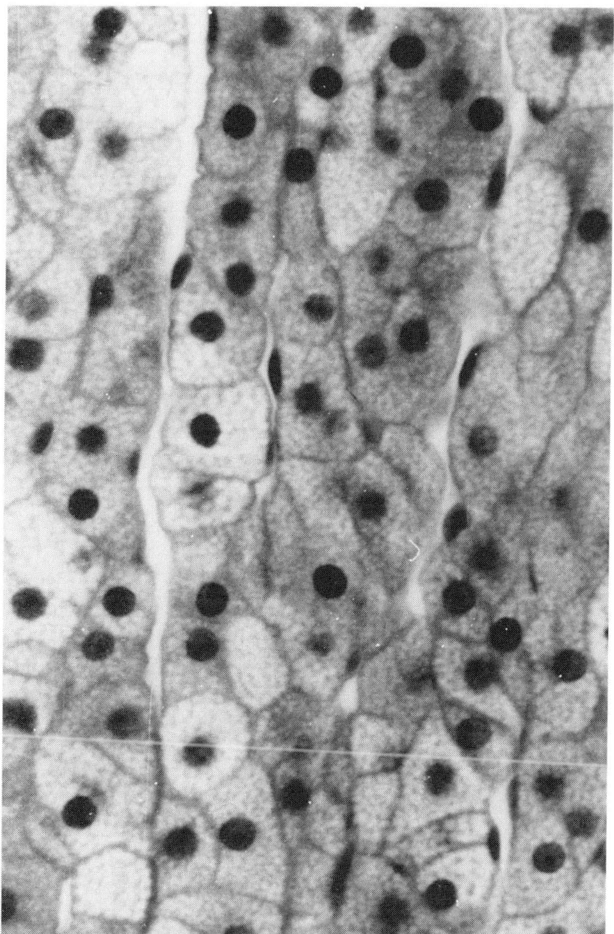

Figure 15.23. *Cells in the zona fasciculata are arranged in roughly parallel rows and have a vacuolated appearance due to the dissolution of lipid droplets during histologic processing. Hematoxylin and eosin (×870).*

Medulla

The endocrine cells of the adrenal medulla are modified postganglionic sympathetic neurons, the secretory activity of which is regulated by preganglionic sympathetic innervation. When treated with fixatives containing chromium salts, the large cells stain dark brown, consequently they are often referred to as **chromaffin cells**. Chromaffin cells belong to the APUD system of endocrine cells (see p. 302).

The polyhedral or columnar chromaffin cells are arranged in irregular cords and clusters, separated by a dense network of sinusoidal capillaries. Parasympathetic ganglion cells may occur singly or in clusters among the chromaffin cells (Fig. 15.25).

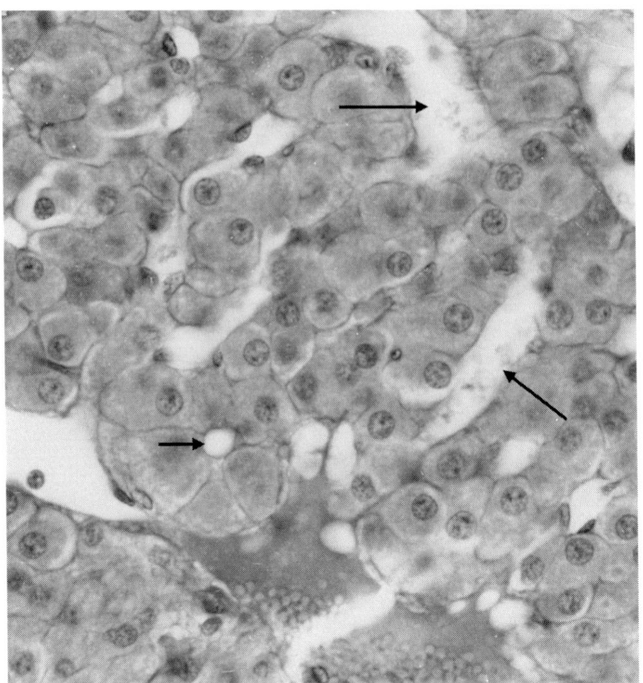

Figure 15.24. *Irregular cords of polyhedral cells are characteristic of the cortical zona reticularis; note the wide sinusoidal capillaries (arrows). Hematoxylin and eosin (×700). (From Dellmann H-D. Veterinary histology: an outline text–atlas. Philadelphia: Lea & Febiger, 1971.)*

Two types of chromaffin cells are distinguished, epinephrine cells and norepinephrine cells. Approximately 80% of the cells are **epinephrine** cells. They have less affinity for chromium salts and contain (in addition to numerous mitochondria) abundant rER and Golgi complex and less dense secretory granules than the norepinephrine cells.

The **norepinephrine** cells give a stronger chromaffin reaction, and their secretory granules are more dense than those of epinephrine cells.

In horses, cows, sheep, and pigs, the medulla is subdivided into two distinct zones: an outer zone made of large epinephrine cells, and an inner zone of clusters of small polyhedral norepinephrine cells (Fig. 15.25).

The main nerve supply consists of exclusively preganglionic sympathetic nerve fibers that end in the medulla, synapsing with the medullary cells. A few nerve fibers terminate on adrenal cortical cells.

FUNCTIONS

Cortex

The zona glomerulosa produces primarily aldosterone, a mineralocorticoid, which maintains the electrolyte level in extracellular body fluids by controlling

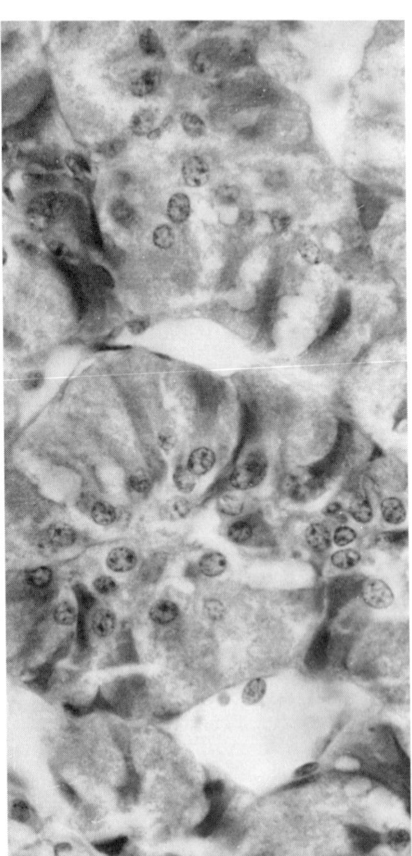

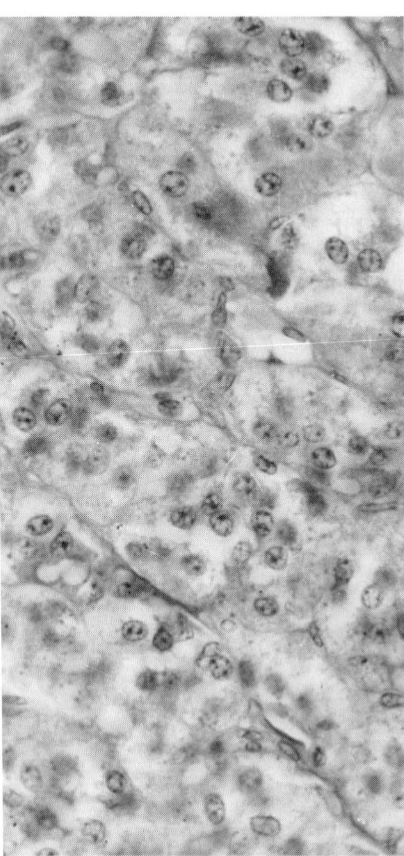

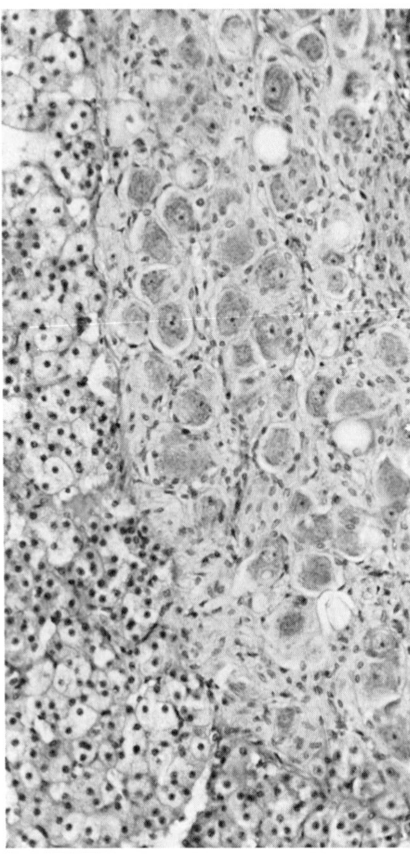

Figure 15.25. *In cows, large epinephrine cells are located in the outer zone (**A**), whereas smaller norepinephrine cells are present in the inner zone (**B**) of the adrenal medulla; they may coexist with groups of nerve cells (**C**). Hematoxylin and eosin (**A, B**: ×615; **C**: ×180).*

the retention and the excretion of sodium and potassium by the kidney tubules. Secretion of aldosterone is regulated primarily by the renin-angiotensin system (see Chapter 11.) and is largely independent of the adenohypophysis. Hypophysectomy alters neither the function nor the structure of the zona glomerulosa.

Both the zona fasciculata and the zona reticularis are involved in the production of the glucocorticoids (cortisol and corticosterone), which participate in protein, fat, and carbohydrate metabolism. They decrease the number of circulating lymphocytes and eosinophils and have anti-inflammatory effects. Glucocorticoid secretion is controlled by hypothalamic CRH and adenohypophysial ACTH, the release of which is influenced by a wide variety of internal and external factors, such as stressors, and by a negative feedback control by glucocorticoids. Hypophysectomy causes atrophy of the zonae fasciculata and reticularis and a decline in their secretory activity.

Medulla

Chromaffin cells are modified postganglionic sympathetic neurons, the secretory activity of which is under the direct control of acetylcholine released from preganglionic sympathetic nerve terminals. Norepinephrine and epinephrine are released under both physical and psychologic stress. They act on adrenergic receptors, especially in the heart, and blood vessels of the lung, viscera, and skin. They activate glycogenolysis in the liver and skeletal muscle, thus increasing blood glucose levels.

ENDOCRINE CELL GROUPS

Pancreatic Islets

STRUCTURE

The endocrine cells of the pancreas are clustered in pancreatic islets. These structures are variously shaped, generally spherical or ovoid, and intermingled with the exocrine pancreatic tissue. The islet cells are arranged in irregular anastomosing cords composed of five different cell types: A(α), B(β), C, D (δ), and F cells.

A cells contain secretory granules insoluble in alcohol that have a positive immunohistochemical reaction for glucagon and stain brilliant red with Masson's trichrome method and Gomori's aldehyde-fuchsin (Fig. 15.26). A cells have the fine structural characteristics of typical protein-secreting cells; their electron-dense secretory granules are concentrated at the vascular pole of the cell. The nucleus is generally deeply indented or lobulated. A cells represent approximately 5 to 30% of the islet population; in pigs, their number decreases from approximately 50% in the newborn animal to between 8 and 20% in the adult. In horses, the A cells are preferentially located in the center of the islets; in cattle, they tend to be arranged at the periphery. The pancreatic islets of the uncinate process in dogs are devoid of A cells.

B cells contain secretory granules soluble in alcohol that stain dark orange with Mallory's trichrome and deep purple with Gomori's aldehyde-fuchsin stain (Fig. 15.26) and have a positive immunohistochemical reaction for insulin. B-cell fine structural characteristics are similar to those of A cells, but the secretory granules contain crystalloids of variable shapes in all domestic mammalian species except horses. Generally, the nucleus is spherical and smaller than that of A cells. B cells are by far the most numerous cells in the pancreatic islets, comprising approximately 60 to 80% of the total islet cell population (up to 98% in sheep). They predominate in the periphery of the pancreatic islets of horses and in the center of the islets in cattle.

C cells are nongranulated or sparsely granulated cells that are considered to be immature precursor cells to the other types of islet cells. They do not give any positive LM staining reaction and can be identified unequivocally only with the electron microscope.

D cells are of relatively rare occurrence (approximately 5% in dogs) and are located mainly in the periphery of the islets. They synthesize somatostatin.

In addition, a heterogeneous population of small granulated cells occurs, which are considered precursors to a variety of cells that produce various gastroentero-pancreatic hormones (e.g., pancreatic polypeptide, vasoactive intestinal polypeptide, and cholecystokinin-pancreozymin [CCK]). In dogs, cells that produce pancreatic polypeptide (F cells) have been identified.

FUNCTIONS

Insulin, the hormone synthesized and secreted by the B cells, facilitates cellular uptake of glucose; it reduces the blood glucose level by facilitating the uptake of glucose by skeletal muscle and adipocytes and by inhibiting the release of glucose from the liver. Absence or insufficient secretion of insulin causes **diabetes mellitus**, a severe disturbance of carbohydrate metabolism, characterized by hyperglycemia and glycosuria. Concurrently, glycogen stores in the liver and other tissues are depleted. An excess of insulin may result in a rapid decrease of the blood glucose level and subsequent convulsions and death, unless the effect is counteracted by the administration of glucose.

Glucagon, the secretory product of pancreatic A cells, counteracts the effect of insulin by breaking down liver glycogen and increasing the blood glucose level.

Somatostatin is synthesized in D cells and has an inhibitory action on the secretion of insulin and glucagon. Pancreatic polypeptide, synthesized by canine F cells, stimulates gastric secretion and inhibits intestinal motility and bile secretion.

Other Groups of Endocrine Cells

Other groups of endocrine cells in the hypothalamus, heart, testis, and ovary have been dealt with elsewhere. The reader is referred to the appropriate chapters.

SINGLE ENDOCRINE CELLS

Throughout the organism, single endocrine cells occur that are characterized by the uptake of amine pre-

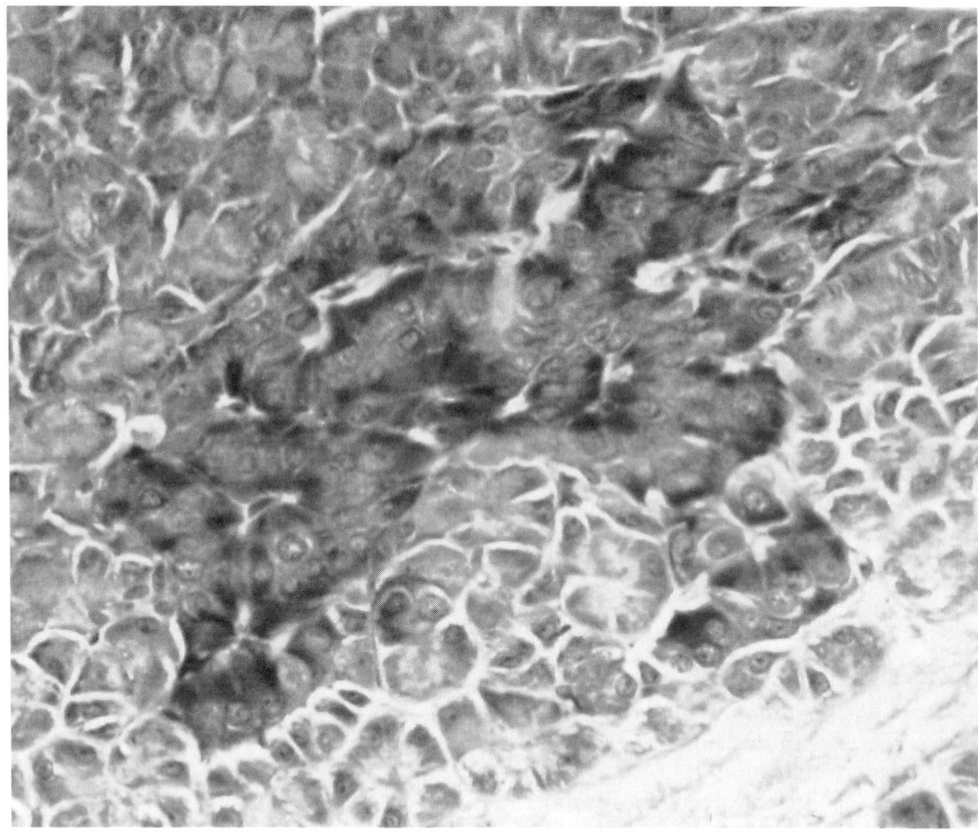

Figure 15.26. *In this canine pancreatic islet, a few intensely red stained A cells are interspersed among the many dark blue B cells. Aldehyde-fuchsin (×105).*

cursors and their subsequent decarboxylation in the process of amine or peptide hormone synthesis. Therefore, these cells are referred to as **APUD cells** (**a**mine **p**recursor **u**ptake and **d**ecarboxylation). APUD cells include the following diverse cells: endocrine cells in the mucosa of the respiratory and gastrointestinal systems; epinephrine- and norepinephrine-secreting cells in the adrenal medulla and paraganglia; chemoreceptors in the carotid body; and thyroid parafollicular cells (C cells), pancreatic islet cells, juxtaglomerular cells, corticotropes and melanotropes in the adenohypophysis.

Some APUD cells derive from neural crest tissue (e.g., adrenal medullary and paraganglionic cells, C cells, and endocrine cells in the gastrointestinal and respiratory systems); they are considered to be modified neurons and are referred to as the **diffuse neuroendocrine system**.

REFERENCES

Bhatnagar AS, ed. The anterior pituitary gland. New York: Raven Press, 1983.

Hadley ME. Endocrinology. Upper Saddle River, Prentice Hall, 1996.

Harris GW, Donovan BT, eds. The pituitary gland. Berkeley: University of California Press, 1966.

Holmes RL, Ball JN. The pituitary gland. A comparative account. New York: Cambridge University Press, 1974.

Motta PM, ed. Ultrastructure of endocrine cells and tissues. Boston: Nijhoff, 1984.

Müller EE, MacLeod RM, eds. Neuroendocrine perspectives. Amsterdam: Elsevier, 1982.

Norris DO. Vertebrate endocrinology. San Diego: Academic Press, 1997.

Relkin R, ed. The pineal gland. New York: Elsevier, 1983.

Van Blerkom J, Motta PM, eds. Ultrastructure of reproduction. Boston: Nijhoff, 1984.

16

Integument

NANCY A. MONTEIRO-RIVIERE

GENERAL CHARACTERISTICS

Skin is a complex, integrated, dynamic organ that has functions that go far beyond its role as a barrier to the environment (Table 16.1). The skin, or integument (derived from the Latin word meaning **roof**), is the largest organ system of the body and consists of an epidermis and a dermis (Fig. 16.1).

The epidermis is a keratinized stratified squamous epithelium derived from ectoderm and is the outermost layer of the skin (Fig. 16.2). It undergoes an orderly pattern of proliferation, differentiation, and keratinization, the processes of which are not completely understood. The epidermis can become specialized to form various skin appendages, such as hair, sweat, and sebaceous glands; digital organs (hoof, claw, nail); feathers; horn; and specialized glandular structures. The epidermis is composed of two primary cell types based on origin, the keratinocytes (stratum basale, stratum spinosum, stratum granulosum, stratum lucidum, and stratum corneum) and the nonkeratinocytes (melanocytes, Merkel cells, and Langerhans cells). The epidermal lay-

Table 16.1.
Functions of Skin

Environmental barrier
Diffusion barrier
Metabolic barrier
Temperature regulation
Regulation of blood flow
Hair and fur
Sweating
Immunologic affector and effector axis
Mechanical support
Neurosensory reception
Endocrine (e.g., vitamin D)
Apocrine/eccrine/sebaceous glandular secretion
Metabolism
Keratin
Collagen
Melanin
Lipid
Carbohydrate
Respiration
Biotransformation of xenobiotics

ers can be classified in layers above the basement membrane to the outer surface as follows: stratum basale (basal layer), stratm spinosum (spinous or prickle layer), stratum granulosum (granular layer), stratum lucidum (clear layer), and stratum corneum (horny layer).

The dermis or corium is of mesodermal origin and consists of dense irregular connective tissue. It lies beneath the basement membrane and extends to the hypodermis.

Beneath the dermis is a layer of loose connective tissue, the hypodermis (subcutis), which is not part of the skin but rather the superficial fascia seen in gross anatomic dissections. The hypodermis with elastic fibers aids in binding the skin to the underlying fascia and skeletal muscle.

In general, the basic architecture of the integument is similar in all mammals. Differences exist, however, in the thickness of the epidermis and dermis between species and within the same species in various regions of the body. Because dermatologic, cutaneous pharmacologic, and toxicologic studies use skin from different animal species and body sites, species differences in cutaneous structure must be taken into consideration.

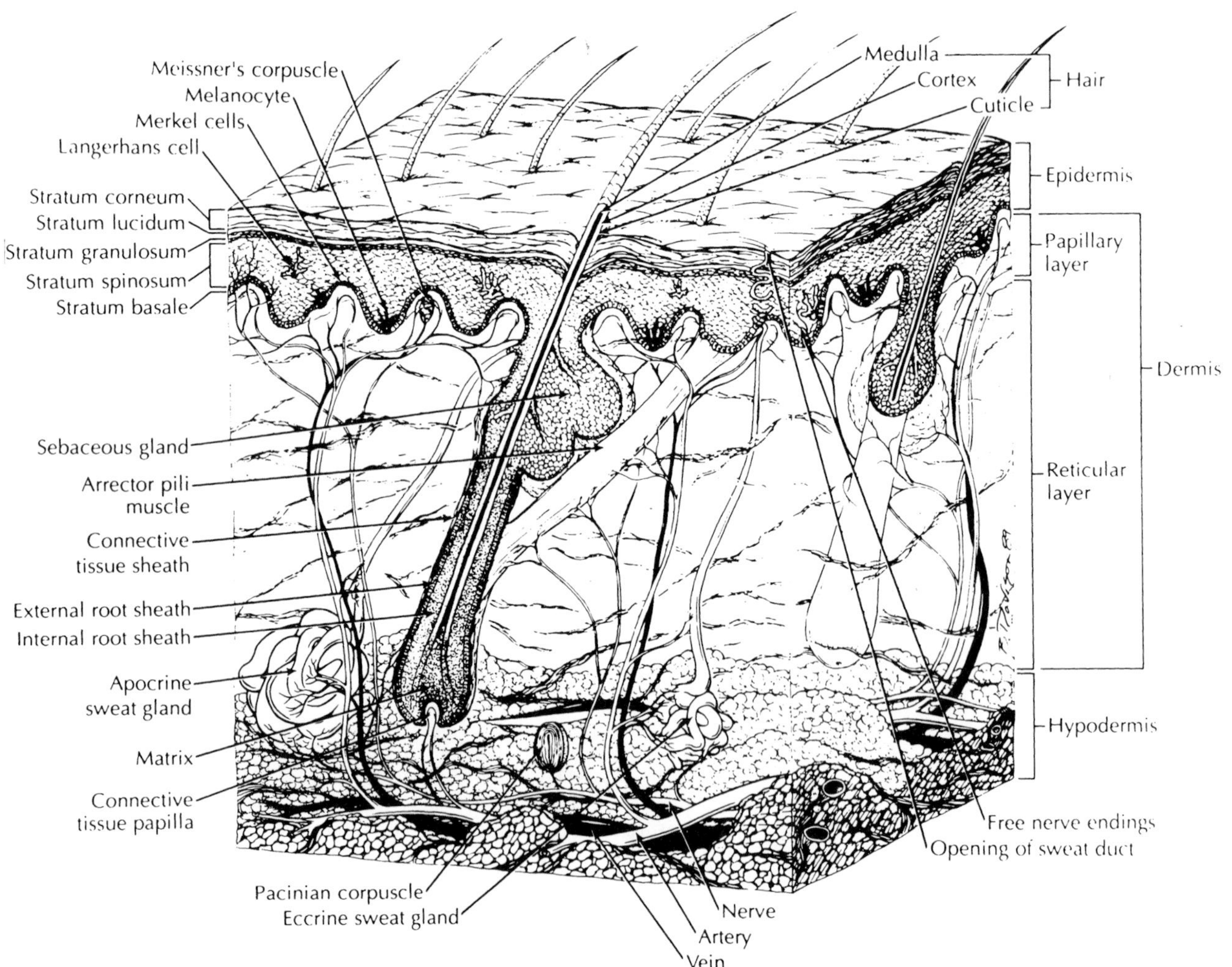

Figure 16.1. *Schematic drawing representing the structure of the integument found in typical skin in various regions of the body. (From Monteiro-Riviere NA. Comparative anatomy, physiology, and biochemistry of mammalian skin. In: Hobson DW, ed. Dermal and ocular toxicology: fundamentals and methods. Boca Raton, FL: CRC Press, 1991.)*

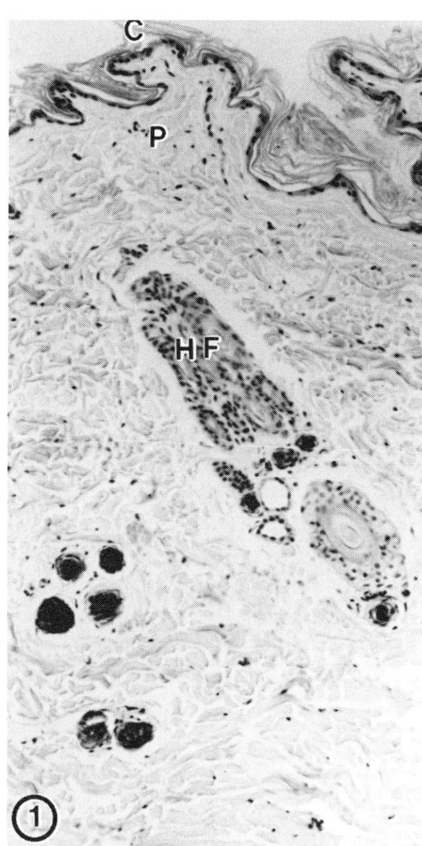

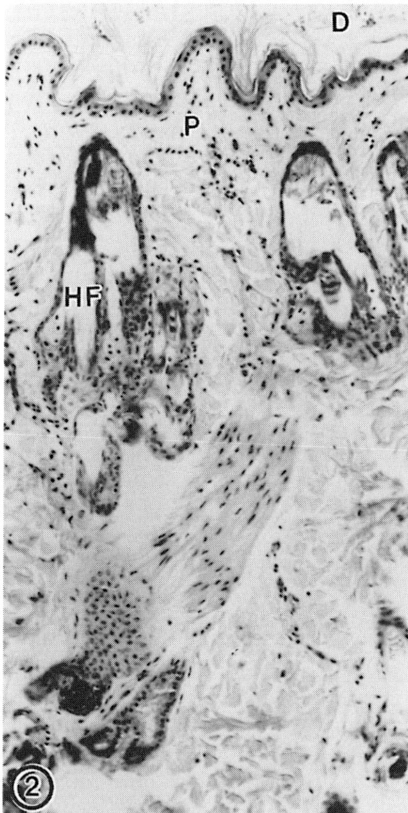

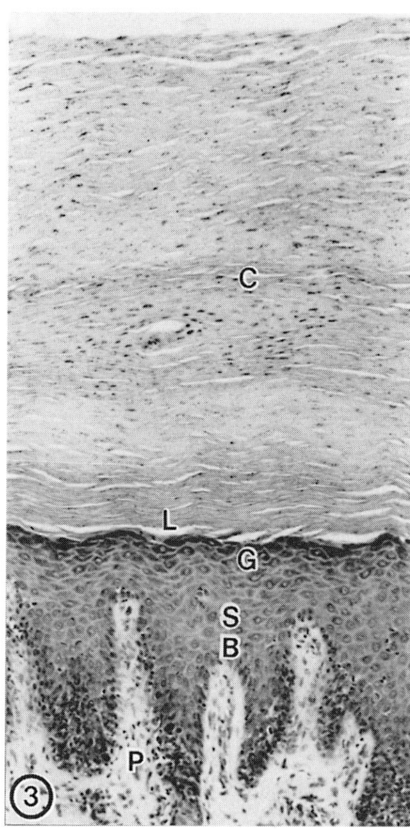

Figure 16.2. *Epidermis (cat). **1.**, Thin skin with one to two viable cell layers, abdomen region. **2.**, Skin with thin epidermis with hair follicle cluster (HF), lumbar region. **3.**, Foot pad with thick stratum corneum. Stratum disjunctum (D); stratum corneum (C); stratum lucidum (L); stratum granulosum (G); stratum spinosum (S); stratum basale (B); superficial papillary layer of the dermis (P). Hematoxylin and eosin (×120).*

Usually, the skin is thickest over the dorsal surface of the body and on the lateral surfaces of the limbs. It is thinnest on the ventral side of the body and medial surfaces of the limbs. In regions with a heavy protective coat of hair, the epidermis is thin; in nonhairy skin, such as that of the mucocutaneous junctions, the epidermis is thicker. On the palmar and plantar surfaces, where considerable abrasive action occurs, the stratum corneum is thickest (Fig. 16.2.3). The epidermis may be smooth in some areas but has ridges or folds in other regions that reflect the contour of the underlying superficial dermal layer (Figs. 16.2.1, 16.2.2, 16.2.3).

EPIDERMIS

The epidermis is a keratinized stratified squamous epithelium comprising keratinocytes forming several layers and nonkeratinocytes.

Epidermal Keratinocytes

STRATUM BASALE

The **stratum basale** (stratum germinativum) consists of a single layer of columnar or cuboidal cells that rests on the basal lamina (Fig. 16.3). The cells are attached laterally to each other and to the overlying stratum spinosum cells by desmosomes and to the underlying basal lamina by hemidesmosomes. The nucleus is large and ovoid and occupies most of the cell. These basal cells are heterogeneous functionally. Some basal cells can act as stem cells, with the ability to divide and produce new cells, whereas others primarily serve to anchor the epidermis.

STRATUM SPINOSUM

The succeeding outer layer is the **stratum spinosum**, or "prickle cell layer," which consists of several layers of irregular polyhedral cells (Figs. 16.2.3 and 16.4). Desmosomes connect these cells to adjacent stratum spinosum cells and to the stratum basale cells below. Tonofilaments are more prominent in this layer than in the stratum basale. The large intercellular space usually seen in this layer is a shrinkage artifact, which occurs in preparing the sample for light microscopic study. The uppermost layers of the stratum spinosum contain small membrane-bound organelles known as lamellar granules.

STRATUM GRANULOSUM

The third layer is the **stratum granulosum**, which consists of several layers of flattened cells lying parallel to

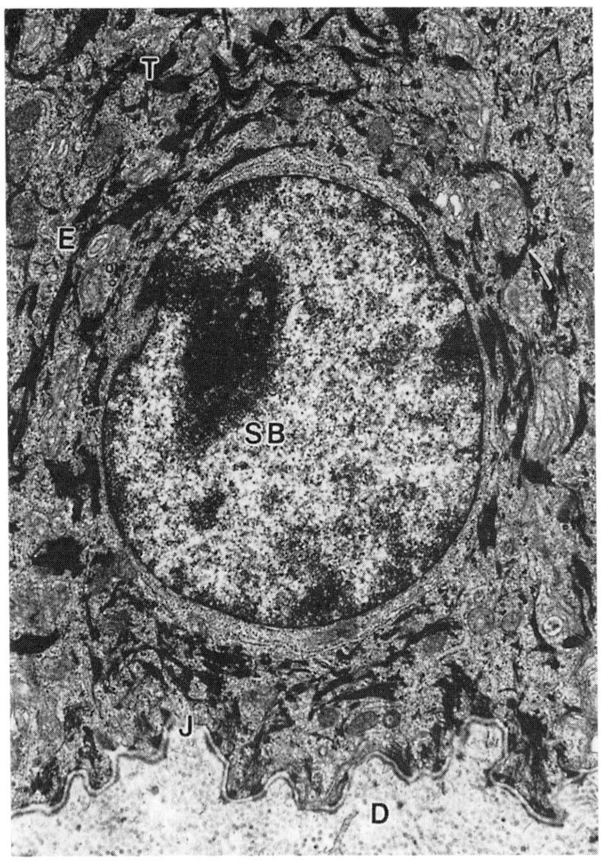

Figure 16.3. *Transmission electron micrograph of pig skin. Area depicting the epidermis (E), dermis (D), epidermal–dermal junction (J), stratum basale cell (SB), tonofilaments (T), and desmosome attachments (arrow) (×10,700).*

the epidermal–dermal junction (Figs. 16.2.3 and 16.5). This layer contains irregularly shaped, nonmembrane-bound, electron-dense **keratohyalin granules**. These granules contain profilaggrin, a structural protein and a precursor of filaggrin, and are believed to play a role in keratinization and barrier function. Another characteristic feature of the stratum granulosum is the presence of the **lamellar granules** (Odland bodies, lamellated bodies, or membrane-coating granules). These granules are smaller than mitochondria and occur near the Golgi complex and smooth endoplasmic reticulum (sER). Higher in the epidermis, these granules increase in number and size, move toward the cell membrane, and release their lipid contents by exocytosis into the intercellular space between the stratum granulosum and stratum corneum, thereby coating the cell membrane of the stratum corneum cells (Fig. 16.5). As one can now appreciate, the term "membrane-coating granule" is appropriate. The major components of lipids are the ceramides, cholesterol, fatty acids, and small amounts of cholesteryl esters and hydrolytic enzymes such as acid phosphates, proteases, lipases, and glycosidases. The content and mixture of lipids can vary between species.

STRATUM LUCIDUM

The **stratum lucidum** (clear layer) is only found in specific areas of exceptionally thick skin and in hairless regions (e.g., plantar and palmar surfaces, planum nasale) (Fig. 16.2.3). It is a thin, translucent, homogeneous line between the stratum granulosum and stratum corneum. This stratum consists of several layers of fully keratinized, closely compacted, dense cells devoid of nuclei and cytoplasmic organelles. Their cytoplasm contains protein-bound phospholipids and eleidin, which is a protein that is similar to keratin but has a different staining affinity.

Figure 16.4. *Transmission electron micrograph of the stratum spinosum layer of pig skin. Area shows the nuclei of two stratum spinosum (SS) cells attached by desmosomes (arrows) (×23,500).*

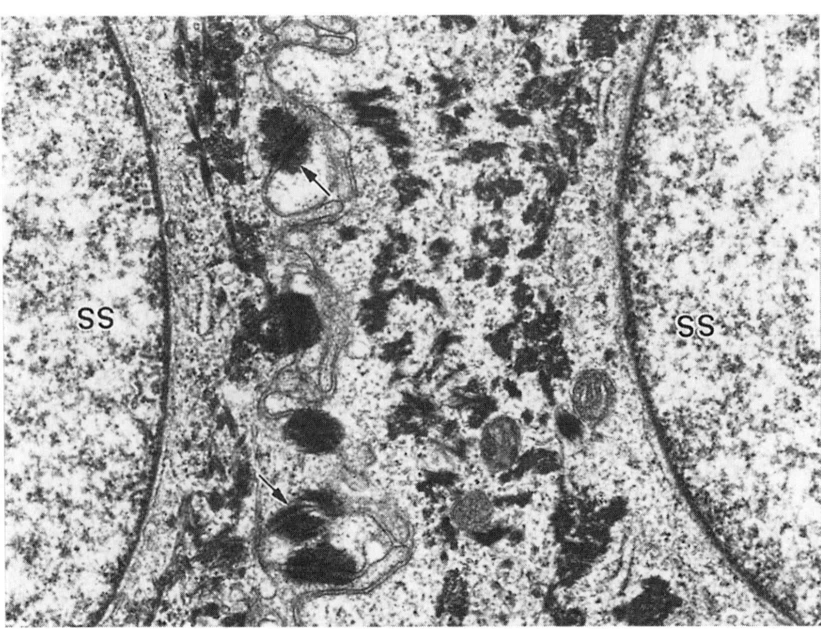

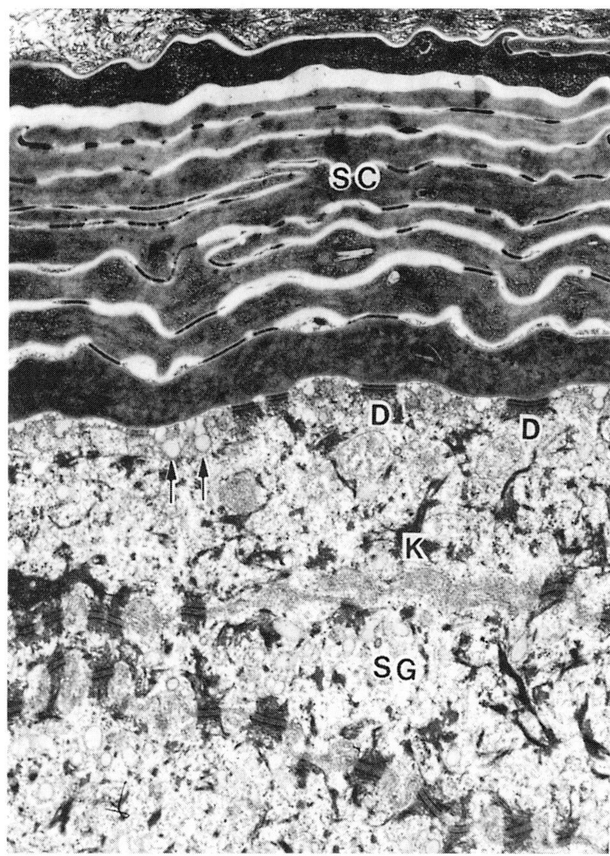

Figure 16.5. *Transmission electron micrograph of the upper stratum granulosum (SG) and stratum corneum (SC) of pig skin. Membrane-coating granules or lamellar bodies (arrows) are present in the stratum granulosum layer, with some fusing to the plasma membrane to release their contents. Keratohyalin granules (K) and numerous desmosomes (D) are present (×14,900).*

STRATUM CORNEUM

The **stratum corneum** is the outermost layer of the epidermis and consists of several layers of completely keratinized dead cells, which are constantly being shed. This layer appears clear and contains no nuclei or cytoplasmic organelles (Figs. 16.2.1, 16.2.2, 16.2.3, and 16.5). The most superficial layers of the stratum corneum that undergo constant desquamation is referred to as the **stratum disjunctum**. The stratum corneum cell layers vary in thickness in different areas (i.e., abdomen versus back) of the body and between species. The stratum corneum cells are highly organized and stacked one upon another to form vertical interlocking columns and having a flattened tetrakaidecahedron shape. This 14-sided polygonal structure provides a minimum surface:volume ratio, which allows for space to be filled by packing without interstices. This spatial arrangement found in hairy skin helps one to understand that transepidermal water loss is a function of the integrity and permeability of this layer. The intercellular substance derived from the lamellar granules is present between the stratum corneum cells and forms the intercellular lipid component of a complex stratum corneum barrier, which prevents both the penetration of substances from the environment and the loss of body fluids. The keratinized cells are surrounded by a plasma membrane and a thick submembranous layer that contains a protein, involucrin. This protein is synthesized in the stratum spinosum and cross-linked in the stratum granulosum by an enzyme that makes it highly stable. Therefore, involucrin provides structural support to the cell, thereby allowing the cell to resist invasion by microorganisms and destruction by environmental agents, but does not seem to regulate permeability.

Keratinization

Keratinization is the process by which epidermal cells (keratinocytes) differentiate. After the basal epithelial cells undergo mitosis, they migrate upward. The volume of the cytoplasm increases and the differentiation products (tonofilaments, keratohyalin granules, and lamellar granules) are formed in large amounts. The tonofilaments and the amorphous material, keratohyalin, form a meshwork. As the cellular contents increase, the nuclei disintegrate and the lamellar granules discharge their contents into the intercellular space coating the cells. The remaining organelles such as mitochondria and ribosomes disintegrate, and the flattened cells become filled by filaments and keratohyalin, which then arranges itself into bundles. The final product of this epidermal differentiation and keratinization process is the stratum corneum, which consists of protein-rich cells containing fibrous keratin and keratohyalin surrounded by a thicker plasma membrane coated by the exterior lipid matrix. This forms the commonly known "brick and mortar" structure in which the lipid matrix acts as the mortar between the cells, which are the bricks.

Epidermal–Dermal Junction

The **epidermal–dermal junction** (or skin basement membrane zone) is a complex and highly specialized structure recognized with the light microscope (periodic acid-Schiff stain) as a thin, homogeneous band. When viewed with the transmission electron microscope, however, the epidermal–dermal junction consists of four components: *(a)* the cell membrane of the basal epithelial cell, which includes the hemidesmosomes; *(b)* the lamina lucida (lamina rara); *(c)* the lamina densa (basal lamina); and *(d)* the sub-basal lamina (sublamina densa or reticular lamina) with a variety of fibrous structures (anchoring fibrils, dermal microfibril bundles, microthreadlike filaments) (Fig.16.6). The basement membrane has a complex molecular architecture with numerous components that play a key role in adhesion of the epidermis to the dermis. The macromolecules that are ubiquitous components of all basement membranes include type IV collagen, laminin, entactin/nidogen, and heparan sulfate proteoglycans. Other basement membrane components such as bullous pemphigoid antigen (BPA), epidermolysis bullosa acquisita

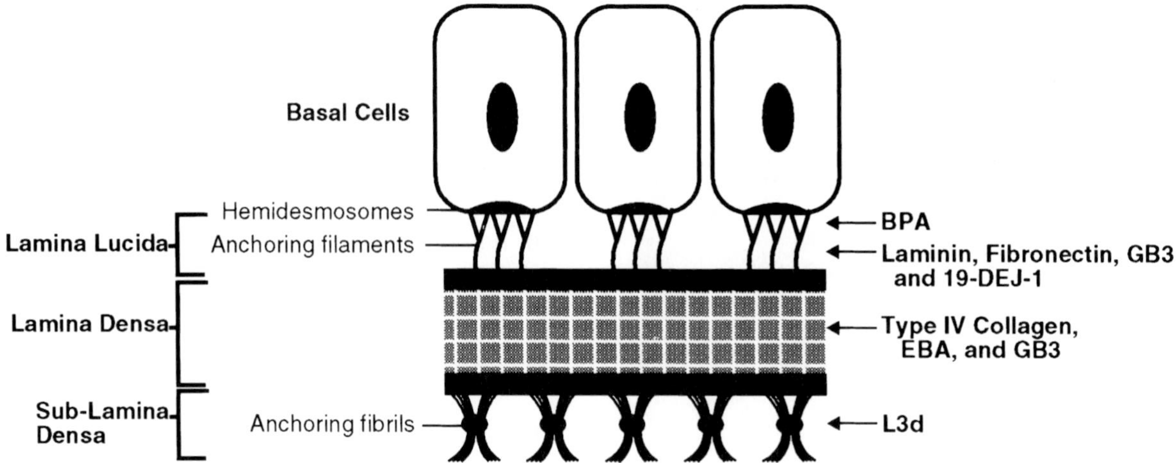

Figure 16.6. *Schematic of the basement membrane of skin depicting the precise location of the macromolecular components. (From Monteiro-Riviere NA, Inman AO. Indirect immunohistochemistry and immunoelectron microscopy distribution of eight epidermal-dermal junction epitopes in the pig and in isolated perfused skin treated with bis (2-chloroethyl) sulfide. Toxicol Pathol 1995;23:313–325.)*

(EBA), fibronectin, GB3, L3d, and 19DEJ-1 are limited in their distribution to the epithelial basement membrane of skin. The basal cell membrane of the epidermal–dermal junction is not always smooth. It may be irregular, forming fingerlike projections into the dermis. The basement membrane *(a)* plays a role in maintenance of epidermal–dermal adhesion, *(b)* acts as a selective barrier between epidermis and dermis by restricting some molecules and permitting the passage of others, *(c)* influences cell behavior and wound healing, and *(d)* serves as a target for both immunologic (bullous diseases) and nonimmunologic injury (friction- or chemical-induced blisters).

Epidermal Nonkeratinocytes

MELANOCYTES

Melanocytes are derivatives of the neural crest and are located in the basal layer of the epidermis (Fig. 16.1). They also occur in the external root sheath and hair matrix of hair follicles, in the sweat gland ducts, and in sebaceous glands. Melanocytes have several dendritic processes that either extend between adjacent keratinocytes or run parallel to the dermal surface. The melanocyte has a spherical nucleus and contains typical organelles (ribosomes, endoplasmic reticulum, Golgi, etc.). The cytoplasm is clear except for pigment-containing ovoid granules, which are referred to as melanosomes. The **melanosomes** impart color to skin and hair. The dark brown pigment is called eumelanin, and the yellow red is called pheomelanin. The enzyme tyrosinase is needed to produce melanin within the melanocytes, and the reaction involves the following series of steps, in short: tyrosine→dopa→dopaquinone→melanin. Albino animals lack tyrosinase; therefore, they cannot produce melanin, even though they have a normal number of melanocytes. After melanogenesis, the melanosomes migrate to the tips of the dendritic processes of the melanocyte; the tips then become pinched off and phagocytized by the adjacent keratinocytes. They remain as discrete organelles surrounded by a membrane or can become aggregated and surrounded by a membrane to form a melanosome complex. Melanosomes are randomly distributed within the cytoplasm of the keratinocytes, although they often become localized over the nucleus, thereby forming a cap-like structure that presumably protects the nucleus from ultraviolet radiation (Fig. 16.7). Skin color is determined by several factors, such as the number, size, distribution, and degree of melanization of melanosomes.

MERKEL CELLS

Merkel cells are located in the basal region of the epidermis in both hairless and hairy skin. Their long axis is usually parallel to the surface of the skin and, thus, perpendicular to the columnar basal epithelial cells above (Figs. 16.1 and 16.8). The nucleus is lobulated and irregular, and the cytoplasm is clear and lacks tonofilaments. These cells have a characteristic vacuolated cytoplasm predominantly on their dermal side, contain spherical electron-dense granules, and are connected to adjacent keratinocytes by desmosomes. When associated with axons, this cell becomes a Merkel cell–neurite complex, and specialized areas containing these complexes are known as **tactile hair discs** (Haarscheiben, hair discs, or tylotrich pads). The terminal axon associated with a Merkel cell is derived from a myelinated nerve, but as it approaches the epidermis, it loses its myelin sheath and terminates as a flat meniscus on the basal aspect of the cell (Fig. 16.8). Merkel cells are believed to function as slow adapting mechanoreceptors for touch.

LANGERHANS CELLS

Langerhans cells are most commonly found in the upper spinous layer of the epidermis (Figs. 16.1 and 16.9).

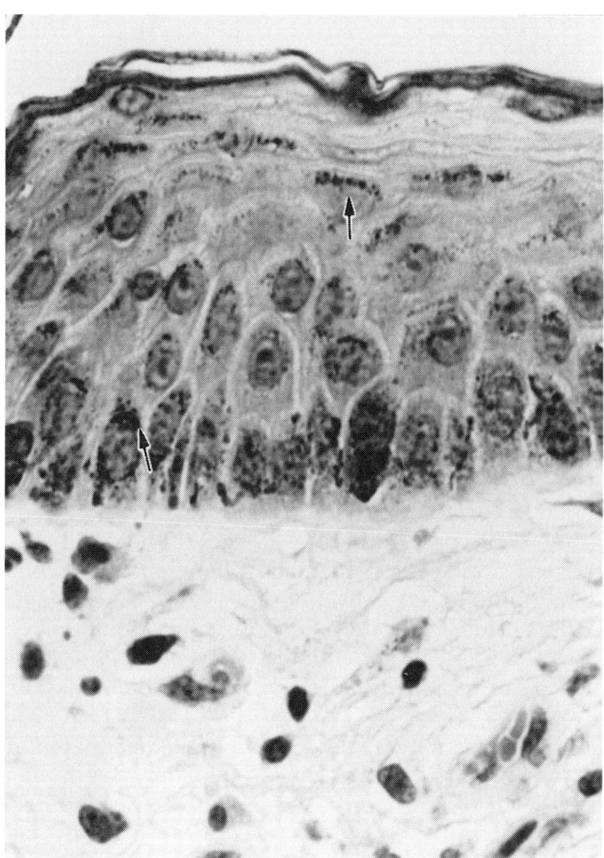

Figure 16.7. *Melanin granules (arrows) highly concentrated in the stratum basale cell layer and forming apical caps in the upper layers of the horse abdominal skin. Hematoxylin and eosin (×800).*

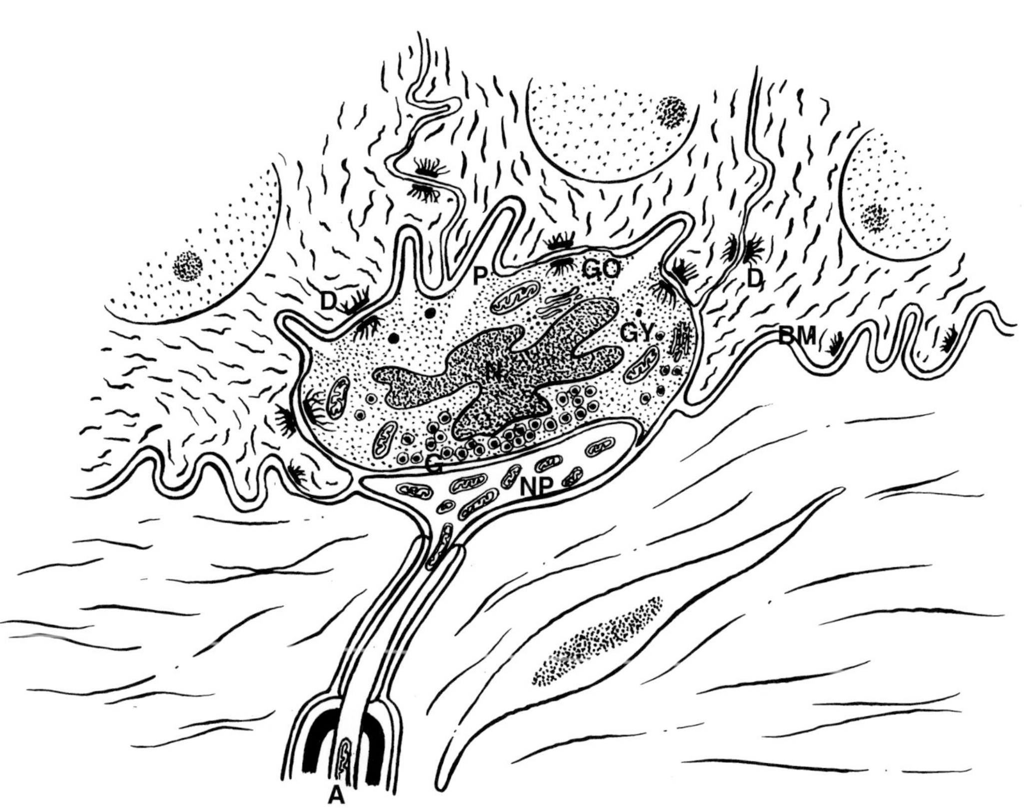

Figure 16.8. *Schematic drawing of a Merkel cell-heurite complex from a foot pad of a cat. Irregular nucleus (N), Golgi (GO), desmosome (D) connecting to adjacent keratinocytes, glycogen (GY), cytoploplasmic process (P), basement membrane (BM), Merkel's cell dense core granules (G), axon (A) and nerve plate or disc (NP).*

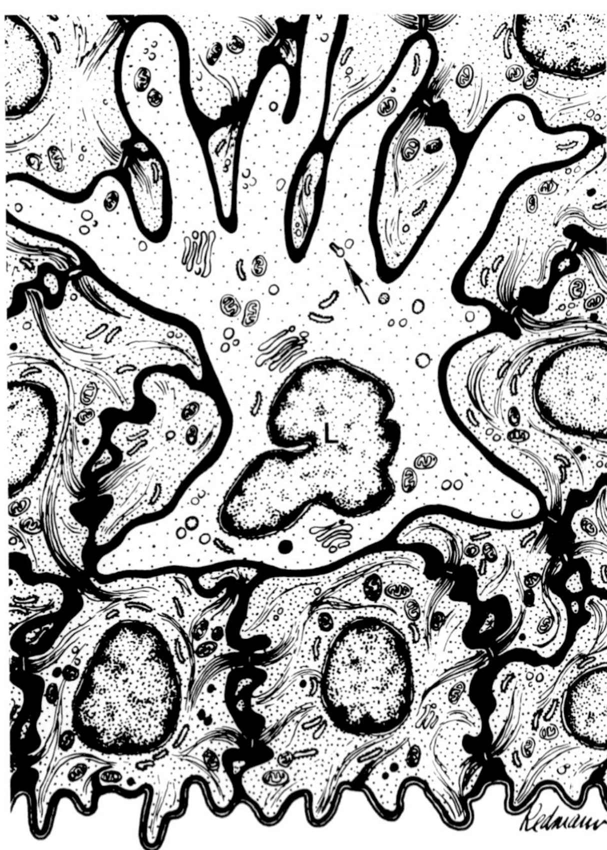

Figure 16.9. *Schematic of a Langerhans cell (L). Heavy black areas represent the intercellular space. The racket shape granules (arrow) can be found in the dendritic processes. Note the idented nucleus and electron lucency of the cytoplasm. (From Monteiro-Riviere NA. Ultrastructural evaluation of the porcine integument. In: Tumbleson ME, ed. Swine in biomedical research. New York: Plenum Press, 1986;1:641.)*

They have also been identified in the stratified squamous epithelium of the upper digestive tract, female genital tract, and sheep rumen. In addition, Langerhans cells are present in dermal lymph vessels, in lymph nodes, and in the dermis. In addition, they have been reported in the lung in fibrotic disorders, mycosis fungoides, atopic dermatitis, and the nondermatologic disorder, eosinophilic granulomatosis. They usually are not apparent in routine sections but may appear as clear cells in the suprabasal epidermis. They can only be positively identified with special stains. Langerhans cells and their granules have been well characterized in rodents and man but rarely have been reported in the domestic species. Langerhans cells with their granules have been identified in the epidermis of adult pigs and cats, but only Langerhans-like cells (no granules) have been seen in the skin of dogs.

At the ultrastructural level, Langerhans cells have an indented nucleus and the cytoplasm contains typical organelles; they lack tonofilaments and desmosomes. A unique feature of this cell is distinctive rod- or racket-shaped granules in the cytoplasm that are known as Langerhans (Birbeck) cell granules. Langerhans cells have long dendritic processes that traverse the intercellular space up to the granular cell layer. Langerhans cells are derived from bone marrow and are functionally and immunologically related to the monocyte–macrophage series. They are capable of presenting antigen to lymphocytes and are considered to be the initial receptors for cutaneous immune responses (delayed-type hypersensitivity).

DERMIS

The **dermis** consists primarily of dense irregular connective tissue with a feltwork of collagen, elastic, and reticular fibers embedded in an amorphous ground substance. The predominant cell types of the dermis are fibrocytes, mast cells, and macrophages. Plasma cells, chromatophores, fat cells, and extravasated leukocytes are often found. The dermis is traversed by blood vessels, lymph vessels, and nerves. Sebaceous and sweat glands are also present, along with hair follicles and arrector pili muscles.

The dermis can be divided into a superficial papillary layer that blends into a deep reticular layer without a clear line of demarcation (Fig. 16.10). The **papillary layer** is the thinnest layer, consists of loose connective tissue, is in contact with the epidermis, and conforms to the contour of the stratum basale. The papillary layer can protrude into the epidermis, thereby giving rise to

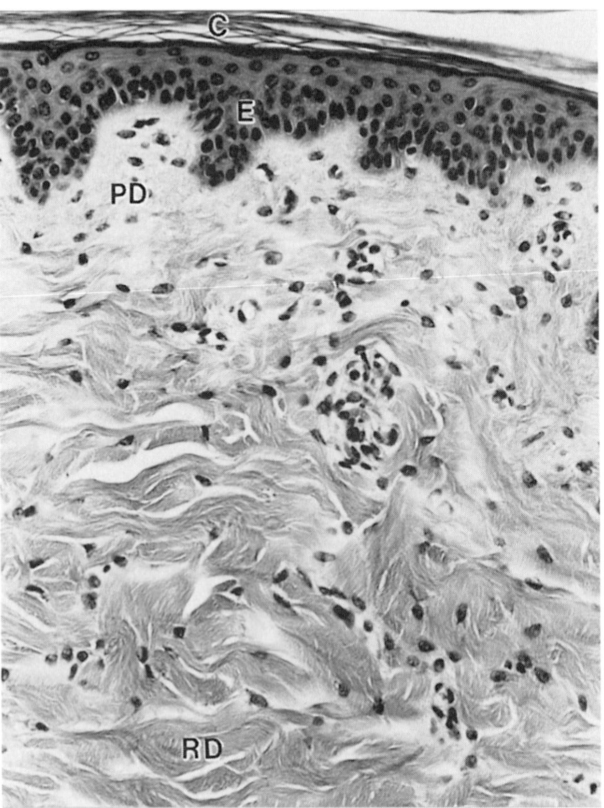

Figure 16.10. *Pig skin from the abdomen region. Epidermis (E), stratum corneum (C), superficial papillary dermis (PD), deep reticular dermis (RD). Hematoxylin and eosin (×250).*

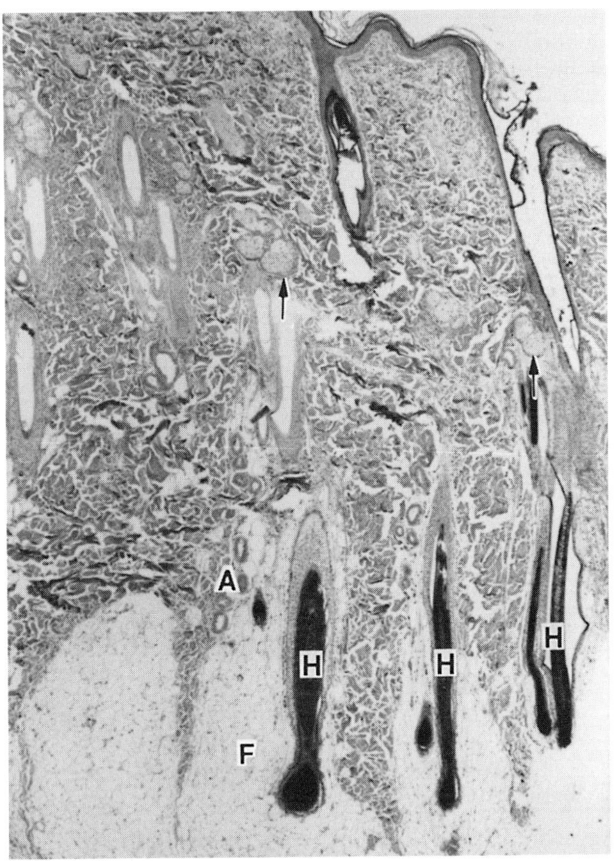

Figure 16.11. *Hypodermis with three large primary hair follicles (H) extending into the subcutaneous fat (F) (dog). Note the sebaceous glands (arrows) and apocrine gland ducts (A). Hematoxylin and eosin (×35).*

the dermal papilla. When the epidermis invaginates into the dermis, epidermal pegs are formed. The **reticular layer** is thicker and consists of dense connective tissue. Connective tissue cells are fewer in the deeper layers of the dermis.

In the dermis, smooth muscle fibers are located near hair follicles and are referred to as **arrector pili**. In addition, smooth muscle fibers are present in specialized areas such as the scrotum, penis, and teat. Skeletal muscle fibers of the cutaneous trunci penetrate the dermis and allow voluntary movement of the skin. Also, skeletal muscle fibers are associated with the large sinus hairs of the facial region.

HYPODERMIS

The **hypodermis** (subcutis) anchors the dermis to the underlying muscle or bone. The loose arrangement of collagen and elastic fibers allows the skin flexibility and free movement over the underlying structures. Adipose tissue is present in this layer and may form small clusters of cells or large masses that create a cushion or pad of fat called the **panniculus adiposus** (Fig. 16.11). Pork bacon and fatback are derived from the panniculus adiposus. Large fat deposits (structural fat) in the hypodermis are characteristic of the carpal, metacarpal, and digital pads, where they act as shock absorbers.

SKIN APPENDAGES

Hair

In domestic mammals, hair covers the entire body, with the exception of the foot pads, hoofs, glans penis, mucocutaneous junctions, and teats of some species. Hair is a flexible, keratinized structure produced by a hair follicle.

The distal or free part of the hair above the surface of the skin is the hair **shaft**. The part within the follicle is the hair **root**, which has a terminal, hollow knob called the hair **bulb**, which is attached to a dermal papilla.

The hair shaft is composed of three layers: an outermost cuticle, a cortex of densely packed keratinized cells, and a medulla of loose cuboidal or flattened cells (Fig. 16.12). The **cuticle** is formed by a single layer of flat keratinized cells in which the free edges, which overlap like shingles on a roof, are directed toward the distal end of the shaft. The **cortex** consists of a layer of dense, compact, keratinized cells with their long axes parallel to the hair shaft. Nuclear remnants and pigment granules are present within the cells. Desmosomes hold the cells firmly together. Near the bulb, the cells are shorter and more oval and contain spherical nuclei. The **medulla** forms the center of the hair and is loosely filled with cuboidal or flattened cells (Fig. 16.12). In the root, the medulla is solid, whereas in the shaft, it contains air-filled spaces. Secondary hairs lack a medulla. The pattern of the surface of the cuticular cells, together with the cellular arrangement of the medulla, is characteristic for each species.

The hair or fleece of sheep is referred to as **fibers**. The three types of fibers are *(a)* wool fibers, tightly crimped fibers of small diameter lacking a medulla; *(b)* kemp fibers, coarse and with a characteristic medulla; and *(c)* coarse fibers of intermediate size relative to wool and kemp fibers. The various breeds of sheep produce wools with different characteristics, and these various kinds of fleece are used for different purposes.

Hair Follicles

STRUCTURE

The hair follicle is formed by growth of the ectoderm into the underlying mesoderm of the embryo. The epithelial downgrowth becomes canalized, and the surrounding cells differentiate into several layers or sheaths that surround the hair root. The follicle is embedded in the dermis, usually at an angle, and the bulb may extend as deep as the hypodermis (Figs. 16.11 and 16.13). The hair follicle consists of four major components: *(a)* internal root sheath, *(b)* external root sheath, *(c)* dermal papilla, and *(d)* hair matrix.

The innermost layer, next to the hair root, is the **internal root sheath**, which is composed of three layers: *(a)*

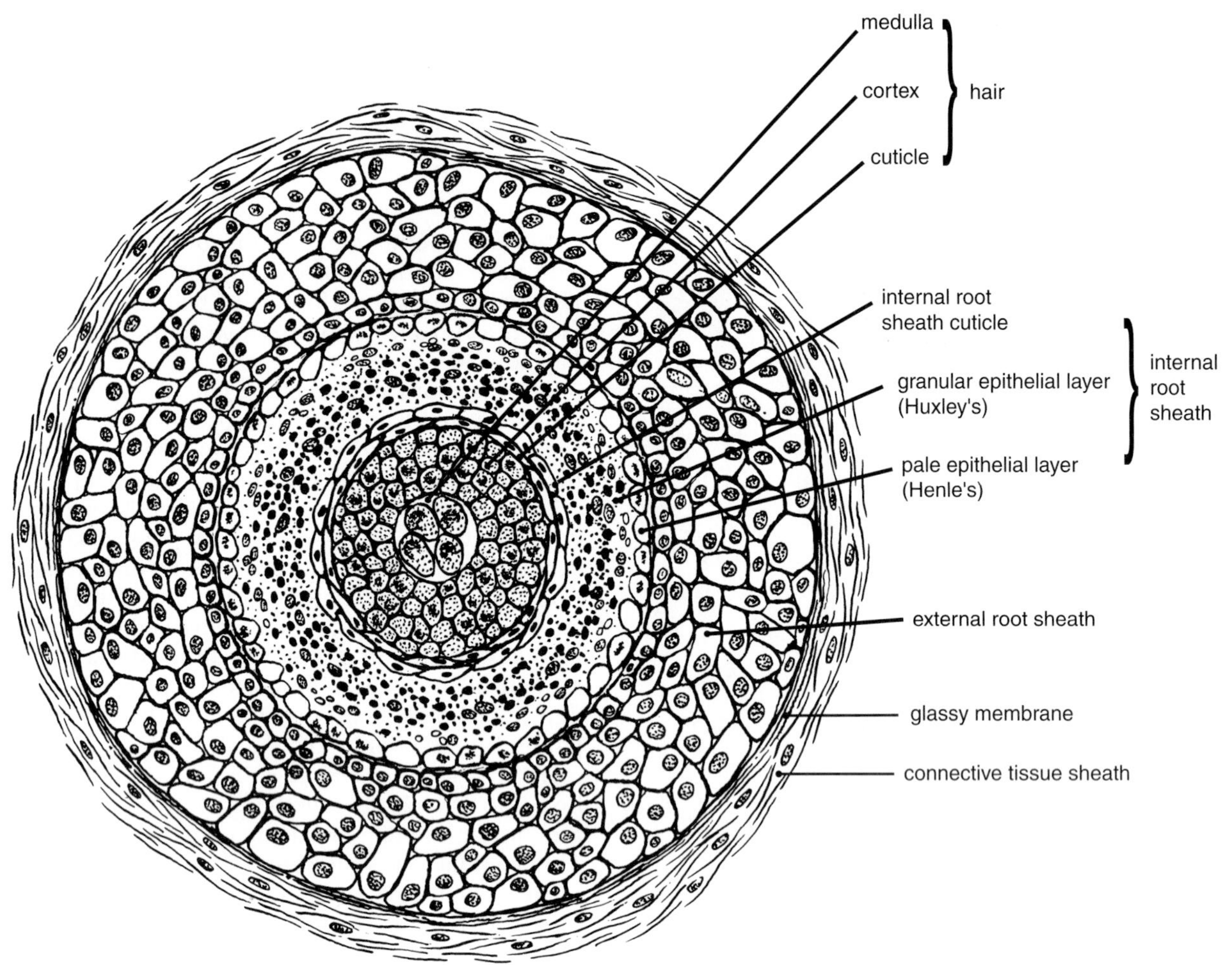

Figure 16.12. *Schematic of an oblique section of a hair follicle.*

internal root sheath cuticle, *(b)* middle granular epithelial layer (Huxley's layer), and *(c)* outer pale epithelial layer (Henle's layer) (Fig. 16.12). The **cuticle** of the internal root sheath is formed by overlapping keratinized cells similar to those of the cuticle of the hair, except that the free edges are oriented in the opposite direction or toward the hair bulb. This arrangement results in a solid implantation of the hair root in the hair follicle. The **granular epithelial layer** is composed of one to three layers of cells rich in trichohyalin (keratohyalin in hair) granules. The **pale epithelial layer** is the outermost layer of the internal root sheath and is composed of a single layer of keratinized cells. Immediately below the opening of the sebaceous glands, the internal root sheath of the large follicles becomes corrugated, forming several circular or follicular folds. The sheath then becomes thinner, and the cells fuse, disintegrate, and become part of the sebum.

The **external root sheath** is composed of several layers of cells similar to the epidermis, with which it is continuous in the upper portion of the follicle. External to this layer is a homogeneous glassy membrane corresponding to the basal lamina of the epidermis (Fig. 16.12). The entire epithelial sheath is enclosed by a connective tissue sheath composed of collagen and elastic fibers richly supplied by blood vessels and nerves, especially in the dermal papilla.

The **dermal papilla** of the hair follicle is the region of connective tissue directly underneath the hair matrix. The cells covering the dermal papilla and composing most of the hair bulb are the **hair matrix cells**. These are comparable to stratum basale cells of regular epidermis and give rise to the cells that keratinize to form the hair (Fig. 16.13). They differ from the keratinocytes of the surface epidermis with respect to the type of keratin produced. The surface keratinocytes produce a "soft" form of keratin that passes through a keratohyalin phase. The cells containing "soft" keratin have a high lipid content and a low sulfur content and desquamate when they reach the surface. The matrix cells of the hair follicle produce a "hard" keratin, which is characteristic of hair, horn, and feather. The keratinocytes do not go through a keratohyalin phase, do not desquamate, and have a low lipid content and a high sulfur content. Hair pigment is derived from the epidermal melanocytes located over the dermal papilla. Gray hair results from the inability of melanocytes in the hair bulb to produce tyrosinase. Hair color is determined by the amount and distribution of pigment and by the presence of air, which appears white in reflected light. Silvery white hair is the result when the pigment has faded and the medulla becomes filled with air.

HAIR CYCLE

In the surface epidermis, the process of keratinization is continuous because of the uninterrupted production of new keratinocytes, but in the hair follicle, the matrix cells undergo periods of quiescence during which no mitotic activity occurs. When the matrix cell proliferation is reinstituted, a new hair is formed. This cyclic activity of the hair bulb allows for the seasonal change in the hair coat of domestic animals. Hair requires approximately 3 to 4 months to regrow after shaving for normal or short coats and up to 18 months for long coats. The length of time varies, depending on the growth stage of the hair follicle.

The period during which the cells of the hair bulb are mitotically active is called **anagen**. After this growth phase, the hair follicles go through a regressive stage, referred to as **catagen**. During this period, metabolic activity slows down, and the base of the follicle migrates upward in the skin toward the epidermal surface, until all that remains of the bulb is a flimsy, disorganized column of cells, or club hair. The hair follicle then enters **telogen**, a resting or quiescent phase in which growth stops and the base of the bulb is at the level of the sebaceous canal. After the resting phase, mitotic activity and keratinization start again in the renewed anagen phase and a new hair is formed. As the new hair grows beneath the telogen follicle, it gradually pushes the old hair upward toward the surface, where it is eventually shed (Fig. 16.14). This intermittent mitotic activity and keratinization of the hair matrix cells constitute the hair cycle which is controlled by several factors, including length of daily periods of light, ambient temperature, nutrition, and hormones, particularly estrogen, testosterone, adrenal steroids, and thyroid hormone.

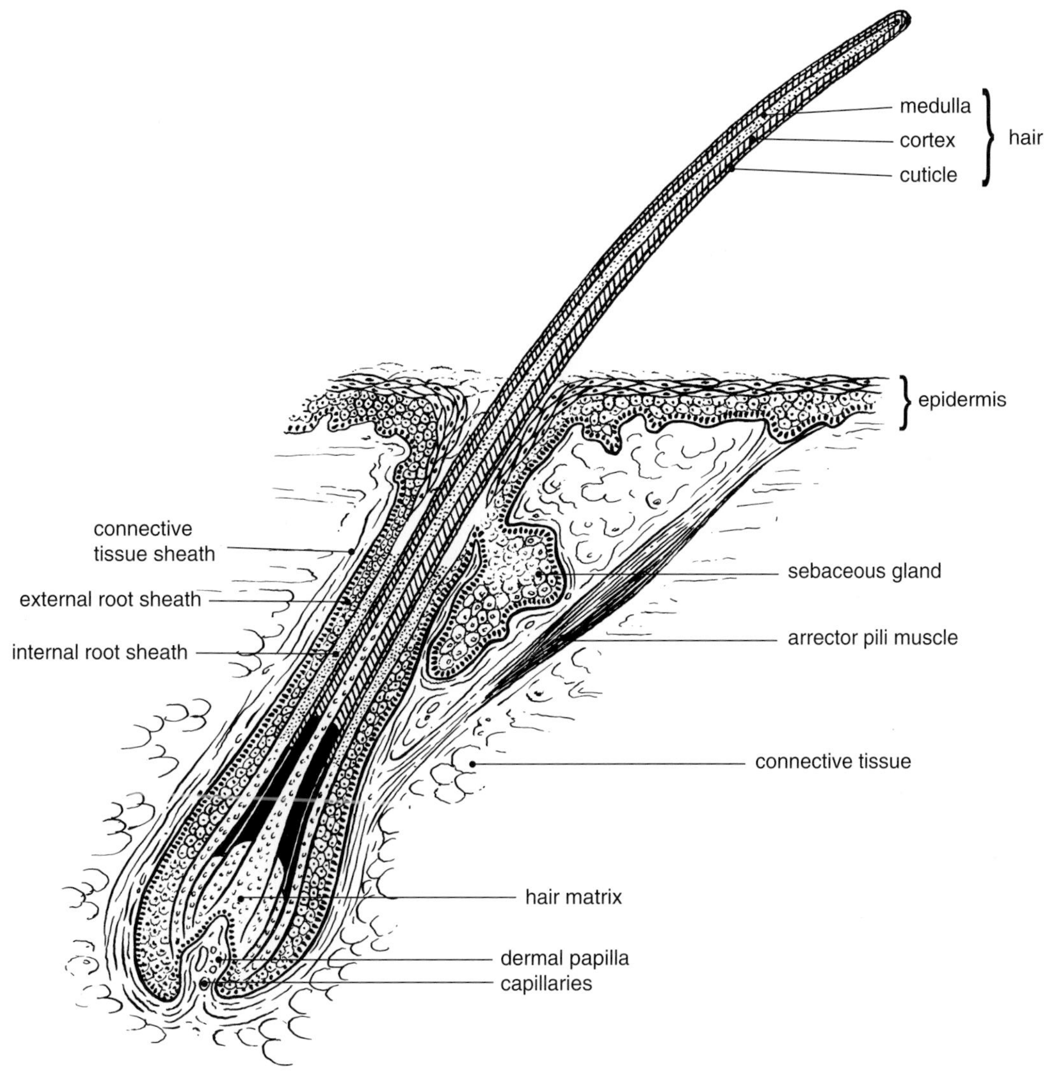

Figure 16.13. *Schematic of a longitudinal section of a hair follicle.*

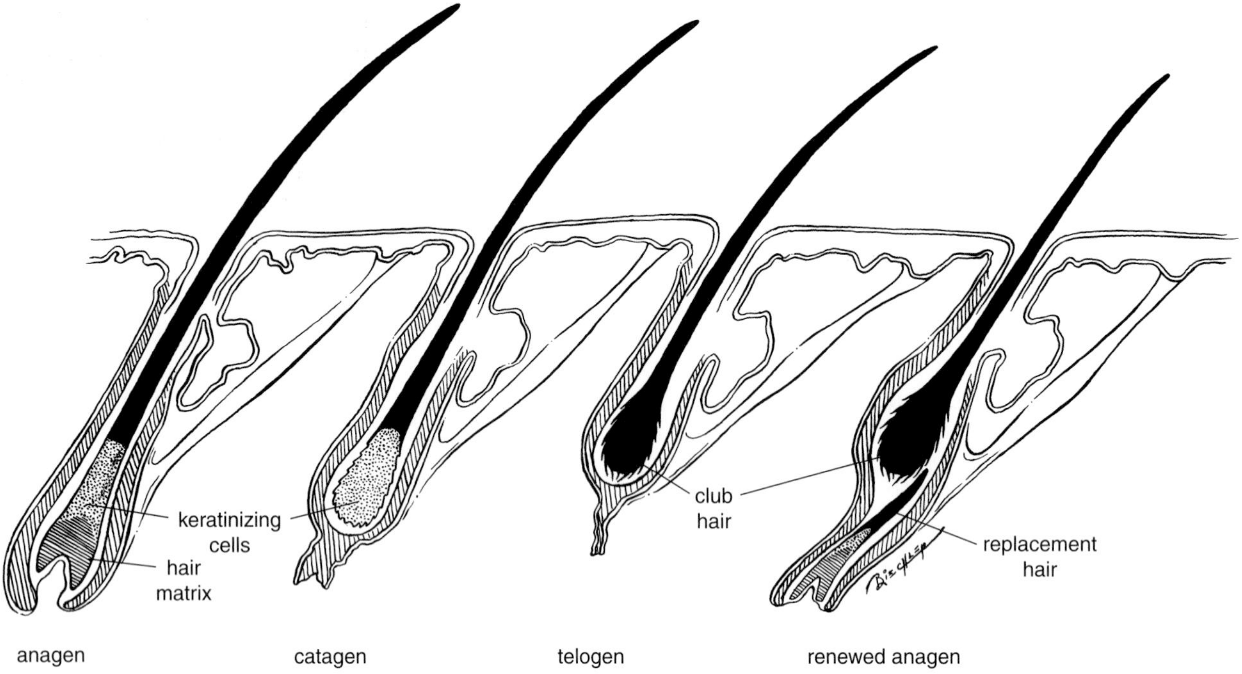

Figure 16.14. *Schematic of the three main stages of hair follicle growth and replacement.*

Associated with most hair follicles are bundles of smooth muscle called the **arrector pili muscle**. This muscle attaches to the connective tissue sheath of the hair follicle and extends toward the epidermis, where it connects to the papillary layer of the dermis (Fig. 16.15). These muscles are anchored by elastic fibers at their insertions and attachments and are innervated by autonomic nerve fibers. The arrector pili muscles are especially well developed along the back of dogs, where they cause the hair to "bristle" when they contract. The contraction of the arrector pili muscles during cold weather elevates the hairs, thus allowing minute air pockets to form in the coat. This dead-air space provides significant insulation that helps to maintain internal body temperature. The contraction of this muscle not only erects the hairs but also may play a role in emptying the sebaceous glands. In addition to the arrector pili muscle, another smooth muscle has been described in pigs, called the **interfollicular muscle**, which spans the triad of hair follicles (Fig. 16.16). It is located midway between the level of the sebaceous gland and the apocrine sweat gland. Upon contraction, the interfollicular muscle draws the three follicles close together into a new relationship, thereby rotating the outer follicles of the triad. Any kind of adjustment of the hair follicle and hair may play a part in thermal regulation, sensory function, emptying of the skin glands, or self defense.

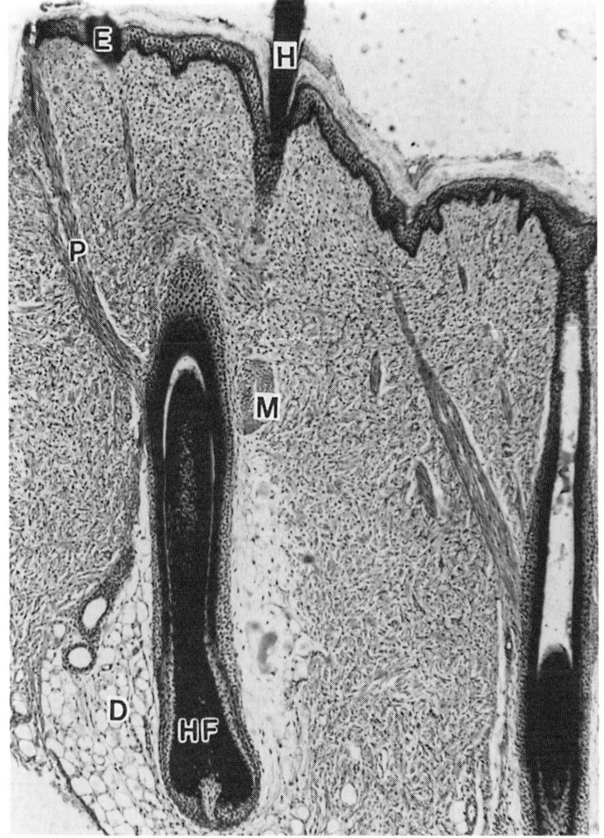

Figure 16.15. *Longitudinal section of a hair follicle (HF) showing an attached arrector pili muscle (P), cross section of the interfollicular muscle (M), epidermis (E), hair (H), and hypodermis (D). Pig, Bodian's protargol (×100).*

TYPES OF HAIR FOLLICLES

Hair follicles are classified into several types. A primary hair follicle has a large diameter, is rooted deep in the dermis, and is usually associated with sebaceous and

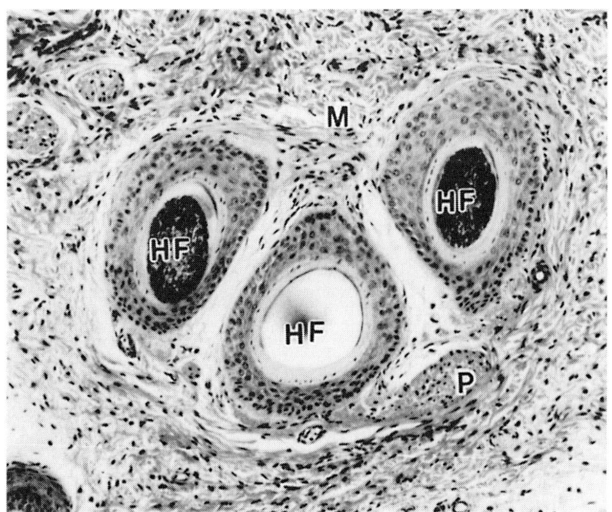

Figure 16.16. *Hair follicle triad (pig). Note the hair follicles (HF) occurring in groups of three, typical of young pigs. The interfollicular muscle (M) and arrector pili muscle (P) can be seen. Hematoxylin and eosin (×140).*

sweat glands and an arrector pili muscle (Fig. 16.11). The hair that emerges from such a follicle is called a **primary hair** (guard hair). A secondary follicle is smaller in diameter than a primary follicle, and the root is nearer the surface. It may have a sebaceous gland but lacks a sweat gland and an arrector pili muscle. Hairs from these follicles are **secondary**, or underhairs.

Follicles with only one hair emerging to the surface are called **single** or **simple follicles. Compound follicles** are composed of clusters of several hair follicles located in the dermis. At the level of the sebaceous gland opening, the follicles fuse and the various hairs emerge through one external follicular orifice. Compound hair follicles usually have one primary hair follicle and several secondary hair follicles.

Many differences exist in the arrangement of the hair follicles among the domestic animals. Horses and cattle have single hair follicles that are distributed evenly. Pigs have single follicles grouped in clusters of two to four follicles; clusters of three are most common in young pigs (Figs. 16.16 and 16.17). This cluster is usually surrounded by dense connective tissue. The compound follicle of dogs consists of a single large primary hair and a group of smaller secondary underhairs (Fig. 16.18). A diversity of hair types are found in different breeds of dogs. For example, in the German Shepherd, a greater number of secondary hairs exist, whereas in the short-coat breeds like the Rottweiler and terriers, a greater number of primary hairs are present. Primary hairs usually emerge separately, whereas as many as 15 secondary hairs may emerge from a single opening. Compound follicles occur in clusters of three, with a slightly larger center follicle. The arrangement of the follicles in cats consists of a single large primary (guard) hair follicle surrounded by clusters of two to five compound follicles (Fig. 16.19). Each compound follicle has three coarse primary hairs and six to 12 secondary hairs. The skin of sheep has hair-growing regions, such as the face, the distal part of the limbs, and the pinna of the ear, and has wool-growing regions that cover most of the body. The hair-growing regions contain mostly single follicles, whereas the densely covered wool-growing regions have many compound follicles. The typical follicle cluster contains three primary follicles and several secondary follicles. In goats, the primary follicles occur in groups of three; three to six secondary follicles are associated with each group.

Sinus or **tactile hair follicles** of the head are highly specialized for tactile sense like the vibrissae (whiskers) of a cat. They are very large single follicles characterized by a blood-filled sinus between the inner and outer layers of the dermal sheath (Fig. 16.20). The sinus is divided into an upper annular sinus (nontrabecular, not separated by connective tissue) and a lower cavernous sinus (trabecular, separated by connective tissue). In horses and ruminants, the annular sinus is traversed by fibroelastic trabeculae throughout its length. In pigs and carnivores, however, in the upper portion of the sinus hair follicles, the inner layer of the dermal sheath thickens, forming a sinus pad, and this pad is surrounded by an annular sinus free of trabeculae (Fig. 16.21). Skeletal muscles are attached to the outer sheath of the follicle, allowing some voluntary control. Numerous nerve bundles penetrate the outer sheath and ramify in the trabeculae and inner dermal sheath.

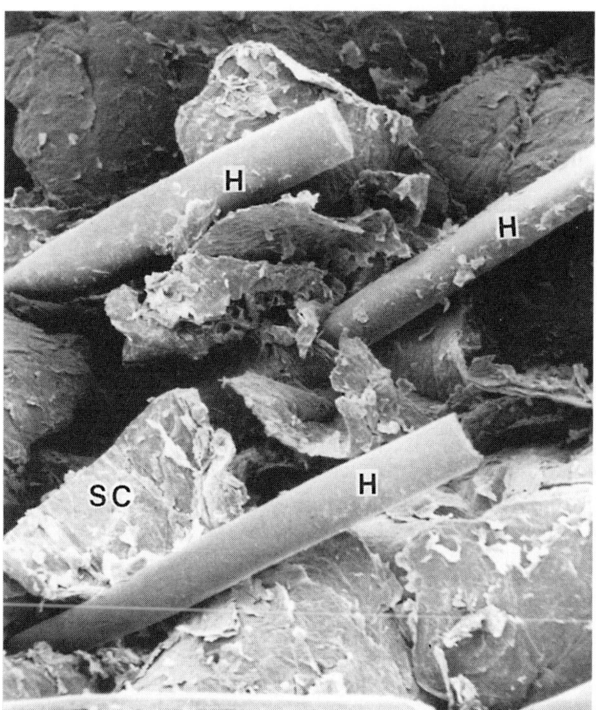

Figure 16.17. *Scanning electron micrograph of pig skin depicting hairs (H) occurring in groups of three emerging from the stratum corneum. Note the flaky appearance of the stratum corneum (SC) cells (×60). (From Monteiro-Riviere NA. Comparative anatomy, physiology, and biochemistry of mammalian skin. In: Hobson DW, ed. Dermal and ocular toxicology: fundamentals and methods. Boca Raton, FL: CRC Press, 1991.)*

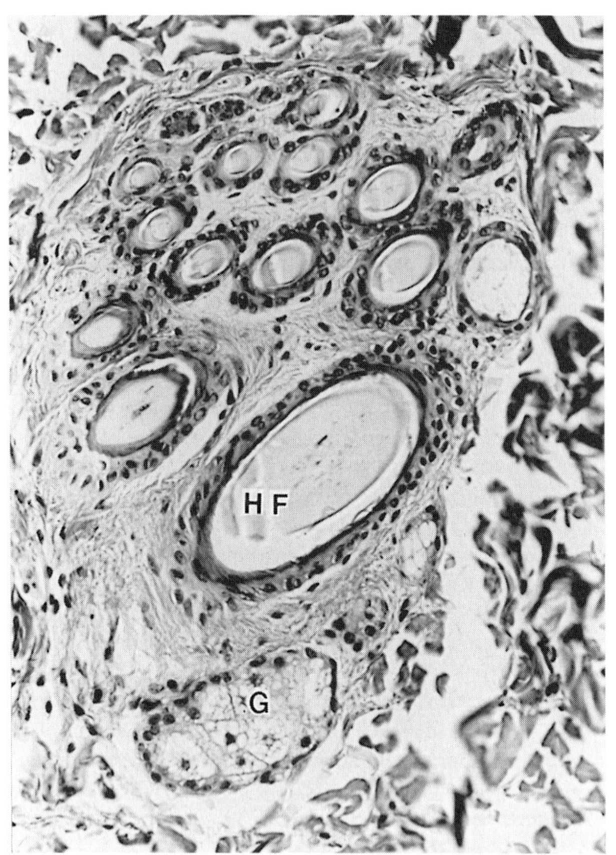

Figure 16.18. *Compound hair follicle (dog). Primary hair follicle (HF) and sebaceous glands (G). The other round structures are all secondary follicles. Hematoxylin and eosin (×120).*

Skin Glands

SEBACEOUS GLANDS

Sebaceous glands may be simple, branched, or compound alveolar glands that release their secretory product, sebum, by the holocrine mode. They are most frequently associated with hair follicles, into which their ducts empty to form the pilosebaceous canal of the hair follicle (Fig. 16.22). In certain hairless areas, such as the anus, the teat of horses, and the internal layer of the prepuce of some species, sebaceous glands empty directly onto the skin surface through a duct lined with stratified squamous epithelium. The **secretory unit** consists of a solid mass of epidermal cells, enclosed by a connective-tissue sheath that blends with the surrounding dermis. At the periphery of the glandular mass, a single layer of low cuboidal cells rests on a basal lamina. Most of the mitotic activity takes place in this layer, and as the cells move inward, they enlarge, become polygonal, and accumulate numerous lipid droplets. The cells near the **duct** contain pyknotic nuclei. The sebum is derived from the disintegration of the epithelial cells and passes into the lumen of the hair follicle through a short duct lined with stratified squamous epithelium. Sebum, an oily secretion containing a mixture of lipids, acts as an antibacterial agent and, in hairy mammals, as a waterproofing agent.

Many areas of the body of certain species have especially well-developed accumulations of sebaceous glands, some of which are associated with sweat glands. These sites include the infraorbital, inguinal, and interdigital regions of sheep, the base of the horn of goats, anal sacs of cats, and the prepuce and circumanal region of dogs, and are described later in this chapter. Some areas of the skin, such as the foot pads, hoofs, claws, and horn, lack sebaceous glands.

SWEAT GLANDS

Based on their morphologic and functional characteristics, sweat (sudoriferous) glands are classified into two types: **apocrine** and **merocrine** (eccrine). The apocrine type is the most extensively developed in the domestic mammals. The structure of apocrine sweat glands varies considerably among species, and whether the apocrine mode of secretion occurs in all sweat glands designated as apocrine and in all domestic species is uncertain. Nevertheless, the term apocrine is retained, primarily for didactic reasons.

The **apocrine sweat glands** are simple saccular or tubular glands with a coiled secretory portion and a straight duct. The secretory portion has a large lumen

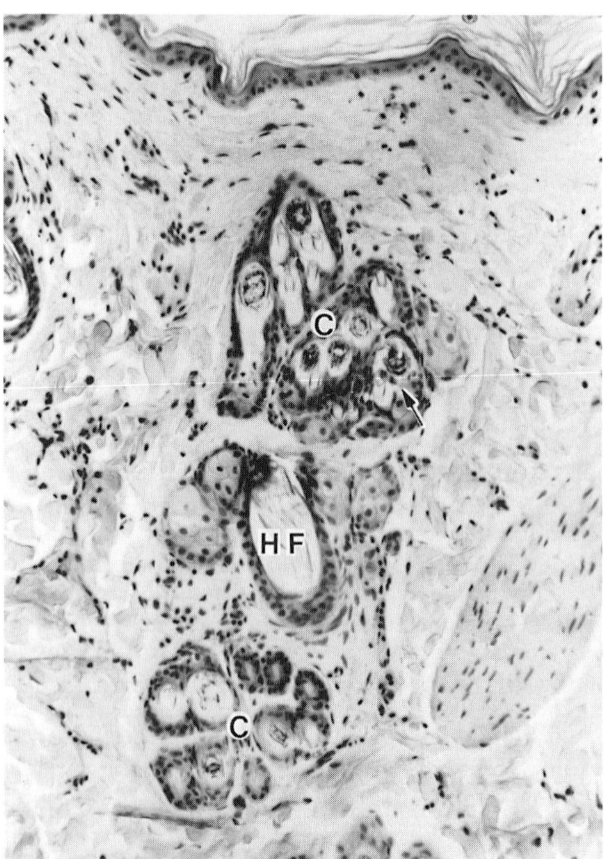

Figure 16.19. *Hair follicle cluster (cat). Primary hair follicle (HF) surrounded by groups of compound follicle clusters (C) that contain primary and secondary hairs (arrow). Hematoxylin and eosin (×160).*

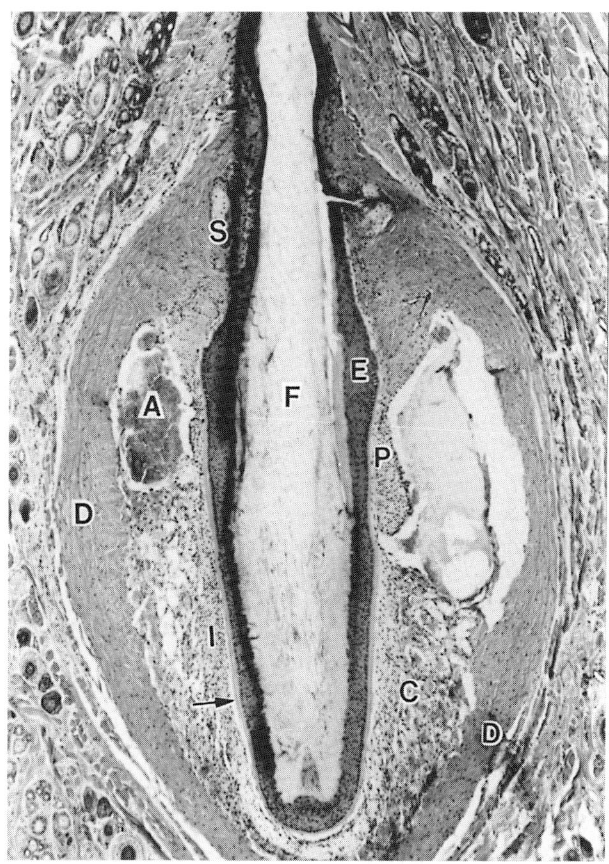

Figure 16.20. *Sinus hair follicle (cat). Outer layer of the dermal sheath (D); inner layer of the dermal sheath (I); upper annular sinus filled with blood (nontrabecular) (A); cavernous blood sinus with trabeculae (C); glassy membrane (arrow); external root sheath (E); hair (F); sinus pad (P); sebaceous glands opening into the pilosebaceous canal (S). Hematoxylin and eosin (×50).*

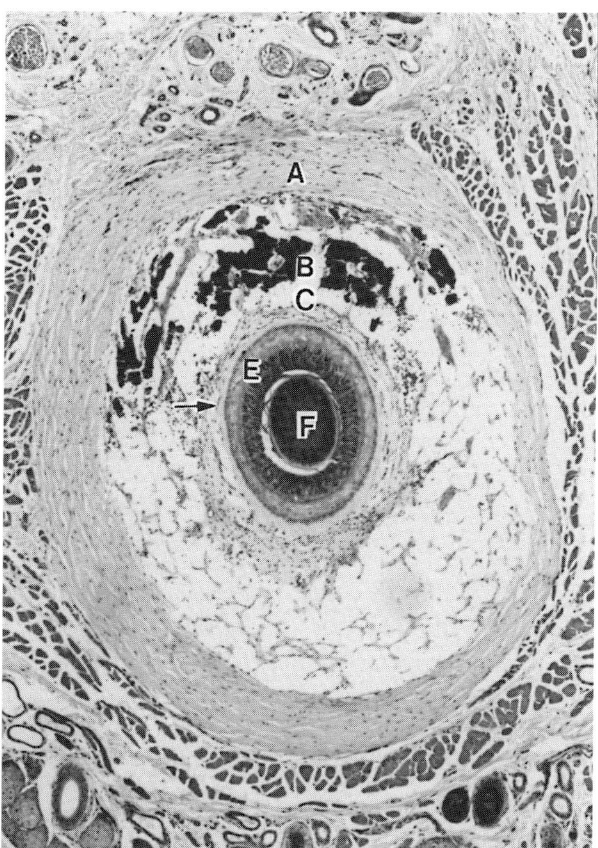

Figure 16.21. *Cross section of a sinus hair follicle (cat). Outer layer of the dermal sheath (A); cavernous blood sinus with trabeculae (B); inner layer of the dermal sheath (C); glassy membrane (arrow); external root sheath (E); hair (F). Hematoxylin and eosin (×60).*

lined with flattened cuboidal to low columnar epithelial cells, depending on the stage of their secretory activity (Fig. 16.23). The cytoplasm may contain glycogen, lipid, or pigment granules. The free surface of cells in apocrine sweat glands has cytoplasmic protrusions, indicative of their secretory activity (Fig. 16.23). Myoepithelial cells are located between the secretory cells and the basal lamina (Fig. 16.23). The duct portion pursues a straight course toward the upper part of the dermis. It has a narrow lumen and two layers of flattened cuboidal cells. Most frequently, the duct penetrates the epidermis of the hair follicle just before it opens onto the surface of the skin. The apocrine glands in the domestic animals are located throughout most of the skin. This characteristic contrasts with their distribution in humans, in which they are mainly in the axillary, pubic, and perianal regions. In horses, these glands secrete abundantly and produce visible sweat during exercise and at high temperature. In other species, the secretion is scant and rarely perceptible. In dogs and cats, the glands may be tortuous or serpentine, and in ruminants, the lumen is dilated, giving the appearance of large saccules. The apocrine glands are least active in goats and cats. The function of apocrine glands is to produce a viscous se-

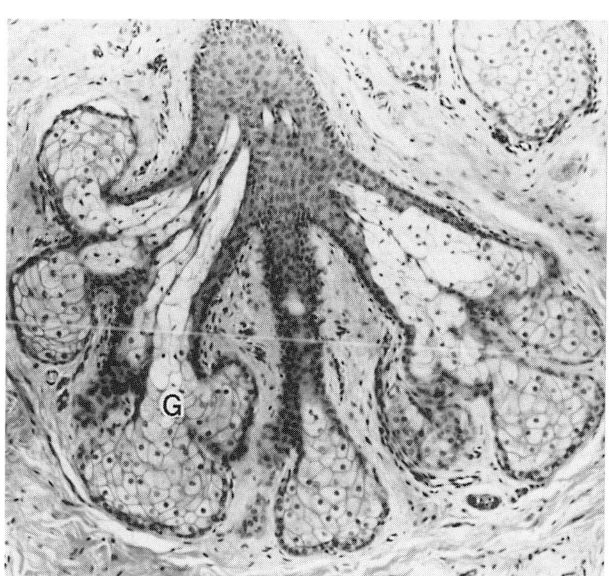

Figure 16.22. *Multilobular sebaceous glands (G) of the labium (horse). Hematoxylin and eosin (×110).*

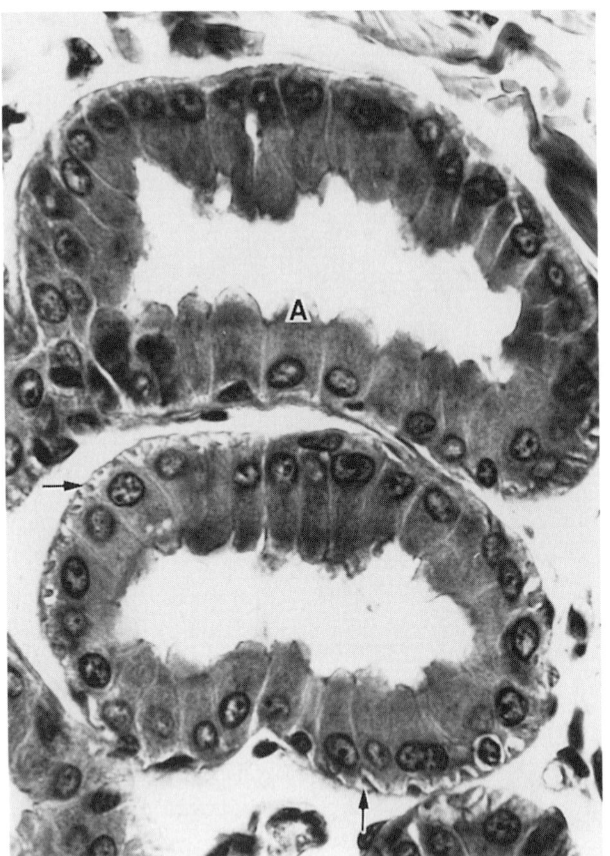

Figure 16.23. *Apocrine sweat glands from a dog, illustrating myoepithelial cells (arrows) and apical secretory caps (A). Hematoxylin and eosin (×660).*

cretion that contains a scent that is related to communications between species, probably as a sex attractant or as a territorial marker.

The apocrine glands are specialized in structure and function in several areas. These special apocrine sweat glands are described later in this chapter.

The **merocrine** (eccrine) sweat **glands** are found mainly in special skin areas, such as the foot pads of dogs and cats, the frog of ungulates, the planum rostrale of pigs, the bovine planum nasolabiale, and the carpal glands of swine. They are simple tubular glands that open directly onto the skin surface rather than into hair follicles. The secretory portion is composed of cuboidal epithelium with two distinct cell types (Fig. 16.24). The dark cells have more ribosomes than the clear cells, and numerous mucin droplets occur in the apical part of the cell. The clear cells lack cytoplasmic basophilia, contain lipid inclusions, and produce aqueous sweat. At the base of these cells, there is an infolding of the plasma membrane, which suggests that they play a role in electrolyte transport. Intercellular canaliculi occur between adjacent clear cells and course from the lumen to the base of the epithelium. Myoepithelial cells are specialized smooth muscle cells that surround the secretory units and aid in emptying the gland of secretion. The duct, which is composed of two layers of cuboidal epithelial cells, is relatively straight and opens directly onto the surface of the epidermis.

BLOOD VESSELS, LYMPH VESSELS, AND NERVES

Terminal branches of the cutaneous arteries give rise to three plexuses: *(a)* the deep or subcutaneous plexus, which in turn gives off branches to the *(b)* middle or cutaneous plexus, which provides branches to make up the *(c)* superficial or subpapillary plexus (Fig. 16.1). The reverse applies for venous return to the cutaneous veins. By this arrangement, all components of the skin are ensured an adequate blood supply. The superficial plexus also furnishes the capillary loops that extend into the dermal papillae when present. Lymph capillaries arise in the superficial dermis and form a network that drains into a subcutaneous plexus.

The nerve supply to the skin varies in different parts of the body. Small subcutaneous nerves give rise to a nerve plexus that pervades the dermis and sends small branches to the epidermis. Several kinds of endings are present: free afferent nerve endings in the epidermis and dermis (encircle hair follicles) and free efferent endings in the hypodermis (at arrector pili muscles, glands, and blood vessels). Large lamellar corpuscles have been observed in the frog of the equine hoof, the

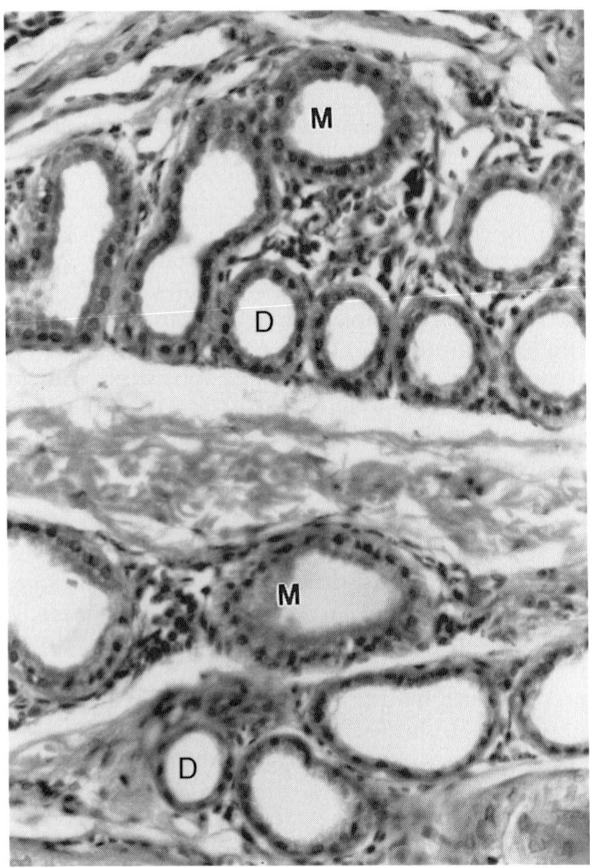

Figure 16.24. *Merocrine sweat glands (M) from the nasolabial plane and ducts (D) (cow). Hematoxylin and eosin (×300).*

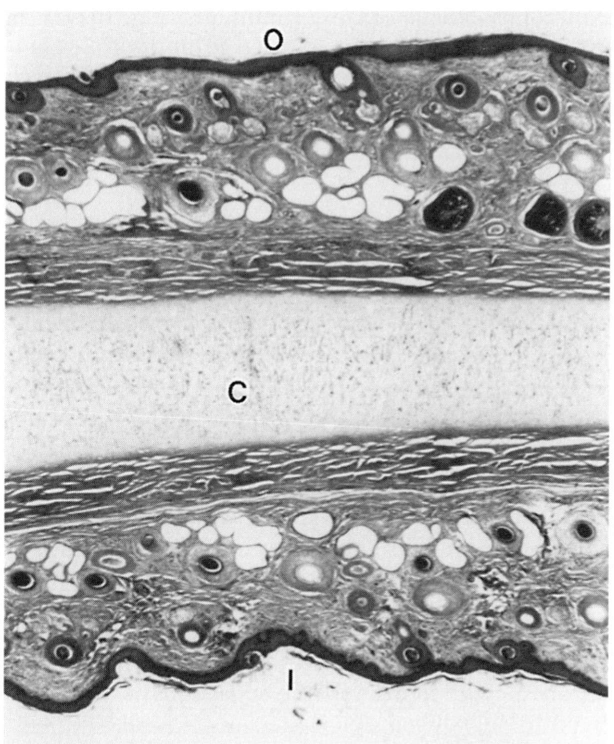

Figure 16.25. *Auricula of the ear (cow). Outer surface (O); inner surface (I); auricular elastic cartilage (C). Hematoxylin and eosin (×30)*

digital cushion of the dog and cat, and the anal sac wall of the cat.

SPECIAL SKIN STRUCTURES

External Ear

The pinna or ear is covered on both sides by thin skin containing sweat and sebaceous glands and hair follicles. The convex surface of the pinna usually has more hair follicles per unit area than does the thinner concave surface (Fig. 16.25). Blood vessels traverse the perforations in the elastic cartilage that forms the core of the pinna. Trauma to or even bending of the cartilage can damage the blood vessels and may cause hematomas on the lateral surface of the cartilage in ears of dogs.

The lumen of the **external auditory canal** is irregular in contour, the result of several permanent skin folds. The skin that lines the canal contains small hair follicles, sebaceous glands, and ceruminous glands. Ceruminous glands are simple coiled tubular apocrine sweat glands. The ceruminous glands open either into hair follicles or onto the surface. They increase in number in the lower third of the meatus. The combination of sebum with the ceruminous gland secretion and the desquamating stratified squamous epithelium forms the cerumen or ear wax. The external auditory canal is supported by elastic cartilage in the outer portion and by bone near the tympanic membrane.

Eyelids

The outermost covering of both upper and lower eyelids is typical skin containing sweat and sebaceous glands and hair follicles (Fig. 16.26). The eyelashes and their associated sebaceous glands (glands of Zeiss) are numerous in the upper lid of all species except cats. In the lower eyelid, the eyelashes are fewer in number in ruminants and horses and are generally absent in cats, dogs, and pigs. Tactile hairs may be present on or near the eyelids. The inner surface of the eyelids, the palpebral conjunctiva, is a mucous membrane and contains lymphatic tissue at its base. Its epithelial covering varies with the area and species from stratified squamous epithelium near the edge of the eyelid to various combinations of columnar, cuboidal, polyhedral, and squamous cells. As a result, it is variously described as stratified squamous, stratified cuboidal, stratified columnar, and transitional or pseudostratified. Goblet cells are often present (Fig.16.27).

The most characteristic feature of the eyelids is the **tarsal glands** (Meibomian glands), which are better developed in the upper lid (Fig. 16.28). They are multilobular sebaceous glands with a central duct, which opens onto the palpebral surface at the margin of the eyelid (Fig. 16.28). These glands are most highly developed in the cat and poorly developed in swine. The tarsal glands are surrounded by the **tarsal plate**, a compact layer of collagen and elastic fibers. Skeletal muscle fibers from the orbicular muscle (orbicularis oculi) penetrate the eyelid, and scattered bundles of smooth muscle fibers are also present.

Apocrine sweat glands, referred to as **ciliary glands** (glands of Moll), open rostrally to the tarsal glands and near the eyelashes or into the follicles of the eyelashes.

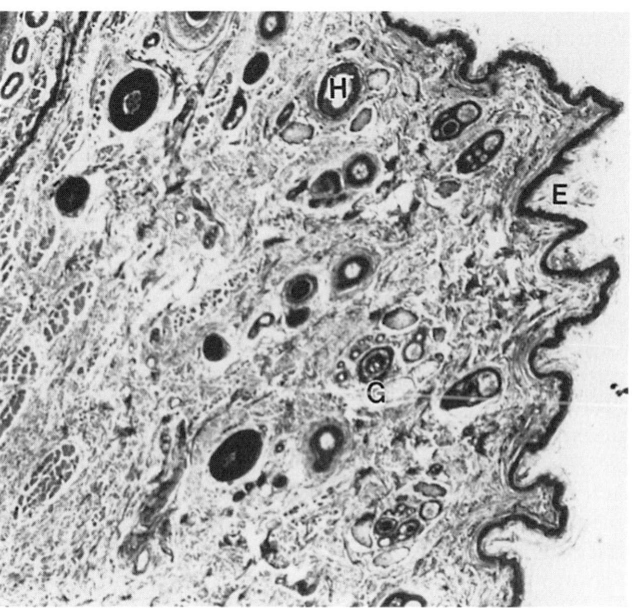

Figure 16.26. *Upper eyelid (dog). External or skin surface (E), numerous eyelashes (hairs) (H), and sebaceous glands (G) are present. Hematoxylin and eosin (×50).*

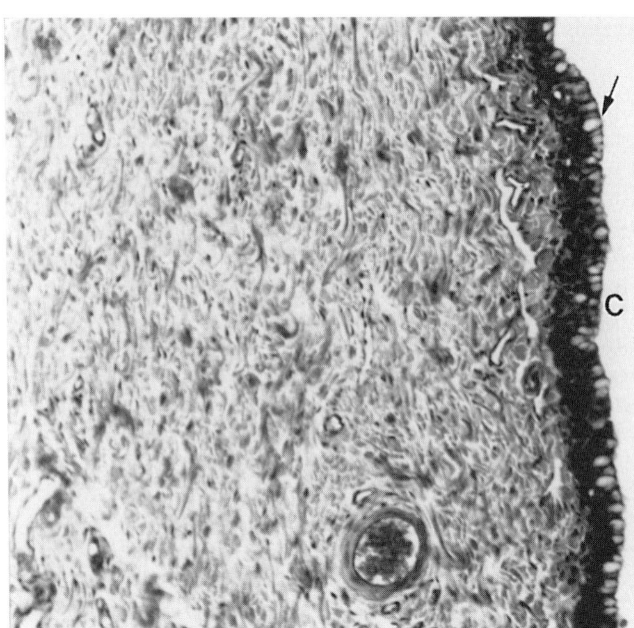

Figure 16.27. *Upper eyelid (dog). Internal or conjunctival surface (C) with pseudostratified epithelium with goblet cells (arrow). Hematoxylin and eosin (×150).*

Unlike ordinary sweat glands, the terminal portions of ciliary glands are only slightly coiled, and the gland lumina are more dilated. They are lined by typical cylindric secretory and myoepithelial cells (Fig. 16.23). Their structure and location are similar in all domestic animals, but their function is obscure.

Infraorbital Sinus

The infraorbital sinus of sheep, located medially and rostrally to the eye, is lined with thin skin that contains few hairs, large sebaceous glands that form a continuous layer around the sinus, and a few peripherally located apocrine sweat glands. The secretions of these glands are responsible for the sticky, yellow fatty substance on the skin.

Nose

The skin around the external openings of the nasal cavity is slightly modified in each species. The planum nasolabiale of the cow has a smooth, thick keratinized epidermis (Fig. 16.29), whereas the planum nasale of dogs and cats is composed of a thick, keratinized epidermis with distinct elevations and grooves. These characteristics provide the basis for identification by nose printing, similar to fingerprinting. Neither sweat nor sebaceous glands are associated with this area. The skin around the nostril of horses is usually thin and contains fine hairs and numerous sebaceous glands. The planum rostrale of pigs has fine hairs sparsely distributed over the surface and numerous large merocrine sweat glands. The planum nasale of small ruminants and the planum nasolabiale of large ruminants (Fig. 16.30) contain no hair follicles but have large merocrine glands (serous) with morphologic characteristics of salivary glands. The secretion from these glands via a duct system aid in keeping the nasolabial plane moist.

Mental Organ

The mental organ of pigs consists of a large spherical mass of apocrine and sebaceous glands with a few tactile hairs located midway between the jaws behind the angle of the chin. Tactile corpuscles (Meissner's) and nerve fibers are present in the dermis and, therefore, are believed to play a role in transmitting mechanical stimuli.

Submental Organ

The submental organ of cats, located in the intermandibular space, is composed of sebaceous gland lobules, each containing a central collecting space. These lobules are surrounded by skeletal muscle. The function of this organ is in olfactory marking. Cats will rub this organ on specific items and the sebaceous scent is transferred to the rubbed object.

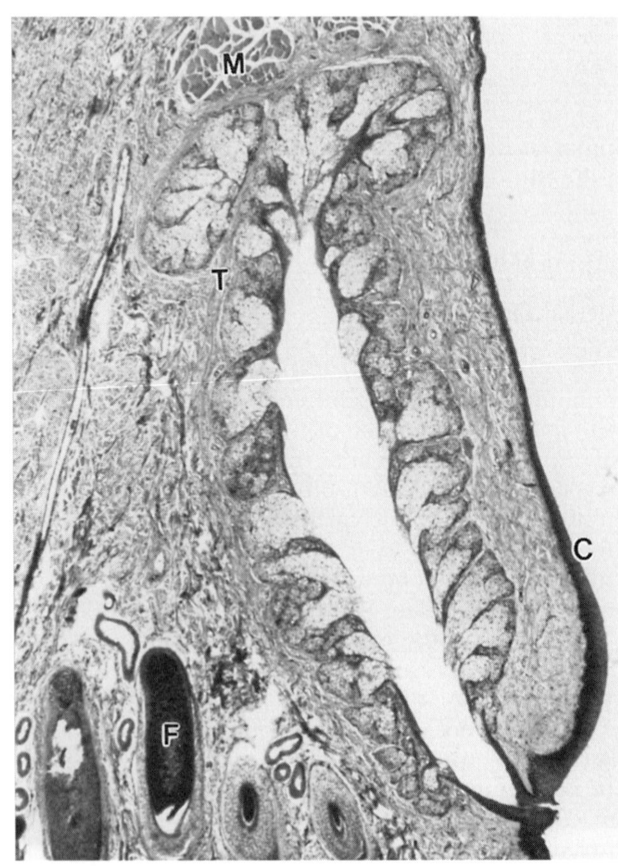

Figure 16.28. *Tarsal gland in the upper eyelid (dog). Multilobular sebaceous tarsal gland in longitudinal section surrounded by the tarsal plate (T), skeletal muscle (M), and hair follicles (F). The conjunctival surface (C) is nonkeratinized stratified squamous epithelium. Hematoxylin and eosin (×40).*

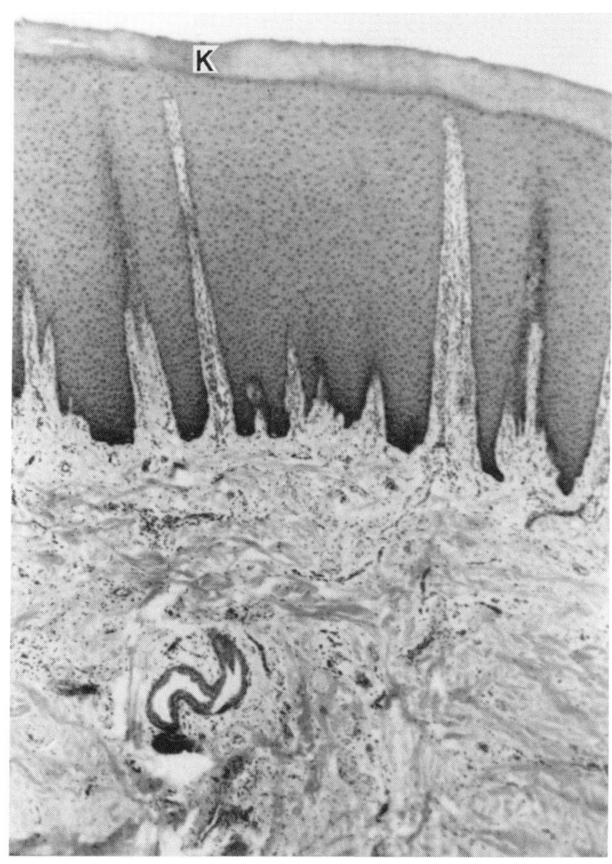

Figure 16.29. *Planum nasolabiale (cow). Notice the thickened keratinized epithelium (K). Hematoxylin and eosin (×50).*

Carpal Glands

The carpal glands of pigs are accumulations of numerous lobules of densely packed merocrine sweat glands on the medial surface of the carpus. They open to the skin surface through three to five diverticula lined with stratified squamous epithelium. Each lobule is drained by a duct lined with a bilayered cuboidal epithelium, which pursues a tortuous course through the dermis and epidermis and then opens into a diverticulum.

Interdigital Sinus

The interdigital sinus of sheep is located between the digits just above the hoofs. The opening of the sinus is at the dorsal tip of the interdigital space. The skin of the sinus contains a few hair follicles, associated sebaceous glands, and numerous large apocrine glands collectively referred to as the **interdigital glands**.

Inguinal Sinus

The inguinal sinus of sheep is a cutaneous diverticulum in the inguinal region of both sexes that contains scattered small hair follicles, sebaceous glands, and apocrine glands.

Scrotum

Generally, scrotal skin is thinner than skin on other parts of the body. Sebaceous and apocrine sweat glands are present but differ in size and number in various species. Boars have only a few small apocrine sweat glands in the scrotal skin, whereas stallions have large sebaceous and well-developed apocrine sweat glands. The amount of pigment varies with species and breed. Short, fine hair is characteristic of all species. The tunica dartos is a unique layer of smooth muscle and fibroelastic connective tissue associated with the dermis of the scrotum. These muscle fibers play an important role in the regulation of testicular temperature.

Anal Sacs

The anal sacs (sinus paranales) of domestic carnivores are paired cutaneous diverticula, the ducts of which open into the anal canal at the level of the anocutaneous junction (Fig. 16.31). The ducts and sacs are lined by stratified squamous epithelium. Both sebaceous and apocrine sweat glands occur in cats (Fig. 16.32), but dogs have only large apocrine sweat glands. The anal sac duct of dogs is prone to occlusion, which results in anal sac engorgement with secretory material and detritus. The infection that frequently follows this occlusion necessitates either

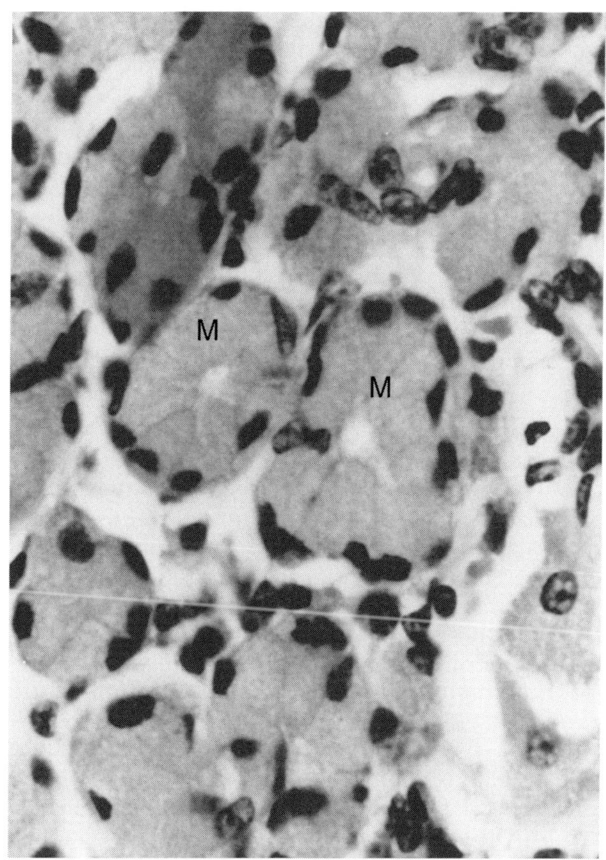

Figure 16.30. *Merocrine (mucous) glands (M) of the nasolabial region (cow). Hematoxylin and eosin (×780).*

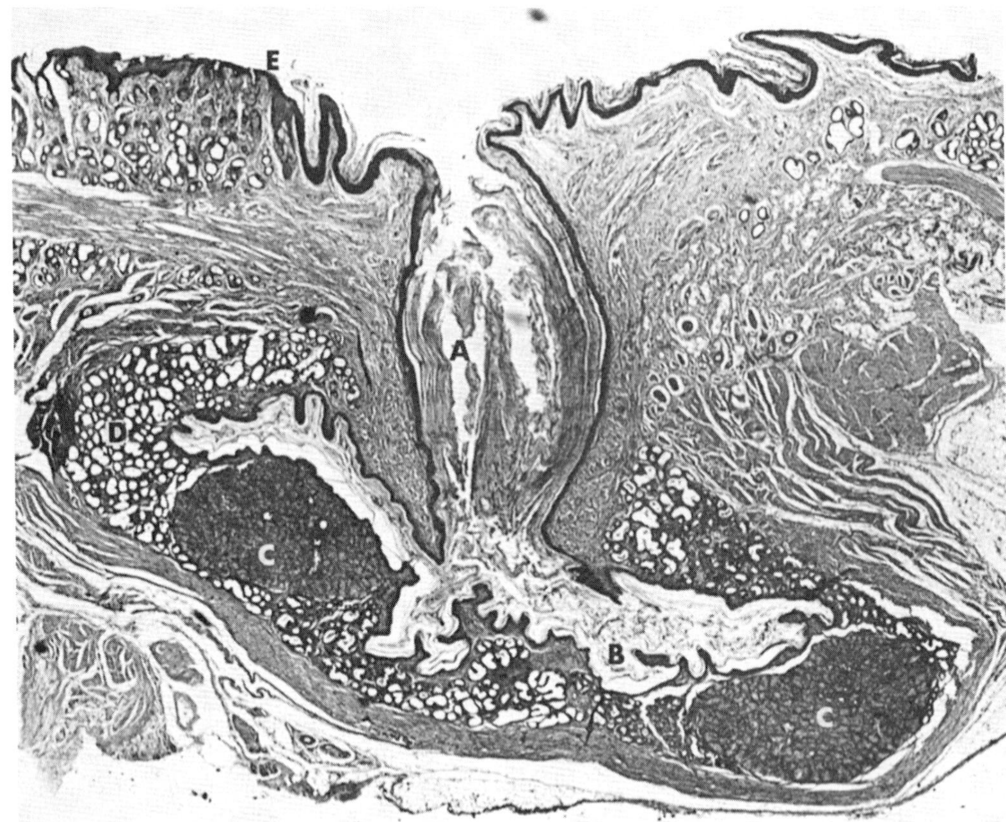

Figure 16.31. *Anal sac and associated glands (cat). Duct (A) and lumen (B) of the anal sac filled with keratinized epithelial fragments and secretory material. Sebaceous gland masses (C); apocrine anal sac glands (D); linea anocutanea (E). Hematoxylin and eosin (×17). (From Greer MB, Calhoun ML. The anal sacs of the domestic cat — felis domesticus. Am J Vet Res 1966;27:773.)*

the expression of the content of the sac or the surgical removal of the sac. This problem is rare in cats, probably because the sebaceous glands within the wall of the sac add sufficient amounts of lipid to the secretory material, consequently decreasing the possibility of occlusion of the duct. The secretion of these glands is a brownish and oily fluid that can have a pungent odor with impaction and infection and may function in social recognition in dogs.

Circumanal Glands

The circumanal glands of dogs are lobulated, modified sebaceous glands located around the anus in the cutaneous zone (Fig. 16.33). They extend from the mucocutaneous junction peripherally for approximately 1 to 3 cm in all directions. Similar glands have been described in the skin of the prepuce, tail, loin, and groin. These glands are present shortly after birth, increase in size throughout adult life, and tend to atrophy during or at senility. They are clinically important because they rank third in frequency as the site of all canine tumors.

These glands comprise a superficial and a deep portion. The superficial portion consists of typical sebaceous glands, whereas the deep portion of these glands are ductless and composed of solid, compact masses of cells that resemble closely packed liver cells with intercellular canaliculi (Fig. 16.33). The term **hepatoid** has been used

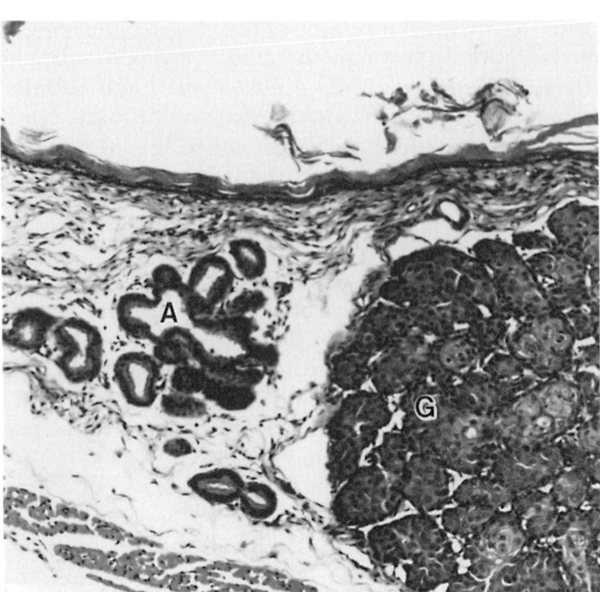

Figure 16.32. *Higher magnification of the anal sac (cat). Note the large apocrine glands (A) and sebaceous glands (G). Hematoxylin and eosin (×120).*

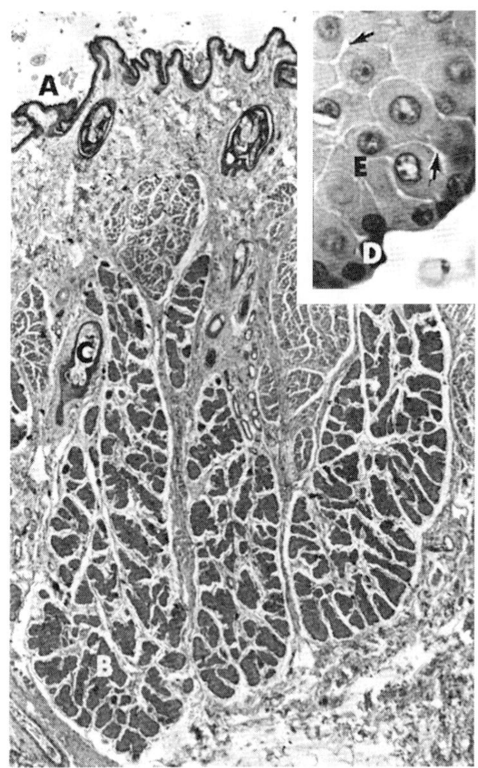

Figure 16.33. *Circumanal glands (dog). Cutaneous zone (A); hepatoid circumanal gland (B); ducts (C). Hematoxylin and eosin (×20). Inset, peripheral cells (D); nonsebaceous gland cells (E); intercellular canaliculi (arrows). Hematoxylin and eosin (×480).*

to describe the glandular parenchyma (cuboidal cells with granular eosinophilic cytoplasm) that make up the main mass of each deep lobule. A precise function for these glands has not been determined; however, it may be involved in the metabolism of a steroid hormone.

Supracaudal Gland

The supracaudal gland (tail gland or preen gland), located in an oval circumscribed area on the dorsum of the tail (3 to 9 cm from base of the tail) in dogs and cats, is an accumulation of large sebaceous glands that empty into single hair follicles (Fig. 16.34). The apocrine sweat glands in this region are rudimentary. The arrector pili muscles are well developed and appear as large bundles (Fig. 16.34). The epidermis above this gland is extremely thin, and the structure of this gland is similar to the superficial portion of the circumanal glands. The secretion may cause a matting of the hair of the region, especially if the glands are overactive. This matting can present a problem in show cats, because the appearance of the hair coat of the tail is affected. The secretion from the large glands may aid in olfactory recognition.

Mammary Gland

Knowledge of the microscopic anatomy of the mammary gland is important to understand the clinical problem of mastitis in large animals and mammary tumors in small animals. Mastitis is inflammation of this gland and is one of the most common and economically significant clinical diseases in the cow. In response to bacterial infection, inflammatory changes occur in the gland with influx of many bloodborne neutrophils.

The mammary gland is a compound tubuloalveolar gland (Fig. 16.35). Groups of tubuloalveolar secretory units form lobules separated by connective-tissue septa.

ALVEOLI

Secretory alveoli are lined by a simple epithelium that varies markedly in height during various stages of secretory activity (Fig. 16.36). Shortly after milking, the alveolus begins a new secretory cycle. At this time, the lumen is partially collapsed and irregular in outline.

The basal portion of the columnar epithelial cells contains a well-developed rough endoplasmic reticulum (rER). The spherical nuclei are located near the center of the cell. Lipid droplets in close association with mitochondria and vesicles filled with micelles of milk protein occur throughout the cell apex. As the secretory cycle continues, the lipid droplets move toward the surface that protrudes into the alveolar lumen. These lipid droplets are released from the cell surrounded by vary-

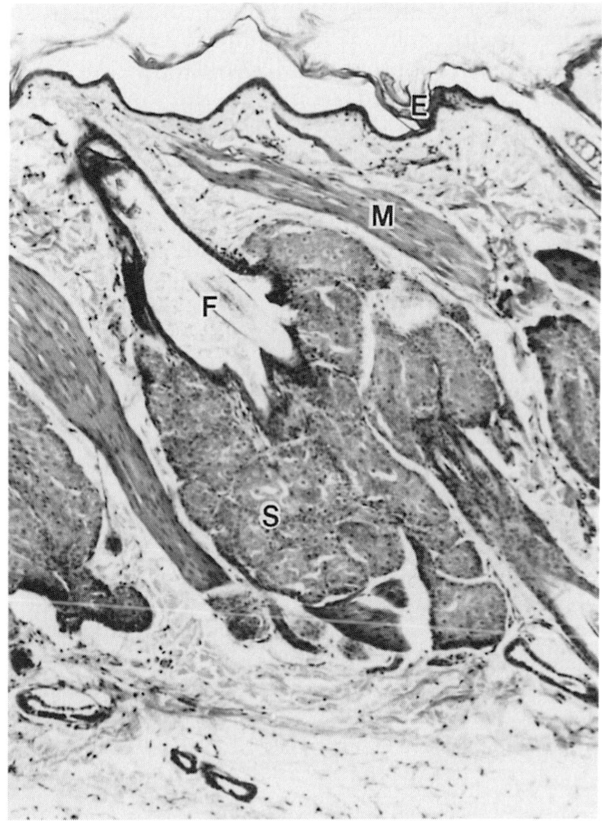

Figure 16.34. *Supracaudal gland region, tail (cat). Thin epidermis (E), sebaceous glands (S) and ducts opening into hair follicles (F), and large bundles of smooth muscle (M). Hematoxylin and eosin (×80).*

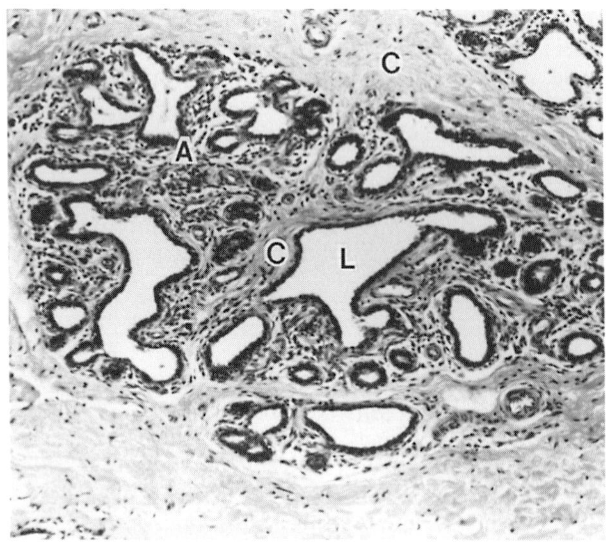

Figure 16.35. *Nonlactating mammary gland (cow). Gland lobules with alveoli (A), large irregular openings represent intralobular duct (L), and loose connective tissue (C). Hematoxylin and eosin (×110).*

ing amounts of cytoplasm, along with the plasmalemma. The protein micelles move toward the surface, where they are released by exocytosis. Milk is thus produced by both apocrine and merocrine secretion. Continuous milk production enlarges the lumen, and adjacent alveoli may fuse partially. At the end of the secretory cycle, the epithelial cells are the low cuboidal type. All the lobules within the gland are not in the same secretory phase at the same time. Some lobules may complete their secretory cycle and be filled with milk before others begin. Therefore, a single histologic section may contain lobules in various stages of activity. Usually, all of the secretory units within a lobule are in approximately the same secretory phase.

Myoepithelial cells contract in response to oxytocin released from the neurohypophysis and thereby force the milk from the secretory units into the duct system. This phenomenon is called **milk letdown**.

INTERSTITIUM

The interstitial tissue of the mammary gland provides important structural support for the secretory units and contains the blood vessels, lymph vessels, and nerves. Each secretory unit is surrounded by loose connective tissue with an extensive plexus of blood and lymph capillaries. Plasma cells and lymphocytes are common, particularly at parturition, when the colostrum is being secreted. The interlobular connective tissue is thick and contains the lobular ducts and larger blood and lymph vessels.

DUCTS

The duct system begins with an intralobular duct, which drains into a lobular duct. This lobular duct, in turn, drains into a lobar lactiferous duct, which is the primary excretory duct for a lobe. The intralobular duct epithelium is simple cuboidal. Spindle-shaped myoepithelial cells may be associated with these ducts. Lobular ducts are lined proximally by a simple cuboidal epithelium and, more distally, by two layers of cuboidal cells. Longitudinal smooth muscle fibers become associated with these ducts as they merge with other lobular ducts to form the large **lactiferous ducts**. The two-layered cuboidal epithelium continues in these larger ducts, and smooth muscle becomes more prominent. Sacculations result from variations in the diameter of the lumen. The constrictions between these sacculations may have an annular fold containing smooth muscle. In ruminants, several lactiferous ducts empty into a lactiferous sinus (gland sinus) at the base of the teat. This sinus is continuous with the teat sinus (teat cistern, cavity of the teat), which opens into the papillary duct (teat canal, streak canal) leading to the external surface of the teat. The papillary ducts of the other domestic mammalian species open separately onto the teat surface; cats have four to seven ducts, dogs have seven to 16 ducts, and pigs and horses have two to three ducts.

TEAT

The **teat** or nipple contains the terminal part of the duct system and is lined with a mucous membrane that

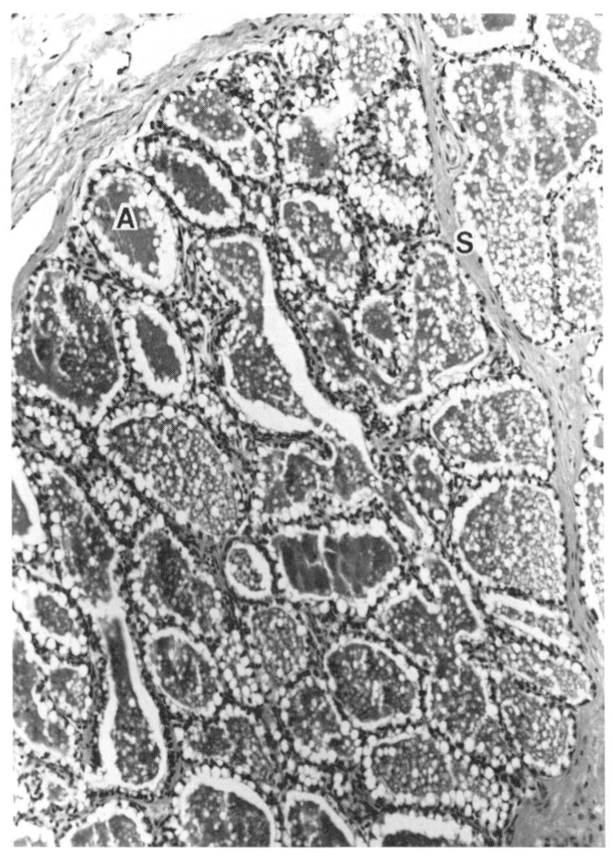

Figure 16.36. *Lactating mammary gland filled with colostrum (sheep). Alveolus (A); interlobular septum (S). Hematoxylin and eosin (×120)*

lies next to the dermis of the skin. The teat of ruminants has a large lumen, the teat sinus, lined by a bilayered cuboidal epithelium. An annular fold of the mucosa extends into the opening between the lactiferous and teat sinuses. The size of this opening is somewhat variable from one animal to another. Occasionally, trabeculae of connective tissue may extend across the opening, resulting in a slowing of the milk flow from the lactiferous sinus to the teat sinus. These trabeculae are called **spiders**, and frequently, veterinarians must cut them surgically.

The lamina propria of the teat sinus may contain small clusters of mammary gland tissue. Smooth muscle bundles oriented parallel to the long axis are prominent in some species and form the boundary between the teat mucosa and the dermis. Numerous blood vessels form a vascular stratum, which becomes engorged with blood during the milking or suckling process; thus, the skin is stretched, resulting in a smooth surface. After milking, when the blood has drained from the teat vessels and the longitudinal smooth muscle has contracted, the teat surface returns to its typical corrugated appearance.

The papillary duct is a small duct lined with a stratified squamous epithelium. Circularly oriented bundles of smooth muscle in the mucosa form a sphincter to hold the milk until it is forced out by milking or suckling.

The skin of the teat in cows and sows is composed of a thick, stratified squamous epithelium and dermis without hair follicles and sweat or sebaceous glands. However, in some domestic species like sheep and goats, the teat may contain fine hairs and sweat and sebaceous glands.

MAMMARY GLAND INVOLUTION

After the lactation period or sudden arrest of suckling or milking, glandular involution begins. The alveoli are distended by accumulated milk and no further secretion occurs until they are emptied. It was once believed that if the secretory product were not removed for several days, the epithelial cells would degenerate and the residual milk in the lumen would be absorbed gradually. However, recent research has suggested less loss of mammary epithelial cells than previously believed. Characteristically, the involuted mammary gland has more interstitial tissue than glandular elements, and isolated clusters of branched tubules with a few small alveoli are all that remain of the parenchyma. They are lined by a low cuboidal epithelium with prominent underlying myoepithelial cells. The connective-tissue septa are thicker, and fat cells may occur singly or in clusters. Lymphocytes and plasma cells are present in significant amounts. Small, dark-staining bodies of casein (corpora amylacea) may be found in the alveoli, ducts, or interstitial tissue.

DIGITAL ORGANS AND HORN

The digital organ consists of a keratinized portion, the underlying dermis, the hypodermis, the bones and associated structures, and the digital pads. The keratinized portion is made of a hard keratin or horn, such as in the hoofs of horses, ruminants, and pigs and the claws of carnivores. The dermis (corium) contains blood vessels and nerves. The hypodermis is absent in the hoof wall, sole, and claw. The bones or phalanges and their ligaments and tendons form the supportive structure of the digital organ. The digital organ in carnivores includes the digital pads, which are thick cushionlike structures that rest on the ground.

Equine Hoof

A knowledge of the structure of the tissues of the hoof is important to the understanding of the pathophysiology of laminitis, the most devastating clinical disease syndrome of the digital organ.

The keratinized portion of the digital organ is composed of three main parts. The **wall** (paries) is that portion that is visible when the foot is placed on the ground. The **sole** (solea) forms the greatest part of the ventral surface of the foot; the **frog** (cuneus ungulae) is a wedge-shaped mass medial and caudal to the sole.

WALL

The wall of the hoof is composed of three layers (Fig. 16.37). From the outside inward, they are the **stratum externum** (tectorium), the **stratum medium**, and the **stratum internum** (lamellatum). Each of these is structurally distinct and is described separately in the following paragraphs.

The **stratum externum** is a thin layer of tubular and intertubular horn, which originates from the germinal layers of the epidermis of the periople, a ring of soft, nonpigmented tubular horn of modified skin above the coronary border of the hoof. Toward the back of the foot, the periople widens into a broad keratinized layer or bulb (heel). The perioplic corium is papillated and continuous with the dermis of skin proximally and the coronary corium distally.

The **stratum medium** consists of tubular and intertubular "hard" horn and is the main supportive structure of the wall, which is arranged in a tubular structure (Fig. 16.38). The horny tubules are solid rods and are oriented parallel to the outer surface of the hoof, and their keratinized cells have a highly ordered arrangement. The cross-sectional profiles of the tubules may be circular, oval, or wedge-shaped and have a central region of loose keratinized cells similar to the medulla of the hair shaft (Fig. 16.39). The cortex of the tubule has three zones. The **inner zone** contains keratinized cells oriented around the medulla in fairly tight coils; the cells of the **middle zone** form loose spirals; and the cells of the **outer zone** form another layer of tight coils. This coiled, springlike arrangement of the cells of tubular horn helps dampen the compression of the hoof when it strikes a hard surface. The intertubular horn fills the spaces between the tubular horn.

The stratum medium is produced by the stratum basale

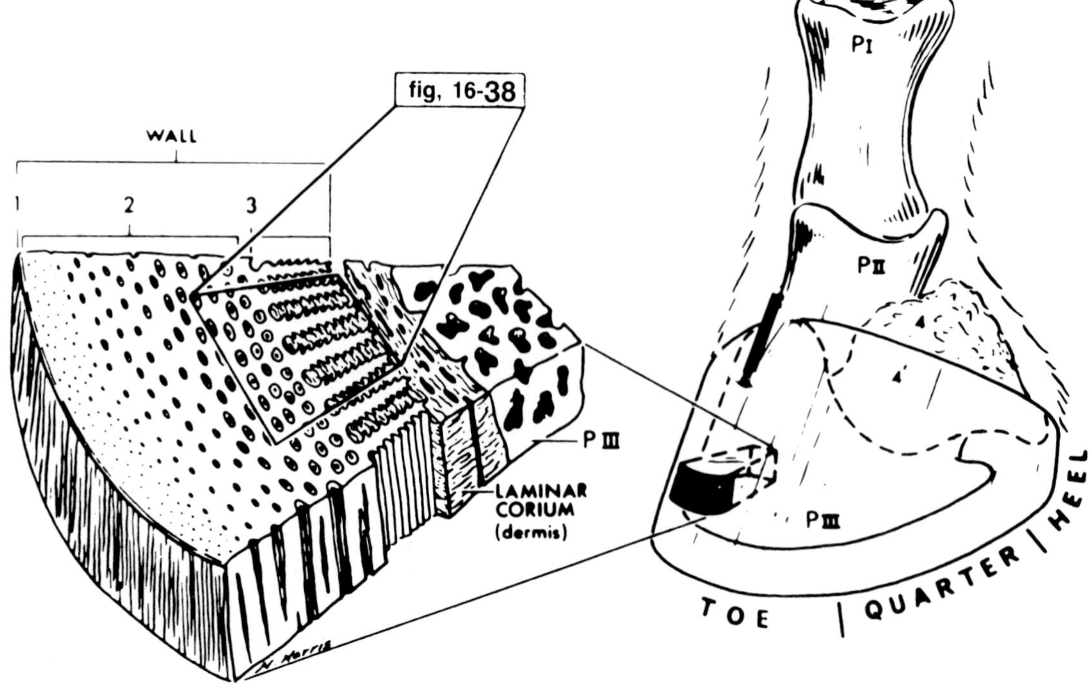

Figure 16.37. *Frontolateral view (equine foot). The wall of the hoof is composed of three layers: stratum externum (1), stratum medium (2), stratum internum (3); proximal (PI), medial (PII), distal (PIII) phalanges; lateral cartilages of the hoof (4) and (4′). (From Stump JE. Anatomy of the normal equine foot, including microscopic features of the laminar region. J Am Vet Med Assoc 1967;151:1588.)*

Figure 16.38. *Wall of hoof (horse) from the area marked in Figure 16.37. Stratum internum (A); stratum medium (B); laminar corium (C); primary lamina (D); secondary laminae (E); tubular horn (F); intertubular horn (G). Hematoxylin and eosin (×38). (From Dellmann HD. Veterinary histology: an outline text–atlas. Philadelphia: Lea & Febiger, 1971:265.)*

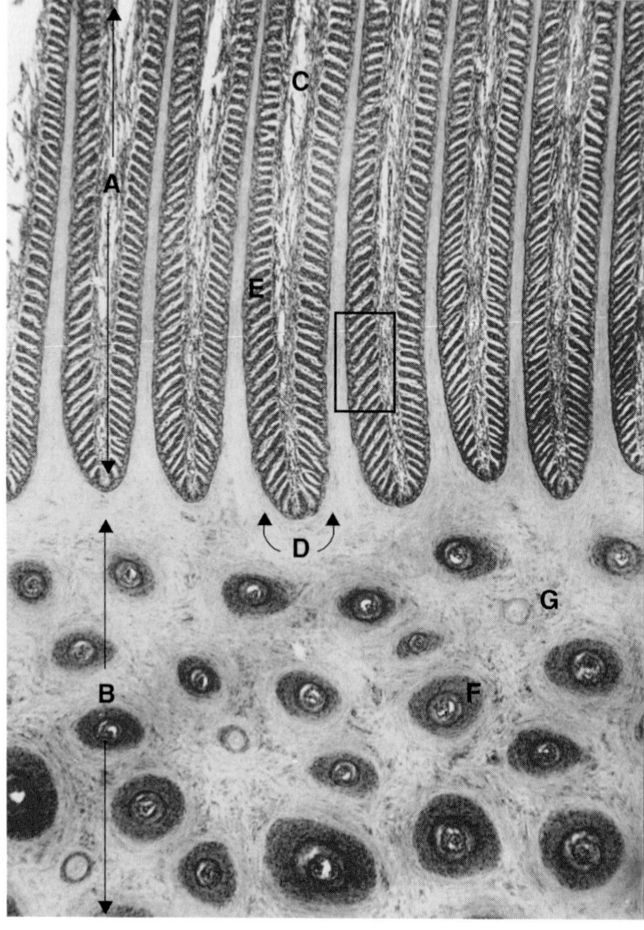

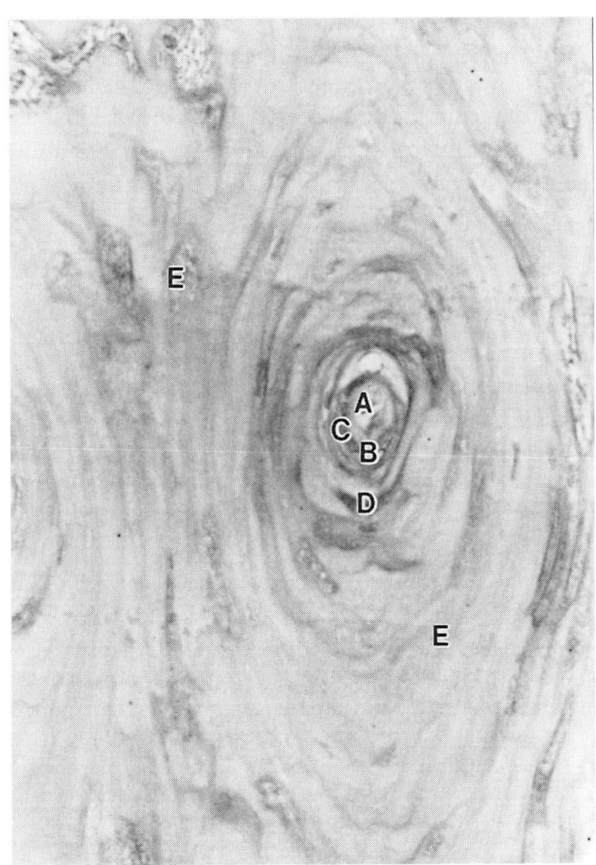

Figure 16.39. *Stratum medium showing the cellular arrangement of tubular horn, hoof (horse). Medulla (A); inner zone of cortex (B); middle zone of cortex (C); outer zone of cortex (D); intertubular horn (E). Hematoxylin and eosin (×250).*

and stratum spinosum of the epidermis lining the coronary groove (Fig. 16.37). This epidermis covers the coronary corium, a bed of vascularized connective tissue with long papillae. The germinal cells covering the tips of the papillae give rise to loose cells of the medulla of the tubule, whereas those over the sides and base of the papillae proliferate to form the keratinized cells of the cortex. The germinal cells covering the interpapillary part of the coronary corium give rise to the intertubular horn. The layers of the intertubular horn consists of hard keratin and helps to hold the tubules together. The deeper connective tissue of the coronary dermis is composed of dense collagen fibers and numerous large blood vessels.

The **stratum internum** (lamellatum) consists of approximately 600 primary, vertically oriented, keratinized laminae extending inward from the stratum medium, with which they are continuous (Fig. 16.38). One hundred to 200 secondary laminae project at acute angles from each primary lamina (Fig. 16.40). These laminae interdigitate with similar laminae of the corium and form a complex epidermal–dermal association that anchors the keratinized hoof to the underlying connective tissue. The primary epidermal laminae are part of the stratum corneum (hard keratin) produced by the stratum germinativum located between the proximal ends of the dermal laminae at the deep edge of the coronary groove. The cells keratinize as they move downward, as those of the stratum medium. The secondary epidermal laminae are composed of stratum germinativum. The stratum basale of each secondary lamina rests on the connective tissue of each secondary dermal lamina, forming the interdigitation between the two laminae. The central core of each secondary epidermal lamina is composed of stratum spinosum, one to three cell layers in thickness, that attaches to the sides of the primary epidermal lamina (Fig. 16.40). The germinal cells of the secondary laminae multiply throughout the length of the laminae only at a rate to keep up with the downward growth of the horny laminae. The wall grows in length at the rate of 6.4 mm per month; 9 to 12 months are required for the hoof to grow from the coronary border to the ground at the toe region. The interdigitation between the nonpigmented wall laminae with the pigmented tubular and intertubular horn of the sole is referred to as the **white line**. A disturbance in the physical and physiologic (nutritional blood supply) influences on various parts of the hoof results in laminitis.

The laminar corium (dermis) fills the space between

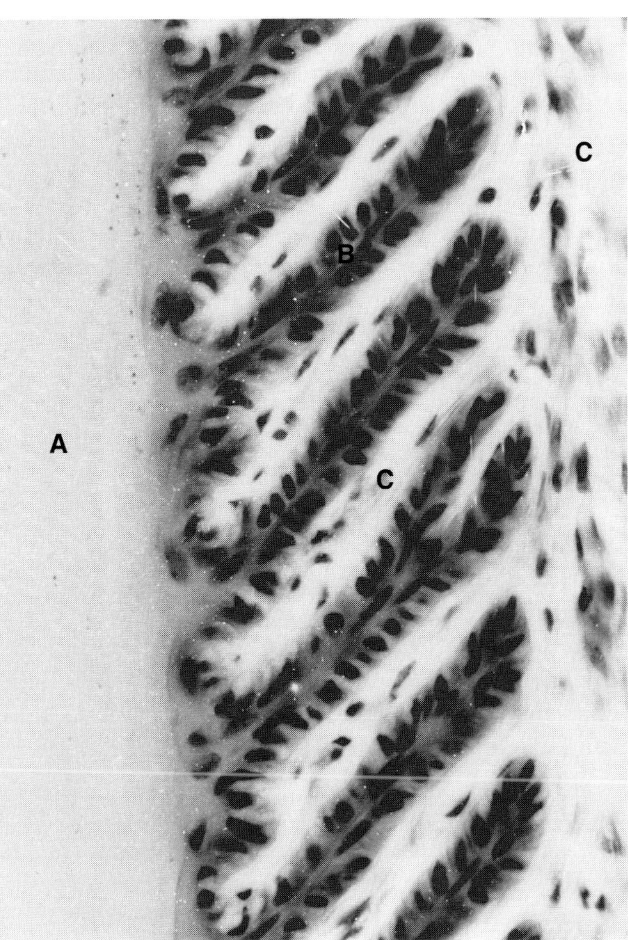

Figure 16.40. *Secondary laminae, hoof (horse). See area marked in Figure 16.38. Primary lamina on the wall (A); secondary lamina (B); laminar corium (C). Hematoxylin and eosin (×435). (From Dellmann HD. Veterinary histology: an outline text–atlas. Philadelphia: Lea & Febiger, 1971:264.)*

the horny laminae of the stratum internum and the bone of the distal phalanx. The corium is composed of bundles of coarse collagen fibers and a massive network of large arteries and veins without valves. This vascular bed helps to dampen the compressive forces transmitted from the hard inflexible hoof to the phalanx.

SOLE

The sole is composed of tubular and intertubular horn. Its superficial layers are not firmly attached and can be peeled off in the form of small flakes. The corium (dermis) of the sole bears long papillae, the epidermal covering of which gives rise to the tubular horn of the sole. It blends with the periosteum of the ventral surface of the distal phalanx.

FROG

The frog is composed of keratinized tubular and intertubular horn that is softer than the wall and sole. The corium (dermis) of the frog forms small short papillae. The connective tissue blends with the digital cushion, which is a wedge-shaped mass of collagen and elastic fibers among masses of fat that acts as a shock absorber. Branched coiled merocrine sweat glands occur chiefly in the part that overlies the central ridge of the frog.

Ruminant and Swine Hoofs

The digital organs of ruminants and pigs are similar to those of horses, with a few exceptions. The stratum internum and corresponding laminar corium consists of only primary laminae. The sole consists of a narrow rim next to the angle of inflection of the wall. There is no frog, but a prominent bulb of soft thin horn that is continuous with the skin makes up a large part of the ventral surface of the hoof.

Claw

The claws or nails of dogs and cats are specialized structures that are continuous with the epidermis and dermis and consist of shields of hard keratin that cover the distal phalanges and possess a wall and a sole (Fig. 16.41).

The **wall** or **claw plate** covers the coronary corium and the wall corium. It is thickest in the area of the dorsal ridge and gradually thins out along the side. Its thin ventral margins extend beyond the junction of the wall with the sole. The epidermis of the dorsal ridge forms a few short laminae that interdigitate with similar dermal laminae.

The epidermis of the **sole** is thick and produces a softer form of keratin than that of the wall. A stratum granulosum and a stratum lucidum are present.

The dermis of the claw is composed of dense irregular connective tissue that forms a thick ridge over the dorsal surface of the distal phalanx. It is rich in blood vessels and prone to hemorrhage if the nail is cut too short.

The claw fold is a fold of skin, similar to the periople of the hoof, that covers the claw plate for a short distance on its dorsal and lateral margins. As the plate grows, it carries with it a thin layer of keratinized cells.

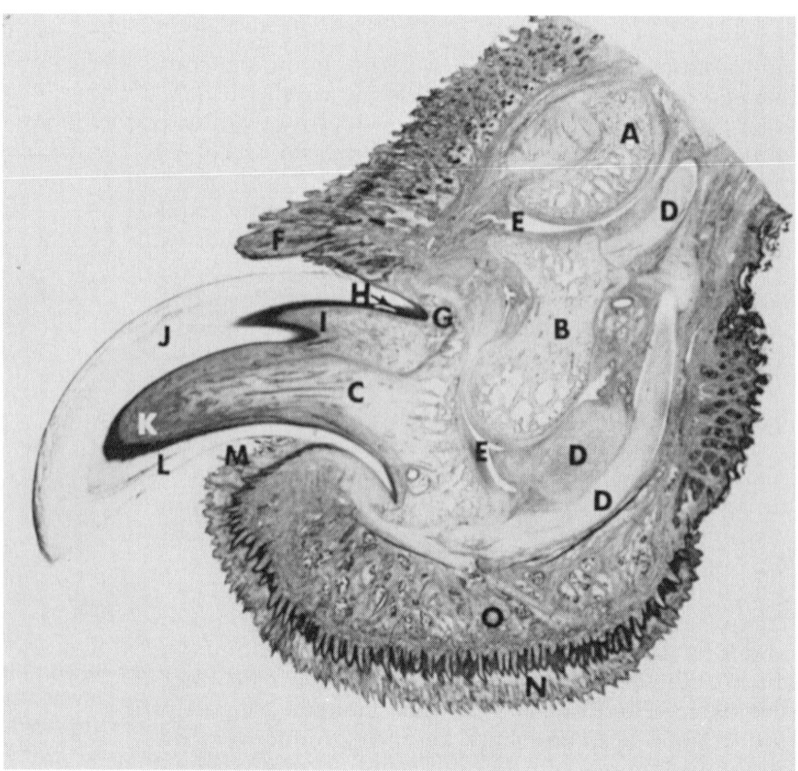

Figure 16.41. *Claw (dog). Proximal phalanx (A); middle phalanx (B); distal phalanx (C); tendons (D); joint cavities with accompanying joint capsules and articular cartilages (E); fold of skin overlying claw (F); ungual crest (G); nonkeratinized epidermal layers of the claw (H); dorsal ridge (I); stratum corneum of the claw epidermis (J); dermis (K); sole (L); limiting furrow between the sole and digital pad (N); dermis of the digital pads with clusters of coiled merocrine sweat glands and fat (O). Hematoxylin and eosin (×4). (From Adam WS, Calhoun ML, Smith EM, et al. Microscopic anatomy of the dog: a photographic atlas. Springfield, IL: Charles C. Thomas, 1970.)*

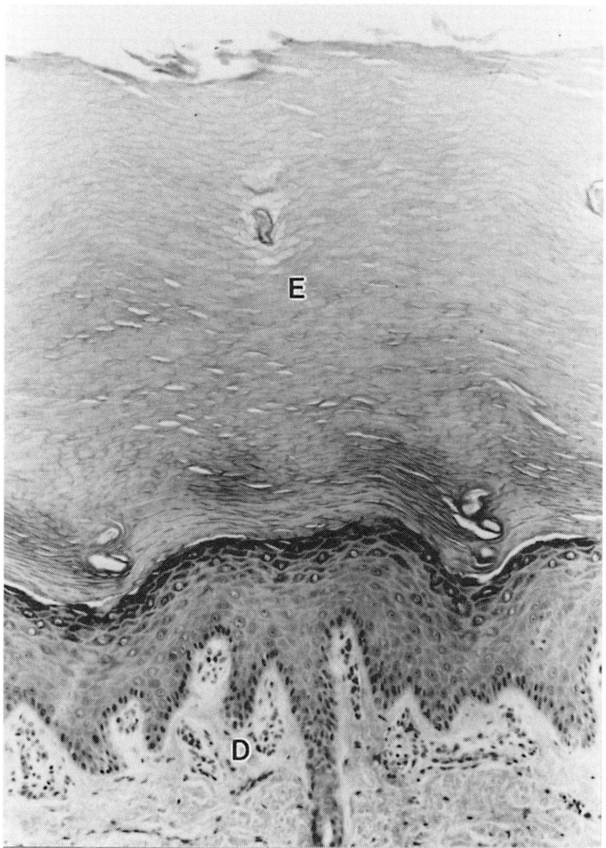

Figure 16.42. *Foot pad (cat). The keratinized epidermis (E) is smooth and the dermis (D) is papillated. Hematoxylin and eosin (×125).*

This layer of cells is produced by the epidermis of the inner surface of the claw fold.

Digital Pads

The digital pads of the dog and cat are covered by a thick hairless epidermis that contains all cell layers, including a stratum lucidum. The surface is smooth in the cat (Fig. 16.42) and roughened by keratinized conical/rounded papillae in the dog (Fig. 16.43). The dermis has prominent papillae that interdigitate with the epidermal pegs and contains coiled merocrine sweat glands that extend into the digital cushion, the hypodermis. Subcutaneous masses of adipose tissue are separated and enclosed by collagen and elastic fibers.

Chestnut and Ergot

The equine supracarpal and tarsal chestnuts and the ergot at the flexion of the fetlocks have a thick epidermis composed of tubular and intertubular horn interdigitating with long dermal papillae (Fig. 16.44). Arrector pili muscles, glands, and hairs are absent in both of these structures.

Horn

Horns of the ruminant species are actually growths from the cornual processes of the frontal bone of the skull. The horns are covered by a hard keratinized epidermis, a dermis, and a hypodermis.

The epidermis has a thick stratum corneum composed of hard tubular and intertubular horn. A thin outermost layer of soft keratin, the epikeras, forms at the root of the horn and is similar to the epidermis of the periople. It desquamates as keratinized scales, similar to the stratum externum of the hoofs. The dermis is papillated and, together with the thin hypodermis, fills the space between the epidermis and the periosteum of the bone.

AVIAN INTEGUMENT

The avian **epidermis** is composed of stratified squamous epithelium that is similar to but thinner than that of mammals (Fig. 16.45). The epidermis of feathered skin consists of only a few cell layers (Fig. 16.46), whereas unfeathered skin is much thicker. The terminology of the epidermal cell layers is different from that in mammals. There is a stratum basale, a stratum intermedium (actually stratum spinosum), a stratum transi-

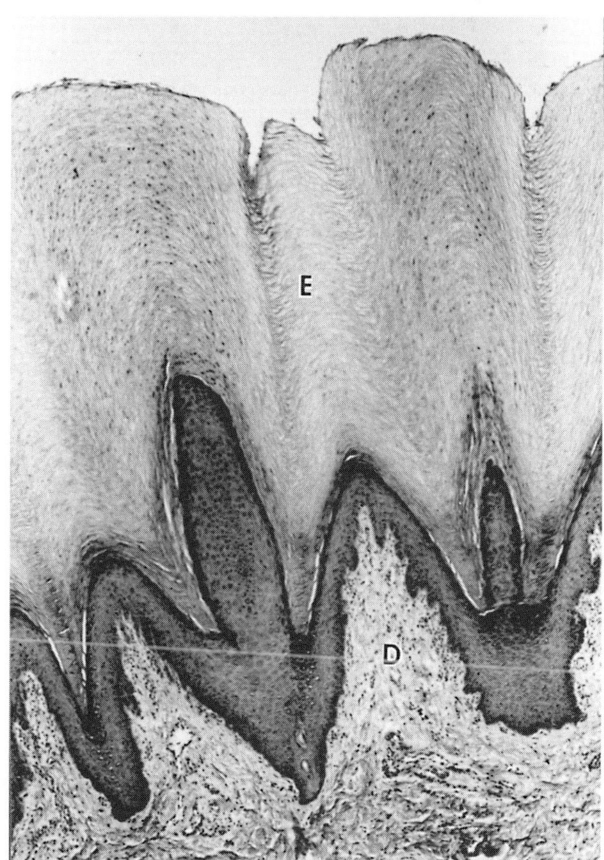

Figure 16.43. *Foot pad (dog). The keratinized epidermis (E) is rough in the dog and the dermis (D) is papillated. Hematoxylin and eosin (×50).*

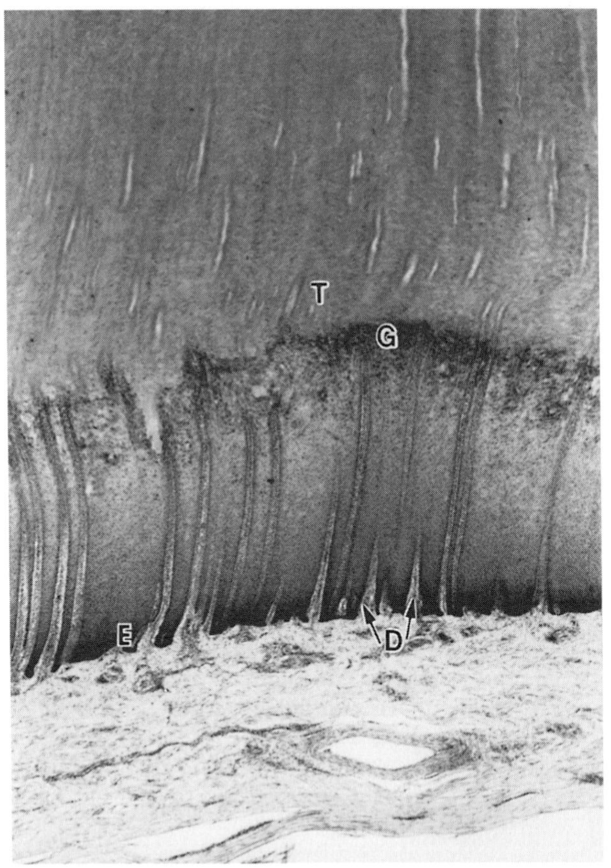

Figure 16.44. *Chestnut (horse). Epidermal papillae (E); stratum granulosum (G); dermal papillae (D), and horny tubules (T). Hematoxylin and eosin (×25).*

tivum (actually stratum granulosum but lacks keratohyalin granules), and a stratum corneum. The term **stratum germinativum** is also used to represent all the cell layers except for the stratum corneum. The avian integument is sometimes referred to as an organ of lipogenesis because of the extensive amount of lipid found in the epidermal cells in most avian species. The epidermis synthesizes triacylglycerols, phospholipids, wax esters, free fatty acids, and monoglycerols, and diacylglycerols.

The skin of birds, unlike that of mammals, is completely aglandular, with the exception of the uropygial gland or preen gland. This gland is a bilobed structure (Fig.16.47) that lies dorsally at the base of the tail and opens through a papilla to the surface of the skin. This gland is considered to be analogous to the sebaceous gland in mammals because it produces a fatty and oily substance that is released by the holocrine mode of secretion and is regulated by hormonal influences (Fig. 16.48). The combination of both the uropygial gland sebum and the lipid from the epidermal cells acts as an antibacterial agent, prevents the feather keratin from drying out, and acts as a waterproofing agent.

Feathers are similar to hair follicles and are of epidermal origin and develop within the follicle (Fig. 16.46). The feather consists primarily of keratin and remains in the follicle until it is plucked or molted and then a new feather develops in its place. Interfollicular muscles are common in birds and are believed to play a significant role in governing the radiative heat load by adjusting the angle of the feather.

The dermis and hypodermis (subcutis) are subdivided into the stratum superficiale (superficial layer); stratum profundum (deep layer), which includes the stratum compactum (dense layer) and the stratum laxum (loose connective tissue containing fat, large vessels, smooth muscle, and follicles); and lamina elastica (elastic lamina of the dermis). In addition, several smooth muscles with elastic tendons are associated with each feather follicle, and cutaneous striated muscles function in voluntary movement of the skin in response to stimuli.

The avian plantar skin does not possess all cell layers like the plantar skin of dogs and cats. It lacks a true stratum granulosum layer and has a thick smooth surface consisting of ridges of keratin (Fig. 16.49).

The comb, paired wattles, and ear lobes consist of a double layer of skin with numerous blood vessels in the dermis. During mating, the vessels become congested, thereby giving a bright red appearance to the comb and wattles.

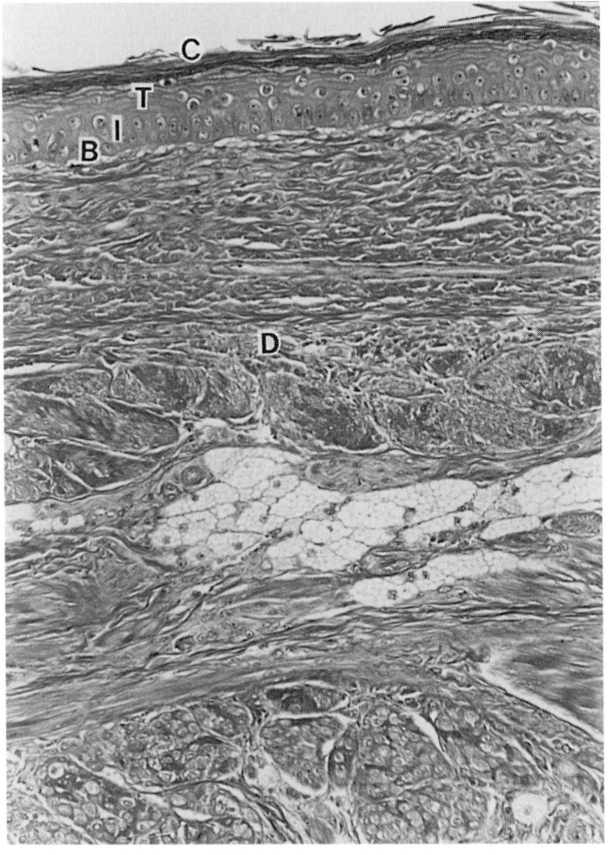

Figure 16.45. *Unfeathered chicken skin. Note the stratum basale (B), stratum intermedium (I), stratum transitivum (T), and stratum corneum (C) cell layers. The dermis (D) and subdivided layers can be seen. Hematoxylin and eosin (×250).*

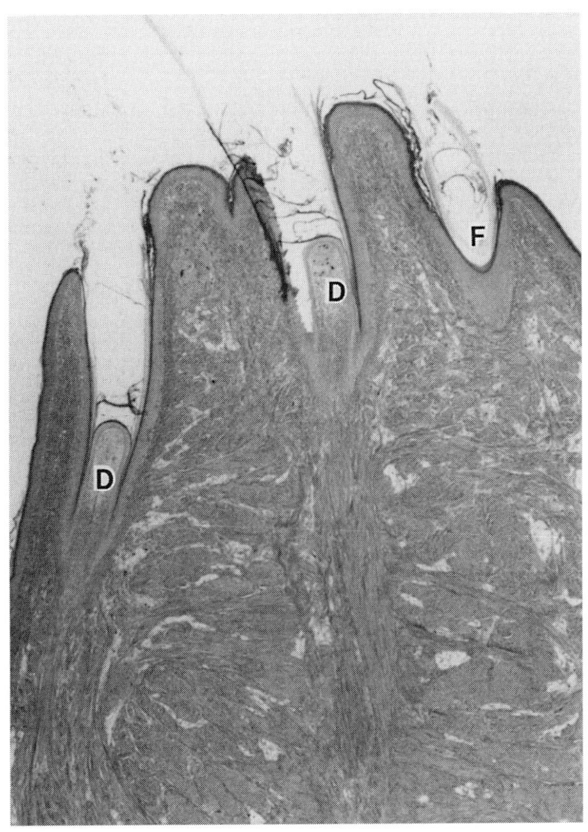

Figure 16.46. *Feathered chicken skin. Note two developing follicles (D) and a mature follicle (F). Hematoxylin and eosin (×35).*

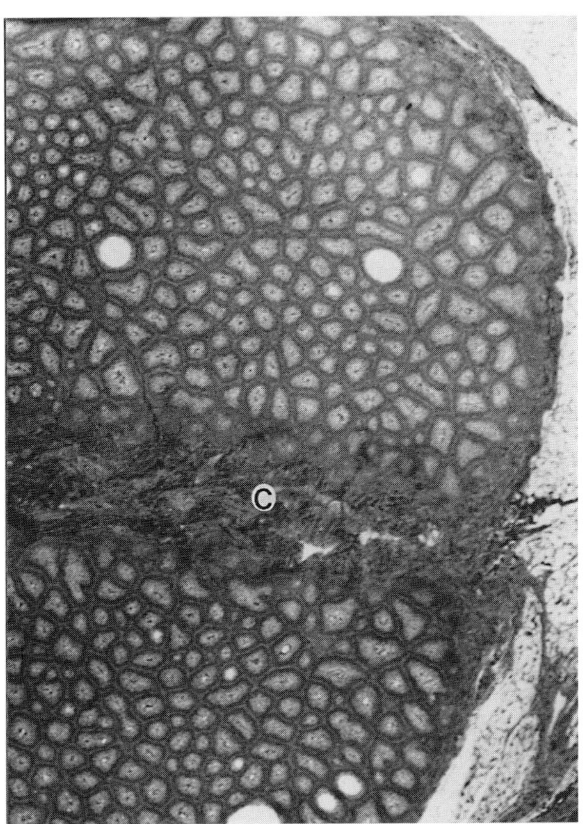

Figure 16.47. *Uropygial gland. Note the bilobed structure separated by connective tissue (C) Hematoxylin and eosin (×35).*

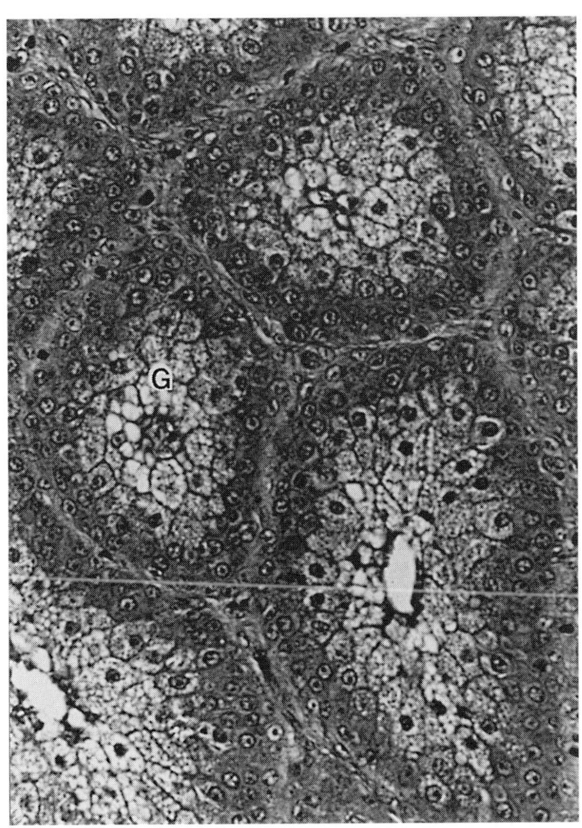

Figure 16.48. *Higher magnification of the uropygial gland in Figure 16.46. Note the large sebaceous glands (G). Hematoxylin and eosin (×350).*

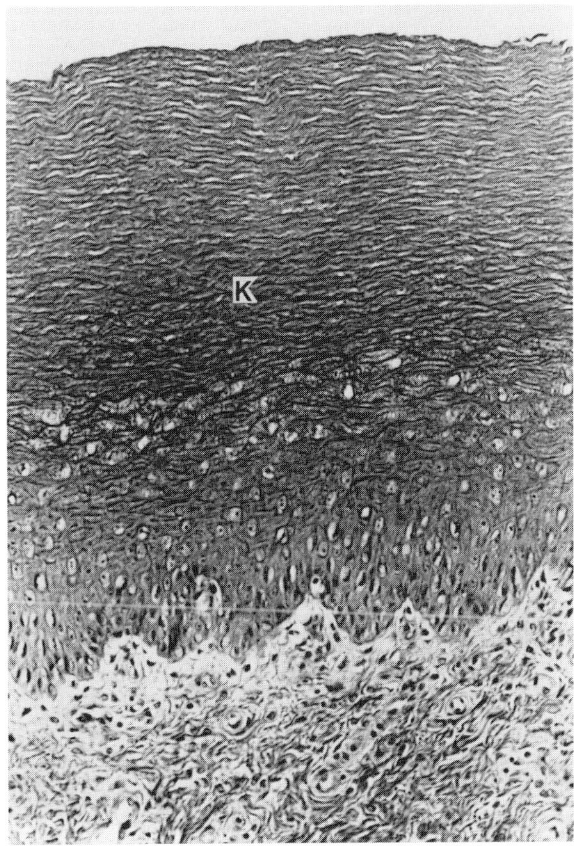

Figure 16.49. *Avian plantar skin. Note that the thickened keratinized region (K) is smooth. Hematoxylin and eosin (×250).*

REFERENCES

Anderson RR. Mammary gland. In: Larson BL, ed. Lactation. Ames, IA: Iowa State University Press, 1985:3.

Briggaman RA. Epidermal-dermal junction: structure, composition, function and disease relationships. In: Moshnell AN, ed. Progress in dermatology, part II. Evanston, IL: Dermatology Foundation, 1990:1.

Budras KD, Hullinger RL, Sack WO. Light and electron microscopy of keratinization in the laminar epidermis of the equine hoof with reference to laminitis. Am J Vet Res 1989;50:1150.

Elias PE. Epidermal lipids, barrier function, and desquamation. J Invest Dermatol 1983;80:44s.

Hodges RD. The integumentary system. In: The histology of the fowl. New York: Academic Press, 1974:1.

Lavker RM, Sunt TT. Heterogeneity in basal keratinocytes: morphological and functional correlations. Science 1982;215:1239.

Lucas AM, Stettenhein PR. Avian anatomy. Integument. Agricultural Handbook 362, part II. Washington, DC: U.S. Department of Agriculture, 1972.

Marcarian HQ, Calhoun ML. The microscopic anatomy of the integument of the adult swine. Am J Vet Res 1966;27:765.

Menton DN. A liquid film model of tetrakaidecahedral packing to account for the establishment of epidermal cell columns. J Invest Dermatol 1976;66:283.

Monteiro-Riviere NA. Comparative anatomy, physiology, and biochemistry of mammalian skin. In: Hobson DW, ed. Dermal and ocular toxicology: fundamentals and methods. Boca Raton, FL: CRC Press, 1991:3.

Monteiro-Riviere NA. Ultrastructural evaluation of the porcine integument. In: Tumbleson ME, ed. Swine in biomedical research. New York: Plenum Press, 1986;1:641.

Monteiro-Rivere NA, Stromberg MW. Ultrastructure of the integument of the domestic pig (sus scrofa) from one through fourteen weeks of age. Anat Histol Embryol 1985;14:97.

Monteiro-Riviere NA, Bristol DG, Manning TO, et al. Interspecies and interregional analysis of the comparative histologic thickness and laser Doppler blood flow measurements at five cutaneous sites in nine species. J Invest Dermatol 1990;95:582.

Monteiro-Riviere NA, Inman AO. Indirect immunohistochemistry and immunoelectron microscopy distribution of eight epidermal-dermal junction epitopes in the pig and in isolated perfused skin treated with bis (2-chloroethyl) sulfide. Toxicol Pathol 1995;23:313.

Smith JL, Calhoun ML. The microscopic anatomy of the integument of the newborn swine. Am J Vet Res 1964;24:165.

Stromberg MW, Hwang YC, Monteiro-Riviere NA. Interfollicular smooth muscle in the skin of the domesticated pig (sus scrofa). Anat Rec 1981;201:455.

Talukdar AH, Calhoun ML, Stinson AW. Sweat glands of the horse: a histologic study. Am J Vet Res 1970;31:2179.

Webb AJ, Calhoun ML. The microscopic anatomy of the skin of mongrel dogs. Am J Vet Res 1954;15:274.

Wolff-Schreiner EC. Ultrastructural cytochemistry of the epidermis. Int J Dermatol 1977;16:77.

17

Eye

H. DIETER DELLMANN

The eye is located in the bony orbit, along with extraocular muscles, ligaments, adipose tissue, blood vessels, nerves, and glands. The lacrimal apparatus, the eyelids, and the third eyelid provide protection to the eye. The globe consists of three tunics that enclose compartments containing refractive media.

The three tunics of the eye are (Fig. 17.1): *(1)* the **fibrous**, or outer tunic (tunica fibrosa bulbi), which is in turn subdivided into *(a)* the sclera, the white tough posterior portion of the globe, and *(b)* the cornea, the transparent portion of the fibrous tunic, which bulges slightly in the center of the rostral pole of the eye; *(2)* the **vascular**, or middle, tunic (tunica vasculosa bulbi), also referred to as the uveal tract, composed of *(a)* the choroid, *(b)* the ciliary body, and *(c)* the iris; and *(3)* the **neuroepithelial**, or inner, tunic (tunica interna bulbi) with *(a)* an optic portion, the retina, containing the sensory receptors and *(b)* a blind portion that is epithelial in nature and covers the ciliary body and the posterior surface of the iris.

The anterior compartment is filled with aqueous humor and is located between the cornea and the vitreous body. It is further subdivided into *(a)* the anterior chamber (camera anterior bulbi) located between the cornea and the iris and *(b)* the posterior chamber (camera posterior bulbi) located between the iris and the vitreous body and containing the lens. The posterior compartment (camera vitrea bulbi) of the eye, located between the lens and the retina, is filled with the vitreous body.

FIBROUS TUNIC

Sclera

The sclera is a layer of dense irregular connective tissue that protects the eye and maintains its form (shape). Thickness of the sclera varies in different parts of the eye and among species. Bundles of collagen fibers containing a few elastic fibers and elongated fibroblasts, as well as melanocytes in some areas, are arranged parallel

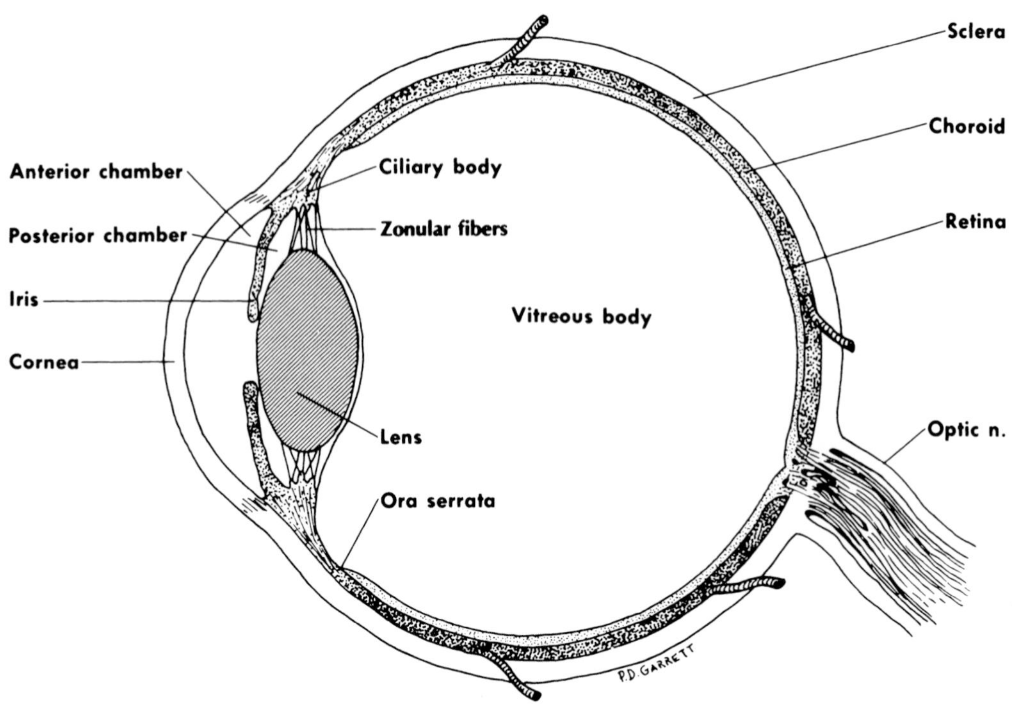

Figure 17.1. *Schematic drawing of a longitudinal section through the eye.*

to the surface of the globe. These bundles are intricately interwoven and arranged predominantly in an equatorial direction near the junction between sclera and cornea, the so-called limbus, and around the optic nerve. In the other portions of the eye, meridional bundles predominate. In the layer of the sclera adjacent to the choroid, elastic fibers predominate, and fibroblasts and melanocytes are more numerous; this layer is referred to as the **lamina fusca sclerae**.

A firm attachment to the sclera is provided for the tendons of the extrinsic eye muscles through the interweaving of tendon and scleral fibers. The optic nerve leaves the eye through numerous perforations in a disk-like area referred to as the **area cribrosa sclerae**.

Cornea

The transparent cornea is a convex–concave lens, thicker at the center than at the periphery, and with a smaller radius of curvature centrally than peripherally. Because the cornea also has a radius of curvature smaller than that of the sclera, it is more curved than the sclera.

The cornea is composed of five layers: *(a)* anterior epithelium, *(b)* subepithelial basement membrane, *(c)* substantia propria, or stroma, *(d)* posterior limiting lamina (Descemet's membrane), and *(e)* posterior epithelium (corneal endothelium).

ANTERIOR EPITHELIUM

The anterior (corneal) epithelium is nonkeratinized stratified squamous, between four and 12 layers in thickness (Fig. 17.2). The epithelial cells are tightly packed, interdigitate profusely, and adhere through numerous desmosomes. The numerous microvilli on the surface of the superficial cells function to retain the tear film on the corneal surface. Numerous free nerve endings are present among the epithelial cells. The regenerative capability of injured corneal epithelium is pronounced; mitotic divisions, along with cell movements, ensure a rapid return to normal of injured epithelium. An intact epithelium is necessary for maintenance of corneal transparency.

SUBEPITHELIAL BASEMENT MEMBRANE

The subepithelial basement membrane consists of a basal lamina and a layer of reticular fibers. Frequently, this layer can be distinguished with the light microscope (Fig. 17.2). It should not be confused with the anterior limiting lamina (Bowman's membrane), a modified outermost layer of the substantia propria that is present only in primates.

SUBSTANTIA PROPRIA

The corneal substantia propria, or stroma, consists of varying numbers (approximately 100 in the cat) of collagen fiber layers or lamellae (Fig. 17.2). Within one layer, the fibers are always parallel with the corneal surface; in successive layers, the fibers cross each other at right angles. Adjacent lamellae are held together firmly by fibers that deviate from their parallel course. Occasional elastic fibers are observed at the periphery of the cornea.

The predominating cell type of the corneal substantia

propria is the fibrocyte, located mainly between the collagen layers rather than within them. These cells are elongated and branched, with little cytoplasm (Fig. 17.2).

The amorphous ground substance stains metachromatically owing to the presence of sulfated glycosaminoglycans (chondroitin sulfate, keratan sulfate). The ground substance plays an essential role in the transparency of the cornea by maintaining an optimal degree of hydration; excessive water content causes opacification of the cornea.

POSTERIOR LIMITING LAMINA

With the light microscope, the posterior limiting lamina appears as a highly refractile, thick amorphous layer that gives a positive periodic acid-Schiff (PAS) reaction (Fig. 17.2). At the fine structural level, the lamina consists of two regions: an anterior zone and a posterior zone. The anterior zone is composed of collagen fibrils (wide-spaced collagen type VIII), arranged in a regular, hexagonal array. The posterior zone is adjacent to the corneal endothelium and consists of basal lamina material.

POSTERIOR EPITHELIUM

A simple squamous epithelium of flat hexagonal cells covers the caudal surface of the cornea (Fig. 17.2). The cells interdigitate heavily and contain numerous mitochondria and pinocytotic vesicles. The epithelium functions in the maintenance of the transparency of the cornea; defects in the epithelium cause edema and opacification of the cornea, which disappear rapidly after regeneration of the epithelium. Epithelial regeneration occurs through increased mitosis in the vicinity of the wound.

Corneoscleral Junction (Limbus)

At the limbus, the sclera overlaps the cornea. The corneal epithelium gradually changes into conjunctival epithelium, which rests on a lamina propria of loose connective tissue. The characteristically layered collagen fibers of the substantia propria assume a more irregular arrangement, become associated with elastic fibers, and are continuous with the equatorial bundles of the sclera. The posterior limiting lamina splits and is continuous with the connective-tissue trabeculae of the corneoscleral trabeculae. The posterior epithelial cells become flatter and larger and surround these trabeculae.

The only blood vessels supplying the cornea are located at the level of the limbus because the normal cornea is completely devoid of blood vessels. The corneal nerves originate from a marginal dense nerve

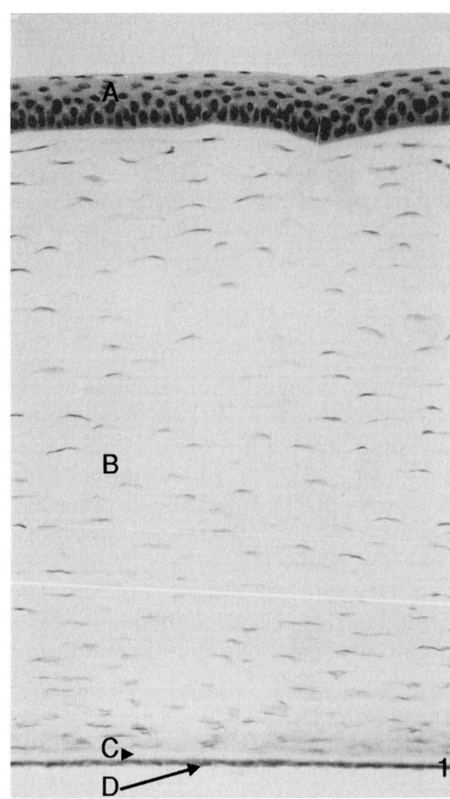

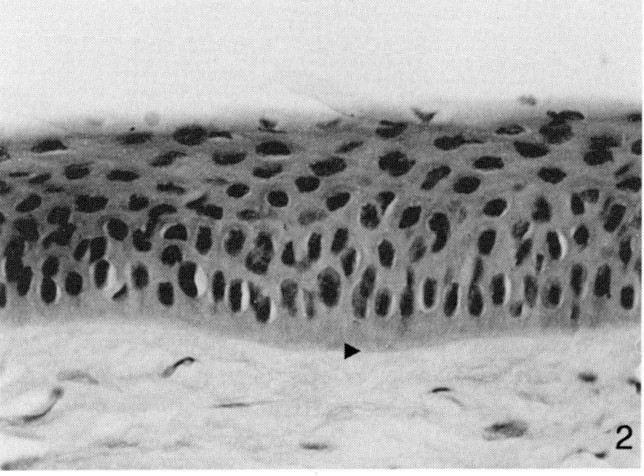

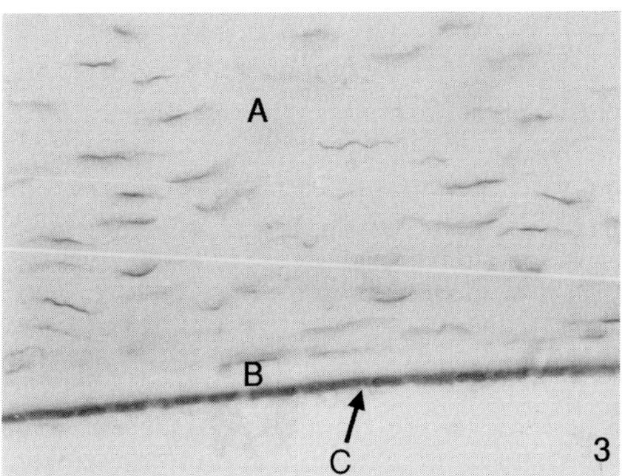

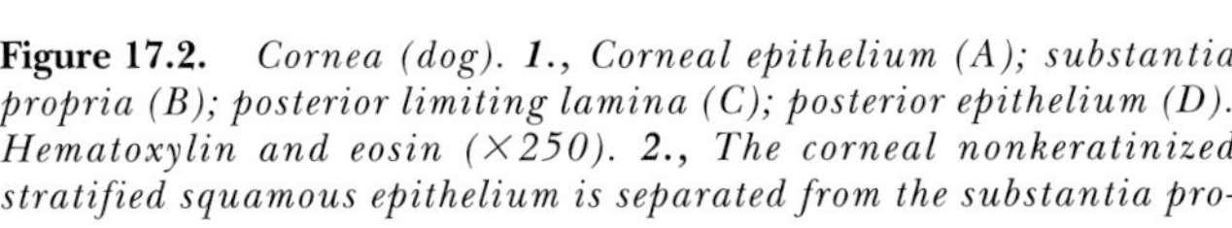

Figure 17.2. *Cornea (dog). **1.**, Corneal epithelium (A); substantia propria (B); posterior limiting lamina (C); posterior epithelium (D). Hematoxylin and eosin (×250). **2.**, The corneal nonkeratinized stratified squamous epithelium is separated from the substantia propria by a rather thick basement membrane (arrow). Hematoxylin and eosin (×500). **3.**, Substantia propria with fibrocytes and collagen fibers (A), the posterior limiting lamina (B), and the posterior epithelium (C). Hematoxylin and eosin (×500).*

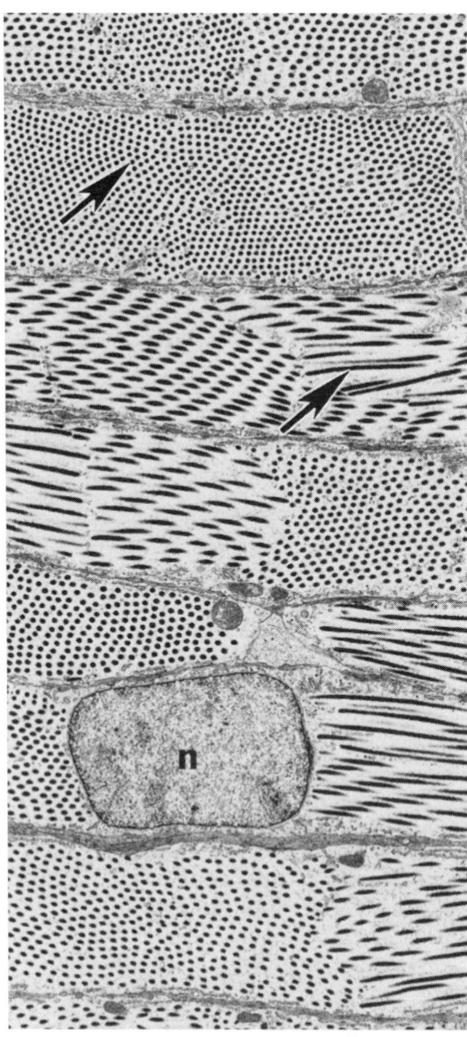

Figure 17.3. *Electron micrograph of the feline tapetum lucidum illustrating the bricklike arrangement of cells and bundles of parallel rods (arrows) oriented in various directions with their long axes perpendicular to the angle of incident light and a tapetal cell nucleus (N) (×3780). (Courtesy of E.J. King.)*

fiber plexus at the same level or from the ciliary plexus of the vascular tunic.

VASCULAR TUNIC

The vascular tunic, or uveal tract, comprises three portions: the choroid, the ciliary body, and the mesenchymal components of the iris.

Choroid

The choroid is a thick, highly vascularized layer that is continuous with the stroma of the ciliary body anteriorly and extends posteriorly around the globe. The outer side of the choroid is connected with the sclera; the inner side is adjacent and intimately attached to the pigmented epithelium of the retina. The choroid is subdivided into five layers as follows.

SUPRACHOROID LAYER

The suprachoroid layer is the most peripheral layer (see Fig. 17.8) of the choroid. It consists of bundles of collagen and some elastic fibers, fibrocytes, and numerous melanocytes.

VASCULAR LAYER

Numerous large arteries and veins, separated by a stroma similar to that of the suprachoroid layer, make up this layer (see Fig. 17.8).

TAPETUM LUCIDUM

The tapetum lucidum is a light-reflecting layer, supposedly increasing light perception under conditions of poor illumination. The tapetum is located mainly in the dorsal half of the fundus of the eye. In herbivores, the tapetum is fibrous, consisting of intermingling collagen fibers and a few fibrocytes. In carnivores, the tapetum consists of a varying number of layers of flat polygonal cells that appear bricklike in cross section (Figs. 17.3 and 17.7). The thickness of the tapetum varies, being multilayered at its center (up to 15 cell layers thick in dogs and 35 cell layers thick in cats) and thinning to a single cell at its periphery. The tapetal cells are packed with bundles of parallel small rods, all of which are oriented with their long axes parallel to the retinal surface. In cats, the rods may be modified melanosomes, and the tapetal cells at the outer periphery (next to the sclera) contain both rods and normally shaped melanosomes. Zinc is associated with the rods in both dogs and cats and may contribute to the reflection of light. Diffraction of light as a result of the spatial orientation of the rods (or of the collagen fibrils in herbivores) is probably responsible for producing the light reflection of the tapetum. In swine, the tapetum is absent.

CHORIOCAPILLARY LAYER

The choriocapillary layer (lamina choroidocapillaris) is a dense network of capillaries immediately adjacent to the pigmented epithelial layer of the retina (see Figs. 17.7 and 17.8). The wide capillaries often deeply indent the pigmented epithelial cells; their endothelium is fenestrated, endothelial nuclei and pericytes are located only toward the choroidal side of the capillaries, and the capillary and pigmented epithelial basal laminae are fused (see Fig. 17.8). Capillaries provide nutrients to the pigmented epithelium and retinal receptor cells.

BASAL COMPLEX

The basal complex (complexus basalis) is also referred to as **Bruch's membrane**. It separates the choroid from the retina. Species variation occurs among domestic animals with respect to the degree of development and thickness of the basal complex. When fully developed, the basal complex consists of the basal lamina of the retinal pigment epithelium, a layer of collagen and elastic fibers, and the basal lamina of the capillaries of the choriocapillary layer. Frequently, and consistently in the area over the cellular tapetum, pigment epithelial and capillary basal laminae are fused (Fig. 17.8).

Ciliary Body

The ciliary body is the direct rostral continuation of the choroid (Fig. 17.1). It begins caudally at the ora serrata, a sharply outlined dentate border that marks the transition between the optic part (pars optica retinae) and the blind or ciliary part (pars ciliaris retinae) of the retina. Rostrally, it is continuous with the iris and participates in the formation of the trabecular meshwork of the iris angle (see p. 339). All layers of the choroid extend into the ciliary body, except the tapetum lucidum and the choriocapillary layer. The ciliary body contains the ciliary muscle and is covered by a bilayered epithelium.

Rostrally, the ciliary body projects **ciliary processes** into the posterior chamber (Fig. 17.1); these form the ciliary crown (corona ciliaris or pars plicata). Ciliary processes have a core of loose connective tissue permeated by a dense network of capillaries. Caudally, the ciliary body is flat and smooth and is referred to as the **pars plana** or orbiculus ciliaris.

CILIARY MUSCLE

The ciliary muscle is located peripherally in the ciliary body. It consists of smooth muscle fibers, which are primarily oriented meridionally in most species. The meridional fibers originate from the corneal stroma, the connective tissue of the trabecular meshwork of the iris angle, and the sclera. They are attached by elastic tendons to the basal complex of the choroid. In addition, radiate and circular fibers are present; the latter predominate in the nasal portion of the ciliary body. Contraction of the ciliary muscle during accommodation reduces tension of the zonular fibers of the lens and the lens becomes more convex, whereas relaxation has the opposite effect.

EPITHELIUM

The ciliary body is covered by two layers of cuboidal epithelial cells of neuroepithelial origin. The outer **pigmented epithelial layer** is continuous with the pigmented epithelium of the retina. It consists of heavily pigmented, simple cuboidal epithelium (Fig. 17.4) on a basal lamina next to the stroma. These cells have deep basal invaginations of the plasma membrane.

The inner **nonpigmented epithelial layer** consists of cuboidal or columnar cells (Fig. 17.4) with a basal lamina, which separates it from the posterior chamber. The basal portions of the cells thus face the posterior chamber. They possess numerous deep plasmalemmal invaginations and associated mitochondria, and extensive rough endoplasmic reticulum (rER) and Golgi complexes are present in the cell apices. The cell apices are joined by zonulae occludentes.

The apical surface of the pigmented epithelial layer and the adjacent nonpigmented epithelial layer are connected through microvillous processes. Desmosomes, gap junctions, and puncta adherentia occur between adjacent epithelial cells within one layer and also between the cell apices of the two layers. These structures are characteristic of actively transporting epithelia and play a role in the transport of aqueous humor.

AQUEOUS HUMOR

The aqueous humor is a thin, clear fluid similar to blood plasma, but it has a considerably lower protein content. The aqueous humor is elaborated by fibrocytes and the capillaries of the ciliary processes and is transported via the epithelial layers into the posterior chamber. This transport is selective in that certain molecules are excluded from transepithelial passage. The aqueous humor flows from the posterior chamber through the pupil to the anterior chamber, where it drains via the iridocorneal angle (described below).

Iris

The iris is located rostrally to the lens and separates the anterior and posterior chambers, which communi-

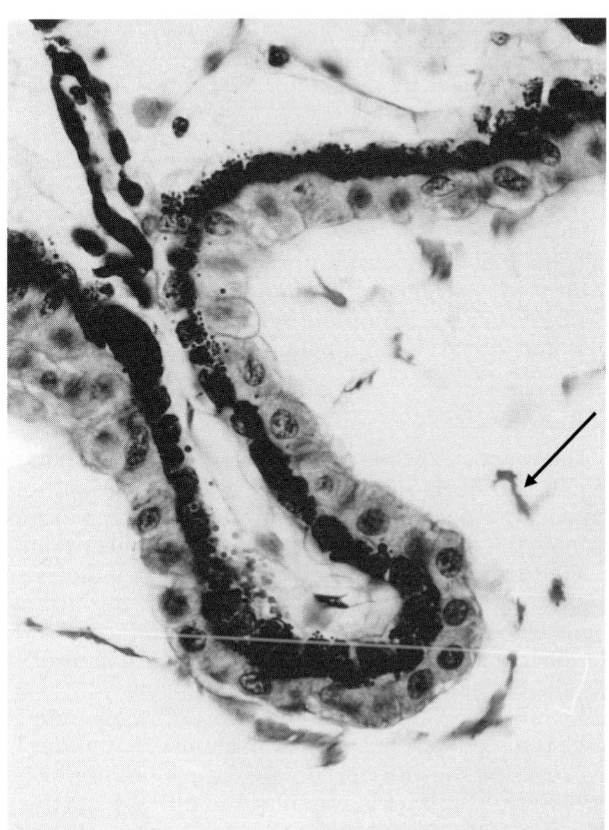

Figure 17.4. *This canine ciliary process is covered by pigmented and nonpigmented epithelial cells. Remnants of zonular fibers (arrows) are present in the posterior chamber. Masson's trichrome (×600).*

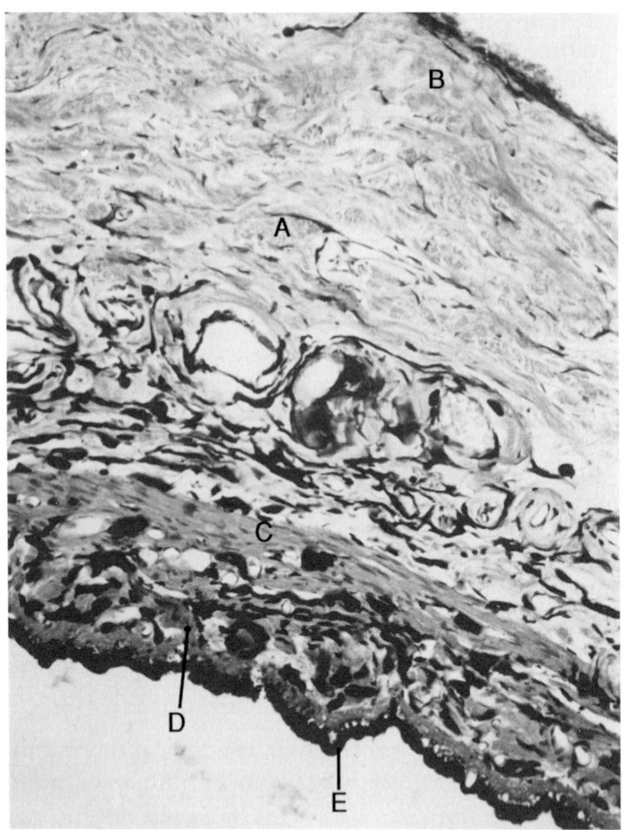

Figure 17.5. *In this canine iris, the stroma (A) is the thickest layer containing many blood vessels and melanocytes; toward the anterior chamber, an avascular anterior limiting layer (B) is present. This section of the iris was taken near the pupillary opening, so that the fibers of the sphincter muscle (C) were cut longitudinally. Dilator muscle (D) and posterior pigmented epithelial cell layer (E). Hematoxylin and eosin (×175).*

cate through the central opening, the **pupil**. The iris consists of a **stroma** of pigmented, highly vascularized loose connective tissue, the **sphincter** and **dilator muscles**, and a bilayered **epithelium**.

STROMA

The stroma of the iris consists of regular, arcuate bundles of collagen fibers supported by highly vascularized loose connective tissue containing many melanocytes, which determine the color of the iris. Spiral collagen fiber bundles derived from several arcuate collagen fiber bundles surround each stromal blood vessel; through this arrangement, blood vessels change their position in synchrony with the fiber bundles during contraction or dilatation of the iris, thereby eluding compression and kinking.

Toward the anterior chamber, fibrocytes separated by large intercellular spaces form an almost continuous lining covering the **anterior limiting layer** (or anterior border layer). This layer is avascular and differs from the remainder of the iris stroma in that it is particularly rich in melanocytes and proteoglycans (Fig. 17.5). It also contains channel-like spaces or crypts that often penetrate deep into the stroma, especially at the pupillary margin, and that communicate with the anterior chamber.

The arterial blood vessels originate from the **major arterial circle** (circulus arteriosus major) at the periphery of the iris and radiate, spirally wound, into the stroma, forming capillary loops in the vicinity of the pupillary margin. The veins have a straighter arrangement than the arteries and return to the base of the iris and the ciliary body.

MUSCLES

Two muscles are present in the iris that regulate the size of the pupil. They are both of neuroepithelial (pigmented epithelium) origin.

The **sphincter muscle** (musculus sphincter pupillae) is composed of a network of smooth muscle cells, circularly arranged near the pupillary margin (Fig. 17.5). The fibers cross each other at acute angles laterally and medially in animals with oval pupils and dorsally and ventrally in animals with slitlike pupils. The arches of the collagen fiber bundles of the iris stroma loop through the muscle network, thus enabling the muscle fibers to act on them. The sphincter muscle receives parasympathetic innervation through the oculomotor nerve (nucleus of Edinger–Westphal; synapses in the ciliary ganglion).

The **dilator muscle** (musculus dilator pupillae) is a partial differentiation of the anterior epithelial layer, a continuation of the pigmented epithelial layer of the ciliary body (Fig. 17.5). Whereas the basal portions of the epithelial cells possess the structural characteristics of smooth muscle cells, the apical portions have retained those of typical pigmented epithelial cells (myopigmentocytes). The dilator muscle is innervated by sympathetic postganglionic neurons in the cranial cervical ganglion.

EPITHELIUM

The posterior pigmented epithelial layer (Fig. 17.5) of the iris is a continuation of the nonpigmented epithelial layer of the ciliary processes, which gradually becomes pigmented toward the base of the iris. Frequently, the epithelial cells are separated by wide intercellular spaces. On its posterior (inner) surface, the epithelium is covered by a basal lamina.

In ungulates, several dark masses, called **iridial granules** (granula iridica), are found at the dorsal (larger granula) and ventral pupillary margins. They are focal proliferations of the two epithelial layers that project into the anterior chamber at the dorsal and ventral pupillary margins.

Iridocorneal Angle

The iridocorneal angle (or iris, filtration, or drainage angle) is a region located at the periphery of the anterior chamber, where the corneoscleral junction, the ciliary body, and the iris converge. Drainage of aqueous humor from the anterior chamber into the blood is extremely important functionally. Structurally, the iridocorneal angle is a meshwork that comprises the pectinate ligament, trabecular meshwork, and trabecular (aqueous) veins.

PECTINATE LIGAMENT

The pectinate ligament consists of numerous long, thin primary and accessory strands extending between the corneoscleral junction and the base of the iris (Fig. 17.6). Each strand comprises a core of collagen fibrils covered by mesothelium (continuous with the corneal endothelium).

TRABECULAR MESHWORK

The **uveal trabecular meshwork** is continuous with the pectinate ligament and is a dense network of mesothelium-covered collagen fibrils, delineating the spaces of Fontana. The uveal trabecular network gradually becomes the structurally identical but tighter-meshed **corneoscleral trabecular meshwork** (adjacent to the cornea and sclera; Fig. 17.6).

VENOUS DRAINAGE

Aqueous humor drains through the pectinate ligament into the trabecular meshwork, where it gains access to **aqueous collecting veins**. It then passes into the

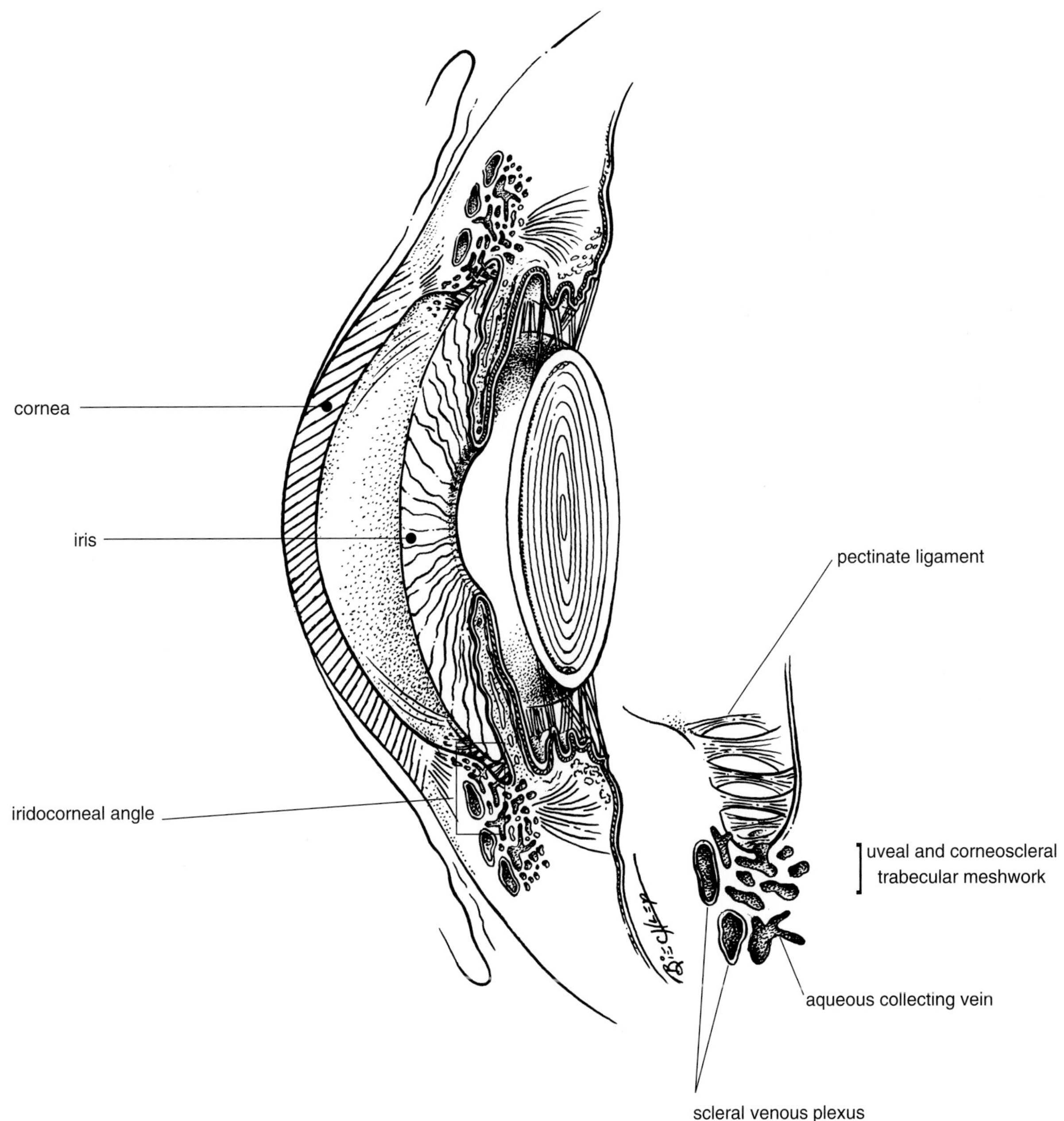

Figure 17.6. *Schematic of the anterior portion of the eye, illustrating the drainage route of aqueous humor from the anterior chamber of the eye (between cornea and iris) through the strands of the pectinate ligament into the spaces of the uveal and corneoscleral trabecular meshworks into aqueous collecting veins and the scleral venous plexus. The inset shows a higher magnification of the rectangular area of the iridocorneal angle.*

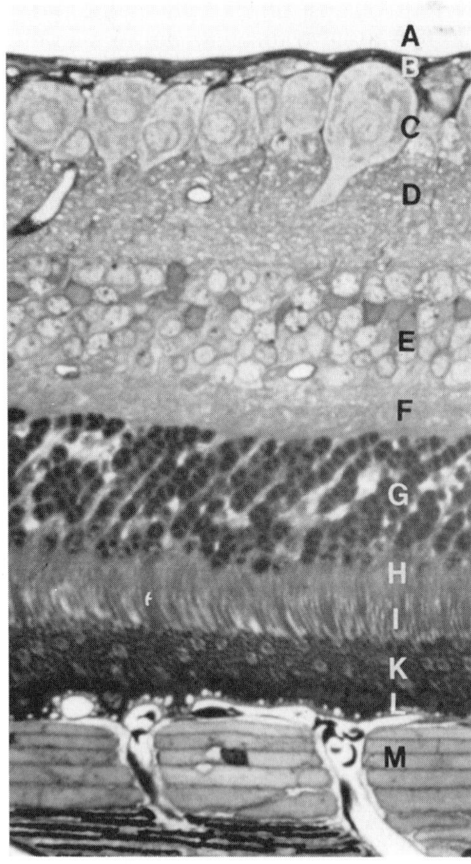

Figure 17.7. *Semithin section through the canine retina and adjacent layers of the choroid at the level of the area centralis. Vitreous body (A); optic nerve fiber layer (B); ganglion cells (C); inner plexiform layer (D); inner nuclear layer (E); outer plexiform layer (F); outer nuclear layer (G); external limiting membrane (H); inner segments of rods and cones (I); outer segments of rods and cones (K); pigment epithelium and choriocapillary layer (L); cellular tapetum lucidum (M). Richardson's stain (×800). (From Hebel R. Entwicklung und Struktur der Retina und des tapetum lucidum des Hundes. Ergebnisse der Anatomie und Entwicklungsgeschichte 45/2. Berlin: Springer Verlag, 1971.)*

scleral venous plexus (plexus venosus sclerae), two to four large vessels located in the sclera, posterior to the limbus (Fig. 17.6). A canal of Schlemm, a circumferential endothelium-lined channel, present in the human eye, is absent in domestic mammals.

NEUROEPITHELIAL TUNIC — RETINA

The retina is the sensory portion, also referred to as the **pars optica retinae**, of the neuroepithelial tunic. The nonsensory portion of this tunic, which begins at the ora serrata, covers the ciliary body and the iris as a double epithelial layer and is also called the **pars caeca retinae**.

Except at the transition toward the ora serrata and at the optic disk, the retina consists of the following layers (Fig. 17.7; see also Fig. 17.8): *(1)* pigment epithelium, *(2)* layer of rods and cones, *(3)* external limiting membrane, *(4)* outer nuclear layer, *(5)* outer plexiform layer, *(6)* inner nuclear layer, *(7)* inner plexiform layer, *(8)* ganglion cell layer, *(9)* optic nerve fiber layer, and *(10)* internal limiting membrane.

The **retinal pigment epithelium** is a simple squamous or cuboidal epithelium resting on a basal lamina (Figs. 17.7 and 17.8). Capillaries of the choriocapillary layer frequently deeply indent the cells. The base of the cell is characterized by deep infoldings of the plasma membrane and associated numerous mitochondria. Cell apices are connected by zonulae adherentes and occludentes. Numerous melanin granules are present, except in the cells overlying the tapetum lucidum. Microvillous apical processes partially surround the outer segments of rods (Fig. 17.8). Several layers of leaflike processes entirely surround the outer segments of cones (Fig. 17.8).

The functions of the pigment epithelium are complex. They include transport of nutrients and metabolites from the capillaries in the choriocapillary layer to the rods and cones, phagocytosis, lysosomal degradation and recycling of the shed outer segments of the photoreceptors, and absorption of light by the melanin.

The **photoreceptive layer** comprises the outer segments, connecting cilia and inner segments of the photoreceptive **rods** and **cones** (first neuron of the visual pathway) forming a distinct layer adjacent to the pigment epithelium (Fig. 17.7).

The **outer segments** consist of stacks of disks surrounded by the cell membrane. The disks are actually flattened membrane spheres, with molecules of visual pigment present in the membranes. Each day, triggered by onset of morning light, short stacks of the oldest disks are shed from the distal ends of the photoreceptors and are subsequently phagocytized by, and degraded in, the retinal pigment epithelial cells. New disks are continually added to the proximal ends of the outer segments. Whereas the rods extend to the apical surface of the pigment epithelium, the cones terminate a certain distance from the epithelial surface. Each outer segment is connected to its inner segment by a **cilium**. The **inner segments** contain the basal bodies of the cilia, as well as many mitochondria.

The rod cells are responsible for vision in dim light, whereas the cone cells function in bright light and are responsible for color vision. Thus, animals who are mainly active at night have retinas with fewer cone cells than those of animals active during the day.

The **external limiting membrane** is formed by zonulae adherentes between processes of adjoining radial glial (Müller) and photoreceptor cells. The microvilli of the radial glial cells project peripherally between the inner segments of the rods and cones (Fig. 17.8).

The **outer nuclear layer** contains the perikarya of the rods and cones (Fig. 17.7). The **outer plexiform layer** is composed of the axon terminals of the photoreceptor cells, i.e., rod spherules and cone pedicles, forming synapses with the processes of the horizontal cells, and the dendrites of the bipolar cells (Fig. 17.8).

As many as four (in dogs) layers of nuclei make up the **inner nuclear layer** (Fig. 17.7), which comprises bipolar, horizontal, amacrine, and radial glial cells. Most of the nuclei in the center of this layer belong to the **rod** and

cone bipolar cells (the second neuron of the visual pathway). Dendrites of the rod bipolar cell contact several rods, and the axon synapses with amacrine and/or ganglion cells (Fig. 17.8). The cone bipolar cells are either midget bipolar cells that contact a single cone or flat bipolar cells in which dendrites contact several cones while their axons synapse with amacrine and ganglion cells. Nuclei located in the outer portion of this layer belong to **horizontal cells**, the processes of which synapse with rod and cone axon terminals in the outer plexiform layer. Nuclei located in the inner portion belong to **amacrine cells**. Their cell processes extend into the inner plexiform layer and establish contact with the dendrites and perikarya of ganglion cells and with the axons of bipolar cells. Amacrine cells also seem to be interconnected (Fig. 17.8). The nuclei of the **radial glial cells** are interspersed among the other nuclei. The radial glial cells are elongated, fibrous astrocytes extending between the internal and external limiting membranes (Fig. 17.8). They provide mechanical support and nutrition to the retina.

The **inner plexiform layer** is the region of synaptic contacts between bipolar and ganglion cells, between amacrine and ganglion cells, and between adjacent amacrine cells.

The **ganglion cell layer** (third neuron of the visual pathway) is composed of large neuronal perikarya. Their axons form a separate layer, the **optic nerve fiber layer** (Figs. 17.7 and 17.8). The axons converge and exit at the optic disk of the retina and form the optic nerve. The **internal limiting membrane** is formed by the expanded processes of the radial glial cells, which unite to

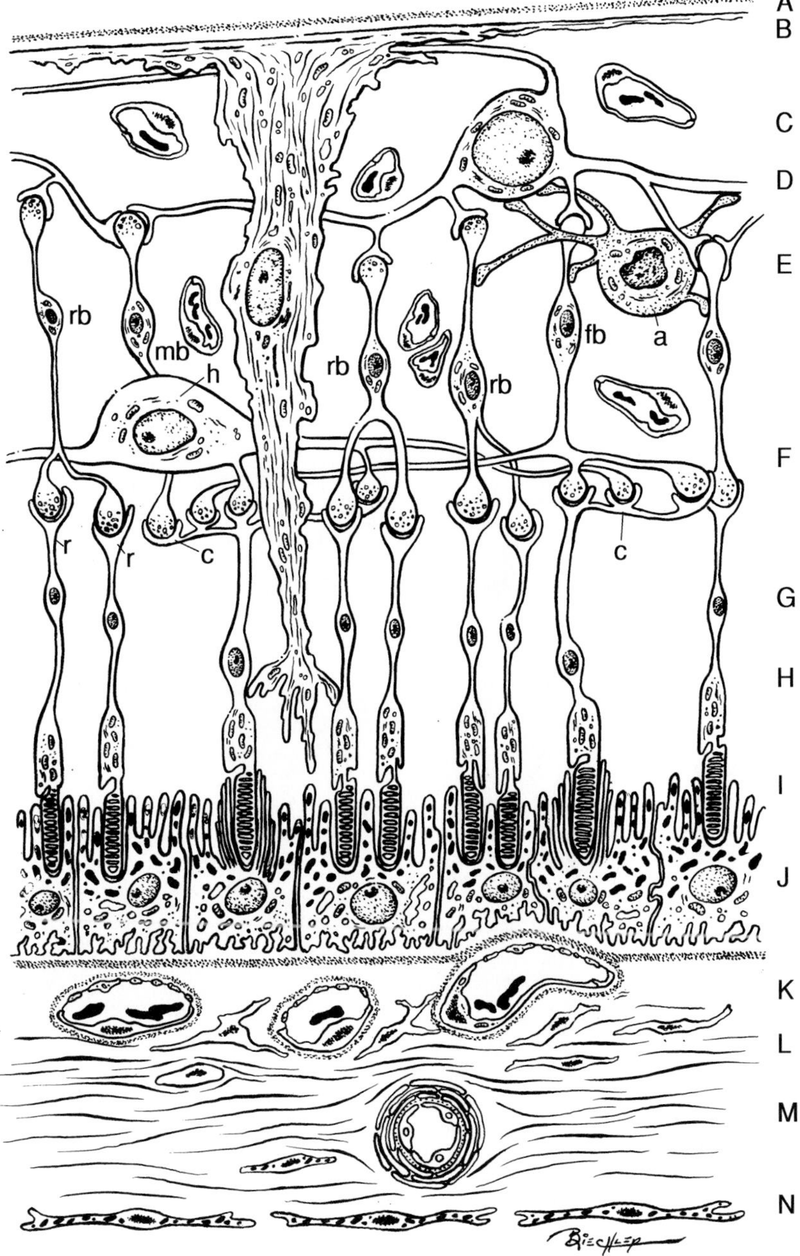

Figure 17.8. *Schematic drawing of the organization of the retina (A–J) and choroid (K–N). Internal limiting membrane (A); optic nerve fiber layer (B); ganglion cell layer (C); inner plexiform layer (D); inner nuclear layer (E); outer plexiform layer (F); outer nuclear layer (G); level of the external limiting membrane (H); layer of outer and inner segments of rods and cones (I); pigment epithelium (J); choriocapillary layer (K); choroid connective tissue, in lieu of tapetum lucidum (L); vessel layer of the choroid (M); suprachoroid layer (N). The rod spherules (r) have synaptic contact with rod bipolar cells (rb), which synapse with ganglion cells. The cone pedicles (c) have synaptic contact with midget bipolar cells (mb), which contact a single cone, and flat bipolar cells (fb), the dendrites of which contact several cones and the axons of which then synapse with amacrine (a) and ganglion cells. Horizontal cell processes (h) contact rod spherules and cone pedicles. Amacrine cells (a) contact the axons of bipolar cells and dendrites and perikarya of ganglion cells. Radial glial cells provide support to the retina; their cytoplasmic processes extend between and around the other cells, and their foot processes participate in the formation of the internal limiting membrane.*

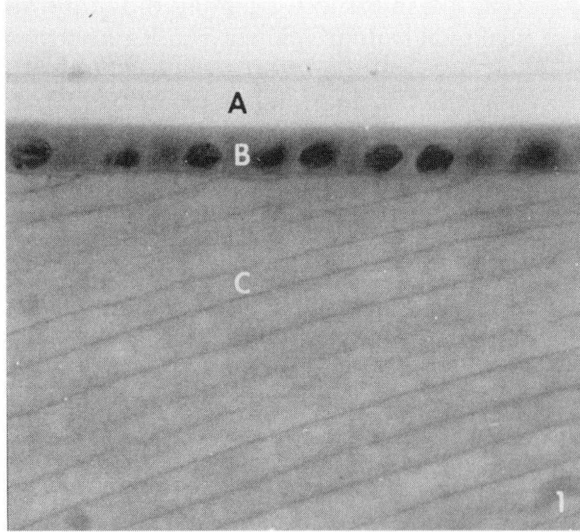

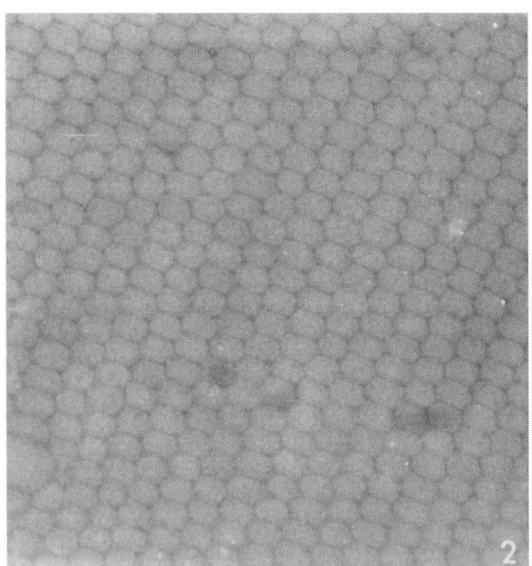

Figure 17.9. *Canine lens. 1., The lens capsule (A) covers the anterior lens epithelium (B) underneath which are the lens fibers (C). 2., Cross section through lens fibers. Hematoxylin and eosin (×660).*

form a continuous layer, analogous to the external glia limitans in the central nervous system (Fig. 17.8), and a basal lamina. Occasional astrocytes, microglial cells, and oligodendrocytes are present in the retina in the inner plexiform, ganglion cell, and optic nerve fiber layers.

The **area centralis retinae** is a small round or oval area of the retina located dorsally and laterally to the optic disk. This area differs from the remainder of the retinae in that it is characterized by an increased number of cones, a thickening of the inner plexiform layer, an increased number of ganglion cells, thinning of the optic nerve fiber layer, and absence of large blood vessels (Fig. 17.7). The area centralis retinae is the area of most acute vision and corresponds to the area of the macula and fovea in primates.

The retinal **vasculature pattern** varies greatly among species. In the holangiotic pattern (cats, dogs, cows, pigs, and sheep), blood vessels occur in the optic nerve fiber layer. Wide capillaries are found at the periphery of the retina, and venules and arterioles are present toward the optic disk (papilla). Numerous capillaries are present in the inner nuclear, ganglion cell, and nerve fiber layers. In the paurangiotic pattern (horses), the vessels radiate only a short distance from the optic disk.

REFRACTIVE MEDIA

Lens and Zonular Fibers

The **lens** is a transparent, biconvex structure that is situated between the iris and the vitreous body and suspended by the zonular fibers to the ciliary body (Fig. 17.6). It consists of the lens capsule, lens epithelium, and lens fibers.

The lens is entirely surrounded by the **lens capsule** (Fig. 17.9), which consists of several layers of collagen fibrils alternating with basal lamina material. It is much thicker on the anterior lens surface than on the posterior surface.

Beneath the anterior lens capsule is the **lens epithelium** (Fig. 17.9), a layer of simple cuboidal epithelial cells. Their bases face the lens capsule and their apices face the lens fibers. At the equator, they elongate and

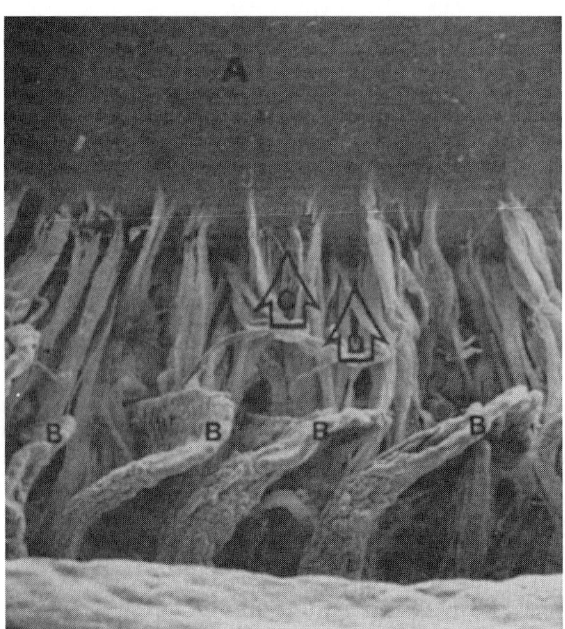

Figure 17.10. *Scanning electron micrograph illustrating a caudal view of ciliary processes and attachment of zonular fibers to the lens (cat). Posterior lens (A); ciliary process (B); posterior zonular fibers (C); anterior zonular fibers (D). Notice that the zonular fibers extend from between the bases of the ciliary processes and aggregate at their lenticular insertion. (From Gelatt KM. Textbook of veterinary ophthalmology. Philadelphia: Lea & Febiger, 1981.)*

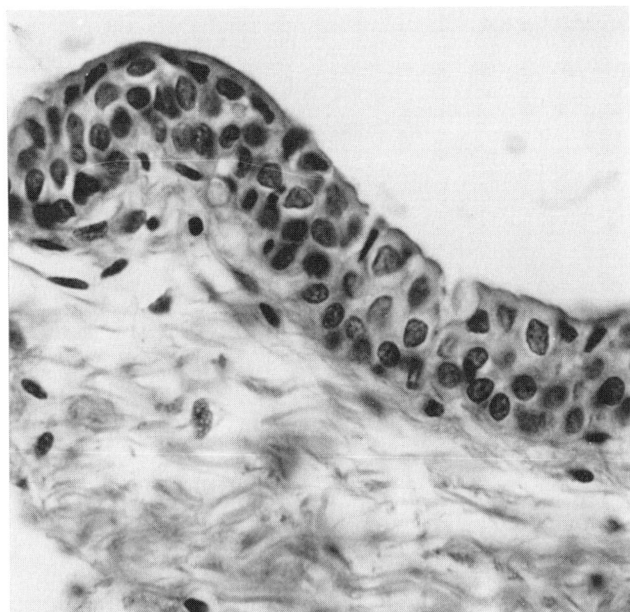
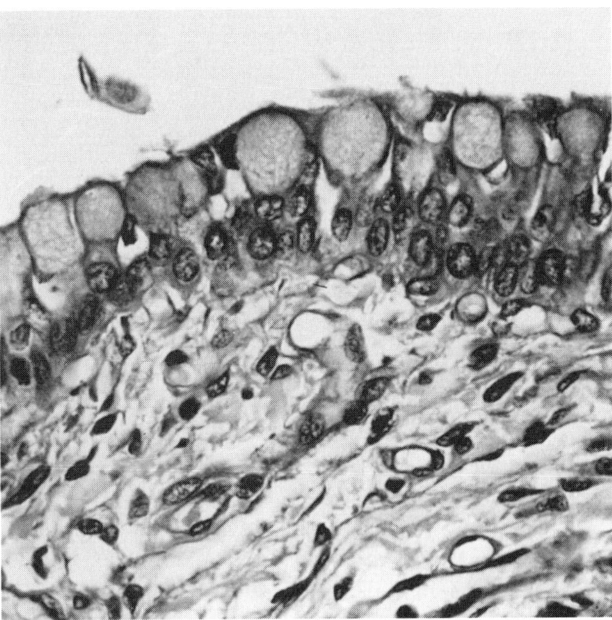

Figure 17.11. *1., Transitional epithelium of the porcine conjunctiva. Hematoxylin and eosin (×540).* **2.,** *Pseudostratified columnar epithelium with many goblet cells of the canine conjunctiva. Hematoxylin and eosin (×540).*

differentiate into **lens fibers**, which make up the bulk of the lens. Through continuous differentiation of lens epithelial cells and addition of fibers, the lens grows throughout life. Fully differentiated lens fibers are U-shaped prism-shaped cells that extend toward the anterior and posterior poles (Fig. 17.9). They lack a nucleus and are virtually devoid of organelles. They interdigitate extensively (especially where fibers from opposite sides of the equator meet to form lens sutures) and are connected through gap junctions and desmosomes.

The **zonular fibers** originate from the ciliary inner limiting membrane, mainly between the ciliary processes and from the pars plana (Figs. 17.4 and 17.11). The fibers are composed of fibrils identical to the microfibrils of elastic fibers (see chapter 3) and are attached to the lens capsule by fusion with its outermost layers.

When the ciliary muscle contracts during accommodation, the zonular fibers slacken, the elastic lens fibers then shorten, and the lens assumes a more spherical shape, focusing the image on the retina.

Vitreous Body

The vitreous body occupies the posterior compartment, the space between the lens and the retina (Fig. 17.1). It is a hydrogel containing 98 to 99% water and is rich in hyaluronic acid and acid mucopolysaccharides. It adheres tightly to the optic papilla and the ora serrata; it also attaches to the internal limiting membrane of the retina and the posterior part (pars plana) of the ciliary body. In most domestic mammals, it is firmly attached to the posterior lens capsule as well; during cataract surgery (removal of the lens), the posterior lens capsule must remain intact to prevent the vitreous body from collapsing and prolapsing forward.

The vitreous body contains a network of sparse collagen fibrils. Fibrils are concentrated peripherally, forming a layer called the **hyaloid membrane** or **cortex**. In the cortex, a few fibrocytes and macrophages are present.

ACCESSORY ORGANS

Eyelids

The eyelids are movable folds of skin that protect the eyes. Their structure is described in Chapter 16.

Third Eyelid and Conjunctiva

The third eyelid is a conjunctival fold fortified by hyaline (ruminants, dogs) or elastic (horses, pigs, cats) cartilage. The **conjunctiva** is a pseudostratified columnar (horses and carnivores) or transitional (pigs, ruminants) epithelium with goblet cells (Fig. 17.10). It is based on a propria of highly vascularized loose connective tissue rich in fibrocytes, lymphocytes, and plasma cells, with some mast cells and macrophages also present. It also may contain solitary and aggregated lymphatic nodules.

The (superficial) **gland of the third eyelid** surrounds the base of the shaft of the T-shaped cartilage plate. It is similar in structure to the lacrimal gland and likewise contributes secretion to the tear film; it is serous in horses and seromucous in all other domestic mammals. Frequently, acinar cells secrete lipid. A deep gland of the third eyelid (Harder's gland) is present in cattle and pigs.

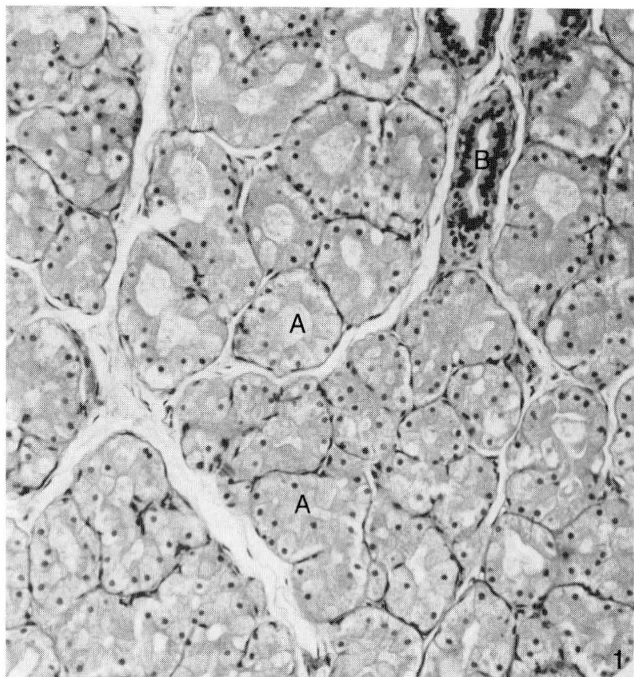

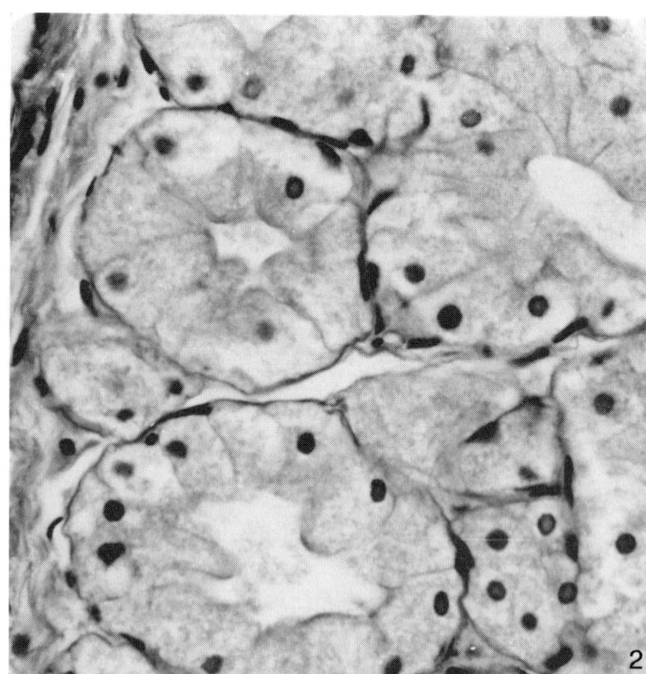

Figure 17.12. *Porcine lacrimal gland. **1.**, Acini (A) and a secretory duct (B). Trichrome (×185). **2.**, The light staining of the acinar cells is due to dissolution of lipid inclusions. Trichrome (×600).*

Lacrimal Apparatus

The **lacrimal gland** is a compound tubuloacinar or tubuloalveolar gland (Fig. 17.12). It is serous in cats and seromucous in dogs and ungulates. The acinar cells frequently contain lipid inclusions and are surrounded by myoepithelial cells (Fig. 17.12).

The intercalated and secretory ducts are lined with simple and stratified cuboidal epithelia, respectively (Fig. 17.12). The lacrimal ductules are lined with stratified cuboidal epithelium.

The glands of the third eyelid (see above) are likewise included in the lacrimal apparatus.

Excess tears accumulate in the lacrimal lake (lacus lacrimalis), a medially located widening of the conjunctiva lined by a stratified squamous and columnar epithelium. They enter the **lacrimal canaliculi**, which are lined with stratified squamous epithelium, through the puncta lacrimalia to reach the lacrimal sac and its continuation, the nasolacrimal duct.

The **nasolacrimal duct** is lined by a stratified columnar epithelium with goblet cells or by transitional epithelium (pigs). It begins with an ampullar widening, the **lacrimal sac**, the propria of which contains lymphatic tissue. Toward the nasal end of the duct, simple branched tubuloacinar mucous (or seromucous in sheep and goats) glands are present.

SPECIES VARIATIONS

Many ocular anatomic and histologic variations occur among species. Among mammals, differences include size and shape of the globe; size and shape of the cornea; thickness of cornea and sclera; point of optic nerve exit; shape and orientation of the pupil; shape and distribution of melanin granules; degree of development of the ciliary muscle; shape, relative size, and color of lens; thickness of various retinal layers; retinal vascular patterns; absence of or location and type of tapetum lucidum; thickness of choroid; and types of lacrimal glands.

The differences between mammals and other vertebrates are much more striking. For example, eyes of birds vary greatly in shape, and their scleras contain cartilage and, in many species, ossicles. In birds and some other vertebrates, such as snakes and lizards, a highly vascular structure called the **pecten** extends from the optic disk region into the vitreous body. Several other differences exist between mammalian eyes and those of other vertebrates. For details of the structure of many nonmammalian eyes and of species differences among mammals, the reader is referred to the listed references.

REFERENCES

Dowling JA. The retina: an approachable part of the brain. Cambridge, MA: Harvard University Press, 1987.

Duke-Elder S. The eye in evolution. Vol. 1, System of ophthalmology. London: Henry Kimpton, 1958.

Fine BS, Yanoff M. Ocular histology, a text and atlas. 2nd ed. Hagerstown, MD: Harper and Row, 1979.

Samuelson DA. Ophthalmic embryology and anatomy. In: Gelatt KN, ed. Veterinary ophthalmology. 2nd ed. Philadelphia: Lea & Febiger, 1991.

Walls GL. The vertebrate eye and its adaptive radiation. Bloomfield Hills, MI: The Cranbrook Press, 1942.

18

Ear

ISAK FOSS
GORDON FLOTTORP

The ear is composed of three divisions: the external ear, the middle ear, and the internal ear. The external ear, structured for sound collection, is composed of the auricle, or pinna, and the external auditory canal. The middle ear consists of the tympanic membrane, the tympanic cavity, and the three auditory ossicles and their associated muscles and ligaments. It is connected to the nasopharynx by the auditory tube. This air-filled cavity containing the ossicles is primarily for sound conduction. The inner ear, consisting of a membranous labyrinth enclosed within the osseous labyrinth in the petrosal part of the temporal bone, is structured for both hearing and equilibrium.

EXTERNAL EAR

The microscopic description of the auricle and the external auditory canal is included in Chapter 16.

MIDDLE EAR

Tympanic Membrane

The thin **tympanic membrane** delimits the external auditory canal from the tympanic cavity (Fig. 18.1). It is covered externally by stratified squamous epithelium and internally by simple squamous epithelium continuous with that of the tympanic cavity. Between these two epithelial sheets is a connective-tissue layer composed of central circularly and peripheral radially oriented collagen fibers. Where the manubrium of the malleus attaches to the tympanic membrane, the connective tissue is somewhat thicker and contains blood vessels and nerves that course along the manubrium and spread radially. Collagen fibers are sparse or even absent in the dorsal portion of the membrane, referred to as the **flaccid** part.

Tympanic Cavity

The air-filled tympanic cavity contains three auditory ossicles (malleus, incus, and stapes) and their muscles and ligaments (Fig. 18.1). The cavity is lined with simple squamous or simple cuboidal epithelium resting on a thin layer of connective tissue. A few epithelial cells have cilia, particularly those on the floor of the cavity.

Auditory Ossicles

The auditory ossicles traverse the middle ear, connecting the tympanic membrane to the membrane of the vestibular (oval) window of the internal ear (Fig. 18.1). These compact bones transmit vibrations across the middle ear cavity. The manubrium of the malleus is firmly attached to the tympanic membrane, and the small hooklike process on the neck of the malleus serves as an attachment for the tensor tympani muscle tendon. The head of the malleus articulates with the incus,

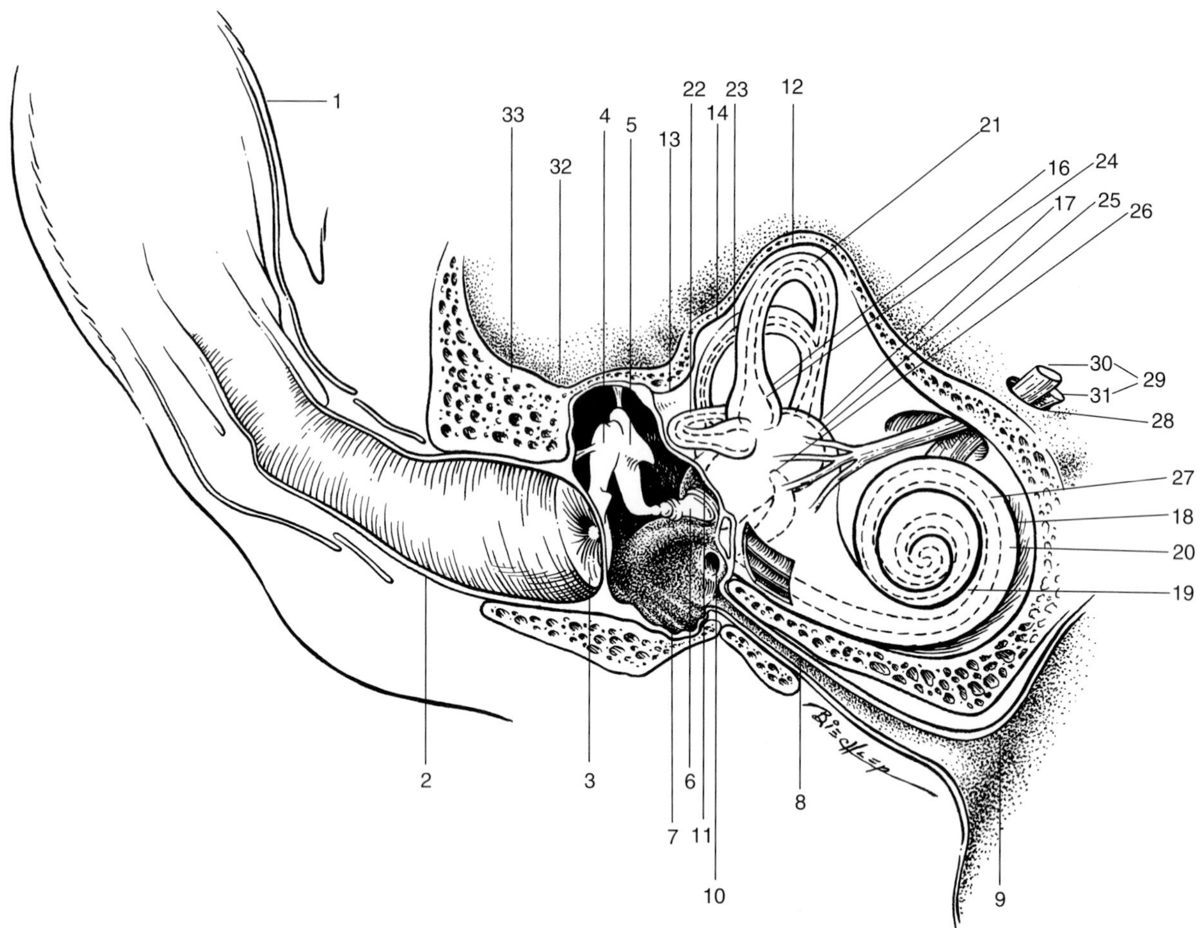

Figure 18.1. *Schematic drawing of the right ear (dog), rostral aspect, showing the external ear with the auricle (1) and external acoustic meatus (2); middle ear with the tympanic membrane (3); auditory ossicles comprising the malleus (4), incus (5), and stapes (6); tympanic cavity (7); auditory tube (8) with connection to the nasopharynx (9), cochlear window (10), and vestibular window (11), where the footplate of the stapes is located; internal ear with the bony labyrinth comprising the anterior (12), lateral (13), and posterior (14) semicircular canals, each with an osseous ampulla (16); the vestibule (17) and the cochlea (18) with the scala vestibuli (19) and the scala tympani (20); membranous labyrinth comprising the anterior (21), lateral (22), and posterior (23) semicircular ducts, each with a membranous ampulla (24), utricle (25), saccule (26), and cochlear duct (27). Moreover, the internal acoustic meatus (28) with the vestibulocochlear nerve (29), comprising the vestibular nerve (30) and the cochlear nerve (31), are depicted, together with the cranial cavity (32) and the temporal bone (33).*

which, in turn, articulates with the stapes. Ligaments hold these synovial articulations in place. The stapedius muscle attaches to the rostral crus of the stapes, and the footplate of the stapes is attached to the vestibular window by an annular ligament. Muscles of the middle ear (tensor tympani and stapedius) are composed of skeletal muscle and function to dampen ossicle movement, protecting the inner ear structures from excessive vibration.

Auditory Tube

The **auditory tube** connects the tympanic cavity to the nasopharynx (Fig. 18.1). It is lined by ciliated pseudostratified columnar epithelium (with goblet cells) resting on loose connective tissue. The tube is surrounded by bone near the tympanum and by an incomplete cartilaginous tube toward the pharynx. The cartilage is hyaline near the bone and contains a gradually increasing number of elastic fibers toward the pharynx. The propria is thin and without glands in the osseous portion and becomes thicker and contains seromucous glands and lymphatic nodules in the cartilaginous part. Aggregated lymphatic nodules are present at the pharyngeal extremity. In the horse, the auditory tube expands ventrally to form the **guttural pouch**, which has the same histologic features as the pharyngeal portion of the tube but lacks a cartilaginous support. The function of the auditory tube is to secure the same air pressure on the two sides of the tympanic membrane. Usually, the auditory tube is closed, but it opens during yawning and swallowing, thus equalizing the air pressure on both sides of the tympanic membrane.

INTERNAL EAR

The inner ear comprises the **bony labyrinth** and the **membranous labyrinth**.

Bony Labyrinth

The bony labyrinth is a system of canals and cavities within the petrous part of the temporal bone. Bone of the labyrinth has the highest content of tricalciumphosphate, $(Ca_2)_3(PO_4)_2$, per volume unit and is therefore the hardest and least compressible bone in the body.

The cavities of the labyrinth include the vestibule, three semicircular canals, and the cochlea (Fig. 18.1). The **vestibule** is a small oval space connecting the cochlea with the semicircular canals located at the medial wall of the tympanic cavity. Three **semicircular canals** (anterior, posterior, and lateral) lie at right angles to each other caudally and dorsally to the vestibule, and all communicate with the utricle. The **cochlea** is a bony tube wound in the shape of a spiral. The **spiral canal** of the cochlea makes several turns around an axis of spongy bone, the **modiolus**. The modiolus is a cone-shaped hollow osseous structure in which the cochlear nerve and its spiral ganglion are located. The number of coils varies from species to species, e.g., dog, 3 1/4; cat, 3; horse, 2 1/4; pig, 4; guinea pig, 4 1/2; cow, 3 1/2; man, 2 3/4. The base of the modiolus forms the rostral part of the internal acoustic meatus, where the cochlear nerve and blood vessels enter the cochlea. The bony canal is partially divided by a hollow bony projection, the **spiral osseous lamina**, which contains the branches of the cochlear nerve to the spiral organ. The width of this lamina is largest at the cochlear window and diminishes toward the apex of the cochlea.

The triangular cochlear duct splits the cochlea into two compartments, above and below (Fig. 18.2). The dorsal compartment, or **scala vestibuli**, extends from the region of the **vestibular window** (oval) to the apex of the cochlea, where it becomes confluent with the ventral compartment, the **scala tympani**, through an opening called the **helicotrema** (Fig. 18.3). The scala tympani ends at the **cochlear window** (round).

The canals and cavities of the bony labyrinth are lined by periosteum. A clear fluid, **perilymph**, fills the **perilymphatic space** between the periosteum and the membranous labyrinth (Fig. 18.3). Perilymph is similar in composition to its main source, cerebrospinal fluid. The fluid is also produced by blood capillaries that are located in the connective tissue of the osseous labyrinth. Perilymph flows from the subarachnoid space through

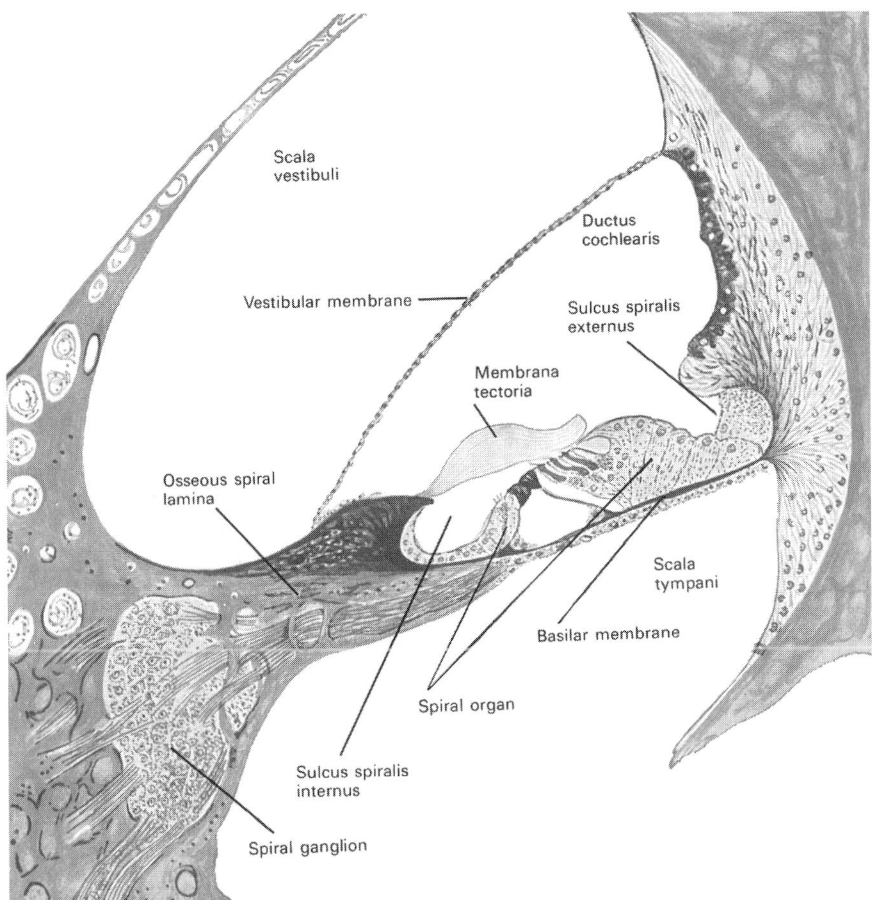

Figure 18.2. *Section through the second turn of the cochlea from a human cochlea. The modiolus is to the left. Mallory's stain. (From Berry MM, Standring SM, Bannister LH. Auditory and vestibular apparatus. In: Williams PL, ed. Gray's anatomy. 38th ed. Edinburgh: Churchill Livingstone, 1995:1367.)*

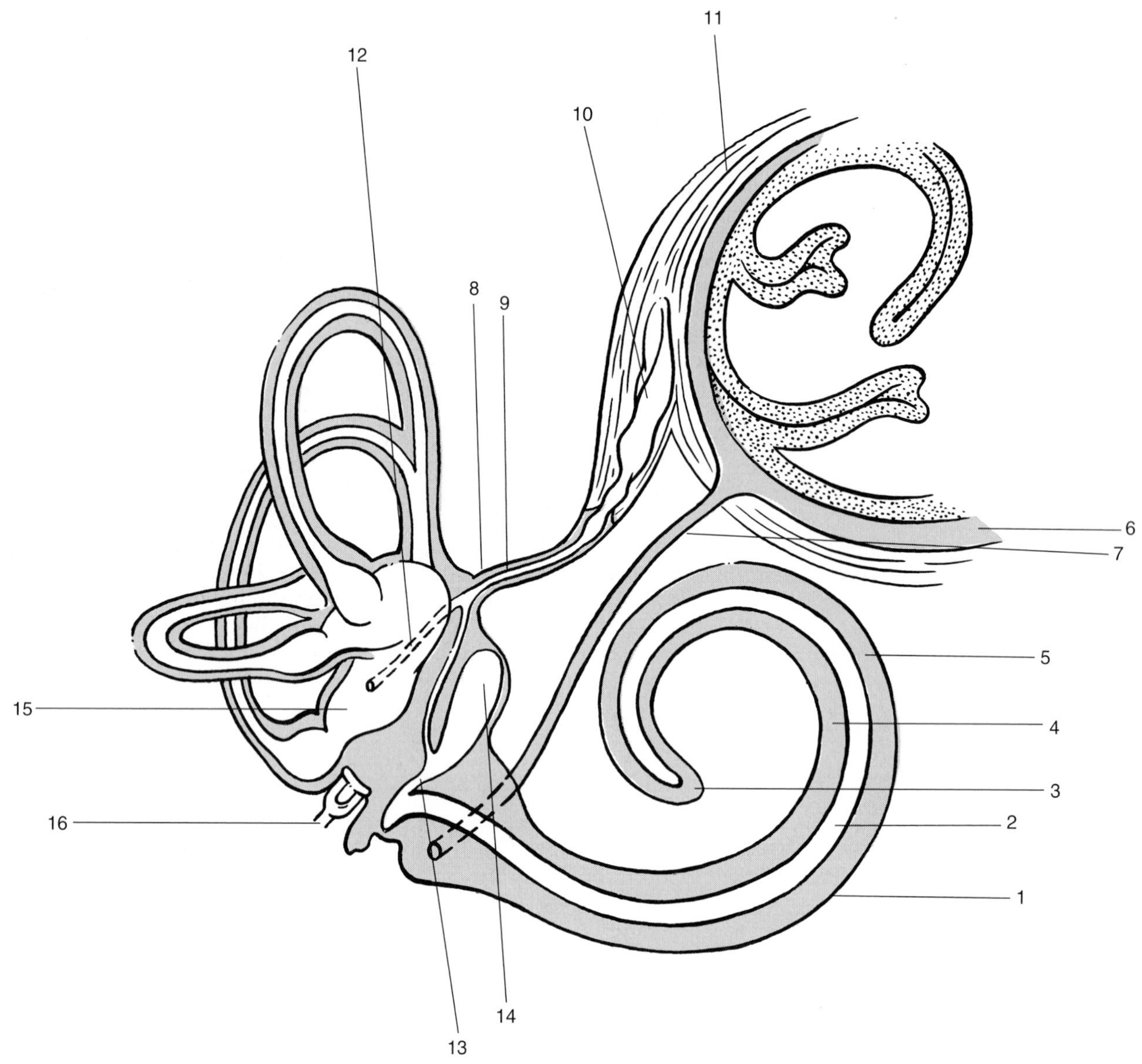

Figure 18.3. *Schematic drawing of the right internal ear with its connections to the cranial cavity, intradural space, and subarachnoidal space (rostral aspect). The cochlea (1) with its contents is drawn uncoiled to show the blind end of the cochlear duct (2) and helicotrema (3), where there is open connection between scala vestibuli (4) and scala tympani (5) at the apex of the cochlea. Note especially that there is open connection between the subarachnoidal space (6), which contains cerebrospinal fluid, and the scala tympani, which contains perilymph. This connection is the cochlear canaliculus (7). The other connection to the cranial cavity is the vestibular aqueduct (8), which houses part of the endolymphatic duct (9) and part of the endolymphatic sac (10). Dura mater (11), the utriculosaccular duct (12), ductus reuniens (13), saccule (14), utricle (15), and stapes in the cochlear window (16) are also seen.*

the cochlear canaliculus into the cavities of the bony labyrinth. The **vestibular aqueduct**, a space surrounding the endolymphatic duct, also contains perilymph.

Membranous Labyrinth

The membranous labyrinth comprises the semicircular ducts, utricle, saccule, cochlear duct, endolymphatic duct, and endolymphatic sac (Fig. 18.3). The membranous labyrinth is lined with simple squamous epithelium and filled with a fluid called **endolymph**, which is more viscous than perilymph. Endolymph is produced by cells adjacent to the cristae ampullares and the macula of the utricle, in addition to the stria vascularis, which is described later in this chapter. The connective tissue underlying the epithelium of the labyrinth is continuous with mesothelium-covered connective tissue trabeculae. The trabeculae span the adjacent perilymphatic space and anchor the membranous labyrinth to the bony wall.

The **semicircular ducts** lie within the semicircular

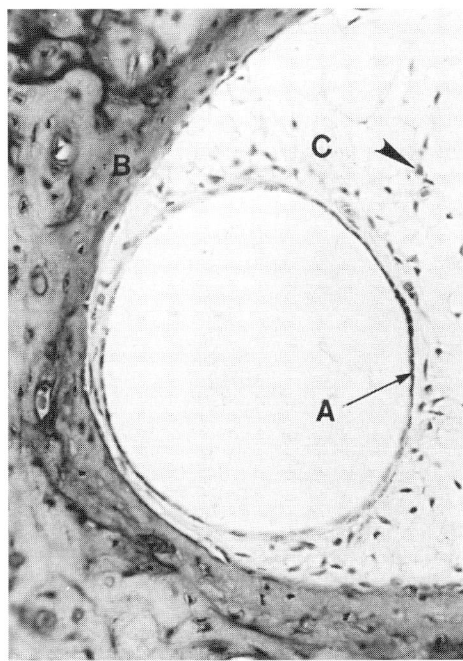

Figure 18.4. *Semicircular canal (cat). The epithelium-lined membranous tube (A) lies within the osseous labyrinth (B). The perilymphatic space (C) contains delicate mesothelium-lined connective-tissue trabeculae (arrowhead). Hematoxylin and eosin (×400).*

canals (Fig. 18.4). Each duct has an enlarged ampullated end, whereas the other end has even dimension. The detailed connection of the ducts with the utricle is shown in Fig. 18.3.

The medial wall of the vestibule has two depressions in which the **utricle** (caudodorsal) and the **saccule** (rostroventral) are housed (Fig. 18.3). These two structures are connected by the **utriculosaccular duct**. The utricle and saccule give off ducts that join to form the **endolymphatic duct**, which terminates as the **endolymphatic sac**. This sac lies partially in the **vestibular aqueduct**, partially intradurally between the two laminae of the dura. Part of the duct is surrounded by the vestibular aqueduct.

The **cochlear duct** is connected to the saccule by a small duct, the **ductus reuniens**, and ends as a blind sac at the apex of the cochlea. The cochlear duct is separated from the scala vestibuli by the **vestibular membrane** (Reissner's membrane) and from the scala tympani by the **basilar membrane** (Figs. 18.2 and 18.5). The vestibular membrane is composed of scant collagen fibers covered with simple squamous epithelium on both surfaces. A basement membrane separates the epithelia from the connective tissue. The basilar membrane is attached to the outer osseous cochlea by the spiral ligament and extends to the spiral lamina of the modiolus. The membrane is composed of collagen fibers embedded in homogeneous ground substance; it increases in thickness as it progresses from the cochlear window to the helicotrema. The basilar membrane varies continuously in width from the cochlear window, where it is narrowest, to the helicotrema, where it is widest, at the ratio 1:1.7. The width is measured from the edge of the osseous spiral lamina to the attachment in the spiral ligament (Figs. 18.2 and 18.5). On the side facing the scala tympani, the basilar membrane is covered with simple squamous epithelium, and the spiral organ of hearing (organ of Corti) is present on the cochlear duct surface.

The third wall of the triangular-shaped cochlear duct contains many blood capillaries and is called the **stria vascularis** (Figs. 18.2, 18.5, and 18.6). It is lined with stratified cuboidal epithelium resting directly (with no basal lamina) on a layer of connective tissue (Fig. 18.7). The epithelium has marginal cells, intermediate cells, and basal cells (Fig. 18.7). The free surface of the marginal cells has short and irregular microvilli. Deep plasmalemma infoldings divide the basal cytoplasm into compartments containing numerous mitochondria. The intermediate cells have many processes that interdigitate with each other and with the marginal cells. These processes also partially surround and isolate each marginal cell from adjacent cells but never reach the endolymphatic surface (Fig. 18.7). Intraepithelial capillaries are present, surrounded by an extremely narrow perivascular space (Fig. 18.7). The stria vascularis contributes to the production of endolymph and regulates its ion content, which has high potassium and low sodium levels. Only the marginal cells are of ectodermal origin, whereas the intermediate and basal cells develop from connective tissue cells in the spiral ligament and are therefore of mesenchymal origin. During maturation of the stria vascularis, the basal lamina below the marginal cells becomes fragmented and gradually disappears. Remnants of the basal lamina can occasionally be identified in the morphologically newly mature stria vascularis.

At the junction of the stria vascularis and the spiral organ, the stratified epithelium changes abruptly to simple cuboidal. This region is called the **spiral prominence** (Figs. 18.2 and 18.5).

The functional divisions of the internal ear are the **vestibular apparatus** and the **auditory apparatus**.

Vestibular Apparatus

The vestibular apparatus includes the organs of equilibrium, composed of the semicircular ducts, saccule, and utricle. Within these structures are specialized neuroepithelial areas, the crista ampullaris, macula utriculi, and macula sacculi, which function to detect motion and maintain equilibrium.

CRISTA AMPULLARIS

The membranous ampulla of each semicircular duct contains the **crista ampullaris**, a structure sensitive to rotatory movements (angular acceleration and deceleration) (Figs. 18.8 and 18.9). The crista ampullaris is composed of a ridge of sensory epithelium resting on thickened connective tissue, which projects into the lu-

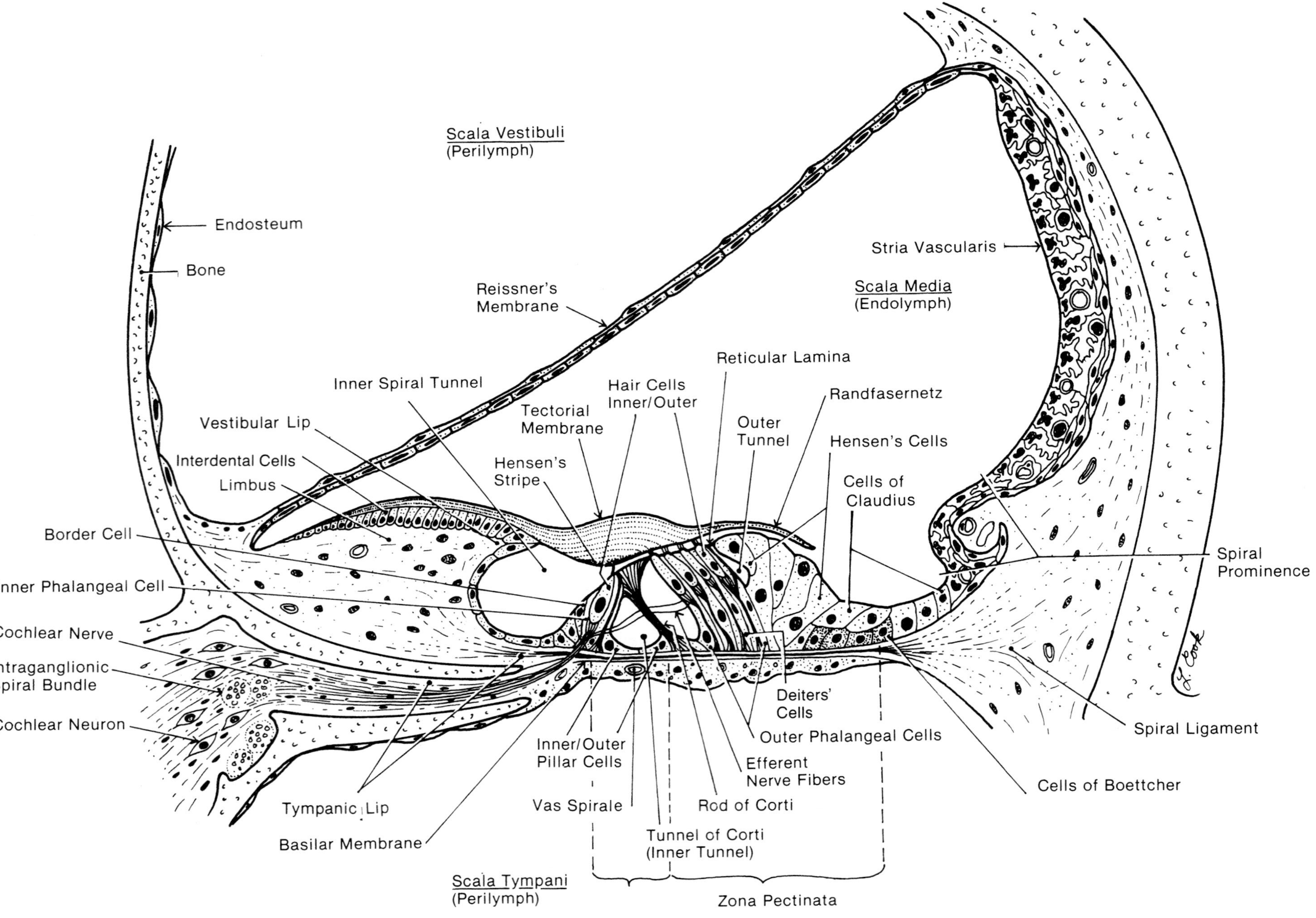

Figure 18.5. *Cochlear duct. This is a diagrammatic sketch showing the cytologic structures of the cochlear duct. (From Schuknecht HF. Anatomy. In: Schuknecht HF, ed. Pathology of the ear. 2nd ed. Philadelphia: Lea & Febiger, 1993:31.)*

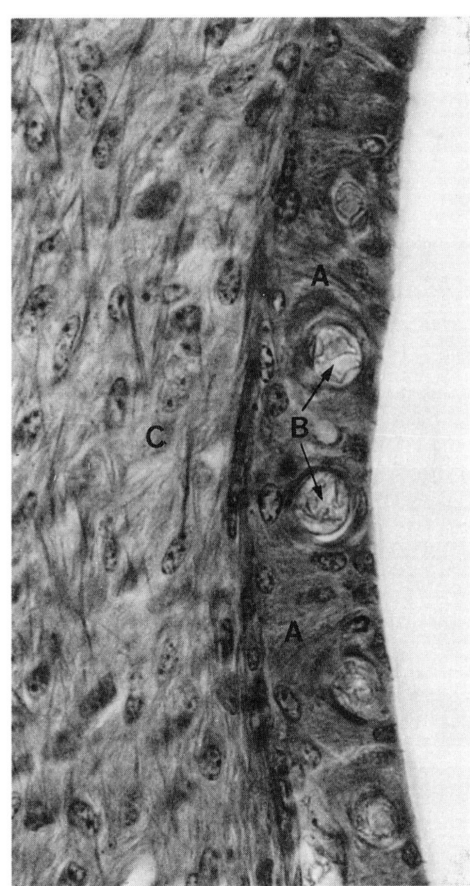

Figure 18.6. *Stria vascularis (guinea pig). This stratified cuboidal epithelium (A) is traversed by numerous capillaries (B) and rests on loose connective tissue (C). Crossmon's trichrome (×600).*

men of the ampulla. The sensory epithelium consists of sensory hair cells and supporting cells. The hair cells project into an overlying gelatinous **cupula**. The cupula contacts the opposite wall of the ampulla and deflects in the direction of fluid movement, much like an elastic diaphragm. This deflection causes the hair bundles to bend. The epithelial cells surrounding the crista are considered sites of endolymph production.

Two types of hair cells (types I and II) are recognized at the ultrastructural level. The type I cell has a narrow neck and a rounded base that fits into a cup-shaped afferent nerve terminal (nerve chalice), which is in contact with efferent nerve fiber endings. These endings, which contain many vesicles, may have an inhibitory function. The type II cell is cylindric and is innervated by both afferent and efferent nerve endings (Fig. 18.10).

In the apical region of each hair cell is a cluster of 40 to 80 stereocilia that contain numerous actin filaments anchored in a complex terminal web of actin filaments called the **cuticular plate** located at the cell apex. The stereocilia are arranged in approximately four to five rows. The length of the stereocilia increases progressively toward one pole of the cell, in which a single **kinocilium** is located. The tip of each stereocilium is linked to its neighbor in the adjacent, taller row by a fine strand called **tip link**. The kinocilium has the typical 9 + 2 microtubule structure; however, it is incapable of independent motion. The stereocilia may tilt toward the side in which the kinocilium is located, making the whole bundle cone-shaped. This arrangement of the stereocilia and the single kinocilium gives each hair cell a functional polarization toward the kinocilium. Whenever the stereocilia bend in the direction described, the afferent nerve fiber in contact with the cell is excited. Conversely, movement in the opposite direction causes inhibition. In the ampullary crista of the lateral semicircular duct, the kinocilium of all the hair cells is facing the utricle, whereas in the ampullary crista of the anterior and posterior semicircular ducts, the kinocilium of all the hair cells is oriented away from the utricle.

The supporting cells are tall and columnar with microvilli. They synthesize the matrix of the cupula and therefore contain numerous secretory vesicles.

MACULAE OF THE UTRICLE AND SACCULE

On the anterior wall of the utricle and on the medial wall of the saccule are receptor organs, the **macula utri-**

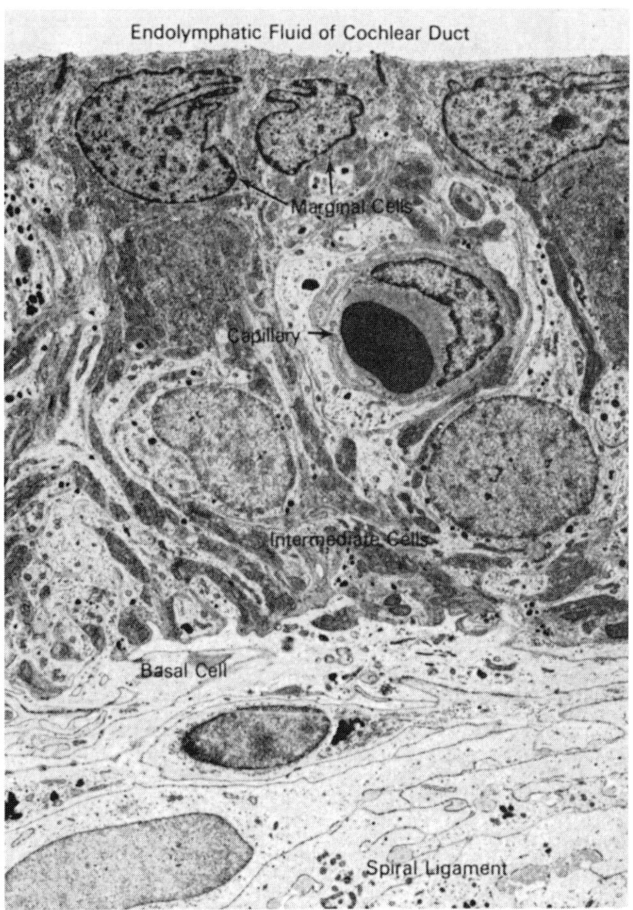

Figure 18.7. *Stria vascularis, transmission electron micrograph (squirrel monkey) (×3752). (From Schuknecht HF. Anatomy. In: Schuknecht HF, ed. Pathology of the ear. 2nd ed. Philadelphia: Lea & Febiger, 1993:31.)*

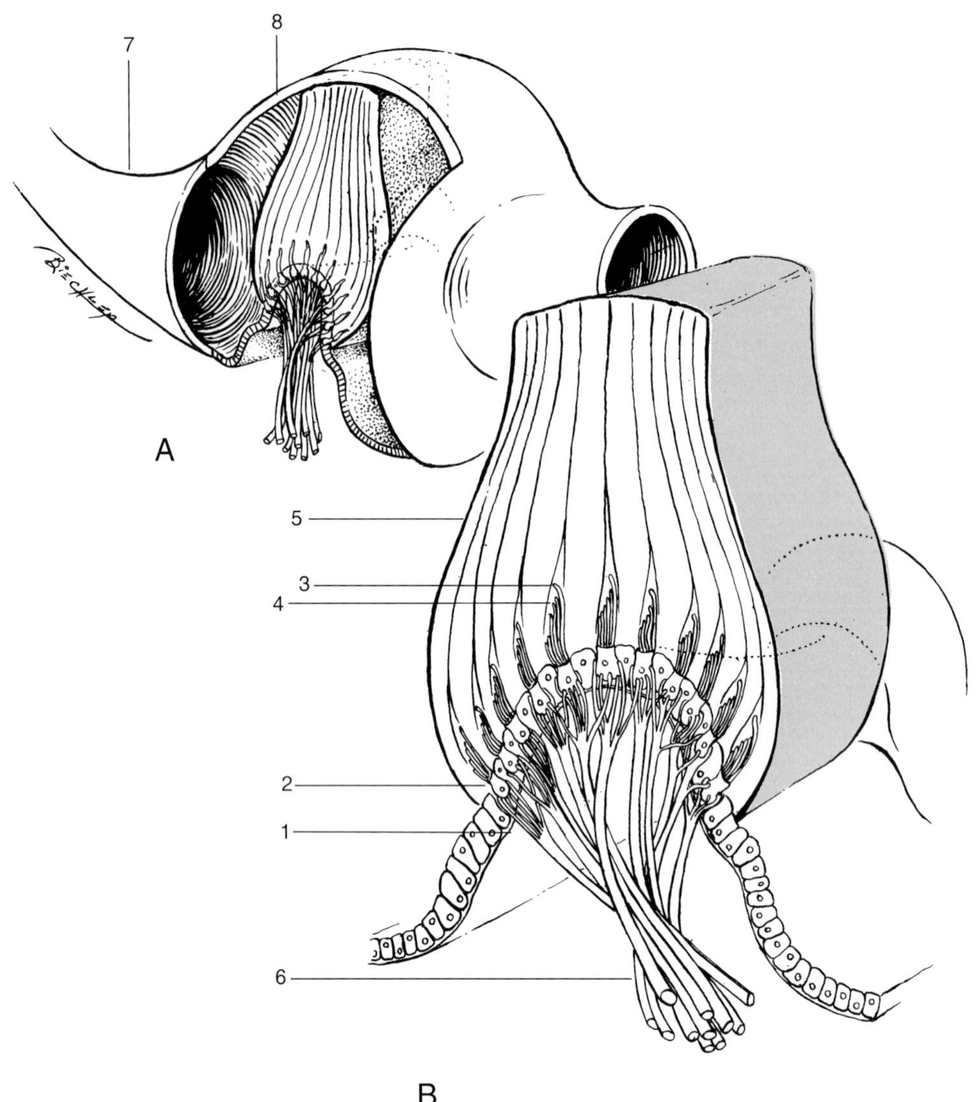

Figure 18.8. *Schematic section of the ampulla of the semicircular duct, showing crista ampullaris (1) containing sensory hair cells (2). Each hair cell has one kinocilium (3) and several stereocilia (4) of different length. On top of the crista ampullaris and the sensory hairs lies the cupula (5), a cup-shaped gelatinous structure that contacts the opposite wall of the ampulla. Ampullary nerve (6), semicircular duct (7), ampulla (8).* ***A.****, Position of the crista ampullaris with the head upright.* ***B.****, Enlarged view of the crista.*

culi and the **macula sacculi**. The macula sacculi is hook-shaped and is oriented vertically when the head is in the normal position. The macula utriculi is kidney-shaped and is oriented horizontally when the head is in normal position. The sensory epithelium of both maculae rests on loose connective tissue containing blood vessels and nerves (Figs. 18.10 and 18.11).

The cells of these receptor organs are essentially the same as those of the crista, i.e., type I and II cells along with the supporting cells (Figs. 18.10 and 18.11). The gelatinous mass into which the hair bundles penetrate has calcium carbonate crystals called **statoconia** on the free surface. Together, they form the **statoconial** (otolithic) **membrane**. Another morphologic difference is that the arrangement of the sensory cells of the macula utriculi is such that the kinocilium of each cell faces toward a stripe, the **striola**, which divides the sensory cell population into two oppositely polarized groups (Fig. 18.10). In the macula sacculi, the hair cell polarization differs in that the kinocilium of each cell faces away from the striola. As in the crista ampullaris of the semicircular ducts, the tip of each stereocilium is connected to its neighbor in the adjacent taller row by a threadlike strand called **tip link**.

VESTIBULAR MECHANISM

With rotation of the head, the endolymph within the semicircular ducts flows through the ampulla. The movement of the fluid displaces the cupula, which then bends the underlying stereocilia of the hair cells of the

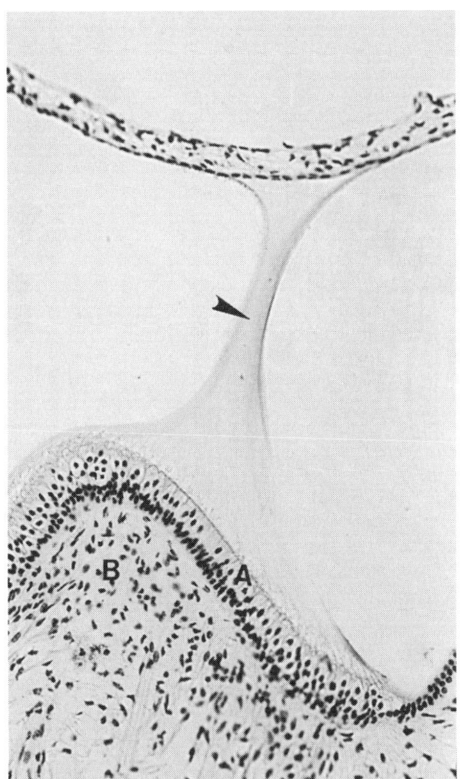

Figure 18.9. *Crista ampullaris (guinea pig). The sensory and supportive cells (A) and the underlying connective tissue (B) form a crest within the ampulla. The gelatinous cupula (arrow) on top of the epithelium extends across to the opposite wall. Hematoxylin and eosin (×400).*

crista ampullaris. As the stereocilia bend toward the kinocilium, the hair cell increasingly stimulates neural impulses in the underlying axons of the vestibular nerve. The neural stimulus decreases as the stereocilia bend away from the kinocilium.

Functionally, macula utriculi and macula sacculi are both receptors that detect the orientation of the head in a gravitational field and control posture, gait, and equilibrium, making the **static labyrinth**. In linear acceleration and deceleration or any change in head position, the heavy statoconia cause shearing forces on the stereocilia of the hair cells. This helps an animal maintain normal posture. Because linear acceleration and deceleration concern movements, both macula utriculi and macula sacculi also belong to the **kinetic labyrinth**. The semicircular ducts belong, however, only to the kinetic labyrinth.

The neural impulses stimulated by the hair cells are transmitted to the brain, where they are interpreted for speed and direction of movement.

Auditory Apparatus

The auditory apparatus comprises the organ of hearing, which includes the scala tympani, scala vestibuli, and cochlear duct. Within the cochlear duct is the epithelial **spiral organ**, which functions in hearing.

SPIRAL ORGAN (ORGAN OF CORTI)

The sensory portion of the organ of hearing is a complex structure that rests on the scala media side of the basilar membrane (Figs. 18.2 and 18.5). This receptor organ has three major components: *(a)* the sensory cells that transform mechanical energy into electrical energy, *(b)* a supportive structure for the sensory cells, and *(c)* the afferent and efferent nerve terminals (Fig. 18.5).

Sensory cells

The sensory cells are in two groups: the **outer hair cells** form a single row adjacent to the inner pillar cells, and the **inner hair cells** lie in three to four rows just outside the outer pillar cells.

The cylindric outer hair cells are slanted toward the inner tunnel (Fig. 18.5). From the apex of each cell, a bundle of approximately 100 stereocilia projects in a W pattern (V or U pattern in some mammals). The stereocilia of each cell form four to five rows of increasing height toward the spiral ligament. Thus, the outer hair cells are morphologically polarized, much like the vestibular hair cells. The longest stereocilia are embedded in the tectorial membrane. The tips of stereocilia are connected to their taller neighbors by means of a threadlike structure, called **tip link**. At the base of the outer hair cells are a few afferent nerve endings and many efferent terminals containing vesicles. Both the inner and outer hair cells have synaptic ribbons where afferent synapses occur.

The inner hair cells are pear-shaped. Each cell has 50 to 60 stereocilia, which form three straight, parallel rows with increasing height toward the spiral ligament. The stereocilia are not embedded in the tectorial membrane; however, the longest stereocilia touch it. As for outer hair cells, tip links connect the tips of stereocilia to their taller neighbors. At the base of these cells are many afferent nerve endings and a few efferent terminals. However, in most cases, the efferent nerve fibers terminate on the dendrites of the afferent nerve fibers (axodendritic synapses). The inner hair cells are almost totally enveloped by **inner phalangeal cells**, and the outer hair cells are almost totally enveloped by **outer phalangeal cells**.

Supporting cells

The cells of the spiral organ include the **border cells**, **inner and outer pillar cells**, **inner and outer phalangeal** (Deiters') **cells**, **outer limiting** (Hensen's) **cells**, and **external supporting** (Claudius' and Böttcher's) **cells** (Fig. 18.5). All these cells have a supportive role.

The columnar border cells rest on the tympanic lip of the spiral limbus, forming a single row on the inner side of the inner hair cells. The inner and outer pillar cells line a prominent triangular space, the **inner tunnel** (Corti's). They have a broad base containing the nucleus and an elongated body packed with tonofilaments that fan out to form the cuticular plate in the cell apex.

The inner and outer phalangeal cells are supportive cells that rest on the basilar membrane and extend up-

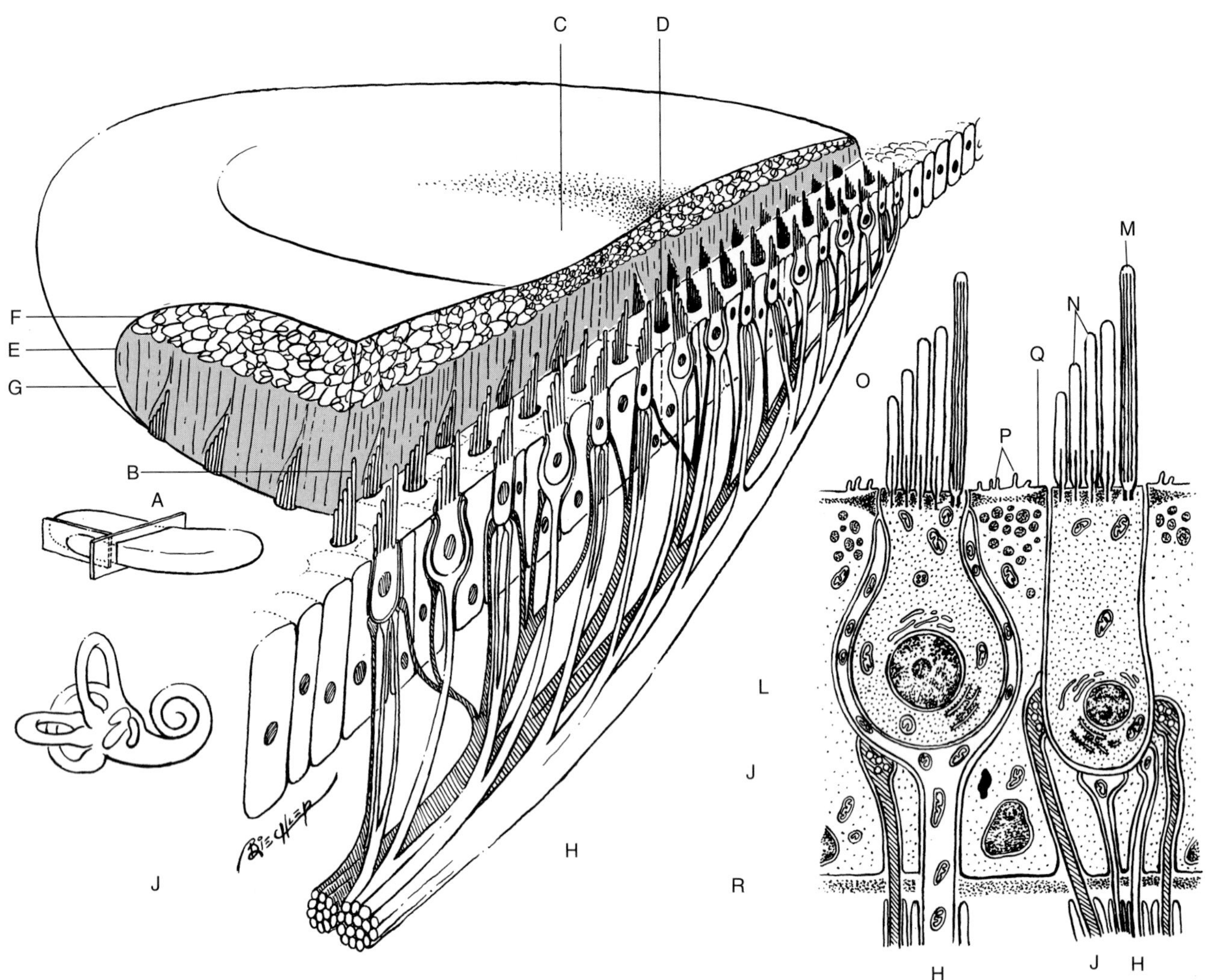

Figure 18.10. *Schematic drawing of macula utriculi illustrates the type I sensory hair cells surrounded by a nerve chalice and the type II sensory cells. The numerous stereocilia (A) and the single kinocilium (B) of each cell form a conelike arrangement; each kinocilium faces the striola (C), represented here as a broken line (D). The statoconial membrane (E) has been cut away to better illustrate the hair cells. Regional differences can be shown concerning the thickness of the crystal layer (F), size of the crystals, structure of the gelatinous substance (G), structure of the sensory hairs, size and density of the sensory cells and distribution of type I and type II cells, localization of the nuclei within the epithelium, and size of the nerve fibers. Note the change in the morphological polarization of the sensory cells in the middle of the striola (D). Afferent nerve fibers are drawn white (H), and efferent nerve fibers are gray hatched (J). In the lower right corner of the figure is a schematic drawing illustrating the general structure of the vestibular sensory epithelium. Type I cell has a constricted neck and a rounded base and is almost completely surrounded by a nerve chalice (L). The more cylindrical type II cell is innervated by bud-shaped nerve endings, which are of two types: sparsely vesiculated, afferent (H) and richly vesiculated, efferent (J). Kinocilium (M), stereocilia (N), cuticle (O), microvilli (P), supporting cells (Q), basal lamina (R). (Modified and redrawn after Lindemann HH. Anatomy of the otolith organs. Adv Otorhinolaryngol 1973;20:405.)*

ward to cradle the base of the hair cells and then send long cytoplasmic processes toward the surface. The phalangeal cells have a bundle of filaments originating from the basal cell membrane and extending to the apex. The phalangeal processes expand into a flat plate held to the hair cells by junctional complexes. The free surface of phalangeal cells and hair cells, with its massive terminal web and intercellular junctions, form the **reticular lamina**, which holds the apical part of the hair cells rigid (Fig. 18.5).

The outer limiting cells and the external supporting cells complete the cellular component of the spiral organ. Hensen's cell is very tall with its nucleus located centrally or close to the cell apex. The cytoplasm is filled almost entirely with cytoplasmic matrix and mitochondria, lipofuscin, and other organelles are scarce. One of the prominent features is the presence of numerous tall microvilli from which dense roots extend into the cytoplasm. The presence of microvilli suggests that these cells may be engaged, to some extent, in fluid absorption. Hensen's cells, Claudius' cells, and inner sulcus cells are similar in their cytoplasmic characteristics, although their sizes and shapes vary. Böttcher's cells are located on the basilar membrane in the basal turn.

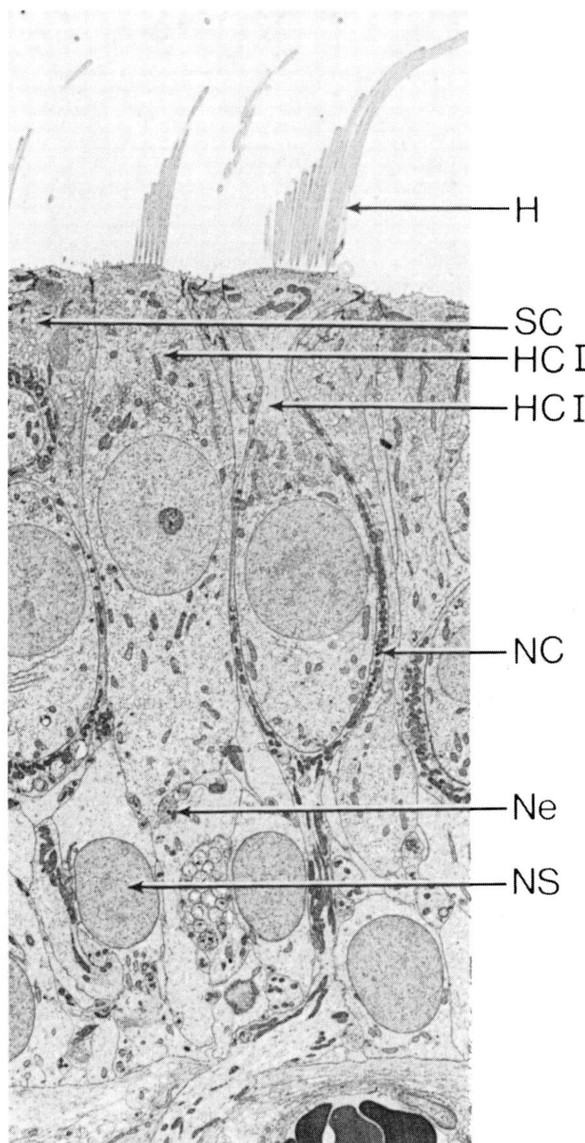

Figure 18.11. *Utricular sensory cells, transmission electron micrograph (cat). The type I and type II sensory cells are separated by supporting cells. H = hairs (stereocilia), SC = supporting cell, HCII = type II hair cell, HCI = type I hair cell, NC = nerve chalice, NE = nerve ending, NS = nucleus of supporting cell (×2331). (From Schuknecht HF. Anatomy. In: Schuknecht HF, ed. Pathology of the ear. 2nd ed. Philadelphia: Lea & Febiger, 1993:31.)*

These cells are found in clusters under the Claudius' cells, and their cell apices do not extend to the endolymphatic surface. Their nuclei are round to oval in shape and show an irregular chromatin condensation. The cytoplasm does not show any unique features and is filled with scattered mitochondria, lipofuscin, microtubules, and ribosomes. These cells interdigitate frequently among themselves. The basal portion toward the basilar membrane is irregular, electron dense at the plasmalemma, and supported by a thick basal lamina. Plasma membrane infoldings toward the Claudius' cells are not extensive. Their function is not known. The outer limiting cells are separated from the outer phalangeal cells by a space, the **outer tunnel**. (Figs. 18.5 and 18.12).

Tectorial membrane

Overlying the spiral organ is the **tectorial membrane**, a gelatinous structure containing glycoprotein and extending from the spiral limbus over the hair cells (Figs. 18.2 and 18.5). The lower surface of this membrane rests on the tips of the tallest stereocilia in each bundle of the inner hair cells, whereas the tallest stereocilia of the outer hair cells are embedded in the membrane. Where the tectorial membrane attaches to the spiral limbus are the **interdental cells**, which apparently secrete the gel-like substance of the membrane.

Spiral ganglion

Fibers from the **spiral ganglion** cells located in the modiolus converge to form the cochlear division of the vestibulocochlear nerve. The peripheral processes of these ganglion bipolar cells course in bundles within the osseous spiral lamina, branch, and terminate in the spiral organ around the base of the hair cells.

AUDITORY MECHANISM

To understand the mechanism of hearing, it is necessary to understand the stimulus, the sound waves. To create sound, vibrations alternately compress the air and then allow it to expand. Successive waves of increased or decreased air pressure travel out from the source. The simplest sound wave, a pure tone, is characterized by frequency and amplitude, which correspond with perception of pitch and loudness (intensity).

The ear is constructed as a receptor of sound waves in air. The outer ear, with the auricle (pinna) and ear canal (meatus), captures sound waves with varying efficiency, depending on the size of the auricle. In mammals, sensitivity of hearing also depends on the ability to either raise or close the outer ear (auricle). Animals raise the outer ear in an attempt to sharpen their hearing or cover the ear canal to block sound and sleep better.

The tympanic membrane acts as a receptor of sound waves in the air. The bridge of the malleus, incus, and stapes transports the received sound energy across the middle ear to the perilymph on the medial side of the stapes footplate. Without the unique middle ear bone chain, only a small fraction of the energy received at the eardrum would be transported to the inner ear. A severed bone chain results in severe hearing loss. The middle ear mechanism not only transports energy from the air to the perilymph in the inner ear but also protects the inner ear against receiving too much energy, which might destroy the hair cells in the spiral organ. When the sound level at the eardrum is approximately 70 to 80 dB, the two middle ear muscles start to contract. Contraction increases as the sound level increases, changing the middle ear adaptation mechanism into a protective mechanism.

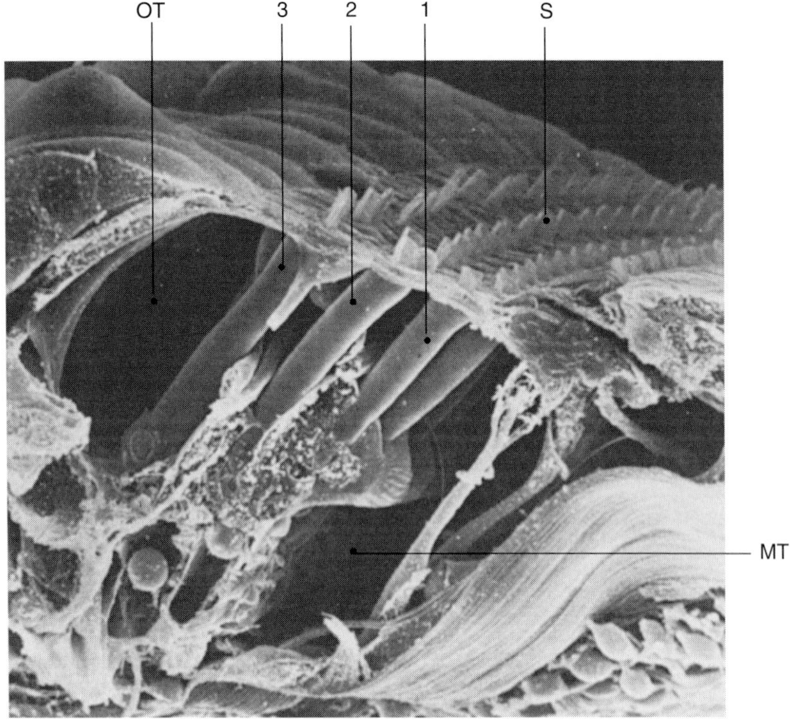

Figure 18.12. *Scanning electron micrograph of the organ of Corti. Outer hair cells: first (1), second (2), and third (3) row. Stereocilia (S), middle tunnel (MT), and outer tunnel (OT). From Weiss L ed. Cell and Tissue Biology, A Textbook of Histology, 6th Ed., p. 1118. Copyright 1988 by Urban & Schwarzenberg, Inc.*

When the ear is exposed to a complex sound (a clang), it breaks down the sound to corresponding pure tones (tonal spectrum). Sound vibrations in the middle ear are transferred by the stapes footplate through the vestibular window to the endolymph of the cochlear duct. These pressure variations in the cochlear fluid cause regions of the basilar membrane to vibrate with different maximum amplitudes, depending on the type of frequencies in the stimulus (Fig. 18.13). The pure tones are formed from the vibrations of the basilar membrane in the inner ear. Residual vibration is released through the cochlear window. The secondary tympanic membrane, covering the cochlear window, vibrates in opposite face to the stapes footplate.

The variation of width, thickness, and elasticity of the basilar membrane allows **tonotopical localization**. Low-frequency sounds cause the basilar membrane to vibrate in the apical end of the cochlea, whereas high frequencies cause vibration in the region close to the cochlear window. Each frequency in the tonal range has a maximal vibration, known as **resonance amplitude**, at a distinct location along the length of the basilar membrane. Hair cells in the spiral organ at the site of maximal vibration are activated by the motion of the membrane.

As described earlier, the hair cells are fixed in the reticular lamina, and the longest stereocilia of the outer hair cells are embedded in the tectorial membrane. Functional evidence suggests that the longest stereocilia of the inner hair cells touch the tectorial membrane. Whenever the basilar membrane is deflected, the reticular lamina is displaced, so that the hairs are moved by a shearing effect against the tectorial membrane. At low vibration amplitudes, only the outer hair cells are stimulated. At greater amplitudes, the inner hair cells are also activated. Stimulation of the outer hair cells results in determination of sound intensity (loudness), whereas stimulation of inner hair cells results in frequency (pitch) determination. The ability of the ear to determine frequency and loudness increases as sound intensity increases to a certain limit. At very high intensity, the ability decreases, probably due to mechanical reasons.

The site of transduction of mechanical energy to electrical signals seems to be the tip of the stereocilia, where the receptor current enters the sensory cell in response to displacement of the hair bundle. The tip links (the stereocilia are connected by filamentous linkages) and the ionic channels situated in the plasma membrane covering the terminal ends of the stereocilia are believed to be involved in the transduction. When pushed in the excitatory direction, tip links are stretched and ionic channels in the stereocilium terminal membrane are in the open state. The channels close when the stereocilium is pushed in the opposite direction. The ionic currents regulate neurotransmitter release at the afferent synapse located at the base of the hair cell. The speed of hair cell response is faster than in any other sensory receptor cells, including neurons. The result is electrical signals that are transferred to the brain via afferent nerve fibers.

The function of the efferent nerve fibers at the base of the hair cells is not yet completely understood. The innervation may have a regulating function in noisy environments, which allows filtering of unwanted sounds

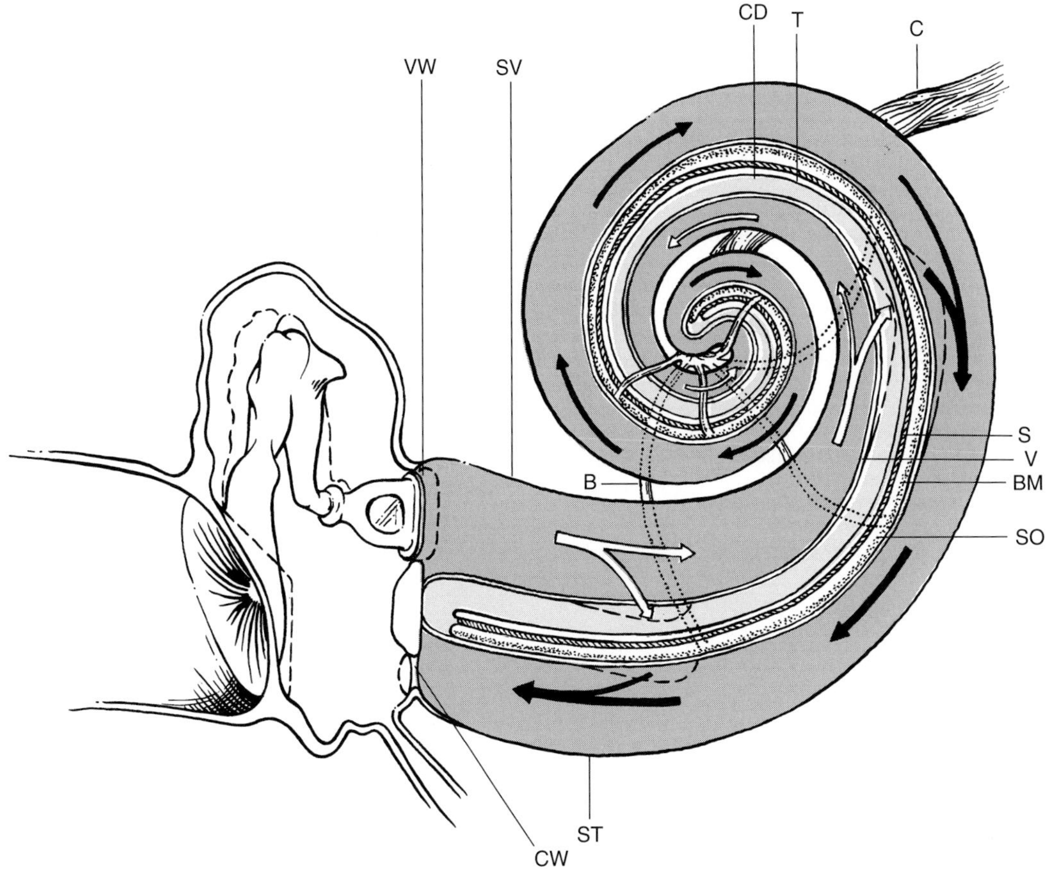

Figure 18.13. *Schematic diagram of events in the stimulation of auditory receptors. The cochlea has been uncoiled to more easily visualize transmission of sound waves and their distortion of the vestibular and basilar membranes of the cochlear duct. Sound waves impinge on the tympanic membrane, causing it to vibrate. The ear ossicles vibrate as a unit — the utmost position of ear ossicles is indicated by stippled lines. The footplate of the stapes moves in and out of the vestibular window, causing increased and decreased fluid pressure in the scala vestibuli. Because fluid is incompressible, this causes distortion of the vestibular and basilar membranes. Short waves (high frequency, high pitch) act at the base of the cochlea. Long waves (low frequency, low pitch) act at the apex of the cochlea. Waves may also travel around the helicotrema at the apex of the cochlea. Impact of the wave on the secondary tympanic membrane, covering the cochlear window, causes it to move in and out at the cochlear window in opposite phase to vestibular window. The white arrows are in the scala vestibuli, and the black ones are in the scala tympani. The thickness of the arrows indicates the strength of increased and decreased fluid pressure. The cochlear nerve (C), with some of its branches (B), vestibular membrane (V), basilar membrane (BM), spiral organ (SO), stereocilia (S), tectorial membrane (T), scala vestibuli (SV), cochlear duct (CD), scala tympani (ST), cochlear window (CW), vestibular window (VW).*

to focus on a particular sound. The efferent system is also believed to play a role in **otoacoustic emissions (OAE)**, the recording of a tone that has radiated into the ear canal from the inner ear in response to a sound stimulus. OAE is currently the most important diagnostic test to determine inner ear status, especially in babies and small children. The existence of OAE in animals has been proven in several species, but diagnostic test results do not agree.

A hearing sensation can also be evoked by vibrations applied directly to the skull, for instance, by pressing a vibrating tuning fork against the mastoid process of the temporal bone. This kind of hearing is called **bone conduction**. The vibrations are transported to the inner ear (cochlea) through the petrous part of the temporal bone. The cochlear window yields more to pressure variation in the cochlear fluid than does the footplate of the stapes in the vestibular window. Thus, **traveling waves** in the basilar membrane occur as for air-conducted sounds. Bone conduction is very important for the perception of self-induced sounds such as human speech and animal vocalization. The pressure waves introduced to the skull also excite the vestibular system.

REFERENCES

Békésy GV. Zur Theorie des Höhrens; die Schwingungsform der Basilarmembran. Physik Zeits 1928;29:793.

Berry MM, Standring SM, Bannister LH, eds. Auditory and vestibular apparatus. In: Williams PL, ed. Gray's anatomy. 38th ed. Edinburgh: Churchill Livingstone, 1995:1367.

Erway LC, Mitchell SE. Prevention of otolith defect in pastel mink by manganese supplementation. J Hered 1973;64:111.

Fay RR. Hearing in vertebrates: a psychophysics databook. Winnetka, IL: Hill-Fay Associates, 1988.

Flock Å. The ear. In: Weiss L, ed. Cell and tissue biology. A textbook of histology. 6th ed. Baltimore: Urban & Schwarzenberg, Inc., 1988:1107.

Flock Å, Wersäll J, eds. Cellular mechanisms in hearing. Proceedings of Nobel Symposium 63. Hear Res 1986;22:1.

Flottorp G. Pure-tone tinnitus evoked by acoustic stimulation: the idiophonic effect. Acta Otolaryngol (Stockh) 1953;43:396.

Flottorp G, Foss I. Development of hearing in hereditarily deaf white mink (Hedlund) and normal mink (Standard) and the subsequent deterioration of the auditory response in Hedlund mink. Acta Otolaryngol (Stockh) 1979;87:16.

Foss I. Development of hearing and vision, and morphological examination of the inner ear in hereditarily deaf white Norwegian Dunkerhounds and normal dogs (black and dappled Norwegian Dunkerhounds). Master's thesis. Ithaca, NY: Cornell University, 1981.

Foss I, Flottorp G. A comparative study of the development of hearing and vision in various species commonly used in experiments. Acta Otolaryngol (Stockh) 1974;77:202.

Friedmann I, Ballantyne J. Ultrastructural atlas of the inner ear. London: Butterworths & Co., 1984.

Gacek RR. Efferent innervation of the labyrinth. Clinical review. Am J Otolaryngol 1984;5:206.

Hudspeth AJ. How the ear's works work. Review article. Nature 1989;341:397.

Kemp DT. Stimulated acoustic emissions from within human auditory system. J Acoust Soc Am 1978;64:1386.

Kimura RS. Distribution, structure, and function of dark cells in the vestibular labyrinth. Ann Otol Rhinol Laryngol 1969;48:542.

Lagardre F, Chaumillon G, Amara R, et al. Examination of otolith morphology and microstructure using laser scanning microscopy. In: Secor DH, Dean JM, Campana SE, eds. Recent developments in fish otolith research. Columbia, SC: University of South Carolina Press, 1995:7.

Metz O. The acoustic impedance measured on normal and pathological ears. Acta Otolaryngol (Stockh) 1946:(Suppl 63):1.

Osborne MP, Comis SD, Pickles JO. Morphology and cross linkage of stereo-cilia in the guinea-pig labyrinth examined without the use of osmium as a fixative. Cell Tissue Res 1984;237:43.

Probst R. Otoacoustic emissions: an overview. In: Pfaltz CR, ed. New aspects of cochlear mechanics and inner ear pathophysiology. Adv Otorhinolaryngol 1990;44;1.

Rabinowitz J. Les effets physiologiques du bruit. Recherche 1991;22(229):178.

Ross MH, Romrell LJ, Kaye GI. Ear. In: Ross MH, Romrell LJ, Kaye GI, eds. Histology: a text and atlas. 3rd ed. Baltimore: Williams & Wilkins, 1995:768.

Schuknecht HF. Anatomy. In: Schuknecht HF, ed. Pathology of the ear. 2nd ed. Philadelphia: Lea & Febiger, 1993:31.

Tortora GJ, Grabowski SR. Auditory sensations and equilibrium. In: Tortora GJ, Grabowski SR, eds. Principles of anatomy and physiology. 7th ed. New York: HarperCollins College Publishers, 1993:487.

Zwislocki J. Theorie der Schneckenmechanik. Acta Otolaryngol (Stockh) 1948;(Suppl 72):1.

Index

Note: Page numbers in *italics* refer to figures; page numbers followed by t refer to tables.